Ending Denial

The Lyme Disease Epidemic
A Canadian Public Health Disaster

Also from KOS Publishing

Corrupt to the Core

Memoirs of a Health Canada Whistleblower

by Shiv Chopra

The Earth's Gift to Medicine

Minerals in Health and Disease

by K.G. Wenzel, MD & R.J. Pataracchia, ND

Healing The Planet One Patient At A Time

by Jozef Krop, MD

Adventures in Psychiatry

The Scientic Memoirs of Dr. Abram Hoffer

Available through the International Society for Orthomolecular Medicine,

16 Florence Ave., North York, ON M2N 1E9 416-733-2117 www.orthomed.org

Available for free downloading on www.kospublishing.com

Dispatches from the War Zone of Environmental Health

by Helke Ferrie

What Part of No! Don't They Understand?

Rescuing Food and Medicine from Government Abuse

by Helke Ferrie

Ending Denial

The Lyme Disease Epidemic
A Canadian Public Health Disaster

A Call For Action From Patients,
Doctors, Researchers, And Politicians

Edited by Helke Ferrie

KOS Publishing

2010

Library and Archives Canada Cataloguing in Publication

Ending denial : the Lyme disease epidemic : a Canadian public health disaster / edited by Helke Ferrie.

Includes bibliographical references.
ISBN 978-0-9811337-1-3

1. Lyme disease—Canada. 2. Lyme disease—Treatment—Canada. 3. Medical policy—Canada. I. Ferrie, Helke, 1948-

RA644.L94E53 2010 362.196'924600971 C2010-901479-0

Published and distributed by
KOS Publishing Inc.
1997 Beechgrove Road
Caledon, ON, Canada L7K 0N3
Tel: 519-927-1049 Fax: 519-927-9542
www.kospublishing.com
Quantity discounts available

Cover and Text Design, Print Production: Beth Crane, WeMakeBooks.ca

Printed and Bound in Canada

THIS BOOK IS DEDICATED TO

Dr. Joseph KUCAN
1946–2009
Dr. Kucan was the driving force that made the *Lyme Action Group* of Ontario a reality. His warmth, humanity, insight, determination, and strength inspired all of us who struggle with the burden of Lyme disease and we all benefitted from his compassion and inspiration.

Gabe MAGNOTTA
1949–2009
Gabe Magnotta, an entrepreneur in the wine industry, was strong enough to take on Ontario's liquor control board and win, but he lost his battle against Lyme disease. His family and his equally determined wife Rossana will not let his death have been in vain.

And to the DOCTORS
who continue to have the courage to treat Chronic Lyme patients in defiance of the political and medical odds.

TABLE OF CONTENTS

FOREWORD

Lyme Disease in Canada

by Terence Young
Member of Parliament (Conservative) for Oakville, Ontario

From the time we can first remember, most of us we were taught to do what the doctor says. Yet, the history of medicine is riddled with commonplace therapies, which greatly increased human suffering with minimal chance of improving human health, and which the medical profession would like everyone to forget. This includes everything from the awful "bleeding" of patients in past centuries, to today's fourth leading cause of death and injury: the over-use of prescription drugs.

How did these harmful medical practices flourish? Doctors refused to search out and accept the best available objective evidence for therapy, and instead based their therapies on the group-think of the day; and they refused to tell patients the real potential risks and benefits of their own therapy, the facts needed to provide truly informed consent, and watch out for adverse effects.

In the twentieth century, a third dynamic made this situation considerably more deadly. Our doctors were increasingly conditioned to put money, prestige, and career ahead of what's best for patients. The Hippocratic oath of two millennia ago, once taken by every graduating medical student, "First Do No Harm," was sacrificed to a new now dominant influence: profitable medical intervention as approved by medical "thought leaders."

As the generous rewards for medical 'thought leaders' and professional authorities grew, they saw fit to defend their own vested interests by killing therapeutic innovation, and attempting to crush the careers of those who practice them. Sadly, this abuse of power has played out on patients with Lyme disease in Canada, who are denied the right to choose truly effective, scientifically-recognized clinical tests to confirm their diagnosis, and the treatment which may be their only chance to reduce their suffering.

If you or someone you love may be suffering from Lyme disease, this book is for you. If you want to know what's wrong with our health care system, this book is for you. If you have wondered why every conversation about our health care system in Canada and the US ends up being about money, this book is for you.

Read it and bear witness to the courage of those who challenge the status quo and truly put patients first. Read it to help protect yourself from the vested interests that have kept doctors and patients in the dark about the true nature of Lyme disease. Read it to understand how blindly doing what the doctor says may be the most dangerous thing you could do for your own health.

Terence H. Young,
M.P. Oakville

PREFACE

Lyme Disease—Emergence of a Disaster

by Jim Wilson

Twenty years ago the first Lyme disease society was formed in Canada. Most Canadians have no idea that Lyme disease has spread unchecked and uncounted for that many years. In 1985, now 24 years ago, Dr. Satyen Banerjee and his wife Maya began seeing Lyme disease in their lab at the British Columbia Centres for Disease Control. Together with Dr. Laverne Kindree, and his daughter Diane, they did extensive field work over the next several years; Lyme disease was discovered throughout BC and the Lyme Borreliosis Society of BC was formed in 1989.

Also in 1989, now 20 years ago, Manitoba reported 93 cases of Lyme disease. Of those, 51 cases had the classic bull's eye rash. Each case was diagnosed by a physician and also formally reported.

One year later, in 1990, the Lyme Disease Association of Ontario was formed by John Scott, a researcher who personally was affected by Lyme disease (see Chapter 2 in this book). They were able to show that Lyme disease is spread randomly by migratory birds who both harbour the disease in their blood and transport infected ticks. This information was published eventually in the Journal of the Canadian Medical Association—almost a decade later, though.

In 1991, 18 years ago, Health Canada held a national conference on Lyme disease for a small group of medical researchers, microbiologists and infectious disease doctors. The result of this conference was to do virtually nothing. Previous and future cases of Lyme disease diagnoses, which had been made and were continued to be made following the global standards of a clinical diagnosis (which are still in effect today), were discounted and reporting basically stopped. The mantra of the federal and provincial governments, led by this small group of researchers and infectious disease doctors was that Lyme disease did not exist in Canada, except perhaps in a couple of locations.

Since then untold thousands of cases have been left to languish as a result of misdiagnosis: Lyme infection is linked to symptoms generally diagnosed as Multiple sclerosis, Parkinson's disease, other motor neuron diseases, chronic fatigue syndrome, Fibromyalgia, colitis, Crohn's disease, psychiatric disorders, Alzheimer's disease, and many others. Many people were given no diagnosis, and told to just accept their fate.

CanLyme has become the central clearing house for all those thousands who have been left to suffer, and the numbers are growing daily.

Since our inception in 2003, CanLyme has been trying to alert provincial and federal governments to the seriousness of this disease. Their collective and scripted response has been, and still is, that Lyme disease is rare in Canada. We are the only country in the northern hemisphere which maintains that Lyme disease is rare—and we just happen to have the highest rates in the world of all those diseases linked to Lyme infection.

From a legislative, legal standpoint our governments are mandated to investigate emerging disease or illness. We have been warning them there is a very consistent set of symptoms seriously affecting the lives of Canadians from coast to coast. In every other country these symptoms are consistent with Lyme disease. In Canada, almost all of these people test negative for Lyme disease, but they are no less sick. These same people test positive for Lyme disease at fully certified and accredited US or European laboratories.

We at CanLyme are recording a unique emerging disease disaster in Canada, and we want it investigated. According to Canadian tests, it is not Lyme disease. I've renamed it as A-R-L-S (Antibiotic Responsive Lyme-like Syndrome). Thousands of Canadians are only getting any quality of life back after an appropriate antibiotic treatment period that just happens to mirror the treatment for Lyme disease. The response to date by governments has been to stress the dangers of antibiotics. This alleged danger pales when compared to the many other drugs used to treat the many symptoms of Lyme disease, or A-R-L-S. It pales when compared to the severity of the disability associated with Lyme disease, or A-R-L-S.

We call upon all political leaders, governments, universities, medical schools, and industry, especially those businesses and government bodies with large contingents of outside workers to urgently support us in our efforts to identify this phenomenon. Live subject and post mortem research is a must. Our laws clearly mandate that governments act immediately on emerging health threats. Their entire effort for 20 years has been to tell doctors and the public that Lyme disease is not a risk in Canada. Well, apparently A-R-L-S is a much higher risk and we demand it be investigated and that government act.

Jim Wilson is the Director and Founder of the Canadian Lyme Disease Foundation, CanLyme www.canlyme.com 250-768-0978

TIMELINE ON LYME DISEASE IN CANADA TO FEBRUARY 2010

Lyme disease is one of seven known human spirochetal bacterial diseases spread by various vectors (e.g. ticks of various species); they all have acute and chronic stages and affect many bodily systems and organs. Some, like syphilis and Lyme, are also transmissible from humans to humans. These diseases are treatable by antibiotics and other drugs. Lyme disease is known as "the great imitator" because it can be one of the causes of Multiple Sclerosis, ALS (Lou Gehrig's Disease), Alzheimer's, Parkinson's, Crohn's, forms of dementia, ADHD, autism (Lyme spirochetes cross the placenta of infected mothers), Scleroderma, rheumatoid arthritis, and heart disease. Known since 1909, evidence shows, Lyme has evolved in all areas: More species of ticks and many animals, as well as migratory birds, now carry the causative spirochete; the spirochete itself has evolved several forms and hundreds of co-infections have emerged; human variations in immune responses now number in the high thirties; co-infections are almost always present; treatment protocols are needed that go beyond the originally useful antibiotics.

Cambridge World History of Human Disease, 1993

Schmidt, G. P. Epidemiology and clinical similarities of human spirochetal diseases, *Rev. Infect. Dis.* 1989, Sept–Oct: 11 Suppl. 6: S1460-9

Public Health of Canada website, last accessed October 14, 2009

1975

Lyme disease was first described in 1909 in Sweden. The American variant was discovered in Lyme, Connecticut in 1975; this variant is linked to a form of joint arthritis first observed in children. Due to the fact that Lyme disease was first identified in its rheumatoid manifestation, the focus in subsequent research tended to be primarily on symptoms consistent with arthritis and the potential relationship between Lyme as an *infectious disease* and Lyme infection as a trigger for an *autoimmune disease*. The controversy that unfolded has roots in this historical accident.

Public Health of Canada website; agreement in medicine; see P. Weintraub, *Cure Unknown,* 2008

1988

Lyme disease becomes reportable in Ontario. However, to date no accurate epidemiological data are known because the knowledge among physicians and the tests available for identifying this infection accurately are not available. Unlike the USA and the EU, Canadian Lyme incidence can only be extrapolated from the US data provided by the Centers for Disease Control.

Public Health of Canada website (item 10): Descriptive epidemiology of Lyme disease in Ontario: 1999–2004—CCDR Vol. 32-21

Dr. S. Banerjee of the Centers for Disease Control in British Columbia confirms 13 cases of Lyme disease, 3 acquired within the province that year.

1989

Lyme Borreliosis Society established in Vancouver, B.C. by Dr. L. and nurse Diane Kindree (first Canadian society of its kind) which funded research conducted by Dr. S. Banerjee of B.C.'s CDC to commence field collection of ticks across B.C. Eventually the results are published in the *Canadian Medical Association Journal.*

See Chapter 2.

1990

The **Lyme Disease Association of Ontario** is founded by John D. Scott who also initiates the first surveys published in various scientific journals, including the *Canadian Medical Association Journal*.

See Chapter 2 by John D. Scott. See www.lymeontario.org

1993

The **Lyme-Borreliosis Support Group** of Manitoba is founded by Elizabeth Wood and her husband Lorne.

1994

The **Infectious Disease Society of America** (IDSA) establishes a two-tiered test protocol at Centers for Disease Control meeting in Dearborn, Michigan: first the so-called ELISA blood test is required, which has an extremely high rate of false negative results, primarily because it was not designed for diagnostic purposes in humans but for surveillance work undertaken by the US Centers for Disease Control. Under IDSA Guidelines, no other, more reliable testing is accepted. Only if a patient has a positive ELISA result, is the Western blot test even allowed for purposes of confirmation. By itself, the Western blot is known to be highly reliable and useful for Lyme diagnosis. The Ontario government has adopted this wholly inappropriate two-tiered protocol. Sources for science on reliable testing began to appear 2001; see below:

For summary of the above see Stricker, R.B. & Johnson, L., Chronic Lyme Disease and the "Axis of Evil," *Future Microbiology*, 2008, 3 (6) editorial

For detailed information see Weintraub, P. *Cure Unknown* and DVD documentary film *Under Our Skin.*

Tylewska, Limitation of serological testing for Lyme borreliosis: evaluation of ELISA and Western blot in comparison, *Klinische Wochenschrift* 114 (13–14): 601–5, 2002

Brunner M. Seronegative Lyme disease: new method of detection of Borrelia burgdorferi antigen complexed to antibody, *Journal of Immunological Methods,* 49 (1-2): 185–19, 2001

J. Burrescano Jr. MD, Diagnostic Hints: Advanced Topics in Lyme Disease: *Diagnostic Hints and Treatment Guidelines for Lyme and other Tick-borne Illnesses*, 16th ed., Sept. 2008

1995

International Lyme Disease Conference held in Vancouver, B.C., arranged and funded by the Lyme Borreliosis Society of B.C.: www.lyme.org/conferences

1996

Lyme Borreliosis Society of B.C. produces a half-hour documentary film entitled "More Than A Tick"; aired many times over a 2-year period on The Knowledge Network.

Lyme Disease Society of Saskatchewan is set up by Melanie Chernipeski.

1997

The Lyme Disease Support Group of New Brunswick is organized by Linda Dochstader in Fredericton.

1998

The *Canadian Medical Association Journal* begins to publish research on Lyme disease in Canada; by 2009 over 30 articles and research papers on Lyme disease, specific to Canada, have appeared, showing increased incidence of the disease-carrying ticks throughout Canada as well as increasing numbers of morbidity in humans. Canada's Public Health authority publishes several hundred such items; yet, evidence shows that practicing doctors seem to be unaware of them and newly developed treatments are generally unavailable.

The high rate of false negatives in testing currently available gives a misleading impression that Lyme is not a significant problem about which physicians need to be knowledgeable. Awareness of physicians treating Lyme encountering difficulties with regulatory authorities in the USA and Canada may also be a deterrent. Although new and more reliable tests have been developed and are available in the US and Europe, they are not available in Canada. Today, Canadians have to pay considerable sums of money to obtain reliable tests in the US or Europe because tests mandated in Canada are usually false negative.

Public Health of Canada website under key-words "Lyme Disease"

Ogden, N.H. et al, The emergence of Lyme disease in Canada, CMAJ Review, CMAJ June 9, 2009, 180 (2) p. 1221-1224.

1999

The **International Lyme and Associated Diseases Society** (ILADS) is founded with the purpose of focusing on all forms of Lyme disease, especially the chronic forms, and to train doctors in evolving treatment methods; protocols are developed which are now used internationally. From 2000–2006 research centers are set up at Columbia University and universities in Connecticut and California to focus on Chronic Lyme and all its varieties. Such centers exist in Europe as well, where many ILADS-trained physicians follow their internationally known protocol.

See website of ILADS and Ontario's CPSO website under key words "Guidelines," go to National Guideline Clearinghouse US; the ILADS guidelines are published in Chapter 10 of this book.

October 1999 a civil jury awarded $1.7 million to a teenager in Maryland, USA, who developed long-term disabilities due to undiagnosed Lyme disease in 1995 when the doctors told his mother she was "a hysterical mom" and refused to test the boy for Lyme infection.

2000

IDSA publishes its first set of guidelines for the treatment of Lyme which are so restrictive in their definition that they exclude most Lyme patients and essentially deny them treatment. In order to force "consensus, the panel refused to accept or consider published information regarding the existence of Chronic Lyme disease and removed a panelist from their panel who dissented from the group's decision to exclude Chronic Lyme disease. Although not consistent with the definition of Lyme disease by the National Institutes of Health, this arbitrarily narrow definition of Lyme disease was published in standard journals and a lively controversy arose throughout the publications and the mainstream media on this development. Canadian government officials had to have been aware of this emerging controversy and should have provided for better testing and treatment options." In the US, a public outcry about the IDSA Guidelines resulted in the establishment of a research department devoted to Chronic Lyme Disease at Columbia University.

The Canadian Medical Association publishes the first detailed report on Lyme disease in Canada on May 30, based on the surveillance research by John Scott.

See Chapter 2 and P. Weintraub, *Cure Unknown*, Connecticut Attorney General press release, May 1, 2008, and Public Health of Canada website

2001

The **Lyme Disease Association** (USA) publishes *Conflicts of Interest in Lyme Disease: Laboratory Testing, Vaccination and Treatment Guidelines*; a 182 page report on the activities of the IDSA guideline panel members, the CDC staff involved with Lyme disease, and the collusion between IDSA and CDC on suppressing proper testing and advancing harmful vaccine projects. This report forms the basis of the 2006 investigation of the IDSA guideline panel by the Attorney General of Connecticut.

2003

The national patient support group, the **Canadian Lyme Disease Foundation (Can-Lyme)** is founded as a registered charity. Based in British Columbia, it supports patients in every province in Canada including Quebec and the Maritimes. CanLyme is dedicated to promoting research that will improve testing and treatment as well as awareness among professionals and the public.

See Preface by Jim Wilson, Director and Co-Founder of CanLyme.

2004

The guidelines of the International Lyme and Associated Diseases Society (**ILADS**) are published which include the diagnosis and treatment of Chronic Lyme Disease as part of their treatment protocols. The ILADS prevention protocol has since been incorporated by the US Environmental Protection Agency (EPA).

See Chapter 10.

2006

March 8–9 the **National Lyme Disease Meeting–Canada** is convened by the Public Health Agency of Canada where Lyme disease experts from both IDSA and ILADS present their data. CanLyme was given 10% of the seats at this conference. CanLyme invited Dr. Daniel Cameron of ILADS and Dr. Nick Harris of IgenX Inc, Dr. S. Donta of IDSA, and lawyer Lorraine Johnson, member of the California Lyme Disease Association. Canada Public Health invited only IDSA members. The report on this conference was not published until January 2008 and none of its recommendations have to date been enacted. Those recommendations are now also out of date.

See Chapters 1 & 4; Chapter 8 contains 2 key articles by Dr. D. Cameron.

National Lyme Disease Meeting March 2006, published by Public Health Agency of Canada.

2006 IDSA formulates new guidelines, which are even more restrictive and continue to ignore the increased volume of contradicting scientific publications, with regard to testing methods recommended and diagnostic interpretations recognized. **Examination by the Attorney General of Connecticut** shows that thousands of internationally published articles on the various forms of Lyme disease had been ignored once again; these new guidelines again explicitly deny the existence of Chronic Lyme Disease. These are the guidelines cited as the basis for Canadian government policy on Lyme, as Canada arbitrarily chose to adopt these guidelines as their authority for public health policy. The story of how this anti-trust investigation began, what its terms of engagement are, in which ways the IDSA guideline panel was compromised, and what significance it has for the practice of medicine is found in L. Johnson (a lawyer) and R.B. Stricker (ILADS Lyme expert physician), "Attorney General forces Infectious Disease Society of American to redo Lyme guidelines due to flawed development process," *J. of Medical Ethics*, 2009, vol. 35: 283 ff.

See Chapter 1.

Wormser, G. P. et al, The Clinical Assessment, Treatment and Prevention of Lyme Disease, Human Granulocytic Anaplasmosis, and Babesiosis: Clinical Practice Guidelines by the Infectious Disease Society of America, 2006, November 1, *Clinical Infectious Disease*, 43: 1089–1134

2007 Canadian Public Health Laboratory Network guidelines for the diagnosis of Lyme borreliosis, published in the *Canadian Journal of Infectious Disease and Microbiology* (vol. 18, No. 2).

2007

An anti-trust investigation of the IDSA Guideline Committee and its members is initiated by the Attorney General of Connecticut. This was caused by Lyme patients proving that these guidelines effectively had the force of law in denying access to treatment and insurance/disability coverage. This action was reported on the medical literature and mainstream media and should have been known in Canada and communicated to infectious disease doctors.

See Chapter 1 for sources and discussion

2008

The US Centers for Disease Control declare Lyme disease an emerging epidemic with tens of thousands of new reported cases annually.

See maps following Preface by Jim Wilson

On **May 1, 2008 announcement by the Attorney General of Connecticut** of findings from the anti-trust investigation into financial conflicts of interest and procedural improprieties involving panel members who authored the 2006 Lyme Guideline. The Chair of that panel (Dr. Gary Wormser) held a bias against the existence of Chronic Lyme disease and was allowed to pick liked-minded panelists. This panel then blocked the appointment of scientists and physicians with divergent views. This investigation also uncovered systemic bias regarding the choice of supporting literature. An agreement was reached compelling the IDSA with supervision coordinated by the Attorney General's office, to select a conflict-of-interest-free new panel to re-assess and revise the guidelines and hold public hearings airing the full spectrum of medical information, including that on Chronic Lyme Disease, which was wholly excluded from the 2006 Guidelines.

The press release from the Attorney General's office with a summary of the investigation's findings regarding the IDSA was also provided to all MPPs of Ontario at the November 2008 press conference in Queen's Park's Media Studio. This was also published in many medical journals and on the websites of all relevant medical organizations.

In **June, 2008,** ***Cure Unknown—Inside the Lyme Epidemic*** **by Pamela Weintraub** is released (Weintraub was the editor of *Discover* magazine, editor-in-chief of OMNI Magazine, associate editor of *Psychology Today*, and a Chronic Lyme patient, along with her entire family who also were ill with Lyme for years). This book describes in detail the inappropriate re-definition of Lyme designed to exclude its most devastating chronic form, and the conflicts of interest involving diagnostic and treatment protocols. Copies of her book go to every state and federal legislator in the US. It details the American plight of Lyme patients and Lyme-literate doctors caught between the rigid views of the IDSA and the patient-centered approach of ILADS. (*Cure Unknown* wins the prestigious American Medical Writers Association award for best book of 2008.)

In **June, 2008,** the **Lyme Action Group** (LAG) is founded by Ontario patients suffering from Chronic Lyme Disease (as diagnosed by international and US-based laboratories; some finally found doctors using the international ILADS protocols, some members still have not found a treating physician).

On **June 23**, the **College of Physicians and Surgeons of Ontario** (CPSO), who regulate physicians in this province, initiates an investigation under Schedule 2, Section 75 a of the RHPA that may lead to a disciplinary hearing, into the practice of ILADS-trained Dr. Jozef Krop of Mississauga. The investigation is at first intended to be general and provided ***no*** specific grounds; later the investigation is changed to relate specifically and only to his diagnosis and treatment of Lyme Disease. Dr. Krop is not given an opportunity to refute very serious misinformation contained in the information intended to prove that "reasonable and probable grounds" exist for this investigation. The CPSO takes 20 charts of Lyme patients only from Dr. Krop's office. The CPSO is informed of the fact that Dr. Krop is an ILADS-trained physician and that the Connecticut Attorney General's findings discredited the IDSA guidelines to which the CPSO appears to adhere; nevertheless, the CPSO investigation continues because of its acceptance of the original complaint against Dr. Krop by an Ontario infectious disease expert, who follows the IDSA, and who reported him for a supposedly invalid diagnosis—namely Chronic Lyme. The ongoing investigation sends a chilling message that intimidates other physicians.

See Chapters 1 and 7.

Late June, the **documentary film *Under Our Skin*** is released. It describes the plight of patients suffering from Chronic Lyme Disease in America, the frequent denial of treatment due to the IDSA/ILADS controversy, the problem with the tests, the targeting of doctors, and the exponentially increasing incidence of Lyme Disease on the American continent; it wins 5 North American awards and one international one. Copies are provided to all State and federal legislators in the US.

On September 4, Congressman Frank R. Wolf, writes to the Inspector General Daniel R. Levinson of the US Department of Health and Human Services, requesting that a formal inquiry be made into the US Centers for Disease Control for their exclusive association with the IDSA and their lack of inclusion of ILADS in information and policy matters. The investigation is pending now.

November 7, LAG holds a press conference in Queen's Park, sponsored by MPP M. Kwinter, at which Chronic Lyme disease patients speak who were either cured or have had their lives drastically improved through the ILADS protocol; they describe the painful odyssey which for years brought them up against infectious disease doctors in Ontario completely unfamiliar with Lyme Disease, unwilling, or unable to treat it. The press kit contained much of the above-cited information and a number of copies of the documentary film were circulated.

In December LAG starts the process of an Ontario-wide petition to the Ontario Government asking for proper tests, treatment, physician education, and safety of the blood supply.

LAG commences correspondence with the Canadian Blood Services (CBS). Since 2003, the CBS website lists Lyme as a disease transmissible through blood transfusions. LAG wants to know why CBS is not screening donors for tick-borne diseases (TBD) using the same mandatory protocols, which are the standard in Europe and since 1994 in the US. CBS asserts that Lyme is not transmitted through transfusions and that it is merely a "theoretical risk." LAG provides the up-to-date research showing that, indeed, the causative Lyme bacterium survives blood transfusion procedures, like all other spirochetal infections are known to do. With respect to Lyme disease, its danger to the blood supply was demonstrated in the late 1980s through research published by the International Red Cross. Many other tick-borne organisms have furthermore been conclusively shown to be spread by blood transfusions, sometimes with fatal results. Published reports of this exist in the scientific literature on transfusions, both in Canada and world-wide.

See Chapter 4

Sometime in 2008—date unknown—the US Centers for Disease Control changed the case definition for Lyme disease. The two-tiered test (e.g. ELISA first, which causes the many false negatives, followed by the confirmatory Western blot only if the ELISA was indeterminate or positive) is abandoned for the single-tier test: www.cdc.gov/ncphi/disss/nndss/casedef/lyme_disease_2008

Nobody in government noticed. Canadian authorities continue to insist they are following the CDC in the US, when they are not even aware the CDC criteria are changed.

2009

The Dr. E. Murakami Cente for Lyme Research, Education and Assistance is established.

January 14, LAG writes formally to the Premier of Ontario, the Minister of Health, and the Attorney General (see package No 1) with copies provided to the entire Ontario Legislative Assembly; the letters are accompanied by supporting evidence from medical and government-based sources and copies of the documentary film *Under Our Skin*. The Attorney General of Connecticut's press release was enclosed also.

In February, LAG informs the Prime Minister of Canada and all federal MPs of the fact that Canada's blood supply must be assumed to be contaminated with Lyme-causing spirochetes. Action is requested for Canada to be in line with other jurisdictions in this regard especially because the federal government passed Bill C-11 into law, which identifies Lyme-causing bacteria as requiring special attention to protect the public from them. On May 29, the federal Minister of Health also informs LAG that contamination of the blood supply by TBD is merely "a theoretical risk." Both CBS and the federal Minister of Health ignore the published evidence to the contrary.

On February 5, Ontario's Ministry of Health informs lawyer Lisa Constantine that testing for Lyme Disease is based on a March/April 2007 publication entitled "The Laboratory Diagnosis of Lyme borreliosis: Guidelines from the Canadian Public Health Laboratory Networks." It reveals that Canada *chose* to use the IDSA testing protocol of 1994 and follow the 2006 IDSA Guidelines, although deficits in both are acknowledged in that publication. Those Canadian laboratory guidelines make ***no reference*** to the 2004 ILADS guidelines. The Ministry seems to disregard that the IDSA guidelines were set aside by the Connecticut Attorney General 9 months prior to this letter, and that those Canadian guidelines have not been updated after the US CDC changed their criteria in 2008.

The Leaders of the Opposition parties (Conservative and NDP) responded rapidly to LAG's letter of January 14. They stated that they have contacted the Premier, the Minister of Health, and the Attorney General asking for action.

On March 16, Premier Dalton McGuinty responds to LAG's January 14 submissionexpressing his concern about the blood supply's integrity and informing LAG that he has asked the Minister of Health and Long-Term Care to respond directly to LAG's concerns.

During the period of January—July LAG members make appointments with many Ontario's MPPs; the meetings get mixed reactions and no action has been taken so far.

The April 1 issue of the ***Journal of the American Medical Association*** (JAMA) publishes an **editorial** and **lead article on the abuse of medical guidelines in all** medical disciplines by giving them the unwarranted appearance of the force of law in a constantly evolving field of science; JAMA's editors are joined by the editors of leading medical journals in recommending the abolition of medical guidelines.

The *Journal of Medical Ethics* (vol. 35) article by Johnson & Stricker is published and the far-reaching implications were discussed with the Minister's Policy Advisor in June—see below. It was also submitted to the Legislature's Social Policy Committee in October.

See Chapter 1

On May 28 the Minister of Health of Ontario, Hon. D. Caplan, writes LAG indicating to LAG that the Canadian Blood Services operates at arm's length from provincial governments and abdicates his responsibility for intervention. In fact, every province can initiate changes to the national blood supply, as LAG pointed out in the correspondence with CBS.

May 29 CBS removes Lyme Disease from the list of diseases transmissible by blood transfusion from it website; it does not have the authority to do this unilaterally—the rest of the world still lists Lyme as potentially transmissible by blood transfusion. However, the relevant literature on Lyme and risks re transfusions remains on CBS's website.

May–Sept In the US, **17 States** enact legislation, regulations, or programs designed specifically to educate and/or **protect doctors treating Chronic Lyme disease**, and the **US federal government tables two bills** (congressional and Senate) to promote education, research, recognition and treatment of Lyme Disease **in all** its forms in the US.

As a result of LAG's January 14th letters to the Ontario government, on June 3 a LAG delegation, accompanied by the president of Canada's national CanLyme organization Jim Wilson, meet with the Senior Policy Advisor to the Minister of Health, Ms Shabnum Durrani, and provides extensive information on Lyme Disease in Canada and gaps in services in Ontario. The urgent requests made are: **1.** Need for appropriate and current testing (we provided appropriate contacts). **2.** Education for doctors in Ontario (we provided an appropriate contact from McMaster University). **3.** Securing the safety of the blood supply. **4.** Protective legislation for physicians diagnosing and treating Lyme according to a variety of available protocols (proof of protective legislation in other jurisdictions was also provided). LAG provides copies of both the book by Weintraub and the documentary film to Ministry of Health. The Connecticut Attorney General's press release and the Medical Ethics article are emphasized.

July 17 The Minister of Health, Hon. D. Caplan, writes to LAG member, Justice Bruce R. Shilton (a Chronic Lyme patient), responding to the latter's request for help on April 22. The Minister fails to address the questions posed in that letter and merely defends the use in Ontario of the antiquated and inappropriate Lyme testing procedure. Justice Shilton's reply of August 12 summarizes the points the Minister failed to address and which are of primary relevance to all Lyme patients in Ontario.

US Congress allocates funds to the Centers of Disease Control specific to the issues of "chronic" Lyme disease research, public awareness etc. These funds were allocated on July 17, 2009 by the House Appropriations Committee and on July 30, 2009, by the Senate Appropriations Committee.

See www.wolf.house.gov/LYME and Chapter 1.

July 30 the Connecticut Attorney General-ordered hearings on the reassessment of the IDSA guidelines are complete and placed on all the relevant websites. The public portion of the reassessment is complete.

On August 28, following up on the suggestion of the Minister of Health's Senior Policy Advisor, a LAG delegation meets with the Director of Ontario's Public Health Department, Nina Aaron, and some of her staff. LAG is informed, that Public Health cannot do anything to make proper testing available but can assist with public and physician education within the limits of their mandate. The Director provided the charts and data in summary form on the Public Health department's most recent research (not yet published) into the presence of Lyme Disease-carrying spirochetes and vectors from Ontario and Canada; they show an exponential increase.

On September 11, LAG member Dr. Douglas Wilson (a Chronic Lyme patient), Prof. Emeritus of McMaster Medical School and a foremost authority on physician education in Canada regarding smoking cessation, discusses Lyme education with Nina Aaron, Director of Public Health Ontario. He is told such educational projects are done through the Health Standards division and she would try and get them interested.

On **September 17, the third annual Wall of Hope event** takes place in front of Queen's Park and MPP France Gelinas formally receives the petition started in November 2008 and presents it the same day in the Ontario Legislature. It contains over 1,400 signatures. The event was featured in the media extensively.

See Hansard for that day.

John D. Scott published an article entitled First Isolation of Lyme Disease Spirochete, Borrelia burgdorferi, from Ticks Collected from Songbirds in Ontario, Canada (*North American Bird Bander*, July–Sept. 2009)

October 5, representatives from LAG and ILADS-trained Ontario physician Dr. Jozef Krop make submissions on bill 179 before the Ontario Legislature's Standing Committee on Social Policy. They support the introduction of a College supervisor in RHPA's Section 5.01 and comment on the need for increased procedural protections to prevent misuse of College investigatory and disciplinary powers to arbitrarily enforce inappropriate standards of practice in new and emerging areas of medicine. LAG asked for protective legislation similar to that in some US jurisdictions to specifically protect physicians' ability to provide appropriate care for patients with Chronic Lyme disease. Dr. Krop's presentation also refers to physicians in other emerging areas of medicine being subjected to inappropriate investigatory and discipline process by the CPSO. He includes the 2001 *Glasnost Report* containing examples (e.g. AIDS, Multiple Chemical Sensitivity, Fibromyalgia and Chronic Fatigue Syndrome, stomach ulcers, now known to be caused by bacteria, and now Lyme Disease.)

The Ontario Society of Physicians for Complementary Medicine (OSPCM) make a submission on Bill 179 emphasizing the need in new and emerging areas of medicine to have assessments done by peers who have the relevant expertise during College investigations and to have additional procedural protection added to the RHPA to prevent unfair treatment in the disciplinary processes.

The full account is available in Hansard

In October, the US Environmental Protection Agency (EPA) **accepted the ILADS-supporting Lyme Disease Association of America as an EPA member organization** and links directly to the LDA website for information on Lyme prevention. The US Federal Drug Administration (FDA) acknowledges the limitations of the two-tiered testing protocol mandated by the 2006 IDSA Guidelines (now set aside by the Connecticut Attorney General, but still mandated in Canada) and approved a new test for Lyme disease, emphasizing that the diagnosis must be first and foremost a clinical diagnosis.

Also in October Ontario's *W5* television program aired the Lyme disease issues in a special program.

October 23–25, two Chronic Lyme patients of particular interest attended the annual international ILADS conference: the person who is the subject of the internationally acclaimed documentary film (enclosed) *Under Our Skin* and who was diagnosed with Multiple Sclerosis, and Dr. Dave Martz featured in the book *Under Our Skin,* who had advanced symptoms of ALS (Lou Gherig's Disease). Both are perfectly healthy now and back to work after many years of serious illness. They both were cured by the ILADS treatment protocols. Dr. Martz also presented at the conference on ALS caused/triggered by Lyme infection.

On November 9, John D. Scott wrote to the Hon. D. Matthews, Minister of Health and Long-Term Care, asking her to put into action what he and his colleagues have published for the past decade in the *Canadian Medical Association Journal* on the prevalence of Lyme disease in Canada. The response received in December 2009 did not engage with the issues presented and was essentially a non-response.

December 4, the Canadian Blood Services meet with Lyme Action Group members in Toronto to discuss LAG's concerns which centre on the need to change the donor interview for purposes of ruling out tick-borne disease pathogens being transferred into the blood supply.

On **December 30 Mr. Gabe Magnotta of Ontario's Magnotta Winery, dies from complications of Chronic Lyme disease**; this resulted from the lack of appropriate tests when he first became ill; finally diagnosed correctly in the US, his health had deteriorated too far to avoid the complications that killed him.

2010

In early January LAG finally received the **official response from the Ontario government to the September 17, 2009, Petition signed by almost 1,500 people.** The response did not engage ***at all*** with the specifics in that Petition. A 10-page, detailed analysis of this non-response with a presentation of the actual, verifiable facts, was sent by LAG to the Hon. D. Matthews, Minister of health and Long-Term Care on January 26. Copies were sent to all Ontario MPPs and the media.

February 1, 2010, Dr. Donald E. Low, Medical Director, Infectious Disease Branch, Ontario Agency for Health Protection and Promotion, informs CanLyme that Ontario (and the rest of Canada) follows the US CDC criteria for testing. He seems unaware that the criteria changed in 2008 and that the criteria used in Canada are still based on the IDSA despite the fact that their guidelines were set aside after an anti-trust investigation in 2009.

On February 3, LAG made a formal written presentation to the Ontario Standing Committee on Finance and Economic Affairs in which the details of the waste of public funds were outlined with respect to Medicare in general and the fallout from inappropriate tests in particular.

Also on February 3, the letter by the **Attorney General of Connecticut** to the **IDSA guideline review panel** is made public, under US freedom of information legislation. The letter indicates that "In anticipation of the Review Panel's issuance of the Final Report [on the validity of the IDSA 2006 Guidelines for diagnosis and treatment of Lyme disease], members of my staff recently visited the office of your local counsel to view minutes and records pertaining to the Review Panel's voting … my staff **discovered that the Review Panel failed to conduct the principal voting required** … on whether each [guideline] recommendation in the 2006 Lyme disease guidelines are justified by the medical/scientific evidence." Instead of conducting this vote, the majority vote, which called for a complete re-write of the 2006 guidelines, was suppressed in the recorded results.

Recommended Resources

C. Carroll, *Lab 257*—The *Disturbing Story of the Government's Secret Germ Laboratory*, Harper, 2005

P. J. Langhoff, *The Baker's Dozen and the Lunatic Fringe—Has Junk Science Shifted the Lyme Disease Paradigm?* Allegory Press, 2008

S. Phillips, MD, *Chronic Lyme Disease—An Evidence Based Review,* May 17, 2008 Lecture at the University of New Haven, CT, available on DVD www.unh-lyme.org

Under Our Skin—There's No Medicine for Someone Like You, Documentary, Open Eye Pictures, 2008—winner of 5 film festival awards, nominee for 2009 Oscar, available on DVD from www.underourskin.com

K. Vanderhoof-Forschner, *Everything You Need To Know About Lyme Disease and other Tick-Borne Disorders*, Wiley, 2nd ed., 2003.

P. Weintraub, *Cure Unknown—Inside the Lyme Disease* Epidemic, St. Martin's Press, 2nd ed., 2009.

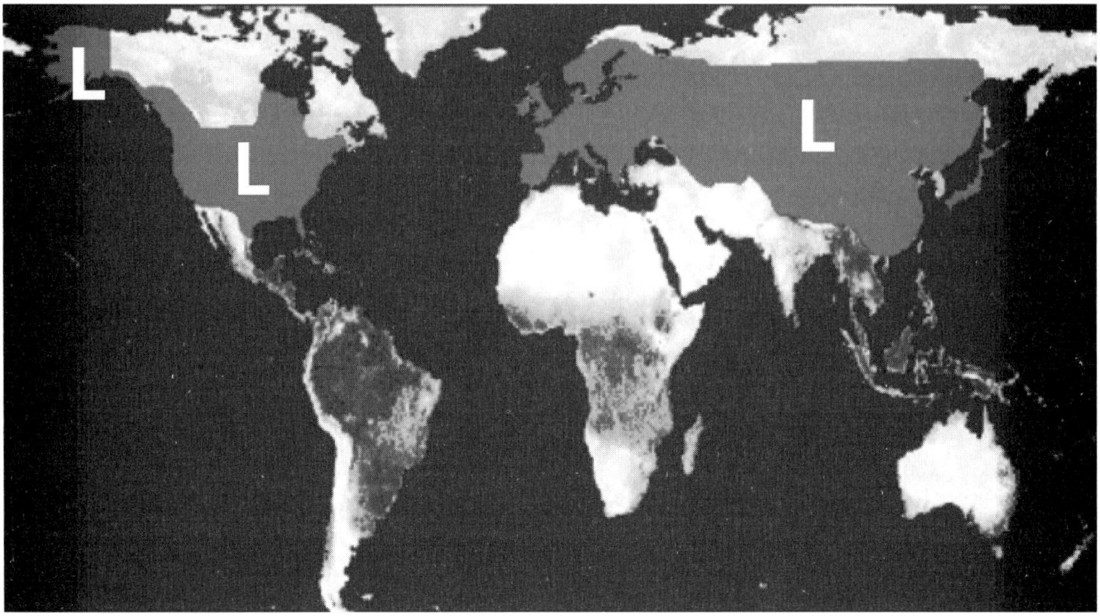

Lyme Disease World Map 2008.

Source: World Health Organization, http://geo.arc.nasa.gov/sge/health/sensor/diseases/lyme.html

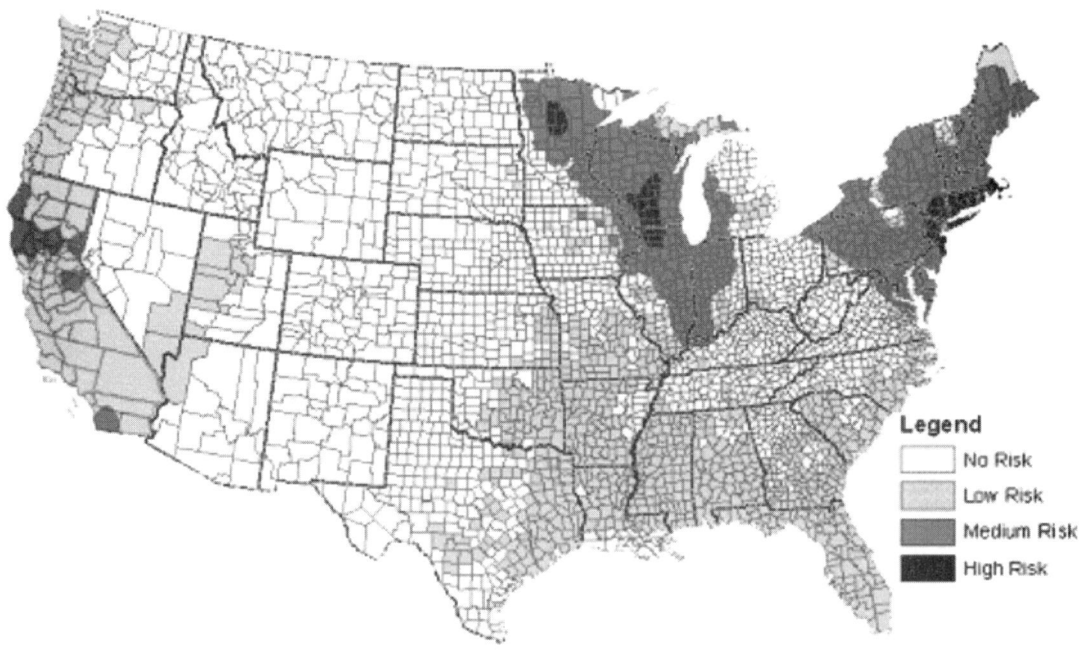

U.S. Maps and Statistics, Lyme Disease Risk.

Source: Dept of Epidemiology and Publich Health, Yale School of Medicine. *Journal of Medical Entomology* 2006 Mar;43(2):166–76.

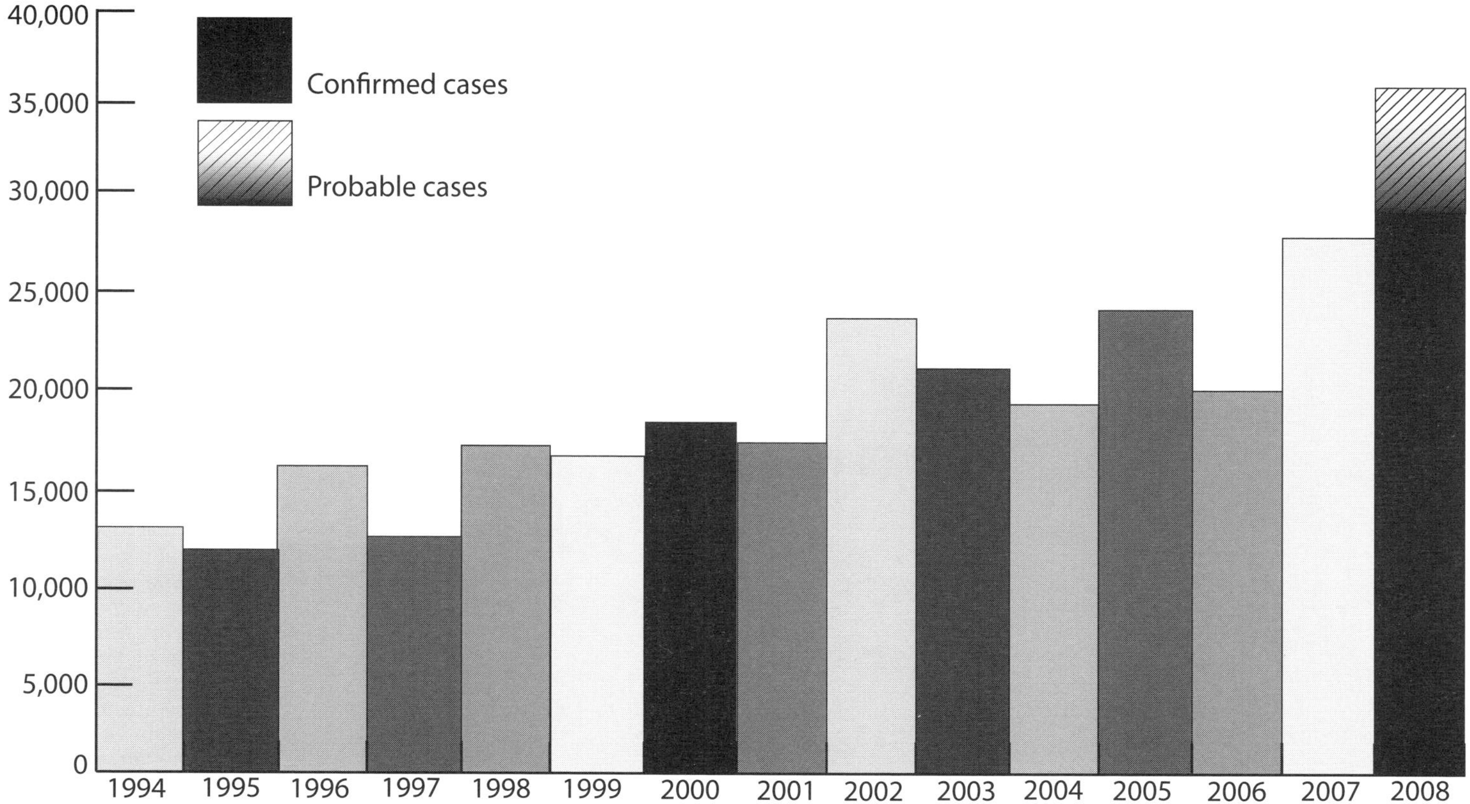

Reported Cases of Lyme Disease by Year, United States, 1994–2008.

State health departments reported 28,921 confirmed cases and 6,277 probable cases of Lyme disease to CDC in 2008. This represents a 5% increase in confirmed cases compared to 2007.

The definition and reporting of probable cases was initiated in 2008 based on revisions to the national surveillance case definition.

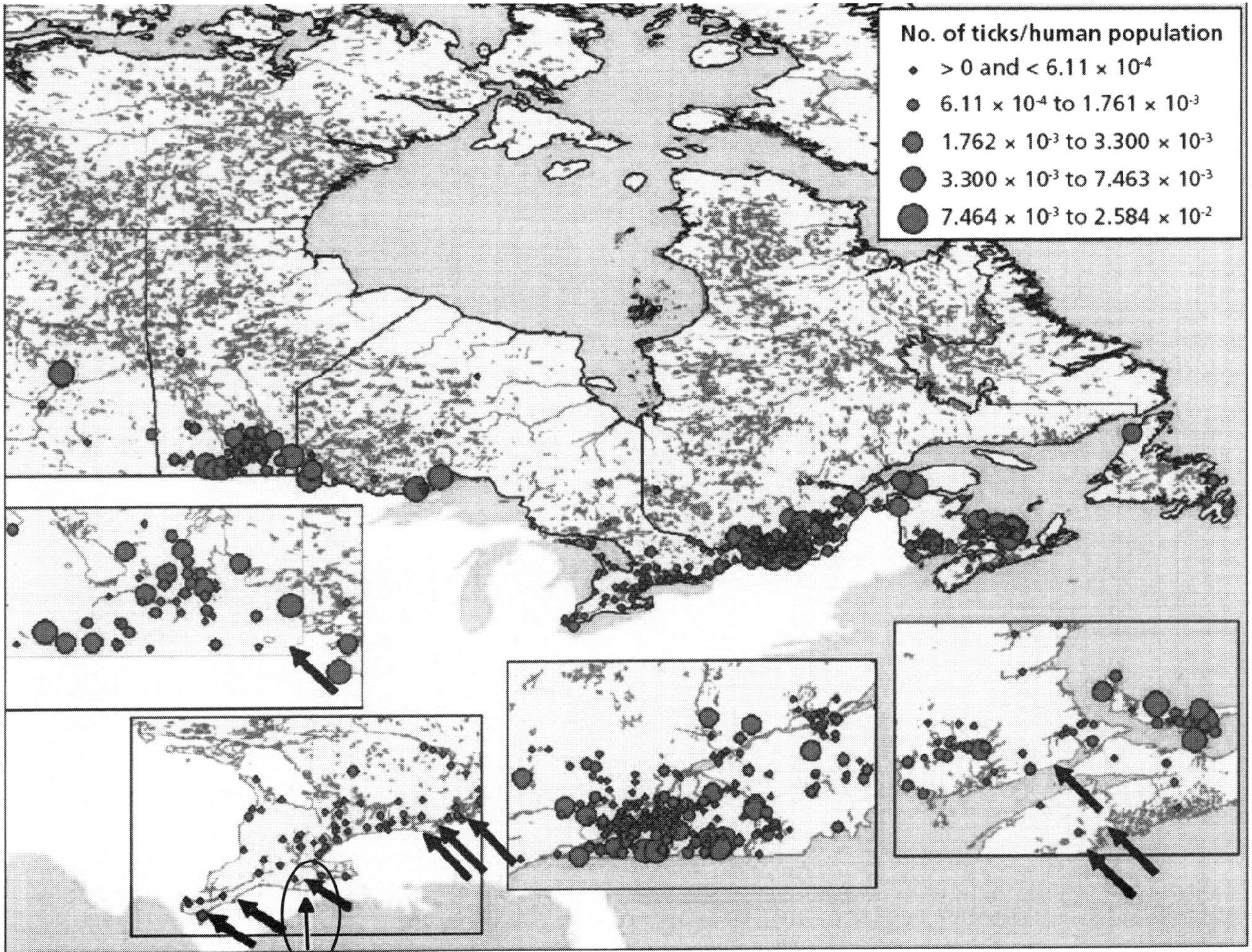

The distribution of *Ixodes scapularis,* reflecting information submitted to provincial and federal public health agencies from January 1990 to December 2003 and to the Lyme Disease Association of Ontario for 1993 to 1999 (circles are centred on the centroid of the census subdivision from which the reports were submitted). Census subdivisions where resident populations of *I. scapularis* are currently known to occur are indicated by arrows, and the cemus subdivision containing the only *I. scapularis* population that was known in 1991 is indicated by the circled arrow.

Source: CMAJ, June 9, 2009, 180(12) Reproduced, with permission, from the Entomological Society of America.

LYME DISEASE IN CANADA

1

THE NATIONAL THEATRE OF THE ABSURD

By Helke Ferrie

> "As we know, there are known known's. There are things we know we know. We also know there are known unknown's. That is to say, we know there are some things we do not know. But there are also unknown unknowns, the ones we don't know we don't know."
>
> —*Donald Rumsfeld*

What This Book Is About And Why You Need To Read It

The principles and values of Public Health are being violated in Canada today on an unprecedented scale by what seems to be the determined decision of the government, regulatory institutions, most of the medical profession, and the public health system to ignore the threat and the available methods of diagnosis and treatment for Lyme disease.

This illness is caused by the bacterium known as *Borrelia burgdorferi,* so called after the Swiss scientist Willy Burgdorfer who discovered its North American variant in the 1980s. These bacteria, and their related co-infections that invariably travel with them, are transmitted by the bite of an infected tick the size of a pinhead. The various species of this tick feed mostly on deer, but now they are known to transmit their resident *B. burgerferi* to migratory birds, mice, domestic pets, and other animals. In humans these bacteria can cause an acute inflammatory disease that can become chronic. Lyme can cross the placenta and blood brain barrier.

Once people are bitten by an infected tick (the most frequent form of transmission), about 60–80% develop a rash around the bite area known as erythema migrans (EM). This rash will rarely appear if the form of transmission was not from a tick bite or a tick species that happens not to cause such a rash. Left untreated, the late manifestation of Lyme disease is characterized by attacks, over weeks or months, of joint swelling, sometimes developing into chronic arthritis. Over time, as Chronic Lyme disease develops, the brain and the central nervous system usually become involved; symptoms include lymphocytic meningitis, cranial neuritis, facial palsy, headaches which are often extreme forms of migraine, muscle weakness, unsteady gait, overwhelming fatigue, stiff and painful neck; often the heart becomes involved and the patient may develop outright myocarditis. Eventually, all organs and bodily systems may be attacked, and treatment becomes extremely difficult at that advanced stage. (See chapter 8.)

Part of the exponential increase in Lyme disease incidence is a function of a process well-known in medical geography; it charts disease occurrence in terms of geographic patterns and findings show that since the beginning of the 20th century, the North American deer population has increased, due to urbanization and reduction in hunting, from an estimated maximum of about 500,000 animals to the current 30 million. In the US and Europe, Lyme disease has increased by more than 100% since 1992. Where accurate data are kept (not in Canada!), it is known that Lyme incidence annually outpaces AIDS and cancer combined. In its acute form it is effectively treatable. Left untreated—*only* because of the suppression of information on reliable diagnosis and clinically proven treatments—it is a devastating chronic illness that now is affecting thousand of Canadians annually. Most of them have no idea what they actually contracted and that it is treatable. Very few know and desperately seek medical help, usually without success in this country.

This book is about this incomprehensible failure of our governments, federal and provincial, and our medical education system to deal rationally with an emerging infectious disease. This failure becomes outright absurd when considering the extraordinary and effective measures the system was able to muster within days when faced with SARS, West Nile virus, or flu epidemics—actual or imagined. Chronic Lyme disease is known as "the Great Imitator," as Syphilis was once called—also caused by a spirochetal bacterium that invades all organs and systems. Lyme is our modern syphilitic epidemic. Once the Lyme spirochete (spiral shaped) and its companion bacteria infest the body they can trigger responses recognized as rheumatoid arthritis, Fibromyalgia and chronic fatigue syndrome, Multiple Sclerosis, Lou Gehrig's disease (ALS), Parkinson's and Crohn's diseases, and scleroderma; in a pregnant woman they can invade the developing brain and central nervous system of the fetus and can cause autism or result in a child born with Chronic Lyme disease. Incidentally, Multiple sclerosis has suddenly increased in Canada by more than 50% in the last 10 years—in tandem with the increase of Lyme in North America.

The concept of Public Health implies a fundamental democracy in medicine. Public Health serves the purpose of making medicine and disease-preventive measures available to everybody. Wherever people live, they share water, soil, and air, are collectively exposed to pathogens and chemical toxins, all shared in the most intimate, and often invisible and unknown ways. Just as democracy is a *way* of dealing with the current and the emergent, Public Health is intended to deal with the current threats to health and the emerging diseases that must be expected.

When plagues in previous centuries depopulated entire regions of the world, the causes became preventable and treatable only much later; the concept of public health arose in tandem with medical science working to develop prevention and treatment for such infectious diseases. Rather like the idea on which the International Red Cross was founded, public health concepts serve the universal human value of health for everyone. We share this planet and everything on it, and this fact requires careful attention and organization. In fact, Public Health interprets the Constitution of Medicine.

When Lyme disease appeared in North America as a serious threat to the people and animals sharing this continent, that medical constitution, for reasons that can be described as criminal, was subverted. Studying the history of Lyme disease is to face the way medicine can be perverted.

Should you be scared? Yes and no. To be human is to be vulnerable to illness. Being alive means being part of the catastrophe of existence. Bacteria can be dealt with, though. Medical science knows how more often than not. What is far more dangerous than the potential for disease is apathy—and that criminal exploitation of human vulnerability to disease for its own ends. If this book makes you *constructively*—coldly, rationally—angry so as to propel you into action in the defense of yourself and your neighbors, its purpose has been achieved. We must demand that our authorities and institutions do what we mandate them to do, what in the language of our laws is called "to serve and protect the public interest."

Because this book contains key information from the medical literature and the most important testing and treatment protocols (chapter 10), as well as access to the vast literature on Lyme disease, it is like a mini-textbook, which can be understood by both doctors and patients. Take it to your doctor, your MP, your MPP or MLA, your lawyer, your insurance company, or anybody else who dares to deny the existence of Lyme disease in Canada and the existence of Chronic Lyme disease. Here is the proof that objectively verifiable information exists on how to diagnose correctly and treat Lyme disease effectively. Any doctor can learn this information.

Finally, this book contains confirmation that, with regard to Lyme disease, following the dictates of Health Canada and obeying the policies of any medical or regulatory authority that ignores or denies the seriousness of this infectious disease, is morally not justifiable.*

* This book was produced on a non-profit basis by the Lyme Action Group. Neither the authors nor the publisher receive any payment for their work; printing costs were met entirely by public donations, and proceeds are going towards advocacy work.

Waiting For Godot

> "The physician's challenge is the curing of disease, educating the people in the laws of health, and preventing the spread of plagues and pestilences."
>
> —SIR WILLIAM OSLER (1849–1919)

In Samuel Beckett's 1953 play, "Waiting For Godot," the characters wait for many days for somebody to come who never does arrive, causing them escalating anxiety about whether they are at the right spot for the expected meeting, whether it is even the correct day for this meeting, who it is they are supposed to meet and why, and why they are waiting at all for somebody about whom they know nothing. Whenever that mysterious Godot is announced as being just about to appear—which always turns out to be an error—those condemned to this interminable torment of waiting shout: "We're saved!" As this expectation always turns out to be yet another false alarm, they enter the next round of anxiety and bewilderment.

A word that frequently is used in this play was invented by Beckett: "apathia." It combines the meanings of the word *apathy*—by which the characters in the play are tormented—and *aphasia,* describing a neurological problem resulting in the inability to speak. Throughout the entire play, an all-pervading sense of meaninglessness, loss of purpose, helpless resignation, and occasional bouts of red-hot anger suffuse its characters.

Anyone who has suffered through many years of Chronic Lyme disease, or any other chronic illness, has taken up residence in Beckett's play—often to remain there for years until they mercifully die. As Chronic Lyme physician, Dr. R. B. Stricker observes, "The level of disability of patients with Lyme disease is equal to that of patients with congestive heart failure, and there are at least 21 studies [by 2008] documenting death in patients with this potentially devastating tick-borne disease." At its worst, Lyme disease is the experience of *apathia*—a combination of apathy on the part of the medical system and an inability of the patient to engage this system in meaningful, helpful dialogue.

Godot for such a patient, at first, is usually the family doctor, the encounter with whose ignorance is generally tragically real, because the attitude regarding Lyme in this country is effectively one of denial, thus ensuring our doctors know next to nothing about Lyme, and whatever they do know is filtered through a propaganda of denial. Lyme patients report again and again how even infectious disease *experts* at Canadian universities told them that they really don't know anything about Lyme and don't know where to begin.

Lyme disease is first and foremost a clinical diagnosis, meaning the signs, symptoms, possible identification of the tick type involved, and patient history are the definitive basis for a diagnosis by a knowledgeable practitioner. However, the tests that would be helpful to treat immediately and effectively and avoid the chronic stage, are not available in Canada. Traditional blood tests cannot be used because the Lyme spirochete does not remain for very long in the blood stream; helpful tests look for signatures of their earlier presence. (See chapter 10) Instead, Canada mandates a testing algorithm so hopelessly obsolete and unreliable, that all it can do and does produce are mostly false negatives. The word "mandates" means that a doctor *cannot* order internationally known reliable tests according to his or her knowledge and as may be relevant to the individual case! The four decades old ELISA test (still useful for other conditions) is totally inadequate for making a Lyme diagnosis and is known to produce up to 90% false negatives, is the preliminary test *mandated* in Canada by the Canadian Public Health Laboratory Network. According to their 2007 guidelines only a positive or "indeterminate" result from this useless test permits the doctor to request a second one—a confirmatory test called the Western blot; all negative ELISA results (most of which miss the presence of the spirochete) are regarded as infallible. Those who have actually a positive infection, go on to become the chronic patients and do not get the necessary treatment. By itself, the Western blot—minus the ELISA, which prevents access to accurate assessment—could be useful, especially the second generation Western Blot now available (see chapter 10).

The most serious shortcoming of these Canadian guidelines is the complete omission of any mention of the existence of and the research published by the International Lyme and Associated Diseases Society (ILADS); their members are trained especially to diagnose and treat the chronic manifestations of Lyme disease. They teach at leading universities, publish in the top professional journals the world over, train doctors in new diagnostic and treatment methods, develop preventive protocols, and treat thousands of Lyme patients often with exceptional success.

The obsolescence of those 2007 Canadian guidelines is further highlighted when one considers that the Centers for Disease Control in the US changed their criteria for Lyme disease in 2008. The revised criteria no longer exclusively require only the ELISA test first, to be followed by the confirmatory Western blot under restricted circumstances. The by-passing of that formerly prerequisite ELISA is now one option—***but Canada hasn't noticed!*** (www.cdc.gov/ncphi/disss/nndss/casedef/lyme_disease_2008)

As recently as February 1, 2010, Dr. Donald E. Low, Medical Director, Infectious Disease Branch, Ontario Agency for Health Protection and Promotion, asserted in a letter to CanLyme that those 2007 Canadian Public Health Laboratory Network guidelines on Lyme diagnosis "follow the testing guidelines of the US Centre for Disease Control," adding that "these guidelines are followed by all provincial Public Health Laboratories in Canada." He made the same statements on the Andy Barrie CBC Metro Morning radio show on January 12, 2010. And in perfect lock-step, the response to LAG's September 17, 2009, Petition to the Ontario Government, was met with the same reply on November 19, 2009. Everybody copies somebody else's information and nobody checks if it is still accurate. Finding the original source is often impossible in this bureaucratic labyrinth—the elusive Godot must be in charge here.

What is even more alarming is the fact that these Lyme-causing bacteria have 15 known genospecies and over 100 strains in just North America, but this mandated testing algorithm only tests for a *single strain*. But it gets even worse: in the 2007 Canadian Public Health Laboratory Network (CPHLN) guidelines for Lyme diagnosis, one finds the need for a "pretest," which totally ignores just about everything that is known to modern medicine about the behavior of infectious diseases: infectious pathogens, being carried by animals and people, by definition know no geographical boundaries. Living things move wherever they want, and what starts as an endemic area, as shown in the World Health Organization map reproduced following CanLyme's Jim Wilson's preface to this book, spreads literally all over the world, if not stopped.

This "pretest" requirement advises in those medically absurd guidelines that even our hopelessly inadequate and antiquated blood testing methods "*for Lyme disease should not be undertaken without a thorough appreciation of the* ***geographic and seasonal setting*** *in which the diagnosis is being considered, as well as an assessment of the* ***likelihood that a specific symptom or symptoms complex is not due to Lyme disease.***" (Emphasis added.) To make sure the treating physician knows how to doubt and then dismiss a patient with clear Lyme symptoms, while simultaneously increasing the illusion that Lyme is helpfully restricted geographically and seasonally, the guidelines continue: "*... the low pretest likelihood of Lyme disease greatly increases the chance of a* ***false-positive*** *result; such false-positive results are often difficult to discount by either the ordering physician or the patient, and these results often lead to unnecessary treatment.*" Oh really? It would be nice to have, for the sake of confirmation, just one documented case of an "unnecessarily treated" person who turned out not to have Lyme after all. Doctors monitor their patients when taking antibiotics and would very quickly notice that no improvement is taking place. There certainly are plenty of cases that require treatment—that host of false-*negatives*.

Well! This is how infectious disease facts become fantasies. No proper surveillance data are gathered; such data cannot be gathered with tests that are known to be mostly ***false negative***; the most authoritative data on tick infestations known to carry this spirochete, some published in the *Canadian Medical Association Journal*, are largely ignored because they are only about ticks—they don't really provide direction on their health implications and direct guidance on what to do about all those people who must be presumed to have become infected. Those medically absurd guidelines amount to a dismissal of fully understood bacterial behavior, which is all-pervasive, inter-continental, and inter-species.

Indeed, we are all trapped in a nation-wide theatre of the absurd. It is close to a miracle that dedicated Canadian researchers, clinicians, and persistent patients have been able to bring out enough facts about Lyme disease in Canada to enable the authors of this book to tell us what is really going on.

Medical Regulation Vs. the Patient

> "In departing from any settled opinion or belief ... the final break is made, as a rule, by some individual who sees with his own eyes, and with the instinct of genius for truth, escapes from the routine in which his fellows live... But he often pays dearly for his boldness."
>
> —Sir William Osler (1849–1919)

The family doctor's ignorance is frequently mixed with a perfectly reasonable fear: treating Lyme patients in Canada, especially advanced cases with Chronic Lyme, may cost a doctor his or her license (see chapter 6 and 7). This is due to the fact that the regulatory authorities in Canada, the provincial Colleges of Physicians and Surgeons, can enforce this national policy of Lyme denial *and* the use of that obsolete testing process. For the CPSO, Chronic Lyme disease may not be a "recognized diagnosis."

The Colleges also frequently cite the dangers of "unnecessary antibiotics," even though it is internationally known that the serious problem of antibiotic resistance is due to its prophylactic use in food-producing animals; they receive low levels of antibiotics over long periods of time due to the overcrowded conditions in which they are kept; they also receive them for the purpose of sudden weight-gain just prior to slaughter, thus causing a saturation of the food supply with antibiotics as well as increasing the rate of cancer in the people who eat that antibiotic-laced meat. In Europe the use of these drugs in this manner was outlawed in the 1980s, causing antibiotic resistance generally to drop dramatically. For a full treatment of this issue nationally and internationally, and clarification of the misconceptions with regard to antibiotic use in humans, the reader is referred to Health Canada scientist Dr. Shiv Chopra's recent book *Corrupt to the Core—Memoirs of a Health Canada Whistleblower*, KOS, 2008.

For a physician to recognize Chronic Lyme disease as a reality—which he or she will undoubtedly do, if reading the full spectrum of the available research or attending an international conference on Lyme—can result in being charged with "failing to maintain the standard of practice" in Canada. Since the federal public health authorities align themselves with the views of the now discredited guidelines of the Infectious Disease Society of America (IDSA—to be described in detail in this chapter in the next section), so do the provincial counterparts and, of course, the medical licensing authorities, the provincial Colleges of Physicians and Surgeons.

Practicing medicine in Canada requires a doctor to be a member of such a provincial College. These colleges trace their existence back to King Henry VIII who created the first College of Physicians for the city of London in 1518. In North America, this system of self-governing colleges began in the late 18th century and in the US was established by a Supreme Court order in 1888.

These professional, self-governing bodies are mandated to uphold the standards of their profession and have the right to discipline their members. They must follow Common Law procedural obligations of many centuries' standing, and these are specifically based on the principle of "natural justice." This principle goes back to the Romans who established that some legal principles are "natural," or self-evident, and did not require a statutory basis, such as the right to be heard (*audi alteram partem*). Natural justice is the basis for procedural fairness, the protection of the rights of individuals involved in disciplinary tribunals so as to enhance public confidence in the process, and today implies that the rights and freedoms enshrined in the Charter are not violated.

In Ontario, where a majority of Canada's doctors work, the CPSO is one of the 26 health professions colleges which all are empowered by statute (Regulated Health Professions Act and the Health Professions Procedural Code) to regulate and discipline their members in accordance with this provincial legislation and the Canadian Constitution.

Certainly these principles are generally followed by the CPSO when working to maintain the standard of practice in the province when it comes to the really gross stuff: sexual abuse or harassment of a patient, financial abuse of patients, or other inappropriate behavior, etc. These transgressions of behavioral standards arise in any society, and among members of any profession.

However, when it comes to the CPSO's interpretation of maintaining the standards of medical practice that happens to incorporate something new, violations of the principle of natural justice have been frequent in the past two decades. Indeed, the CPSO has often met new developments in medicine by using their formidable disciplinary powers, under Section 75 of the Regulated Health Professions Act (RHPA), to enforce either status quo standards of practice, or those the CPSO happens to favor.

That this bias includes the apparent intent to quash new and evolving medical practices became evident during the first discipline hearing of Dr. Krop when he was accused of diagnosing and treating Multiple Chemical Sensitivity (see chapter 7). During that investigation documents surfaced showing that clinical success and patient satisfaction were of no relevance. Every effort was made to find a patient who would testify for the prosecution against Dr. Krop. An internal e-mail memo of March 3, 1994, from the CPSO's investigator to the then chief of investigations, Mr. E. Singleton, states: "Interviews have been conducted with potential witnesses. All of whom are very supportive of Dr. Krop. We have been unable to locate others and attempts are continuing in this regard." It later emerged that an estimated 200 patients of Dr. Krop's were sought out for interviews by the CPSO inspectors.

Since no credible patient could be found to help the CPSO convict Dr. Krop, the logical conclusion should have been, that maybe this physician is doing something right and there actually are no "reasonable and probable grounds" to suggest that the standard of practice was violated. Similar cases, involving various branches of medicine, were described in the *Glasnost Report* of 2001. It included a government-ordered review by KPMG analyzing the CPSO's complaints and discipline process, excerpts from the *Toronto Star's* "Medical Secrets" series, which won the prestigious Michener Award,* and large portions of a legal analysis done by Michael Code, then with Sack Goldblatt Mitchell and now a provincial judge. The *Glasnost Report* was submitted to the Ontario Health Professions Regulatory Advisory Council (HPRAC) for a review of the RHPA.

The effect of invoking disciplinary powers to decide whether a new diagnosis or treatment method meets the standards of practice can be extremely detrimental to patients afflicted with such new and emerging condition. During such standards-of-practice trials, the prosecuting CPSO lawyer is frequently on record making statements such as this one taken from the trial of Dr. S. Kooner. The CPSO lawyer,

* See www.michenerawards.ca/english/cribb2008.htm

Donald Posluns, speaking to the discipline panel stated: "The outcome of treatment is not a useful concept … only the standard of practice is to be evaluated. You set the standards in Ontario, you have never heard of the Pan American Allergy Society and its treatment modalities [from which Dr. Kooner had received additional training], therefore you have to find [him] guilty."

Criminal lawyer Michael Code commented in his report on these types of disciplinary hearings at the CPSO: "The proceedings against Dr. Krop [and about 10 others discussed in his report] would, therefore, appear to involve the *Alice in Wonderland* proposition that doctors are to be disciplined on the basis of some pure scientific principle that has no regard for actual harm and no regard for the satisfaction or dissatisfaction of the patients. That CPSO would spend ten long years, from 1988–1999, pursuing this kind of [issue at] enormous expense through endless disciplinary processes, would seem, at a minimum, to show inappropriate judgment and over-zealousness." During a press conference in the Media Studio of Queen's Park, on May 10, 2000, Code exclaimed: "That's [the CPSO's] analytical methodology! That the actual satisfaction of the patients—whether the treatment actually seems to help—is of no value in establishing scientific principles!"

During Dr. Jozef Krop's first disciplinary hearing, which focused on his diagnosis and treatment of Multiple Chemical Sensitivity, one perceived shortcoming was to be a Fellow of the American Academy of Environmental Medicine (AAEM). This time, he is a member of the International Lyme and Associated Diseases Society (ILADS), and again the CPSO absolutely insisted, despite the defense lawyer's repeated objections, on choosing a reviewer who is in no way Dr. Krop's peer, because the inspector is a member of the IDSA, one of the peer reviewers for the IDSA professional journal, and does not treat patients with Chronic Lyme disease. Even more disturbing is the fact that this CPSO-chosen inspector is on record in the *Ottawa Citizen*, September 10, 2005, denying the seriousness of the disease and insisting on the rarity of its incidence in Canada.

There is a truly astonishing irony in this situation—a contradiction so immense as to be incomprehensible—when considering the following: on the CPSO's website doctors are directed to the "Physician's Toolkit" which, in turn, takes them to the "National Guideline Clearinghouse" of the US government; those guidelines are approved for use by the American Medical Association which the Canadian Medical Association recognizes. Taking courses in any of these offered guidelines provide Continuing Medical Education Credits. Under the search item "Lyme disease," the ***first*** guideline that appears is the one from 2001 published by ILADS! The very one from which Dr. Krop obtained his training in the diagnosis and treatment of Lyme disease. (Its current updated edition is reproduced in full in chapter 10.) Furthermore, the **CPSO's own Position Statement** of November/December 2005, published in that issue of the *Members Dialogue* has this to say:

"This statement clarifies the CPSO's position on clinical practice guidelines (CPGs) in order to assist doctors and the public in understanding how the CPSO utilizes CPGs and to outline how it expects CPGs to be utilized by the profession." The statement explains how such guidelines are developed, that they" synthesize large bodies of evidence, information, and professional opinion," that they are meant to "promote best practice" options, but they will have "variable applicability to individual patients." Importantly, "they do not define a standard of care, but may inform a standard of care. CPGs do not establish inflexible protocols for patient care, nor are they meant to replace the professional judgment of physicians.... The College does not view CPGs as rules 'cast in stone', but rather as important resources, which will provide physicians with a range of appropriate options for patient care, based on available research data and professional consensus." It then encourages doctors to "take advantage of educational programs related to CPGs"—as made available on the CPSO's website, as mentioned above.

Finally, it is specifically mentioned that this Position Statement, and the various existing CPGs are used by the CPSO's Executive and Complaints Committees, in the context of "medical inspections and investigations ... to inform standards of care." Well, when the CPSO invoked a Section 75 disciplinary investigation into Dr. Jozef Krop on June 17, 2008, because of the fact that he treats Lyme disease according to the standards established by ILADS, they must have forgotten their own 2005 Position Paper on the matter.

One of the most important legal cases pertaining to standards of practice in Canada's is the famous **Brett case of 1991** (*Brett et al vs. Board of Directors of Physiotherapy*). Justice O'Leary stated in that decision:

> "... Where an alleged misconduct, however, relates to the methods or techniques of the member in performing the very function of the profession, then a different test must apply. If it be misconduct to use methods and techniques that are foreign to or disapproved by the vast majority in the profession, the profession might never progress. In the case of medicine, for example, acupuncture would probably not have become a method of treatment in Ontario... the member cannot be found guilty of professional misconduct if there exists a responsible and competent body of professional opinion that supports that conduct or judgment ... It is not sufficient for a conviction that the disciplinary panel prefer the

opinion of the vast majority over that of the smaller though equally competent and responsible body of opinion that supports the member in his conduct or judgment."

This "Brett defense," as it is often called, is actually explicitly supported by the CPSO's own 2005 Position Statement. Appointing an IDSA-affiliated physician to assess an ILADS practitioner appears to be a contradiction to both natural justice and the CPSO's own position statement. Given the fact that the IDSA guidelines on Lyme disease are now legally compromised and the IDSA has been ordered to redo them, the CPSO's choice of assessor as well as the decision to invoke a Section 75 disciplinary investigation on *this* standards-of-practice conflict, seems—to say the least—confusing and sends an unintelligible message to the doctors of Ontario.

The CPSO, and the colleges in other provinces in Canada, are able to operate in this manner, because the system is *inherently biased* and lacking in transparency. This potential for *systemic* bias allows self-governance to become hijacked by ideas and agendas that have nothing to do with helping sick people. Unlike the independent system of our courts, Colleges conduct hearings at which they are the policy-maker, investigator, prosecutor, jury, judge, executioner, and publicist—all rolled in one under the same roof. We are so used to this, it no longer strikes us as absurd and fundamentally unjust.

The College initiates a Section 75 investigation that may lead to a disciplinary hearing, a process spelled out in the RHPA. This is done according to the College's own views of what constitutes the standard of practice; then the College decides how the trial is run, may or may not provide full disclosure to the accused, and sets up the jury as it pleases (i.e. the discipline panel). Disclosure is controlled by the College; Dr. Krop does not know to this day what actually prompted the first investigation into Multiple Chemical Sensitivity to commence.

The *appearance* of due process is upheld by hearing most of what the defense wishes to be heard but, in my observation of many such hearings, the *substance* of the defense evidence presented is not necessarily considered.

Finally, the College reports on the entire process strictly on its own terms; the reports of disciplinary hearings are anonymous and published in the *Members Dialogue* to be read by all the doctors of Ontario—from which they may take their lessons.

College decisions are rarely overturned in appeal courts, because those address primarily *procedural* matters, not the *substance* of the disciplinary hearing itself. So, if the College decides it does not approve of the diagnosis of Multiple Chemical Sensitivity for reasons it need not explain, the scientific evidence entered as evidence by the defense will be heard but dismissed, as was the case in Dr. Krop's

MCS hearing, as "lacking the authority of acceptable scientific evidence," without offering any published scientific counter-evidence. The College's opinion is generally hard to challenge in an appeal; the courts defer to the professional colleges as being the assumed experts, due to their self-regulatory status, their presumed expertise in the area, and the fact that the panel heard live evidence. The College is further assumed to be acting in accordance with principles of natural justice, because that is what administrative law tribunals are supposed to do. The appeals court, therefore, believes that a fair hearing must have happened and that the facts presented by the defense were not only heard, but actually carefully considered.

In an article I wrote in 2002, entitled "The Kafkaesque Conviction of Dr. Jozef Krop," I quoted from Kafka's famous 1920s novel, *The Trial*, in which the hero is told, "You can't defend yourself against this court, all you can do is confess." The hero replies, "A single hangman could replace this entire court."

Medical Guidelines Vs. the Hippocratic Oath

> "Everyone is entitled to his own opinion, but not to his own fact."
>
> —Patrick Moynihan, US Senator (1923–2003)

The full story of how Lyme disease became the stuff of "cash, prestige, and careerism," as Hillary Johnson puts it, is found in three important publications listed at the end of this chapter: Pamela Weintraub's magisterial *Cure Unknown—Inside the Lyme Epidemic*, which in 2009 won the American Medical Writers Association Book Award. Second, P. J. Langhoff's 2008 *The Baker's Dozen & the Lunatic Fringe: Has Junk Science Shifted the Lyme Disease Paradigm?*, which focuses on the evidence for the systemic conflicts of interest among the panel members of the IDSA when producing their guidelines of 2006. The "lunatic fringe" phrase was used by IDSA panel members to dismiss the Lyme-treating doctors of ILADS. Also of importance is the report published by the US Lyme Disease Association in April 2001, entitled *Conflicts of Interest in Lyme Disease: Laboratory Testing, Vaccination, and Treatment Guidelines* (available on their website). These reports are deeply disturbing. They constitute the darkest and most depressing information I have read in 14 years of medical science writing.

Of course, Lyme disease is not the first ethical cesspool in recent medial history. Hillary Johnson is the author of *Osler's Web,* which explored the way Chronic

Fatigue Syndrome was denied, to the benefit of the interests mainly of the insurance industry and, in the process, destroyed the careers of many doctors willing to help their patients—many of whom, we now know, actually may have had Lyme disease. Hillary Johnson writes about Weintraub's book that *"the more Weintraub investigated, the more virtually everyone with a shred of authority was losing their credibility, from the nation's 'expert' on Lyme disease, Alan Steere, to the psychologist at* [Weintraub's son's] *high school who, advised her to get her son a good haircut instead of nurturing his fantasy that he was too ill to attend school. As Weintraub would see firsthand, the so-called 'objective' scientists were sending an entire disease down the river and over a cliff, for reasons that seemed frequently to have more to do with mere opinion and crass external forces—cash, prestige, careerism—than with scientific erudition."*

Johnson also points out, that even prior to her own investigation of the denial of Chronic Fatigue Syndrome, and the collusion in that denial by the US Centers for Disease Control, the horrific story of the denial of AIDS had unfolded. That famous book by Randy Shilts, *And the Band Played On,* is still the standard work on the subject. Weintraub, Johnson, and Shilts provided *"that unique body of literature ... a trilogy of aggressive investigation into the willfully unchecked spread of infectious disease in the US"*—and all of North America, since in accordance with NAFTA, Health Canada is expected to go along with whatever the US does or fails to do.

All three disasters occurred, Johnson observes, because those financially compromised so-called experts *"imposed a rigid template on an entity they don't fully understand...* [and] *their studies flow from a disease definition, rather than the other way around ... they have generated information about a 'disease model', but not the disease itself."* This description perfectly fits the IDSA's 2006 Lyme disease guidelines—they have nothing useful to say about the reality of the disease and the actual experience of patients who have it. Indeed, Chronic Lyme is dismissed with these words: *"In many patients, posttreatment symptoms appear to be more related to the aches and pains of daily living rather than to either Lyme disease or a tick-borne coinfection."*

Indeed, this same process of denial has also bedeviled Gulf War Syndrome and Multiple Chemical Sensitivity, or Environmental Illness.

The defining characteristic of corruption in modern medicine is the abandonment of the patient's interest. Be it drug safety and toxic side-effects or treatment choices, emerging conditions or the patient's failure to respond to treatment according to statistical norms, chronic pain that won't go away, or symptoms that are reported that don't fit whichever textbook the examining physician last happened to read—the patient's interest is usually the *least* considered element in the process. The patient may be readily sacrificed to "manageable risk" in the interest of maintaining profits, or containing costs. (Understandably, emergency medicine is the most reliable part of the medical enterprise today.) Dr. Michelle Brill-Edwards, once Canada's top drug regulator at Health Canada, uses the phrase "road-kill on the highway to profit." I am always personally outraged by the phrase "the patient failed treatment," found in patient charts when some regime didn't work as expected. It is the doctor, the system, the drug, the diagnostic process that failed—not the patient. Why does the patient have to conform to budgets, profits, and statistics—especially with an infectious disease that can devastate a society?

In 2002, the US *Annals of Internal Medicine* (vol. 136, no. 3) published simultaneously with the leading medical journals of the world the "Physicians Charter" (recently updated and available on www.professionalism.org), which asserted that doctors must get back to the basics of the Hippocratic oath of 2,500 years ago. The message was clear and, unavoidably crude, although sophisticated prose tried to make it all sound as nice as possible: don't exploit your patients sexually or abuse them financially, don't hurt them, let them chose among available treatments, meet their needs even if they are black, Jews, poor, developmentally delayed, gay or lesbian, in the process of dying, just plain old and frail and befuddled, or don't have any money. Above all, don't betray their confidence and don't lie in your research because somebody offers to pay you for those lies.* This document was prepared by an international team of medical ethicists for the "Medical Professionalism Project" and states at the outset: "*We share the view that medicine's commitment to the patient is being challenged by external forces of change [which] tempt physicians to forsake their traditional commitment to the primacy of patients' interests.*"

Those "external forces" were neatly identified by a senior advisor to insurance giant Kaiser Permanente, Dr. David Eddy, who is quoted in 2000 in the *Journal of the American Medical Association*: "**... whoever controls practice policies controls medicine.**" (Reference 14 in item 3 below.) Primary tools for control over doctors are published practice guidelines, or consensus agreements from regulatory authorities, which define the "standards of practice." Doctors know this and are as frustrated and often as outraged as their patients.**

*German research recently showed that about half of what is published is factually compromised, and in Canada the *Globe & Mail* published statistics showing that more than 80% of our doctors are financially involved with the pharmaceutical industry. (See Ferrie 2004, Section 6 & Ferrie 2008, chapter 3 and sources cited therein.)

**This systemic conflict of interest tends not to arise so much in ordinary daily medical practice and emergency medicine situations; they become dominant in all situations of chronic disease—when treatment and diagnosis are complex, prolonged, unpredictable, and expensive.

Last year, on April 1, 2009, the editors of the world's leading medical journals got together and published an article in the *Journal of the American Medical Association* entitled "Professional Medical Associations and Their Relationship With Industry: A Proposal for Controlling Conflicts of Interest." The editorial in that issue was entitled "Reassessment of Clinical Guidelines—Go Gently Into That Good Night." These statements are calls for radical reform unprecedented in the history of medicine. In the past couple of thousand years one worried about superstitions and charlatans, now we worry about the professionals with a string of important letters behind their names. In the editorial on practice guidelines, the authors state:

> "... too many guidelines have become marketing and opinion-based pieces, delivering directive rather than assistive statements...In one study of 44 guidelines, 87% of the guideline authors had some form of industry tie...guidelines are not patient-specific enough to be useful and rarely allow for individualization of care. Most guidelines have a one-size-fits-all mentality ... If all that can be produced are biased, minimally applicable consensus statements, perhaps guidelines should be avoided completely. Unless there is evidence of appropriate changes in the guideline process, clinicians and policy makers must reject calls for adherence to guidelines. Physicians would be better off making clinical decisions based on valid primary data."

An exhaustive post-mortem of the whole concept of "evidence-based" medicine, which supposedly informs those guidelines, as used, misused, abused, in medicine thereby causing harm patients instead of benefiting their recovery, is found in the 2008 magisterial article by Andrew Miles. He is the editor-in-chief of the *Journal of Evaluation in Clinical Practice* and also is the National Director in the UK of Key Advances in Clinical Practice. This article is co-authored with Michael Laughlin, who teaches applied philosophy at the University of Manchester.

The Lyme disease guidelines produced by the IDSA during the past decade ignored the full range of the existing science—that base of evidence—and did not consider the published clinical evidence on Chronic Lyme disease, the testing procedures known to be useful (such PCR and urine tests), blocked the use of more reliable testing procedures, and ignored the evidence that contradicted their views, no matter where it came from—from colleagues within the IDSA, Lyme patient groups, legitimate and licensed laboratories which had developed FDA approved tests, other recognized medical organizations, and even entire university departments working with Lyme disease.

So influential is the IDSA, by 2006 the US government accepted their denial of the existence of Chronic Lyme as gospel truth, despite the fact that its own National Institutes of Health had validated the severity and reality of Chronic Lyme in formal studies funded by tax money. Insurance companies used the IDSA guidelines to deny coverage, and medical boards used them also to prosecute doctors who treated Chronic Lyme patients for a genuine infectious illness, or resorted to reliable tests.

Even important medical journals were co-opted. *The New England Journal of Medicine* went so far as to criticize the fact that the Attorney General of Connecticut dared to get into this mess and had invoked anti-trust law to clean it up. (The authors of that incomprehensible nonsense were lawyers, not doctors—a fact that reflects poorly on the editorial judgment of that famous journal and on the motives of the authors who ought to be acquainted with legal medicine.)

Undeterred, Richard Blumenthal confronted this Augean stable, and the clean-up process was an impressive undertaking, with all scientific testimony televised live in July 2009. The person appointed to chair this process was Dr. Howard Brody, an expert in medical ethics and the co-editor of an important book on the history of infectious disease, *Cholera, Chloroform, and the Science of Medicine: The Life of John Snow*. In the early 19th century, Snow developed the methods used today to identify and predict epidemics caused by infectious pathogens before such pathogens could even be seen. Dr. Brody has also written extensively on the disastrous influence of the pharmaceutical industry on the practice of medicine.

As stated in the May 1, 2008, press release from the Attorney General's office, announcing the findings of that anti-trust investigation, great care was taken to ensure that the anti-trust investigation was *not* concerned with medical scientific debate as such, range of views on clinical efficacy, or the variety in the methods of practice, but focused on the overt and provable suppression of mainstream published research that contradict the views of the IDSA Lyme guideline panel members. The focus was on procedural issues such as evidence for exclusion of the clinical results and opinions of even their own physician members, or other medical groups, who were exploring new or different ways of diagnosis and treatment with Lyme patients. Finally, the panelists' financial conflicts of interest were found to be so crass and outrageous, that even in these days of corporate profit-focused dominance in medicine, the extent and size of those conflicts was revealed to be astonishing.

Attorney General Blumenthal summarized the review process in a letter to the IDSA dated February 1, 2010: "*As you are aware, during the anti-trust investiga-*

tion of the IDSA, my office uncovered significant procedural deficiencies relative to the IDSA's 2006 Lyme disease clinical practice guidelines. These process deficiencies raised serious questions as to whether the recommendations made in the 2006 guidelines reflected the best available scientific and medical evidence on the subject … … my office and the IDSA negotiated a settlement, which included an Action Plan … the essence [of which] was fairly simple: Step 1 was to establish a stringent procedure for identifying and vetting a completely new review panel …"

At this stage, the first bit of corruption that leaked into the process became evident when the panel excluded, on the grounds of financial conflict of interest considerations, those doctors who made more than $10,000 a year from treating Lyme patients. This was a clever move: any doctor treating a lot of Chronic Lyme patients and who, therefore, actually knew what Chronic Lyme looks like and can demonstrate how it can be effectively treated, was suddenly a pariah expelled into the same group as those IDSA panelists who could be described as having thrown their patients to the wolves while making huge profits from consulting fees with the insurance industry and serve as "experts" to save the industry money. However, once this review process had been ordered by the Attorney General, intervention its progress became practically impossible.

A statement of some sort was expected from this new Review Panel by the end of 2009. Sometime in late January 2010 something happened—it is not clear what—to alert the Attorney General to the possibility of foul play. Maybe Blumenthal has an excellent intuition, having followed the questionable activities of the IDSA Lyme guidelines panels since 1999. In any event, the Attorney General states in his February 1, 2010, letter to the IDSA that *"in anticipation of the Review Panel's issuance of the Final Report, members of my staff visited the office of your local counsel to view the minutes and records pertaining to the Review Panel's voting."*

Blumenthal then reminds the IDSA that *"because my office determined that the IDSA had excluded consideration of divergent evidence and participation of individuals from the 2006 guidelines panel, who held dissenting opinions, the cornerstone of the Action Plan and the 'principle function' of the Review Panel established thereunder, was to look anew and 'make an individual determination whether each of the recommendations in the 2006 Lyme disease guidelines is medically/scientifically justified, in light of all the evidence and information provided"* in those extensive public hearings and through the written submissions during the anti-trust investigation process. He goes on to clarify this further: *"In other words, the Review Panel was assigned the task of determining whether the Lyme disease panel 'got it right' in the first instance for each recommendation."*

After Blumenthal's staff reviewed the records of what happened during those meetings of that Review Panel at the IDSA's lawyer's office, something disturbing emerged. *"During this review my staff discovered that the Review Panel* ***failed*** *to conduct the principal voting required by the agreement and the Action Plan, on whether each recommendation in the 2006 Lyme disease guidelines was justified by the medical/scientific evidence.* ***Instead of conducting this vote,*** *it appears that the Review Panel, with your Vice President of Clinical Affairs present, voted on whether each recommendation warranted one of four actions: (a) no change was required, (b) no change was required, with comment, (c) a revision was necessary, or (d) a re-write was required. These voting parameters do not specifically appear anywhere in the Action Plan .... My staff has notified the IDSA's Vice President of Clinical Affairs and your counsel of the improper voting procedure."*

The change in the voting process, and therefore the scoring process, would favor not making changes in the 2006 guidelines. That's called rigging the vote.

And what exactly was that first recommendation that some member of that new IDSA Review Panel tried so hard to save from oblivion, by simply avoiding those uncomfortable specific instructions they were ordered to follow? The 2006 Lyme testing recommendation, of course! If the full range of medical and scientific information, made available during that anti-trust investigation in public hearings, was to be considered logically and honestly, that unreliable ELISA test, which ensures Lyme patients with false-negatives are screened out and "sent over the cliff," to use Hillary Johnson's words—that test would have to be the very first recommendation to be canned. After that, it's all a cakewalk. Chronic Lyme denial would be impossible to sustain.

The Attorney General ends his letter by telling them to go back and do it right. Again. Given this Attorney General's reputation and record, they had better do so. In any case, humiliation has become inescapable.

Lawyer Lorraine Johnston observes that had the Attorney General not decided to have a quick look-see at this stage, *"the IDSA would have carried out a corrupted process that blatantly violates the agreement—and it might never have been discovered."* Indeed, she is right when stating "*This* [behavior] *turns evidence-based medicine on its head. When the IDSA panel so deliberately violates the voting procedures ... and refuses to comply with the Attorney General's request, there can be only one conclusion: the ability of the IDSA to run this process with integrity is extremely suspect, and any outcome must be viewed critically."*

Either a hell of a lot of money is at stake here for some of the IDSA members or as an organization, or the pride factor has reached a pathological level, or they are scared of some huge liability issues appearing at the horizon. Whatever—as one says today. The truth will out. This is not over and may get a lot worse for the IDSA.

It is necessary to explore how all this affected Canada. First, it must be emphasized that in both the US and Canada, regulatory and government agencies are expected *not* to align themselves arbitrarily with *any* private organization and are *not* to further the views of one organization over all others. In the US there are laws against such arbitrary behavior governing the Centers for Disease Control. Of course they can be ignored, and of course, there the battle rages, too (see Congressman Frank R. Wolf's letter of September 4, 2008, appended to this chapter).

Unfortunately, the Canadian Public Health Laboratories Network guidelines of 2007 align themselves exclusively with the IDSA's 2006 guidelines. Not even so much as a small-font, passing mention of ILADS 2004 guidelines is to be found in the references cited in those Canadian guidelines, nor is there reference to their key research contributions.

The investigation from 2006 to 2008 of the IDSA Lyme disease guideline process by the Attorney General of Connecticut is an event that must be recognized as binding for infectious disease doctors not just in North America, but anywhere in the world. The practice of medicine, like human biology, has no political boundaries. When something in medicine has been discredited—a research finding or a guideline, it applies to everybody on the planet. Canada took no notice so far.

In plain English, this anti-trust investigation can be described as dealing with the effects of lies, greed, and the abuse of power on the practice of medicine and the way these prevented extremely sick patients from getting treatment, or caused them further harm through incorrect treatment.

An anti-trust investigation of this type in medicine is a unique event. Something like this has never happened before. Medical law expert, Lorraine Johnson has pointed out that this legal intervention *"represents the first time that conflicts of interest in the guidelines development process have been addressed using anti-trust theories,"* [e.g. anti-monopoly law]. Applying anti-trust law to medicine, Johnson explains, is warranted *"when a medical society has monopoly power such that its guidelines can take on the force of law, as the IDSA guidelines do."* This is evident in the fact that they are followed by Health Canada as is evident from the Canadian Public Health Laboratory Network guidelines and the insurance industry. Due to this danger of a monopoly opinion, Johnson observes, the IDSA *"has an obligation to ensure that the development process is fair, does not exclude competing points of view, and that its panel is not driven by commercial conflicts of interest."* (See item 3 in this chapter.)

The IDSA members abused their monopoly power to the point of instigating disciplinary action against its own members (and doctors in other medical societies) if they treated Chronic Lyme patients for infection in accordance with published information, such as the ILADS guidelines or other than the IDSA's arbitrarily imposed dictates.

Following the usually fruitless encounter with the family doctor, who is pretty much prevented by this IDSA/ILADS conflict from knowing anything reliable and doing anything useful, the Lyme disease patient's search for Godot usually continues through the land of medical tests. After that predictable fiasco, he or she is shunted from one "expert" to the next, left no choice but to resort to unemployment and disability procedures that are humiliating and often inappropriate, also may endure the loss of family support because the care of Chronic Lyme patients can be a horrendous burden—until total despair descends when the realization dawns, that all those doctors and government authorities tend to follow the rules of their Game. As the subtitle puts it, to that now famous documentary film on Lyme disease, *Under Our Skin*: "There's no medicine for someone like you."

The worst experience for many Chronic Lyme patients can be when somebody suggests that all these bewildering multi-organ and multi-system symptoms are only imagined—after all the tests don't show anything! So, obviously the Godot this patient is waiting for must be a psychiatrist. Janet Sperling, who co-authored chapter 3 with her entomologist husband Felix Sperling from the University of Alberta wrote in an e-mail recently: *"Infectious disease people are determined to make psychiatric diagnoses, although they get angry when psychiatrists state that the patient does not have a psychiatric illness. I love to watch the reaction of doctors [who deny Chronic Lyme as a diagnosis], when I say to them that they should just declare Lyme a psychiatric illness, since psychiatrists are open to complicated illnesses that require long-term treatment. Infectious disease doctors go apoplectic!"*

Ironically, the historical fact is, that it was psychiatrists who in the early 1990s began to take Chronic Lyme disease seriously. Psychiatrist, trained to encounter distressed minds, found the symptoms Lyme patients complained, and which naturally caused patients extreme mental distress as well, involved visible disability and symptoms of severe inflammation together with obvious central nervous system (CNS) problems. The question of whether real, measurable damage was happening to the CNS and the brains of Chronic Lyme patients (as opposed to hypochondriacal delusions) was first asked by Dr. Brian A. Fallon. Today, at Columbia University's Department of Psychiatry he directs the Lyme and Tick-Borne Diseases Research Center from which some of the most important work has come, proving the measurable reality of Lyme's impact on the CNS and the brain. (See item 4 by Dr. Fallon, following chapter 8.)

Chronicity in infectious diseases is not new, nor is CNS involvement. Syphilis, Leprosy, Tuberculosis, AIDS, Hepatitis B and C, Malaria and more all share these properties. Long-term treatment, often with potentially dangerous antibiotics requiring very careful monitoring, is also nothing new in medicine. Indeed, doctors will treat conditions like acne easily with two or more years of antibiotics.

The Lyme-causing spirochetal bacterium *Borrelia burgdorferi* is, however, unique: the syphilis-causing spirochete has only 22 genes; the Lyme-causing one has 132 genes and, as Dr. Robert C. Bransfield, a Chronic Lyme expert, past president of ILADS, and neuro-psychiatrist puts it, this bacterium is so unusual because *"90% of its genes are unrelated to any other known bacteria … it is perhaps the most complex bacteria known."* He observes, that *"syphilis is the dumb cousin"* to Lyme.

This spirochete has the ability to hide in deep tissues and thus becomes invisible in the patient's blood, thereby making direct, traditional blood tests obsolete; 3D imagining of this process was achieved for the first time in 2008. The bacterium rapidly conglomerates in a self-protective cystic form, sheds its outer membrane to evade antibiotic attack (the molecular basis of this so-called L-formation process was published in 2009); it hides effectively from immune and antibiotic attack by creating a camouflage relationship with resident fungi, it passes the blood-brain barrier without difficulty, and it usually appears with other bacteria of various types (the many known co-infections); those often divert medical attention instead of suggesting the presence of the Lyme spirochete as well. Finally, Lyme spirochetes are able to lodge in any and all bodily fluids and thus the disease can become sexually transmissible (see Bach in references). In short, Lyme disease is the perfect bacterial storm.

This is a complex, clever, and very ancient enemy that has become more complex and nasty over time and resistant to treatment (see item 2 in this chapter). Given what medicine knows about infectious disease—historically the very basis of medicine's claim to fame—one would expect the utmost attention to be given to this bacterium. Unfortunately, the vast and usually accurate knowledge about infectious diseases and the amazing available tool kit of tests and antibiotics can also feed the not-so-altruistic tendencies of doctors and policy makers.

Given this spirochete's innate and behavioral complexity, it is not surprising that Lyme has become known in the medical literature as "the great imitator." Depending on what organ or system it invades, it can set off of a host of unpredictable responses known collectively as "idiopathic" diseases (i.e. cause unknown) which are always chronic, ruin the lives of their victims slowly and torturously, cost the state billions in care and more billions in lost revenue from taxes that could have been paid by active, healthy people doing creative work for society. The list of diseases was given in the opening section of this chapter. The reasonable response to these published facts—PubMed has thousands of entries on what was summarized above—*should be* that a differential diagnosis for *all* of these conditions includes testing for Lyme and its co-infections. At the very least this would make fiscal sense, as the Lyme Action Group recently pointed out to Ontario's Standing Committee on Finance and Economic Affairs; almost 50% of the province's budget goes to health care. If even just 10% of all those patients diagnosed with these expensive chronic diseases were cured, or vastly improved, by known Lyme treatment regimes, billions of dollars would be saved and made through the taxes from people no longer disabled.

The current ILADS president-elect, Dr. David Martz, originally an oncologist who wound up in a wheelchair after being diagnosed with the dramatically disabling condition known as Lou Gehrig's Disease (ALS), finally found out he had Lyme and tick-borne co-infections. He now has completely regained his health and runs a Chronic Lyme clinic in the US.

The point of Beckett's play, when applied to health and disease, is that the first step into freedom, or towards finding a cure, is to cease waiting in hope for an external authority—a nebulous savior. Feminist Gloria Steinem used to say that the "personal has become political" and the "political is also always personal." That realization implies the need to become an activist on your own behalf. Today, medicine is politicized to such an extent, that the most genuinely patient-dedicated physician, as well as the most callous profit-oriented careerist, may be enmeshed, with their patients, in a web of conflicting goals, which the patient needs to recognize. Only mouthy patients determined not to succumb to the system will save themselves—and their doctors. Ultimately it is patients who must act to fix this broken system and demand good clinical judgment founded on uncorrupted science.

The good old days, when one believed that "the good doctor knows best," are over. Now, as lawyer Lorraine Johnson explains, *"there is tremendous financial gain in Lyme disease through vaccines* [which so far failed and caused enormous harm before being taken off the market, and which are likely to fail again for well-understood technical and biological reasons], *diagnostic tests* [which have mostly been co-opted to favor vaccine development instead of helpful therapies] *and consulting with insurance companies* [from which doctors recognized as "experts" make literally fortunes]." (Item 3 below).

This is the tragedy of modern medicine. However, patients refusing to wait for Godot open up the possibility of making medicine once again what it should be—science and compassion serving the patient—and no other master.

Lyme Politics

> "By definition, a government has no conscience.
> Sometimes it has a policy, but nothing more."
> —Albert Camus (1913–1960)

When the Lyme Action Group began its awareness campaign in late 2008, doing so by attacking on all fronts in this system simultaneously, it was fully expected that the responses would include "get lost, all is well" letters, replies indicating that LAG is misinformed, or that matters are being attended to progressively and thanking us for our concern. Occasionally, LAG was treated rather respectfully and the concerns voiced engaged with seriously, as was the case with the Canadian Blood Services after the initial polite brush-off (chapter 4).

Somewhat predictably but, nevertheless, appreciated were the responses from Opposition Party members, such as from Ontario's then Progressive Conservative health critic Elizabeth Witmer, who wrote to the Premier, the Attorney General, and the then Minister of Health, asking for action on behalf of Lyme patients. Much appreciated was the pro-active help received from Ontario's NDP health critic, France Gelinas, who tabled in the Legislature LAG's petition signed by almost 1,500 Ontario residents. Liberal MPP Sophia Aggelonitis even visited the new Minister of Health and Long-Term Care, the Hon. D. Matthews, to raise the issues of Lyme in Ontario. Refreshingly, in the federal government, Liberal Opposition member, MP Dr. Carolyn Bennett, took also a pro-active stance and wrote to the Canadian Blood Services on March 23, 2009, demanding the necessary steps to protect the blood supply against tick-borne infectious organisms be taken.

Among the brush-offs the Ontario government's response to the September 17, 2009, petition bearing 1,500 signatures,was painfully disappointing. At the Third Annual Wall of Hope event, held on the lawn in front of Queen's Park, this formal petition was handed to MPP France Gelinas (NDP) who read it into the record that afternoon (see Hansard for that date). The petition requested that " ... *the Ontario Public Health system and OHIP include all currently available and scientifically verified TESTS for Acute and Chronic Lyme diagnosis, to do everything necessary to create PUBLIC AWARENESS of Lyme Disease in Ontario, and to have internationally developed diagnostic and successful TREATMENT PROTOCOLS available to patients and physicians.*" It also informed of the necessity for the government's attention by stating that Chronic Lyme disease "*.... mimics many catastrophic illnesses, such as Multiple Sclerosis, Crohn's, Alzheimer's, arthritic diseases, depression, Chronic Fatigue and Fibromyalgia ... but the scientifically validated diagnostic tests and treatment choices are currently not available in Ontario, forcing patients to seek these in the USA and Europe...*"

When the government's response was made available (only after LAG kept asking for it repeatedly) on January 14, 2010, it simply did not engage with the central issue of the petition at all. It merely informed LAG that proper testing is available, because the currently OHIP covered tests are mandated by the Canadian Public Health Laboratory Network guidelines of 2007—which settles the matter, regardless of 1,500 Canadians informing the Ontario government that reliable test are not available. In other words, the system is so tightly interlocked—from Health Canada down to the Public Health offices—there appears to be no hope of entering into a logical discussion with anybody in the entire system.

To add insult to injury, the following information was passed on to LAG showing that not only is the policy on Lyme disease in Ontario—and the rest of Canada, as the whole country follows those 2007 guidelines on testing—declared perfect by one and all, but in addition this system is further supported by the outright fiction that in Canada treatment for Lyme disease is freely and readily available.

Dated November 26, 2009, one of our members received a letter from the Ontario Health System and Accountability and Performance Division of the Ministry of Health and Long-Term Care. It was a rejection of an application for Out-of-Country Health Services for the treatment of Chronic Lyme disease; this patient originally contracted Lyme disease in Ireland. Due to this lack of available and effective testing and treatment options in Ontario this person became seriously disabled and eventually sought treatment in California by an internationally trained Chronic Lyme disease expert. Improvement was dramatic—until money ran out and an application was made by the responsible family doctor for funds to permit completion of the treatment course. His application was rejected as follows: "*There are several Ontario Infectious Disease Specialists who can diagnose and treat patients with Lyme Disease. A medically necessary consultation with an Ontario specialist should be available in a timely fashion ... treatment of Lyme borreliosis and asso-*

ciated co-infections is performed in Ontario by identical [to the US] or equivalent procedures."

We appear to have entered the realm of science fiction. If there *are* Lyme-literate infectious disease specialists in this province, who are able and willing to treat effectively acute and Chronic Lyme disease, and can do so in "a timely fashion" for those thousands of misdiagnosed chronically ill Lyme patients, we are most anxious to know about them. We do know of some naturopaths who are Lyme-literate; of course, if your dog or horse falls sick with a Lyme infection, the veterinarian will diagnose and treat such animals properly and effectively and in accordance with the latest scientific information.

The response to LAG's Petition concluded with the sage advice *that "everyone [should] take precautions when they are in areas considered at higher risk for contact with ticks .... as the best practice for preventing Lyme disease."* Indeed, that would be a very good idea. But, unfortunately, unlike the approach taken in the US, in Canada signs are rarely posted—if ever—at the entrance to national parks and recreational areas where Lyme-bearing ticks are endemic, especially in the spring and early summer. Those areas have repeatedly been identified in articles published in the *Canadian Medical Association Journal* since the year 2000 and most recently, again, in June 2009. (See maps in this book.) The provincial and national policies on Lyme appear to be not only total denial, but a determined enforcement of that denial.

The single most astonishing and absurd response came from the office of the Hon. Tony Clement, then the federal Minister of Health. This response was not received directly from him, but came to LAG through MP Jack Layton, Leader of the federal New Democratic Party.

The prequel to this event is noteworthy: when the Hon. Tony Clement was running for election to the federal government in 2008, he was approached by Lyme disease patients, and in October went on record at an all-candidates meeting in Lyme-endemic carrying Bracebridge, stating that if re-elected, he would make Lyme disease a top priority and help establish an appropriate policy for the whole country. As soon as he won his seat, he was transferred to a different portfolio.

The federal government introduced Bill C-11, *An Act to promote security with respect to human pathogens and toxins* which was passed into law in 2009; it specifically mentions, among a great many bacteria, viruses and the like, the Lyme-causing pathogen, *Borrelia burgdorferi* as one of the disease agents Canadians must be protected from. This is discussed in more detail in chapter 4.

Meanwhile, the federal NDP was working in various ridings to promote Lyme awareness, especially in B.C. through MP Judy Wasylycia-Leis (NDP Winnipeg

North); she had become aware of the plight of Lyme patients through the national patient support group CanLyme located there, and through provincial MLA David Cubberley (author of chapter 6).

On April 22, 2009, a Chronic Lyme patient received an e-mail from MP Jack Layton, leader of the NDP, in response to a question. His reply included the following statement:

"*... in January of last year [2008] I wrote to [*then*] Health Minister Clement about this very issue, requesting an explanation as to why his department refuses to release results of proficiency tests to the Canadian Lyme Disease Foundation* [founded through the efforts of CanLyme*] that identifies Lyme in the blood—a key to early detection. The Minister's [*Clement*] reply stated the* request for information has been denied on the basis of national security*—the same information he has provided to the Foundation. I cannot understand the basis for this senseless decision to deny the release of information that could benefit so many of the estimated 10,000 Canadians who are bitten* [by Lyme-carrying ticks] *annually and who deserve early detection for effective treatment.*" (Emphasis added.)

What does this mean? The official wording of such a denial is as follows: " ... *access is denied* [because the record] *contains information which could reasonably be expected to be injurious to the conduct of international affairs, the defense of Canada, or any state allied or associated with Canada, or the detection, prevention, or suppression of subversive or hostile activities.*" Can anything be more absurd?

As for the Hon. Tony Clement, he apparently saw the information the government actually has on Lyme as a state secret in January 2008, but by October he had no compunction about making promises that would in actual fact be unfulfillable! The effective national Lyme disease policy would have to be based on that state secret, which is what he told MP Layton ten months earlier! So, either Lyme data at Health Canada are a state secret—something so absurd as to demand a national inquiry—or it is not a state secret, in which case the Hon. Tony Clement has to answer some hard questions.

MP Layton's use of the word "senseless" is certainly dead on. How could proper testing be in conflict with national security? Is this just a case of governmental obfuscation, or did Clement let some cat half-way out of the bag? What comes to mind immediately are the US government reports on experiments for biological warfare purposes involving spirochetal bacteria. That this happened is beyond doubt—what is yet unknown is the connection between the current Lyme disease epidemic and that bio-warfare program. The book on this issue by lawyer Michael

Christopher Carroll, listed below, is based entirely on government records declassified in the 1980s or obtained under freedom-of-information legislation. Is it possible that some dumb nonsense related to that bio-warfare era is still ghosting about in Ottawa and scaring Ministers and bureaucrats? Or might Clement have referred to those tests for Lyme disease that were developed and patented when the Cold War ended, but then were never used because other interests took centre stage, especially vaccine development?

We will probably never know. What we do know today, beyond doubt, is that we can and must do something about Lyme disease now—and leave the bio-warfare story, horrific and true as it might be, to medical historians, and eventually to the often healing and cathartic effect of film and fiction—the visual imagination of Hollywood and the superlative story-telling of John LeCarre.

And this is no flippant dismissal of a possible crime against humanity. Instead, this is an affirmation of a fundamental principle that was once explained to me by one of Canada's leading criminal and constitutional experts, Michael Code (formerly of Sack Goldblatt Mitchell and now a judge in Ontario). Discussing a depressing situation of systemic bias bordering on the criminal in an institution designed to serve the public interest, I expressed my instinctive need to know what on earth would motivate such callous behavior. To which Code replied: " It is not necessary to know the motives of a crime in order to prove it." Past reasons for a present disaster are interesting, but not prerequisite to fixing the mess now.

A perfect example of action that can be taken now and that is practical, ethical, and reasonable comes from Congressman Frank R. Wolf, a member of the US government's powerful Committee on Appropriations—that's the guys who control the nation's budget. His work for Lyme patients has been extraordinary by any measure, and his downright aggressive support for them is truly moving. As mentioned earlier, in the US, there exist rules that prevent the government's agencies, such as the Centers for Disease Control, from aligning themselves preferentially with a private medical organization, such as the IDSA, or any other professional organization. Doing so could unfairly boost such an organization's relative importance in public policy considerations. This could also suppress innovation. As revealed during the anti-trust investigation, the CDC did in fact collude in various ways with the interests of the IDSA. Following this investigation closely, Congressman Wolf decided to ask the Inspector General of the US Department of Health and Human Services to investigate further into this relationship. The response is also reproduced here, and we shall hear in due course how this plays out.

In response to my inquiry, Congressman Wolf replied on January 26, 2010, providing an update on the Lyme situation in the US. The US Committee on Appropriations assigned funds to the CDC for purposes of dealing specifically with Chronic Lyme disease (see full text appended to Congressman Wolf's letter). Congressman Wolf's website (www.wolf.house.gov/LYME) is an excellent source of up-to-date information on Lyme activism in the US.

In closing, I offer the following thought for consideration: the two *least* helpful attitudes in a crisis are first, the "original sin" cop-out. Resorting to it one attempts to understand the current disaster or injustice in terms of its origins (mostly nebulous and always irrelevant) which are sought in genes, bad breeding, God's will, something that went wrong during toilet training, a known or unknown putative traumatic event, a mistake in a ritual performed for the gods, having been snubbed at a high school dance leaving one's ego unable to cope ever since, a questionable election result, a migraine that prevented an important meeting etc. etc. In short, some unfortunate event in the past is blamed for the current mess and paralyzes corrective action, as if written in stone.

The second useless approach is more frequently encountered nowadays, and that's the "conspiracy theory" cop-out. That there are conspiracies and always have been, is beyond doubt. Unfortunately, that's the way social animals may behave—they conspire to achieve something they badly want by banding together. Conspiracies are as much part of everything that happens as gravity. Uncovering them by legal means is occasionally possible, so corrective action can be taken. Undoubtedly, the IDSA Lyme guidelines mess has the rank flavor of conspiracy, as does the Canadian government's support of them.

Neither of those cop-outs are very helpful. The past will not resolve current emergencies, and neither will the paralysis of action engendered by suspecting a conspiracy. The only attitude that is practical, reasonable, ethical, and emotionally sustainable is to stick to the facts and, thereby, serve the needs of those who may benefit from illuminating those facts.

This book is written by people who share that conviction. You will enjoy their courage and their stories. Readers are invited to inform themselves about the facts about Lyme disease and the current medical politics that prevents patients from being tested and treated appropriately. Readers will also learn about doctors who have remained steadfastly true to their calling, which is to be "the friends of humanity," as one of history's greatest physicians, Sir William Osler, defined being a doctor.

Sources and Recommended Reading

Bach, G., MD, *Recovery of Lyme spirochetes by PCR in semen samples of previously diagnosed Lyme disease patients*, presented at the International Scientific Conference on Lyme Disease, April 2001

Bakan, J., *The Corporation—The Pathological Pursuit of Profit and Power*, Viking, 2004

Bransfield, R. C. MD, *An Overview of Neuropsychiatric Lyme Disease*, lecture given July 18, 2008, LDA 7th Tick Borne Diseases Conference, Leicester University UK (download via ILADS website)

Bransfield, R. C., MD, *Chronic Lyme Disease/Tick-Borne Disease: the Controversy,* lecture given July 18, 2008, LDA 7th Tick Borne Diseases Conference, Leicester University UK (download via ILADS website)

Brody, H., *Hooked—Ethics, the Medical Profession and the Pharmaceutical Industry*, Rowman & Littlefield, 2007

Canadian Association of University Teachers, *The Olivieri Report*, Lorimer, 2001

Carroll, M. C., *Lab 257—The Disturbing Story of the Government's Secret Germ Laboratory,* Harper, 2005

Centre for Disease Control, USA: source for Lyme Disease Case Definition 2008: www.cdc.gov/ncphi/disss/nndss/casedef/lyme_disease2008

Chopra, S., *Corrupt to the Core—Memoirs of A Health Canada Whistleblower*, KOS, 2008

Fallon, B.A. *et al.*, Regional Cerebral Blood Flow and Metabolic Rate in Persistent Lyme Encephalopathy, *Archives of General Psychiatry*, vol. 66:544 ff, 2009

Ferrie, H., *Dispatches from the War Zone of Environmental Health*, KOS, 2004

Ferrie, H., *What Part of No! Don't They Understand?—Rescuing Food and Medicine from Government Abuse,* KOS 2008

Glasnost Report—Medicine in Ontario Needs Glasnost—A Report to the Government and the People of Ontario Prepared by Doctors and Patients, 2001

Download the report from www.freedomofchoiceinhealthcare.ca/Articles/GlasnostReport

Glover, W.A. *et al.*, Insights into the Molecular Basis of L-Form Formation and Survival in *Escherichia coli*, *PLoS ONE* vol. 4(10), December 2009

Healy, D. MD, *Let Them Eat Prozac*, Lorimer, 2003

Johnson, H., *Osler's Web—Inside the Labyrinth of the Chronic Fatigue Syndrome Epidemic,* Penguin, 1996

Kassirer, J. P. MD, *On The Take—How Medicine's Complicity with Big Business Can Endanger Your Health*, Oxford University Press, 2005

Langhoff, P. J., *The Baker's Dozen & the Lunatic Fringe: Has Junk Science Shifted the Lyme Disease Paradigm?* Allegory Press, 2008

Lyme Disease Association Inc., *Conflicts of Interest in Lyme Disease: Laboratory Testing, Vaccination, and Treatment Guidelines*, 2001 on www.LymeDiseaseAssociation.org

MacDonald, A.B., Plaques of Alzheimer's disease originate from cysts of *Borrelia burgdorferi*, the Lyme disease spirochete, *Medical Hypothesis*, vol. 67 (3):592f, 2006

McAlister, F. A. *et al. How Evidence-Based Are the Recommendations in Evidence-Based Guidelines?* PLoS Medicine, Vol. 4 (8), August 2007

Miles, A. *et al.* Evidence-Based Healthcare, clinical knowledge, and the rise of personalized medicine, *Journal of Evaluation in Clinical Practice*, Vol. 14:621 ff, 2008

Moriarty, T. J. et al, Real-Time High Resolution 3D Imagining of the Lyme Disease Spirochete Adhering to and Escaping from the Vasculature of a Living Host, *PLoS Pathogens*, vol. 4 (6) June 2008

Moynihan, R & Cassels, A., *Selling Sickness—How The World's Biggest Pharmaceutical Companies Are Turning Us All Into Patients*, Nation Books, 2005

Murakami, E. MD, *The Spread of Lyme Disease*, Lecture given September 28, 2009, at The First Canadian Health Care Conference, available on www.thefirstcandianhealthcareconference.ca

Petersen, M., *Our Daily Meds*, Farrar, Straus & Giroux, 2008

Public Health Agency of Canada, *National Lyme Disease Meeting March 8–9, 2006,* published January 22, 2008 (available online from Public Health Agency Canada)

Robinson, J., *Prescription Games—Money, Ego, and Power Inside the Global Pharmaceutical Industry*, McClelland & Stewart, 2001

Rothman, D.J. et al (11 editors-in-chief of the world's leading medical journals), Professional Medical Associations and Their Relationships With Industry: A Proposal for Controlling Conflict of Interest, *Journal of the American Medical Association*, Vol. 301 (13):1367 ff, April 1, 2009

Samuels, D.S. & Radolf, J. D. eds. Borrelia: *Molecular Biology, Host Interaction and Pathogenesis*, Caister Academic Press, to appear March 2010 (ISBN 978-1-904455-58-5) (textbook)

Schmid, G.P., Epidemiology and clinical similarities of human spirochetal diseases, *Review of Infectious Disease*, Vol. 11, Suppl. 6:S1460f, Sept.-Oct. 1989

Shaneyfelt, T. M., MD, & Cantor, R. M., MD, Reassessment of Clinical Practice Guidelines—Go Gently Into That Good Night, editorial, *Journal of the American Medical Association*, Vol. 301 (8):868 ff, February 25, 2009

Shilts, R., *And the Band Played On—Politics, People, and the AIDS Epidemic*, Penguin, 1988

Smith, R., Medical Journals Are an Extension of the Marketing Arm of Pharmaceutical Companies, *PLoS Medicine*, Vol. 2 (5), May 2005

Smith, R., *The Trouble With Medical Journals*, Royal Society of Medicine Press, 2006

Vinten-Johansen, P. , Brody, H. *et al.* Cholera, *Chloroform, and the Science of Medicine: The Life of John Snow*, Cambridge University Press, 2003

Wagner, W. & Steinzor, R., *Rescuing Science from Politics—Regulation and the Distortion of Scientific Research*, Cambridge University Press, 2006

Weintraub, P. *Cure Unknown—Inside the Lyme Epidemic*, St. Martin's Press, 2nd ed. 2009

Young, T., *Death by Prescription—A Father Takes On His Daughter's Killer: The Multi-Billion-Dollar Pharmaceutical Industry*, Key Porter, 2009

M. Wilton, LLB, The case of Dr. George Gale vs the College of Physicians and Surgeons of Ontario: A legal analysis, *Pain Research and Management—The Journal of the Canadian Pain Society,* Vol. 9 (1) Spring 2004

Documentary DVDs

Money Talks—Profits Before Patient Safety, 2006 www.moneytalksthemovie.com

Phillips, S. MD, *Chronic Lyme Disease—An Evidence-Based Review*, University of New Haven, 2008 www.unh-lyme.org

Under Our Skin—There's No Medicine For Someone Like You, 2008 www.underourskin.com Winner of 5 film festival prizes, 2009 Oscar nominee

For reprint orders, please contact: reprints@futuremedicine.com

Chronic Lyme disease and the 'Axis of Evil'

Perspective
Future Microbiology

Raphael B Stricker[†] & Lorraine Johnson
[†]Author for correspondence ▪ 450 Sutter Street, Suite 1504, San Francisco, CA 94108, USA
▪ Tel.: +1 415 399 1035 ▪ Fax: +1 415 399 1057 ▪ rstricker@usmamed.com

Lyme disease is a controversial illness, and the existence of chronic Lyme disease induced by persistent infection with the Lyme spirochete, *Borrelia burgdorferi*, is the subject of continued debate. A recent publication defined the 'Axis of Evil' in this controversy as physicians who treat patients with needlessly prolonged courses of antibiotics, 'specialty laboratories' that perform 'inaccurate' Lyme testing and the internet, which promotes 'Lyme hysteria'. We examine the 'Axis of Evil' components in the context of diagnostic and therapeutic challenges for Lyme disease patients and their physicians, and we present an evidence-based refutation to this misguided view. Despite its virulent nature, the 'Axis of Evil' perspective is a useful starting point to resolve the controversy over Lyme disease.

Lyme disease is a controversial clinical conundrum [1,2]. Over the past decade, two opposing camps have emerged in the battle over this tick-borne illness. One camp is represented by the Infectious Diseases Society of America (IDSA), which maintains that Lyme disease is a rare illness localized to well-defined areas of the world. According to the IDSA, the disease is 'hard to catch and easy to cure' because the infection is rarely encountered, easily diagnosed in its early stage by distinctive clinical features and in more advanced stages by accurate commercial laboratory tests, and effectively treated with a short course of antibiotics over 2–4 weeks [3,4,101,102]. Chronic infection with the Lyme spirochete, *Borrelia burgdorferi*, is rare or nonexistent, and the concept of chronic Lyme disease rests on 'faith-based' opinion rather than 'evidence-based' science [5,101,102].

The opposing camp is represented by the International Lyme and Associated Diseases Society (ILADS), which argues that Lyme disease is not rare because its spread is facilitated by rodents, deer and birds, and can be found in an unpredictable distribution around the world accompanied by other tick-borne coinfections that may complicate the clinical presentation. According to the ILADS, tick bites often go unnoticed and commercial laboratory testing for Lyme disease is inaccurate [1,6]. Consequently, the disease is often not recognized and may persist in a large number of patients, requiring prolonged antibiotic therapy to eradicate persistent infection with the evasive Lyme spirochete [1,6]. A substantial body of evidence from peer-reviewed scientific studies of tick-borne diseases supports this viewpoint [1,2,6].

A recent opinion piece published in the *New England Journal of Medicine* reiterates the belief that chronic Lyme disease does not exist, and even if it does, the risks of prolonged antibiotic therapy outweigh any benefits [7]. A subsequent letter published in the same journal praises the article for defining the 'Axis of Evil' that threatens the Lyme world: first, physicians who administer extended antibiotic therapy to Lyme patients without justification; second, 'specialty laboratories' that offer inaccurate Lyme test results; and third, of course, the internet, which provides misinformation about Lyme disease to gullible and frightened patients [8].

The opinion piece and letter reflect the viewpoint of IDSA, which released updated guidelines for the diagnosis and treatment of Lyme disease in 2006 [4]. The IDSA guidelines are so restrictive that the Attorney General of Connecticut launched an investigation into exclusionary practices and commercial conflicts of interest of the IDSA panel members who formulated the guidelines [103]. The investigation found that IDSA failed to screen for conflicts of interest on the part of the guidelines panel [104]. Furthermore, the Attorney General noted that the guidelines committee chairman exhibited bias in selecting a panel of 'likeminded' researchers and blocking the appointment of scientists with divergent views [104]. As a result, the IDSA panel suppressed scientific evidence and ignored the rival ILADS viewpoint in formulating narrow guidelines that fail to acknowledge the possibility of persistent spirochetal infection in patients with chronic Lyme disease symptoms. The resultant guidelines place severe limitations on treatment options for Lyme disease patients because these 'voluntary' guidelines are viewed

Keywords
Borrelia burgdorferi ▪ IDSA ▪ ILADS ▪ internet ▪ Lyme disease

future medicine part of fsg

as a mandatory standard of care by medical societies, government agencies and insurance companies [9,10,104]. As part of its settlement with the Attorney General, IDSA is now being forced to re-evaluate its guidelines with a new panel under the oversight of a specialist in medical conflicts of interest [104].

The tactics used by IDSA and its guidelines panel members in response to the above investigation are highly questionable. A total of 11 members of the IDSA guidelines panel were authors of the *New England Journal of Medicine* article, which appears to provide 'independent corroboration' of the restrictive IDSA viewpoint and exoneration of the authors in the guidelines investigation [7]. The *New England Journal of Medicine* publication failed to disclose this conflict of interest and the overlapping authorship, although other significant commercial conflicts were enumerated [7]. The IDSA panel employed a similar strategy of overlapping authorship in formulating 'corroborating' Lyme guidelines published by the American Academy of Neurology (AAN). The Connecticut Attorney General's investigation found that IDSA portrayed the AAN and IDSA Lyme guidelines panels as 'independent' despite the fact that 'the two panels shared several authors, including the chairmen of both groups, and were working on guidelines at the same time' – practices that violated the IDSA's own conflicts of interest policy [11,104].

The driving force in this controversy, however, stems from the disregard for clinical and scientific evidence inherent in the 'Axis of Evil' comment. First, there is growing scientific evidence that chronic Lyme disease does exist, and that this clinical condition is related to persistent infection with *B. burgdorferi* as shown by microbiological and molecular studies [9,12–26]. Persistent infection occurs in animal models and humans because the Lyme spirochete is able to evade both the host immune response and short-course antibiotic therapy to establish chronic infection in protected tissue sites, much like TB [19–26]. This chronic infection leads to persistent musculoskeletal, neurologic and cardiac symptoms that are the hallmark of chronic Lyme disease. By contrast, the leading theory for persistent symptoms owing to 'post-Lyme syndrome', namely an autoimmune response triggered by the eradicated spirochetal infection, has not been supported by scientific evidence [27]. Thus, persistent infection appears to be at the root of chronic Lyme disease, and it follows that longer treatment with antibiotics would be beneficial in this situation [28]. Two recently published randomized, placebo-controlled trials support the practice of physicians who give extended treatment for chronic Lyme disease [29,30], and an ongoing homecare monitoring study supports the relative safety of this treatment approach with proper patient supervision [31].

The second link in the 'Axis of Evil' is the group of 'specialty laboratories' that provide 'questionable' testing for Lyme disease. Ironically it is the patented commercial Lyme tests that are questionable [32,105]. The two-tier Lyme test system endorsed by the IDSA requires a patented, commercially-available IgG screening immunoassay followed by a patented, commercially-available confirmatory western blot. Although this test system has a very high specificity of 99%, meaning that there are very few false positives, the system has a sensitivity ranging from 8–56% based on recent population studies, meaning that the algorithm has 'coin-toss' diagnostic utility at best and may miss as many as nine out of ten Lyme cases [32–35,105]. By contrast, antibody testing for HIV has a sensitivity of 99.5%, meaning that it misses only one in 200 HIV infections. The insensitive Lyme test system assures that many Lyme patients will go undiagnosed and untreated, a problem compounded by the IDSA mandate that diagnosis requires a positive commercial test result. Hence, the search for more sensitive testing offered by laboratories that have established superior assays for Lyme disease [36] is a direct response to the flawed commercial Lyme tests and the IDSA mandate that diagnosis rests on these flawed tests.

The third link in the 'Axis of Evil' is the internet, which is viewed by the IDSA as an instrument of 'Lyme hysteria'. The simple fact, however, is that treatment failure resulting in persistent symptoms is common under the IDSA guidelines [9,28], and the subsequent physician and insurance industry abandonment of patients who do not fit the IDSA Lyme model is unacceptable in a medically sophisticated society [37,38]. Thus, when the IDSA guidelines fail to improve a patient's quality of life, intelligent patients will seek out other sources of information, such as the internet, which acknowledge the shortcomings of commercial Lyme testing and the failure of standard IDSA treatment protocols. These patients will then seek out open-minded physicians to assure that they are given every viable medical option and every reasonable chance of a good clinical outcome. Educated patients are becoming more vocal in their criticism of the IDSA's position on Lyme disease [39]. As a result of the efforts of these informed patients and the Attorney General's action in Connecticut, the narrow IDSA view of Lyme disease has become untenable.

In summary, the IDSA viewpoint embodied by the recent *New England Journal of Medicine* article represents a formidable impediment for patients with chronic Lyme disease, and the Connecticut Attorney General's investigation has effectively challenged this viewpoint. The solution requires that opposing views must be heard, that good clinical outcomes must be the primary goal of Lyme diagnosis and treatment, and that physicians must be free to exercise discretion in dealing with a complex illness. By adopting these principles, IDSA can start to develop guidelines that avoid the abandonment of patients with chronic Lyme disease. When this occurs, the 'Axis of Evil' will disappear.

Future perspective

The collision between the IDSA's position on Lyme disease, embodied in recent publications, and the Connecticut Attorney General's investigation of how that position was established will result in a re-evaluation of the clinical approach to chronic Lyme disease. This process will lead to acceptance of the ILADS view of persistent infection in chronic Lyme disease and a more rational approach to the diagnosis and treatment of tick-borne diseases.

Financial & competing interests disclosure

RBS serves without compensation on the medical advisory panel for QMedRx Inc. He has no financial ties to the company. The authors have no other relevant affiliations or financial involvement with any organization or entity with a financial interest in or financial conflict with the subject matter or materials discussed in the manuscript apart from those disclosed.

No writing assistance was utilized in the production of this manuscript.

Executive summary

- Lyme disease is a controversial illness. Two medical societies, the Infectious Diseases Society of America (IDSA) and the International Lyme and Associated Diseases Society (ILADS), have developed conflicting guidelines for the diagnosis and treatment of this tick-borne disease.
- Recent publications by IDSA members have impugned the scientific basis of the ILADS viewpoint, attributing that viewpoint to an 'Axis of Evil' involving physicians who treat improperly, 'specialty laboratories' that test inaccurately and the internet, which promotes 'Lyme hysteria'.
- An investigation by the Connecticut Attorney General found that the IDSA suppressed scientific evidence and had significant conflicts of interest in developing its Lyme disease guidelines. An impartial scientific panel will be established to review the IDSA guidelines.
- The discredited 'Axis of Evil' comment affords an opportunity to examine the conflicts at the root of Lyme disease diagnosis and treatment.

Bibliography

Papers of special note have been highlighted as:
- of interest
•• of considerable interest

1. Stricker RB, Lautin A, Burrascano JJ: Lyme disease: point/counterpoint. *Expert Rev. Anti-Infect. Ther.* 3(2), 155–165 (2005).

•• **Point by point refutation of the Infectious Diseases Society of America (IDSA) position on Lyme disease.**

2. Harvey WT, Salvato P: 'Lyme disease': ancient engine of an unrecognized borreliosis pandemic? *Med. Hypotheses* 60, 742–759 (2003).

• **Excellent review of major controversies in Lyme disease diagnosis and treatment.**

3. Steere AC, Taylor E, McHugh GL, Logigian EL: The overdiagnosis of Lyme disease. *JAMA* 269, 1812–1816 (1993).

4. Wormser GP, Dattwyler RJ, Shapiro ED *et al.*: The clinical assessment, treatment, and prevention of Lyme disease, human granulocytic anaplasmosis, and babesiosis: clinical practice guidelines by the Infectious Diseases Society of America. *Clin. Infect. Dis.* 41, 1089–1134 (2006).

5. Sigal LH, Hassett AL: Contributions of societal and geographical environments to 'chronic Lyme disease': the psychopathogenesis and aporology of a new 'medically unexplained symptoms' syndrome. *Environ. Health Perspect.* 110(Suppl. 4), 607–611 (2002).

6. Cameron D, Gaito A, Harris N *et al.*: Evidence-based guidelines for the management of Lyme disease. *Expert Rev. Anti-Infect. Ther.* 2(Suppl. 1), S1–S13 (2004).

7. Feder HM Jr, Johnson BJ, O'Connell S, Shapiro ED, Steere AC, Wormser GP: Ad Hoc International Lyme Disease Group. A critical appraisal of 'chronic Lyme disease'. *N. Engl. J. Med.* 357, 1422–1430 (2007).

8. Drapkin MS: An appraisal of 'chronic Lyme disease'. *N. Engl. J. Med.* 358, 430 (2008).

9. Johnson L, Stricker RB: Treatment of Lyme disease: a medicolegal assessment. *Expert Rev. Anti-Infect. Ther.* 2(4), 533–557 (2004).

•• **Encyclopedic review of the Lyme controversy, with excellent summary tables.**

10. Stricker RB, Johnson L: Lyme disease: a turning point. *Expert Rev. Anti-Infect. Ther.* 5(5), 759–762 (2007).

• **Critique of IDSA clinical trials for chronic Lyme disease.**

11. Stricker RB, Johnson L: The American Academy of Neurology Lyme guidelines: through the looking glass. *South Med. J.* 101, 672 (2008).

12. Preac-Mursic V, Weber K, Pfister HW *et al.*: Survival of *Borrelia burgdorferi* in antibiotically treated patients with Lyme borreliosis. *Infection* 17, 355–359 (1989).

13. Liegner KB, Shapiro JR, Ramsay D, Halperin AJ, Hogrefe W, Kong L: Recurrent erythema migrans despite extended antibiotic treatment

with minocycline in a patient with persisting *Borrelia burgdorferi* infection. *J. Am. Acad. Dermatol.* 28(2 Pt 2), 312–314 (1993).

14. Preac-Mursic V, Pfister HW, Spiegel H *et al.*: First isolation of *Borrelia burgdorferi* from an iris biopsy. *J. Clin. Neuroophthalmol.* 13, 155–161 (1993).
15. Battafarano DF, Combs JA, Enzenauer RJ, Fitzpatrick JE: Chronic septic arthritis caused by *Borrelia burgdorferi*. *Clin. Orthop. Relat. Res.* 297, 238–241 (1993).
16. Nocton JJ, Dressler F, Rutledge BJ, Rys PN, Persing DH, Steere AC: Detection of *Borrelia burgdorferi* DNA by polymerase chain reaction in synovial fluid from patients with Lyme arthritis. *N. Engl. J. Med.* 330, 229–234 (1994).
17. Bayer ME, Zhang L, Bayer MH: *Borrelia burgdorferi* DNA in the urine of treated patients with chronic Lyme disease symptoms. A PCR study of 97 cases. *Infection* 24, 347–353 (1996).
18. Nocton JJ, Bloom BJ, Rutledge BJ *et al.*: Detection of *Borrelia burgdorferi* DNA by polymerase chain reaction in cerebrospinal fluid in Lyme neuroborreliosis. *J. Infect. Dis.* 174, 623–627 (1996).
19. Frey M, Jaulhac B, Piemont Y *et al.*: Detection of *Borrelia burgdorferi* DNA in muscle of patients with chronic myalgia related to Lyme disease. *Am. J. Med.* 104, 591–594 (1998).
20. Oksi J, Marjamäki M, Nikoskelainen J, Viljanen MK: *Borrelia burgdorferi* detected by culture and PCR in clinical relapse of disseminated Lyme borreliosis. *Ann. Med.* 31, 225–232 (1999).
21. Breier F, Khanakah G, Stanek G *et al.*: Isolation and polymerase chain reaction typing of *Borrelia afzelii* from a skin lesion in a seronegative patient with generalized ulcertating bullous lichen sclerosus et atrophicus. *Br. J. Dermatol.* 144, 387–392 (2001).
22. Phillips SE, Harris NS, Horowitz R, Johnson L, Stricker RB: Lyme disease: scratching the surface. *Lancet* 366, 1771 (2005).
23. Phillips SE, Burrascano JJ, Harris NS, Johnson L, Smith PV, Stricker RB: Chronic infection in 'post-Lyme borreliosis syndrome'. *Int. J. Epidemiol.* 34, 1439–1440 (2005).
24. Ekdahl KN, Henningsson AJ, Sandholm K, Forsberg P, Ernerudh J, Ekerfelt C: Immunity in borreliosis with special emphasis on the role of complement. *Adv. Exp. Med. Biol.* 598, 198–213 (2007).
25. Stricker RB, Johnson L: Persistent *Borrelia burgdorferi* infection after treatment with antibiotics and anti-tumor necrosis factor-α. *J. Infect. Dis.* 197, 1352–1353 (2008).

■■ **Overview of treatment failure in animal models of chronic Lyme disease.**

26. Hodzic E, Feng S, Holden K, Freet KJ, Barthold SW: Persistence of *Borrelia burgdorferi* following antibiotic treatment in mice. *Antimicrob. Agents Chemother.* 52, 1728–1736 (2008).

■ **Elegant demonstration of treatment failure in a mouse model of Lyme disease.**

27. Stricker RB, Johnson L: Searching for autoimmunity in 'antibiotic refractory' Lyme arthritis. *Mol. Immunol.* 45, 3023–3024 (2008).

■ **Lack of data to support autoimmunity in 'post-Lyme syndrome'.**

28. Stricker RB: Counterpoint:long-term antibiotic therapy improves persistent symptoms associated with Lyme disease. *Clin. Infect. Dis.* 45, 149–157 (2007).

■■ **Evidence for longer antibiotic treatment in chronic Lyme disease.**

29. Fallon BA, Keilp JG, Corbera KM *et al.*: A randomized, placebo-controlled trial of repeated IV antibiotic therapy for Lyme encephalopathy. *Neurology* 70, 992–1003 (2008).

■■ **Evidence for longer antibiotic treatment in chronic Lyme disease.**

30. Cameron D: Severity of Lyme disease with persistent symptoms. Insights from a double blind placebo controlled clinical trial. *Minerva Med.* 99, 489–496 (2008).
31. Stricker RB, Green CL, Savely VR, Chamallas SN: Safety of intravenous antibiotic therapy in chronic Lyme disease. *J. Invest. Med.* 56, 190 (2008).
32. Stricker RB, Johnson L: Lyme wars: let's tackle the testing. *BMJ* 335, 1008 (2007).

■■ **Poor sensitivity of commercial Lyme testing.**

33. Tilton RC, Sand MN, Manak M: The western immunoblot for Lyme disease: determination of sensitivity, specificity, and interpretive criteria with use of commercially available performance panels. *Clin. Infect. Dis.* 25(Suppl. 1), S31–S34 (1997).
34. Binnicker MJ, Jespersen DJ, Harring JA, Rollins LO, Bryant SC, Beito EM: Evaluation of two commercial systems for the automated processing, reading and interpretation of Lyme western blots. *J. Clin. Microbiol.* 46, 2216–2221 (2008).
35. Santino I, Berlutti F, Pantanella F, Sessa R, del Piano M: Detection of *Borrelia burgdorferi sensu lato* DNA by PCR in serum of patients with clinical symptoms of Lyme borreliosis. *FEMS Microbiol. Lett.* 283, 30–35 (2008).
36. Ma B, Christen B, Leung D, Vigo-Pelfrey C: Serodiagnosis of Lyme borreliosis by western immunoblot: reactivity of various significant antibodies against *Borrelia burgdorferi*. *J. Clin. Microbiol.* 30, 370–376 (1992).
37. Amerling R, Winchester JF, Ronco C: Guidelines for guidelines. *Blood Purif.* 25, 36–38 (2007).

■ **Review of problems with medical guidelines.**

38. Krumholz HM: Guideline recommendations and results: the importance of the linkage. *Ann. Intern. Med.* 147, 342–343 (2007).
39. Holmes KD: An appraisal of 'chronic Lyme disease'. *N. Engl. J. Med.* 358, 429 (2008).

Websites

101. Kolata G: Lyme disease is hard to catch and easy to halt, study finds. *New York Times* (2001). http://query.nytimes.com/gst/fullpage.html?res=9A05E0D8113EF930A25755C0A9679C8B63
102. IDSA Website. Frequently asked questions about Lyme disease. www.idsociety.org/lymediseasefacts.htm
103. Coyle M: Antitrust scrutiny of Lyme guidelines. *Natl Law J.* (2007). www.law.com/jsp/nlj/index.jsp
104. Connecticut Attorney General's Office. Attorney General's investigation reveals flawed Lyme disease guideline process, IDSA agrees to reassess guidelines, install independent arbiter (2008). www.ct.gov/ag/cwp/view.asp?a=2795&q=414284

■■ **Stunningly stark assessment of the IDSA Lyme guidelines development process.**

105. Stricker RB, Johnson L: Lyme disease debate: facts or fiction. *BMJ Rapid Response*. www.bmj.com/cgi/eletters/335/7628/1008

Affiliations

- Raphael B Stricker, MD
  450 Sutter Street, Suite 1504,
  San Francisco, CA 94108, USA
  Tel.: +1 415 399 1035;
  Fax: +1 415 399 1057;
  rstricker@usmamed.com
  and,
  International Lyme & Associated Diseases Society, PO Box 341461, Bethesda, MD 20827-21461, USA
- Lorraine Johnson, JD, MBA
  International Lyme & Associated Diseases Society, PO Box 341461, Bethesda, MD 20827-21461, USA
  Tel.: +1 323 461 6184;
  Fax: +1 323 461 6143;
  lbjl@pacbell.net

Available online at www.sciencedirect.com
SCIENCE DIRECT®

Medical Hypotheses (2003) **60**(5), 742–759

doi:10.1016/S0306-9877(03)00060-4

'Lyme disease': ancient engine of an unrecognized borreliosis pandemic?☆

W. T. Harvey, P. Salvato

Diversified Medical Practices, Houston, Texas, USA

Summary Unexpectedly we have found large numbers of chronically ill *Borrelia burgdorferi* PCR- and seropositive patients in Houston, Texas, a zoonotically 'non-endemic' area. In order to understand this finding prior to sufficient data availability, we chose to examine critically currently accepted but troublesome 'Lyme disease' concepts. Our method was to analyze each foundation 'Lyme disease' premise within the context of available medical and veterinary literature, then to reconstruct the disease model consistent with the preponderance of that data. We find the present conceptualization of the illness seriously truncated, with a high likelihood of two distinct but connected forms of human *B. burgdorferi* infection. The yet-unrecognized form appears to have a broader clinical presentation, wider geographic distribution, and vastly greater prevalence. We conclude that 'Lyme disease' currently acknowledges only its zoonosis arm and is a limited conceptualization of a far more pervasive and unrecognized infection state that must be considered a global epidemic.

INTRODUCTION

'No part of the aim of normal science is to call forth new sorts of phenomena; indeed those that will not fit the box are not seen at all'. Thomas Kuhn: *The Structure of Scientific Revolutions* (1).

In 2000, Paul Ewald advanced the hypothesis that evolutionary biology principles, if followed faithfully, predict that infection likely underpins many current illnesses without known etiology, perhaps via a single agent (2). Here we present evidence that may identify one such agent.

Twenty-six months ago, our practice began to test chronically ill patients with multi-system presentation for *Borrelia burgdorferi* (*Bb*) infection. Our criteria further included suspicion of protracted infection and inability to otherwise find a diagnosis. About a third of initial tests were positive via CDC Western blot criteria or serum/urine PCR; however, repeat testing eventually revealed that most are positive. We had not expected these results, as we are in Southeastern Texas, a 'non-endemic' region. (The prevalence of *Borrelia*-infected ticks in Texas is about 1–2%.) (3–5).

Concurrently, we recognized a striking similarity in symptoms and signs of test-positive individuals to other untested patients of ours. Most fit within the presentation criteria of 'late, disseminated Lyme disease' but with some prominent differences. We began antibiotic treatment of all test-positive patients, and most, regardless of presentation, began noticeable improvement within 3 to 6 months.

Since no history of erythema migrans (EM) rash or illness following tick bite was reported by these patients, and most had been ill for many years with similarly ill family members, we set out to understand what we were confronting. Our experience did not match the CDC case definition or the epidemiological evidence for late 'Lyme

☆We have no competing financial interests and have used no grants in creating this paper.

Received 16 July 2002
Accepted 11 November 2002

Correspondence to: **W.T. Harvey** MD, MS, MPH, 3826 Princeton Park Court, Houston, TX 77058, USA. Pager number 713-990-8791,
Phone: 281-461-9866 or Cell: 281-451-8556; Fax: 1-713-961-3085;
E-mail: wth928@aol.com

disease'. To resolve this conundrum, we concluded that our best initial strategy was to derive our own conclusions by careful assessment of all available relevant data.

METHOD

We began by examining the present conceptualization of 'Lyme disease' for comprehensiveness and accuracy. We chose the US Centers for Disease Control and Prevention (CDC) 'surveillance case definition' of 'Lyme disease' as the current standard model of human *Bb* infection. We next isolated what we believed to be the linchpin premises supporting that model, examining each against available pertinent National Library of Medicine (NLM) medical and veterinary *Bb* data. Each premise was addressed independently with relevant data categorized and summed. We then derived a modified illness model of human *Bb* infection by combining the reassessed premises. Finally, we examined this newly-derived illness model within the context of current medical nosology and the realities of contemporary clinical medicine for plausible fit and superior predictability potential.

FINDINGS

Semantics: 'Lyme disease' examined

The origin and conceptualization of 'Lyme disease'

'Lyme disease' is the label given to a human illness first recognized in Old Lyme, CN in 1975 (6). The initial cases resulted from a zoonosis present in local vertebrate reservoirs/hosts and transferred incidentally to humans via an arthropod vector, *Ixodes scapularis* (6–10). The responsible agent was later identified as *B. burgdorferi*, a spirochetal bacterium, with human disease considered to result exclusively from the genospecies cluster *B. burgdorferi sensu lato* (*Bbsl*). (7,11). Globally, the species presently within this cluster include *B. burgdorferi sensu stricto* (*Bbss*), *B. afzelii*, *B. garinii*, *B. lonestari*, and possibly *B. valaisiana* (12,13).

As the knowledge base expanded internationally in the subsequent 26 years, the zoonosis-only conceptualization of 'Lyme disease' persisted with emphasis on acute and early stages. The exclusive focus on zoonosis resulted in a major portion of resources being concentrated on reservoir and vector prevalence (14). The 1975 conceptual model reached 'standard-of-care' status little changed with publication of the CDC 'case classification' in 1997 (15).

'Lyme disease' as defined by the CDC: the prevailing view

The CDC initially published case definitions for Public Health Surveillance in October, 1990. For the first time, uniform criteria were available to be used in case reporting that included 'Lyme disease' (16). The full CDC criteria for 'Lyme disease' were published in the May, 1997 MMWR (CDC Morbidity and Mortality Weekly Report) for surveillance purposes and included clinical description, laboratory diagnostic criteria, confirmed case classification, and relevant definition of terms (15). We refer the reader to the referenced MMWR for the complete surveillance criteria, all contained under the title: 'Lyme Disease (Revised 9/96) clinical description'. More extensive descriptions of the illness presentation, course, epidemiology, and diagnosis may be found in subsequent CDC sources (17,18). We included these in our synthesis of the most comprehensive current conceptualization of 'Lyme disease', but considered the 1997 'surveillance case definition' as authoritative.

The foundation premises of the 'Lyme disease' model

Following are what we consider to be the foundation premises used to create and support the present internationally endorsed conceptualization (model) of 'Lyme disease' believed to represent all human *Bb*-induced illness. (All illness models incorporate a set of premises derived from numerous observations, assumptions and definitions by inductive reasoning. Collectively, the premises deductively create a conceptual framework that constitutes the model. The model is then used deductively to derive diagnosis and treatment.) We state each premise separately, then compare to the available published data. (We reviewed 951 peer-reviewed papers and 13 books to cover what we deemed the relevant literature.) A re-summarization completes the process. Assessment of these 13 premises constitutes the body of our argument.

Before examining the premises which we believe support the concept of *'Lyme disease'*, we stress that our use of this label will be limited to its presently defined conceptual boundaries. The CDC defines *'Lyme disease'*, exclusively as a zoonotic illness. Congenital and gestational transfer cases have been disregarded for reasons not evident to us. This limited perspective is the first important illness-model error that will further compound as we examine its premises.

The 13 premises are grouped into five general areas: Initial Clinical Presentation (1–3), Testing/Confirmation (4–5), Pathogen Transfer, (6–9), Course and Outcome (10–11), and Distribution and History (12–13).

Premise 1: The erythema migrans rash consistently heralds initial *B. burgdorferi* infection

In most early and many recent studies, the presence of an EM rash is presumed to consistently verify *initial* human inoculation of *Bbsl* via tick (17). This assumption is, in fact, the foundation of many important conclusions reached about 'Lyme disease' despite numerous papers that acknowledge secondary EM lesions occur (15,17).

Available data do not support the EM rash to be dependable for diagnosis. The EM rash may follow initial tick inoculation (primary), or it may occur months to years later (secondary) (19–28). The rash also frequently fails to appear following tick inoculation (26). It is not known to be a marker in gestational or congenital *Bbsl* transfer (13). Baranton's recent data show that some Lyme-derived *Bbsl* variants do not cause EM lesions (29).

Premise 2: *Borrelia burgdorferi* infection is sub-clinical in some infected humans with assumed benign outcome

Copious data support that *B. burgdorferi* infection can be 'sub-clinical' and thus unnoticed in infected individuals (20,30–54) and animals (55,56). The average symptomatic/asymptomatic ratio (S/A) in these studies from endemic areas, primarily using serology for diagnosis, is close to 1:1, much as Steere first noted in 1986 (57). The S/A ratio in 'non-endemic' areas may be similar or higher (58). Notably, no recent 'Lyme disease' study referenced by the CDC considers the asymptomatic state to be significant (17,18).

The question of whether sub-clinical cases activate or fail to activate at some future date is intriguing. Lack of sufficiently prolonged longitudinal follow-up in available studies fails to provide an answer. Baranton's recent data, however, show differing pathogenicity among *Bbsl* species, lending support to the reality of some prolonged innocuous sub-clinical infections although study design limits insight into ultimate outcome (59). When prolonged longitudinal outcome has been considered, several studies do support reactivation among patients (31,33,36,37,41,43,49,53,57,60).

Premise 3: Arthritis is a primary late musculoskeletal 'Lyme' infection sequela, where 'late' in CDC parlance is vague

Objective joint swelling is a 'late Lyme disease' symptom criterion (15). This frequently-documented standard, however, was derived primarily from data limited to patients meeting strict 'Lyme disease' requirements, necessitating vector inoculation for inclusion and recent enough for high antibody levels (6,61–69). False-seronegative individuals would have necessarily been rejected, possibly including those with low antibody levels and those infected by sexual, congenital or gestational routes. Further, we find no concise or consistent definition of 'late' in published 'Lyme disease' definition criteria, obfuscating the time when arthritis might be expected to appear (17,18).

In our 'non-endemic' region, we have rarely seen rheumatic joint presentation in our 455 seropositive or PCR positive patients. Many have migratory and intermittent *arthralgias*, however, and most have been ill far longer than one year. We find no data to support our clinical experience, however, likely because our patients fall outside the 'Lyme disease' inclusion criteria.

Premise 4: Humans with late stage 'Lyme disease' show high antibody levels and high numbers of Western blot test bands

The data support this position when applied strictly to presently defined 'Lyme disease' (17,70). These data do not address non-zoonotic transfer cases. An exhaustive review addressing 'Lyme disease' antibody data may be found in a recent work by Gardner (13). IgG and IgM response curves are reproducible within reasonably consistent ranges (8,71–74). Of note, however, referenced patients were studied only a limited number of months following initial vector inoculation, most less than a year (25,72,75–78).

We found no study characterizing immune reactivity to *Bbsl* in untreated patients from non-endemic regions and where symptoms have been present for one year to decades. Consistently, most serious studies have examined and tested only patients from limited geographic areas where high tick infection rate and acute human disease coincide. The immune reaction of infected patients not meeting 'Lyme disease' criteria have fallen outside rigorous scrutiny.

Gardner and others have shown conclusively that a group of *Bbsl*-infected humans was not inoculated transdermally but rather acquired their disease congenitally or gestationally (13,79–81). How might their antibody picture appear? Gardner's exhaustive review of antibody production following gestational *Bbsl* transfer is instructive. In her Table 11-8, 72% of neonates with tissue-verified borreliosis did not produce antibodies in sufficient quantity to be seropositive (13). Review of normal human fetal and neonatal antibody production in general reveals as well lagging IgG and IgM antibody levels to age one year (graph data, P46) (82). Beyond one to three years, we find no clarifying data.

Premise 5: Serologic testing to verify spirochete viability in late 'Lyme disease' cases is reliable

Numerous potential problems confound conclusions from the available in-vivo serology data (37,83–86). Terms such as 'symptomatic' are typically defined within the case definition of *early* (We assume much less than one year after inoculation) 'Lyme disease'. The presumed presence of *B. burgdorferi* in the human host is dependent on a strong history of vector inoculation and the subsequent (early) pattern of antibody response. Other requirements imposed for 'proof of infection' include endemic area residence, length of tick attachment, or recent memory of EM-like rash. High background seropositivity in 'non-endemic' areas is dismissed as 'false' without adequate proof. Studies are also insufficiently longitudinal. The extensive data linking serologic outcome with spirochete presence in the host limit this connection to relatively early 'Lyme disease' and thus exclude late and all non-zoonotic patients.

Once *Bbsl* disseminates in the host, other immune-related factors apply that have not been sufficiently addressed in the 'Dearborn criteria' defining seropositivity (87). Pleomorphism, variable antigen presentation, immune avoidance, individual immune variance, host-derived enzyme cloaking, immune complex sequestration, and antibody inaccessibility to spirochete-privileged sites argue against sustained or consistent immune response (88–92). Recent findings by Wang and Hilton suggest the presence or absence of *Bb* antibody production is associated with unique individual HLA specificities of the Class II (93). Eighteen of 44 (41%) variously symptomatic patients were found seronegative where infection was verified by PCR to Osp A in cerebrospinal fluid or mononuclear cells.

Other data support serology test uncertainty: (1) Seronegativity does not prove absence of a viable *Bb* infection (45,90,93), which is consistent with the principle that negative findings cannot be used to prove lack of positivity. (2) Antibodies may exist minimally or rarely in very late *Bbsl*-infected humans (90). (3) Culture and histological methods have been used extensively by veterinarians, and provide substantial data supporting the inaccuracy and insensitivity of serology in identifying living *B. burgdorferi* in non-human subjects (51,52,60,94–98). (4) By "similarity", the presence of antibodies to *T. pallidum* generally means the presence of spirochetes (99). An evolutionary biology perspective is further to the point. Any persistent pathogen (relevant if *Bbsl* survives into late illness) must effectively escape the immune system. An example is *Chlamydia pneumoniae* infection where antibodies appear only when the agent is causing active pneumonia, yet the organism persists primarily unnoticed and undetected (2).

Bbsl prevalence data are rife with a mixture of asymptomatic seropositive as well as symptomatic seronegative findings (43–45,49,53,65,90,100–107). Many presumptions have been used to rationalize this data. Curiously, none have considered the possibility that the subject pools may include a high number of intra-human transfer cases.

In summary, the preponderance of available data cast serious doubt on the validity of current serology criteria for diagnosing viable human *Bb* infection.

Premise 6: The presumed US human 'Lyme disease' agent is limited to one species of Bbsl: *B. burgdorferi sensu stricto* (*Bbss*)

Until very recently, the presumed sole United States (US) human 'Lyme disease' agent is the species *Bbss*. The preponderance of available data, based on the assumption that all *B. burgdorferi* human infection is zoonotic, supports this assumption (29,59). James has now published evidence, however, that *Borrelia lonestari* infects humans in the US via the vector *Amblyomma americanum* (12). *Borrelia valaisiana* has also been found to infect humans in two US cases (13).

Bbss was the first species to be identified shortly after discovery of the disease in the Northeastern US. Because the illness was immediately assumed solely a zoonosis, this assumption resulted in the tendency to look for other possible species and strains less among ill humans than in vectors and animal reservoirs. Such a 'self-fulfilling' assumption built into the 'Lyme disease' model may have helped assure that the only species identified until recently would be the prevailing regional endemic zoonotic species. Our Houston clinical experience of numerous patients with *Acrodermatits chronicum atrophicans* (ACA), typically found in *Borrelia afzelii*, support the likelihood that other *Borrelia* genospecies cause human disease within the US.

Premise 7: 'Lyme disease' is exclusively a vector-borne (primarily arthropod) illness

To date, the vector considered primary for transmission of *Bbsl* to humans is the arthropod (17) likely related to its role in the initial 1975 recognition of 'Lyme disease' in humans (6). Many arthropod species have been found infected with *Bbsl* and causal transfer established (13). The tick has been studied in North America exhaustively, having the characteristics of a highly effective vector: long life, vertebrate blood meal feeding, and bacterial transovarial passage (13). Its role in 'Lyme disease' is assured, because it is the vector in what is considered exclusively a zoonosis.

Data are available, however, that expand the possible diversity of *Borrelia* vectors worldwide beyond the arthropod. Other possible carriers include the flea (108,109), mosquito (110–112), fly (111), and mite (113). Related enzootic cycles have been only rarely examined, although some data link non-arthropod vectors with animal hosts (110,112–114). We suggest that early, sustained myopic focus on the arthropod as sole vector in the spread of 'Lyme disease' within the zoonosis context likely delayed early consideration of other enzootic cycles as well as non-zoonotic *Bbsl* transfer directly between humans.

We propose the human may well be the most likely 'vector' for *Bbsl* transfer to other humans. The label 'Lyme disease' has become, by convention, a semantic boundary that excludes consideration that an infectious agent responsible for a zoonosis may also exist independently as a *non-zoonosis*. CDC-defining criteria do not address human congenital transfer and in at least one reference deny without proof that sexual transfer occurs (17). This mindset assures that *Bbsl* cases falling outside 'Lyme disease' criteria have not been considered in most research, nor reported to local health agencies.

Premise 8: Congenital (vertical) transmission between humans does not occur

The CDC position on intra-human *Bbsl* transmission is that 'Lyme disease bacteria are not transmitted from person-to-person' (17). Current human and veterinary data make this position indefensible (79,80).

Schlesinger and MacDonald reported the first human congenital transfer cases of *Bbsl*. Gardner provided the initial and now most recent exhaustive review of available human gestational transfer cases (13,81). Her credible supporting studies utilized histological, PCR, or culture identification of *Bb* in both mother and newborn or aborted fetus. She reviewed 263 *Bbsl*-infected cases and summarized the birth outcomes. If mothers are untreated, Gardner notes the high percentage of negative pregnancy outcomes along with symptomatic, as well as seemingly asymptomatic, neonates. Indirect data supports the possibility of human congenital *B. burgdorferi* transfer (95,96,115), including similarity to other spirochetal diseases such as *Treponema pallidum* (116–118).

Contrary data suggest that congenital human (24,119–122) and congenital animal (123–126) transfer does not occur. Use of the 'Lyme disease' model for these studies (with inclusion criteria of EM rash, tick attachment history, or endemic region residence) necessarily excludes congenital transfer, which obviates their conclusions (15). Most of the human data were based on simple surveys of birth outcome, without satisfactory proof of spirochetal absence (likely a current impossibility). The contrary veterinary data appear credible and employ a search for spirochetes by culture or histological methods. These data support animal species that exhibit congenital transference and those that may not, which suggested species-specific transfer differences.

Not unexpectedly, we find no serious or credible epidemiological studies that have attempted to identify the true *rate* of human congenital *Bbsl* transfer. The only method we have of estimating congenital human *Bb* transfer is by other intra-human illnesses. Transfer rates of Cytomegalovirus and Toxoplasmosis range from 14% to 59% (127). The congenital transfer rate of *Treponema pallidum* has been reported as high as 68% in one cohort of *treated* infected mothers (116).

There is evidence to support the possibility that *Bb* may present clinically differently in congenitally infected versus vector-inoculated humans, and a review of similar chronic trans-placental diseases in humans is instructive (82,127). Common in congenital infection are 'silent' transfer, differential neonate illness presentation, and a negative effect on later immune competence. The general principles of neonate immune function, adult immune function, and transplacental transfer of pathogens provide further insight into the relationship between trans-placental agents and a new and developing immune system (13). This information collectively suggests that silent or atypical birth presentation may be common, possibly resulting in delayed or complete lack of recognition of the transfer.

Premise 9: Sexual (horizontal) transfer between humans does not occur

The CDC position on sexual intra-human *Bbsl* transmission is that it does not occur (17).

We find no study that addresses sexual transmission of *Bb* among humans; conversely, we find no study supporting that it does *not* occur. Inferential data, however, suggest the possibility of human sexual transfer. The data come from sound veterinary studies (96,98,115), the finding of *Bb* in human semen and breast milk (128,129), and by similarity to *Treponema pallidum* where sexual transfer is abundantly documented (117,130,131).

Our clinical experience strongly suggests that predictable, possibly inevitable *Bbsl* transfer between sexually active couples occurs. The preponderance of infected spouses we have tested to date also exhibit positive serology or PCR for *Bbsl* presence.

Premise 10: 'Lyme disease' is not considered a persistent infection, implying self-limited outcome

Most CDC-referenced studies support this assumption. There is insufficient or no follow up after initial diagnosis or treatment in these studies, however, to support this position. Extensive use of unsupported presumptions is troubling as well. The latter include labeling patients with persisting or recurring disease characteristics as 'reinfected' without serology or tissue evidence, or presuming lack of infection because subsequent positive antibody tests do not meet 'Lyme disease' inclusion criteria (patients were not from 'endemic' areas, etc.) (17,18).

Substantial data support the probability that human *Bbsl* infection can persist indefinitely. This state may obtain even when treatment is provided according to 'standard guidelines' (52,90,132–135). The supporting rationale for persistence is summarized as follows: (1) Latency and relapse are widely observed *Bb* phenomena (13,89,91,100,136,137). (2) Symptoms frequently re-emerge following therapy (89,94,100,137). (3) Many mechanisms of potential survivability have been found in the highly complex and adaptable *Bb* organism (138–141). (4) An inert survival state is implied by the lengthy time to grow viable spirochetes from EM incubated cultures (43,142). (5) Animal models support extensive survival of *Bb* in tissue despite lack of detectable presence in body fluids (51,52). (6) Cyst forms have been found in-vivo to transfer infection directly without reversion to spirochete form, suggesting a possible alternative mechanism for silent transfer (143). (7) Recent *T. pallidum* data unexpectedly support prolonged human spirochetal infection despite use of standard treatment protocols (144).

Premise 11: Long-term 'Lyme disease' sequelae are autoimmune-induced or the result of past infection damage

This premise is a corollary of premise 10, where long-term infection sequelae are used to rationalize lack of infection persistence. Very few 'Lyme disease' CDC-referenced studies conclude that long-term sequelae are a result of chronic infection (17,18). Several hypotheses, nevertheless, have been advanced to address the nature of 'late' sequelae. Autoimmune effect is one proposed mechanism derived from indirect evidence (145–147). Another is anatomic damage assumed induced by *Bbsl* in earlier infection (148). Both positions are hypothetical and use unsupported assumptions.

On the other hand, substantial data suggest that late sequelae are the result of persistent infection (see Premise 3). We believe this large number of published studies supporting that a high probability of persistent *Bbsl* infection casts doubt on the above two mechanisms as primary determinants of pathology. They may, we believe, be included *within the context of persistence* as potential contributory mechanisms of ongoing pathology.

A search for other clinical outcomes of prolonged *Bb* infection in published data yields no clear answer. The CDC position in 2001 is limited to a few sentences: 'Infrequently, Lyme disease morbidity may be severe, chronic, and disabling. An ill-defined post-Lyme disease syndrome occurs in some persons following treatment for Lyme disease. Lyme disease is rarely, if ever, fatal.' (17). Most published research avoids comment on long-term sequelae (149).

Because of the present dearth of relevant data, we propose use of another perspective to address the question of sequelae from late active *Borrelia* infection. Late effects differing from early effects is used as a rationale that, because of this difference, support that active infection no longer exists. Examination of other persistent infections contradicts this argument. Many infections often present with dissimilar acute and late effects. Examples are Chicken Pox later appearing as 'Shingles', and 'strep throat' manifesting eventually as Rheumatic Fever. Some chronic infections have no acute phase. An example is the virus HHV-8 later manifesting as Kaposi's Sarcoma. Thus, there exists the possibility in late *Bbsl* infection of not recognizing the presentation.

Asymptomatic patients with late infection may also be easily overlooked, and assumed non-infected (20,30–54). Further, ill patients presenting with disseminated symptoms without meeting defined 'Lyme disease' endemicity criteria are also at serious risk of not being considered *Bbsl* infected.

Premise 12: Lyme disease is geographically constrained to areas of high zoonosis prevalence, mostly in North America and Eurasia

Gardner has comprehensively summarized international 'Lyme disease' distribution data (13). The resulting map concentrates illness primarily into a Northern Hemisphere temperate zone belt covering most of Europe and the United States. Expectedly, maps of zoonotic endemicity overlie the illness maps faithfully. We conclude a high likelihood that 'Lyme disease' is constrained to areas of high zoonotic endemicity simply because endemic area occurrence is an inclusion criterion. This illustrates the circularity of creating a predicted disease outcome by limiting its definition.

An extensive search of published literature reveals that distribution of human borreliosis may be much broader than described, practically is essentially globally disseminated. *Bbsl* presence in humans, other vertebrate reservoirs or both, have been reported from over thirty countries on six continents and several islands (5,22,54,55,58,110–112,114,150–179). Failure to document the full geographic extent of the organism may stem from simple lack of public health resources in most countries or lack of recognition of the disease in humans. We find no credible studies of human *Bbsl* infection prevalence conducted outside 'endemic' zoonotic regions.

Premise 13: 'Lyme disease' is a contemporary human illness

Bbsl was first acknowledged as a human pathogen in the US medical literature from 1982 to 1983 (7–9,11). The limited historical data that address earlier human infection do so indirectly by examining reservoir (*Peromyscus*, Massachusetts, 1894) or vector (*Ixodes ricinus*, Germany, 1884) infection using museum DNA evidence(163,180), or disease categorizations based on skin manifestations of unknown etiology (26,30,172,181–185).

Data from outside the 'Lyme disease' zoonosis model vaguely suggest the possibility that *Bbsl* is not a recent pathogen in nature, including human infection. Isolated papers examining *Bb* dissemination address such possibilities as: (1) The birth of the pathogen as a trans-kingdom mutation from African Swine Fever virus (186). (2) European 'Lyme disease' gradient rising from West to East (22). (3) Extensive presence of *Borrelia garinii* and *afzelii* in Eurasia (13). (4) Extensive presence of the spirochete (Garinii and Afzelii only) in Northeast Asia (Vladivostok) in a common Ixodid vector providing opportunity for Siberian-Alaska land bridge transfer 10,000–30,000 BC (187). (5) A recent hypothesis that *Bbsl* may be the protective agent of juvenile and adult arthritis in Louisiana Tchefuncte Indians between 500 BC and 300 AD (187,188). (6) Documented human presence in central and southern South America. (7) *Bb sensu stricto* main genospecies in North America (18). (8) Evidence for spread of *Bb sensu stricto* from the Western hemisphere to Europe after 1492 (189). Together, we suggest these data hint at a possible but unexamined circum-global dissemination of the pathogen over many human generations.

We believe the global occurrence of *B. burgdorferi* and its many strains provides the strongest evidence to support the likelihood that *Bbsl* has been present in nature and in humans for centuries to millennia. Protracted existence of the spirochete, if validated, would provide strong support for broad intra-human spread that began some indefinite time following early vector-to-human transfer.

Re-synthesis of premises by 'preponderance of data' weighting

'Lyme disease' was the label initially given to the illness conceptualization (disease model) of human *Bb* infection. The model congealed about 20 years ago as a zoonosis principally from locally available information. Subsequent worldwide data appear to have been gathered within the contextual boundaries of this initially conceived model. We find that the preponderance of this data support the conclusion that the zoonotic model was, and remains, incomplete, and includes only a portion of all *B. burgdorferi* infected humans. The data suggest there may exist a much larger unrecognized pool of *Bbsl*-infected individuals sustained by persistent intra-human transfer that we provisionally call 'Epidemic Borreliosis'. A summary comparing these two populations is shown in Table 1.

Clinical diagnosis of long-infected patients has been inconsistent and puzzling, specifically regarding the signs of EM rash and arthritis. The erythema migrans rash, initially considered the herald lesion for infection, actually occurs both sporadically in initial inoculation and later as secondary lesions. Its absence alone is thus of no value in rejecting a diagnosis, although its presence alerts to the probability of infection. A symptomatic state may be present or absent in the initial presentation, where absence of symptoms can mask the presence of a non-pathogenic strain. Arthritic joints are considered common in disseminated zoonotic *Bbsl*, but paradoxically, only intermittent and migratory joint pain is described in very late borreliosis.

Laboratory tests are presently reliable for supporting a diagnosis of recent vector-transferred 'Lyme disease' but seem highly unreliable if the transfer was zoonotic more than a year earlier, or was congenital. In these cases where antibodies are likely sparse, serology is valid only when positive. Negative results are necessarily inconclusive and may be seriously misleading, regardless of symptoms. The argument supporting 'false positive' serology, when based on zoonosis criteria, is invalid if *Bbsl* infection is widespread from prolonged intra-human transfer.

The pathogen responsible for 'Lyme disease' is a limited subset of the genospecies *B. burgdorferi*. Until recently, only one human pathogen had been identified in the continental United States: *B. burgdorferi sensu stricto (Bbss)*. The exclusive position of this species likely arose from limiting the early search for vectors to the geographic region where 'Lyme disease' was initially discovered. Given the global diversity of species such as *Borrelia afzelii* and *garinii*, the reality of intra-human transfer, and the probability of prolonged infection, we expect extensive regional diversity of *Bbsl* species in humans both in endemic and non-endemic regions of the earth. We propose that anticipating other species will improve identification by broadening the carriers tested to humans as well as zoonotic vectors and reservoirs.

Transfer of *Bbsl* to humans occurs via both zoonotic vectors ('Lyme disease') and other humans. Congenital transfer is fact. Animal data support that sexual transfer can occur, and other data suggest its possibility. 'Lyme disease' reservoirs and vectors may be even more globally widespread than currently modeled, increasing the probability of broader and historically longer inoculation of *Bbsl* into the human population. The finding of *Bbsl* in

Table 1 Comparison of proposed illness characteristics

	'Lyme disease'[a]	Epidemic Borreliosis[b]
What is the initial disease presentation?		
Erythema Migrans (EM) rash	Frequent but inconsistent	Secondary; occasional
Symptoms present if 'early'	None to flu-like	In neonates: none to fatal
Symptoms present if 'late'	None to multi-organ	None to multi-organ
Joint symptoms if 'late'	Arthritis	Arthralgias[c]
Cardiac signs if 'late'	High-degree block	Arrhythmias, T-waves unstable[c]
Typical illness length at initial presentation	<1 year	<2 years
How is the infection diagnosed?		
Number of Bb species	One (region-specific)	Many (non region-specific)
Serum antibody levels	High and constant	Low or occasional
Accuracy of serology	Accurate	High number of false negatives
Relationship of serology to region of diagnosis	Direct	None
Usefulness of EM rash	Alerts to recent inoculation	Announces infection presence
Usefulness of arthritis	Suggests 'late' infection stage	Suggests zoonosis transfer
How is the disease conferred to humans?		
By Zoonotic Vector?	Yes	No
Congenitally?	No	Yes (proven)
Sexually	No	Yes (not studied)
Regional?	Yes: endemic areas	No: anywhere
What is the disease course & outcome?		
Self-limited?	Defined as likely	No; likely lifelong infection
Latent?	Yes	Yes
Activate or reactivate?	No by assumption	Yes
Considered long-term sequelae	Autoimmunity/residual damage	Infection persistence/(mechanisms not elucidated)
Asymptomatic seropositive patient infection status	Considered infected only if from endemic region	Infected regardless of region of residence
What other epidemiological factors pertain?		
Primary worldwide vector	Arthropod	Human
Bbsl presence in human population (time)	Not addressed	Millennia
Distribution in humans	Confined to endemic areas	Worldwide, diffuse

[a] *'Lyme disease'* – All human cases of human *Borrelia burgdorferi* infection **within** the defined limits of the CDC case definition (15).
[b] Epidemic borreliosis – all human *Borrelia burgdorferi* infection cases **outside** the CDC case definition of 'Lyme disease'. Includes Zoonosis vector-transferred infections more than one year old and all congenital, gestational and sexual intra-human transferred infections whether symptomatic or asymptomatic.
[c] Author's clinical experience.

virtually all countries where it is sought also implies more uniform global distribution of the infection in humans. We expect regionally endemic 'Lyme disease' cases now to be far fewer than intra-human disease cases (Epidemic Borreliosis), and that many of the latter are unrecognized principally due to mislabeling.

Regardless of initial transfer route, human infection with pathogenic *Bbsl* may persist for life. Symptoms and signs may vary from sub-clinical to extensive and severe, including cycling between these states (33,77,190,191). Clinical sequelae from prolonged infection appear likely and may be cumulative with various mechanisms operant. An unknown number of sub-clinical cases may remain undetected for life, regardless of whether latency persists or unrecognized activation occurs. If lifetime persistence is the rule, then all living, untreated patients infected at any time during their lives remain infected.

The preponderance of all reviewed data suggest that *B. burgdorferi* may have been present in both natural reservoirs as well as in humans via intra-human transfer for centuries or millennia. We propose that this concept, if verified, predicts a much larger current population of congenitally and possibly sexually infected individuals worldwide than infected via zoonotic vectors.

In summary, we propose a significantly modified human *Bbsl* infection illness model that incorporates 'Lyme disease' only as one engine feeding a larger reservoir of chronic, *Borrelia*-infected humans (Fig. 1). We believe zoonosis was the likely source of initial human disease, and continues to contribute newly infected cases. We further propose that vertical and horizontal intra-human transmission over generations has likely had a non-linear amplifying effect on human prevalence. If true, this transmission mechanism now significantly exceeds the contribution of new cases from zoonotic vectors, and has reached pandemic proportion on all continents where humans reside. These conclusions strongly support our clinical experience.

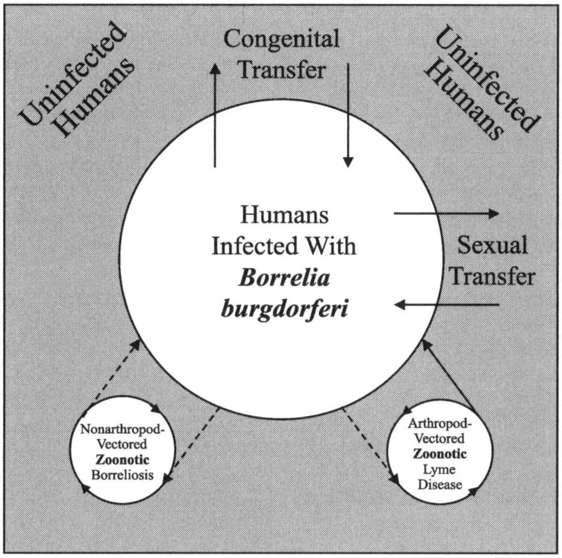

Fig. 1 Revised model of Human Epidemic Borreliosis.

CONCLUSIONS

We propose there are at least two similar and unified, but distinct forms of human *B. burgdorferi* infection: 'Lyme disease', and 'Epidemic Borreliosis' (disease spread directly between humans). Late (more than one year old) zoonotic disease may overlap both forms.

'Lyme disease' is the only presently acknowledged *Bb* illness form, conceptualized as a zoonotic disease where intra-human transfer is considered rare. As defined, 'Lyme disease' is primarily located in limited geographic areas, is clinically recognized relatively early after inoculation, and the reported case numbers are small. Human infection in this model is considered accidental and 'self-limited'.

We propose the existence of a much larger 'non-Lyme' pool of *B. burgdorferi*-infected humans with a clinical presentation of extraordinary variability, global geographic distribution, and far greater prevalence. Transfer is intra-human (congenital and almost certainly sexual) and is initially silent or unrecognized. If not successfully treated, infection is life-long, and latency, late activation, and reactivation are common. Zoonotic cases more than one year old may present similarly. We label this larger pool 'Epidemic Borreliosis'.

Combining both the 'Lyme' and 'non-Lyme' concepts results in a significantly altered model of human *B. burgdorferi* infection. Zoonotic borreliosis is fact and is the milieu within which the complete human disease has existed, perhaps for millennia. Zoonotic transfer was likely the initial route of human inoculation and continues with regularity into the larger pool of infected humans in zoonotically endemic regions. We believe that human endemicity is virtually ubiquitous wherever humans live worldwide and has now reached pandemic proportion. Overlap of these two groups occurs where competent infected vectors exist, but we believe the numbers of 'non-Lyme' cases predominate significantly even here. Infection prevalence has not likely reached numerical stability, since the amplifying effect of congenital transfer, coupled with the current global population expansion, suggests the probability of continuing prevalence rise.

We propose that 'Lyme disease' is a limited conceptualization of a far more pervasive *Borrelia* infection state that is now an unrecognized global epidemic.

DISCUSSION

Our proposed model further challenges many aspects of medical science now believed to be true. Not only does it consign 'Lyme disease' to a minor role in *B. burgdorferi* infection prevalence but supports the idea that a zoonosis can initiate what can later become a vastly more extensive intra-human infectious disease. As a medical model, we find this revised concept works with exceptional success. Until now, the current model has seriously limited our capacity to diagnose and treat many patients. In our patient population, the revised model provides a rational mechanism that far better explains our experience. It effectively resolves the conflicting viewpoints held by clinicians and academicians about what has been labeled 'chronic Lyme disease' and is now allowing us to resolve or minimize illness in most of these patients.

Unexpectedly, the revised model has provided us much more. Most of our patients arrive with a diagnosis from diverse specialty areas but unsuccessfully treated. Use of this reframed model provides rational insight into many of these cases. It provides a successful diagnosis and treatment strategy that, when applied, resolved many patients' symptoms, thus suggesting to us that *B. burgdorferi* may underpin these illnesses as cofactor or origin.

We wondered if all of these 'atypical' *Borrelia*-infected patients might give us a clue to the true magnitude of the infection prevalence. A large number of clinically-similar (to late *Bbsl* infection) medical conditions with unknown etiology exist within the inclusive medical framework. Aaron, reviewing evidence from unexplained medical conditions (chronic fatigue syndrome, fibromyalgia, the irritable bowel syndrome, multiple chemical sensitivities, temporomandibular disorder, tension headache, interstitial cystitis, and the post-concussion syndrome), found substantial clinical overlap (192). Clauw likewise found similar clinical overlap among several of these illness categories, as have others, that include Gulf War Syndrome variants, overtraining syndromes, and numerous 'functional somatic syndromes' (193–197). A single paper by Pachner and Steere written in 1985 provides a credible rationale for most of the neurological symptoms and signs described in these illnesses as well as in human *Bbsl* infection (198). Later papers describe a persistent, infection-based inflammation that may provide the fundamental pathology mechanism (106,145,199–215).

These 'orphan' illnesses that constitute most of our (now) *Borrelia*-positive Houston patients sum to at least a double-digit prevalence in the United States even if we consider only four of these 'chronic syndromes'. Estimates of case-definition fibromyalgia include 2–4% (193,216,217), chronic fatigue syndrome, 0.42% (218), Gulf War syndrome, 4% (219) and multiple chemical sensitivities, 2–5% (220). Vague model boundary limits in these similar 'syndromes' coupled to illness labels where no prevalence data is available make this information unquestionably imprecise. However, when combined with the unknown but finite prevalences of the many other illness categories mentioned above including unknown overlap, however they hint that the combined number is not small.

We wondered whether our proposed model could generate such numbers as the infection rates reported by the CDC support a much lower prevalence (18). When the CDC data are examined using our derived assumptions, however, and a 'zoonosis-only' prevalence is generated, the outcome is 0.6% (Appendix A).

We next generated a crude estimate of the expected background prevalence of 'Lyme disease' in non-endemic regions using the assumptions of Masters (221). The resulting point prevalence is 2% once system stability has been reached. If congenital transfer is added and assumed ongoing for 1000 years, which we think not unreasonable, the point prevalence in 2000 AD becomes 6.5%. If sexual transfer is further added with the same assumptions at a 50% transfer rate, the combined point prevalence becomes 15.5%. Details of this exercise are found in Appendix B.

Another combined prevalence estimate based only on symptoms was generated by one of us in 1993 from an annual medical history form. 2683 employees of a Department of Energy plant were queried regarding 30 common symptoms and signs of late *Bb* infection. Endemicity and EM or tick bite criteria were excluded. 12.8% of the employees met similar symptom criteria. (Appendix C: unpublished data).

These unexpected numbers of possible *Bbsl*-infected patients hidden for decades by mislabeling, fit comfortably within our proposed model and are then not difficult to explain. We propose that where data were not initially available, temporary hypothetical bridges, although dissimilar, were necessarily created by early investigators to fill their model framework gaps. Our proposed model now fills in most such gaps for all these illnesses. It also revises framework elements of other illnesses we had considered unassailable parts of the standard medical paradigm.

We believe failure to recognize the breadth of this infection is readily explainable by inadvertent research errors: (1) most data have been derived only from zoonotically endemic areas, (2) 'validation' rested on inadequate serologic diagnostic methodology, and (3) controls, when used, were useless since half those infected are 'sub-clinical'. Clearly, discovery of the illness in an area of high zoonotic endemicity contributed to early and continuing clinical myopia but was the necessary first step in its recognition.

Other factors contribute to clinical recognition failure. Silent transfer, latency, late activation, and recurrent activation likely combine to create a setting resistant to standard epidemiological detection methods. The pathogen's extreme complexity is another probable contributor. Its adaptability, pleomorphism, genetic diversity, and differential tissue tropism create extraordinary symptom variability. Likewise, activation of numerous latent viruses and opportunistic bacteria from immune depression in late disease may further expand illness complexity. Such varied presentation is not likely to have previously been considered to have a single infectious etiology, thus which excludes *Bbsl* from most differential diagnoses.

We propose that zoonotic transfer combined with human transfer on a global scale for centuries can indeed result in double-digit prevalence.These numbers applied to our model hint at the highly improbable: that the prevalence of all humans infected with *Bbsl* could constitute an even larger percentage of the population by including the sub-clinical cases mostly excluded from epidemiological surveys to date.

The technological solution that can validate our proposed model is a more sensitive and specific laboratory test likely not based on serum antibody presence. We do not offer a specific solution but propose that detection of the organism itself or unique biochemical markers altered by the infection are required. Because of unpredictable latency and inability to use controls, use of Koch's postulate or sophisticated epidemiological methods are no longer adequate in cases such as this and have likely reached the historical limits of their usefulness here (2).

Despite the need for dramatically improved detection methods, there exists even now an instrument capable of recognizing the scope of this illness: the astute clinician willing to carry what Carl Sagan called the 'burden of skepticism' (222). This perspective is an essential medical tool, as the 'system' within which the clinician works requires reframing prevailing cognitive paradigms before unfamiliar ideas can be 'seen' at all (222,223). (The history of medicine, in fact, is built on examples of mindset that delayed recognition or evolution of most illness concepts (224).)

We believe that reliance on familiar models is ultimately the principal reason that what we here term 'Epidemic Borreliosis' remains hidden from the view of science. Our purpose in publishing this newly proposed model is to encourage skepticism by investigators as well as clinicians: to consider the possibility that 'Lyme disease' is an inadequate conceptualization of all human *Bb* infection. We are confident that once considered, others will 'see' what we are finding in clinical practice (223).

We thus propose that 'Lyme disease' is only the herald encounter with a human infectious disease of currently inconceivable proportion. We anticipate that if our model is validated and the proposed high prevalence of *B. burgdorferi* in humans is verified, the conceptual framework of this and many other human diseases will be radically altered.

RECOMMENDATIONS

Our recommendations are based on verifying or disproving the disease model we present here and are derived from the gaps remaining in the data we have reviewed.

The initial task must be to identify all humans infected with *B. burgdorferi*. This likely requires first understanding antibody status in late (beyond 18 months) infections and the pathophysiological mechanisms linking *Bbsl* presence and human disease. Commercial tests to reliably detect living *Bbsl* in humans as well as reservoirs and vectors must then follow to reveal the agent's true worldwide prevalence. Extensive effort will be required to prove or disprove persistence, and to determine all disease entities associated with *Bbsl* infection: whether cause-and-effect, co-factor, or unrelated. Finally, the full extent of epidemiological science must be applied to determine the scope and efficiency of human congenital transfer and to investigate sexual *Bbsl* transfer. Answers will guide development of preventive strategies.

Concurrently, treatment modalities and schedules to eradicate *B. burgdorferi* from all patients regardless of infection route or duration, must be created. If our experience holds, this will be a difficult task, and will require serious and rapid commitment from all nations.

APPENDIX A. DERIVED 'LYME DISEASE' PREVALENCE USING CDC INFECTION RATES

The number of 'Lyme disease' cases reported by the CDC appears unreasonably small compared to our estimates. Within the defined parameters of the current 'Lyme disease' model employed by state and federal public health agencies, 16,273 cases were reported (more likely underreported) in the US in 1999 (0.06% of the population) (17). However, *assuming lifetime prevalence and no treatment*, the 1992–1997 crude mean annual incidence of 5.1 reported cases/100,000 persons/year roughly corresponds to a prevalence of 1,070,000 infections over the 75-year period, 1925–2000 AD (18). This number, likely an underestimate of true prevalence, is nevertheless 0.6% of the period population mean (1963). This suggests that *a 2% true zoonotic-only* stable *Bb* human prevalence may not be unreasonable in the US and, we propose, globally.

APPENDIX B. ESTIMATING THE FULL PREVALENCE OF HUMAN *Bbsl* INFECTION

We used a simple exercise to estimate the possible human *Bbsl* prevalence. Employing complex statistical methods was of no value because insufficient data exists to use precision. We sought only a 'ballpark' number to make the point that the *possibility* of unexpectedly high prevalence exists.

(1) *Assumption 1: Transfer is via Zoonotic vector only.*

- Assume: zoonotic transfer only, one tick bite per decade per human (221), 1% of ticks infected (5), 50% chance of tick-to-human transfer, and prevalence stability.
- Point prevalence = 8 tick bites/lifetime × 1% of ticks infected × 50% chance of infection if bitten × 1/2 (average human at midlife) = PP = 8 (TIR) (CI)/2 = 2%.
- This exercise predicts that 2% of humans are infected with *Bb* in Texas. We propose this number approximates the worldwide background prevalence of humans infected via zoonosis vector transfer regardless of region endemicity.

(2) *Assumption 2: If congenital transfer is combined with vector transfer for at least one millennium.*

- Assume: 2% of the population in 1000 AD was infected via zoonosis only, the prevalence and infection rate are stable, congenital transfer rate is 50%, full population turnover per 100 years, male/female ratio is 1:1, and no congenital transfer occurs before 1000 AD.
- Then 2% of all mothers after 1000 AD are already infected at conception.
- At a 50% transfer rate, 1% of all female newborns will be infected congenitally by 1100 AD.
- These 1% newborn females (1/2% of population) mature and join the 2% infected via zoonotic vectors = 2.5% Infected mothers at 50% transfer rate by 3–4 generations (assume 100 years).
- In the subsequent 100 years after 1000 AD, 2% of population already infected by tick + 1/2% infected congenitally by 1100 AD.
- Every succeeding 100 years, 1/2% more humans will be infected (ignore compounding for simplicity and conservatism): Point Prevalence = 2% + 1/2% $(y-100)/(100) = 2\% + 1/2\%(900/100)$.
- Human point prevalence now = 2% + 4.5% = 6.5% (from 1000 to 2000 AD).

(3) *Assumption 3: If Vector, congenital and sexual transfer are combined for at least one millennium.*

- Assume: Use above assumptions. Add: fathers infect new mothers at a 50% rate, begin in 1000 AD. 2% infected fathers infect 1% more mothers = 3%.
- In 1100 AD all humans born to 2.5% + 1% infected mothers (2% infected fathers infect 98% uninfected mothers at 50% sexual transfer rate).
- Assume 50% rate in congenital transfer continues.
- Using the information in (2), infected humans = 2% + 1.5% (y − 100)/(100).
- Point prevalence now = 2% + 13.5% = 15.5% (from 1000 to 2000 AD).

This exercise has been invoked to demonstrate the possibility that if intra-human transfer is established as common, the numbers of humans presently infected with *Bbsl* may significantly exceed the number of humans infected via zoonotic transfer. The difference is in the stability of the transfer system. Zoonotic systems reach some stability if populations are relatively stable over the short term and exposure remains close to constant. In recent years, the human population has risen rapidly, but so has urbanization with diminished outdoor work and leisure activity. Overall, in the 20th century, we estimate human-vector contact has remained relatively constant. Prior to the 20th century, human-vector contact was more extensive, making our estimates conservative.

Although made possible initially by vector infection, intra-human infection prevalence rises with the passage of time. The latter will rise in absolute numbers as the population size increases. This exercise assumes that human zoonosis infections remain relatively stable. When intra-human transfer occurs extensively, however, prevalence rise can approach geometric progression. Thus, the importance of time in estimating differences in the two types of transmission.

APPENDIX C. OCCUPATIONAL MEDICAL HISTORY SURVEY

In 1993, one of us, while Medical Director of a US Department of Energy facility in a non-endemic state, attempted to estimate the prevalence of chronically ill employees with symptoms similar to late, disseminated Lyme disease. A computerized medical history form was crafted for the required annual medical examination, in which 2683 actively working employees participated. Randomly interwoven in the Review of Systems portion of the questionnaire were 30 questions characteristic of the illness. 'Inclusion' criteria were: 50% of the questions had to be answered in the affirmative, with five questions determined most important: frequent headaches, persistent muscle pain, persistent activity limitation, intermittent and/or migratory joint pain, and any recurrent unexplained neurological symptom such as seizure, vertigo, or focal special-sense phenomenon (e.g., tinnitus or photophobia). There was no follow-on testing for borreliosis.

Active employees (343 (12.8%)) were found to meet our criteria for diagnosis. A random review of 35 (10%) charts selected from this group revealed symptoms had been present from less than a year to nearly 30 years (the full length of employment). A much broader degree of morbidity than in the inclusion criteria was found, with six employees near termination for number of lost workdays due to illness. None of the 35 records revealed a prior diagnosis that might account for the full symptom complex, although the fiscal resources expended on imaging, electronic tests (e.g., EMG, EEG, and EKG), and repeated outpatient visits was considerable. None had been tested for *B. burgdorferi* by any test method.

REFERENCES

1. Kuhn T. In: *The Structure of Scientific Revolutions*, 3rd edn. Chicago, IL: The University of Chicago Press, 1996: 212.
2. Ewald P. In: *Plague Time: How Stealth Infections Cause Cancers, Heart Disease, and Other Deadly Ailments*. New York, NY: The Free Press, 2000: 282.
3. Texas zoonosis diseases. Internet web site ed: Texas department of Health, Zoonosis Control Division, 2000. [Cited 2001 Oct 15]. Available from URL: http://www.tdh.state.tx.us/phpep/dpn/issues/dpn59n10.pdf.
4. Rawlings J. A., Fournier P. V., Teltow G. J. Isolation of *Borrelia spirochetes* from patients in Texas. *J Clin Microbiol* 1987; **25**(7): 1148–1150.
5. Rawlings J. A., Teltow G. J. Prevalence of *Borrelia* (Spirochaetaceae) spirochetes in Texas ticks. *J Med Entomol* 1994: 297–301.
6. Steere A. C. et al. Lyme arthritis: an epidemic of oligoarticular arthritis in children and adults in three connecticut communities. *Arthritis Rheum* 1977; **20**(1): 7–17.
7. Burgdorfer W. et al. Lyme disease-a tick-borne spirochetosis. *Science* 1982; **216**(4552): 1317–1319.
8. Steere A. C. et al. The spirochetal etiology of Lyme disease. *N Engl J Med* 1983; **308**(13): 733–740.
9. Burgdorfer W. Discovery of the Lyme disease spirochete and its relation to tick vectors. *Yale J Biol Med* 1984; **57**(4): 515–520.
10. Davis J. P. et al. Lyme disease in Wisconsin: epidemiologic, clinical, serologic, and entomologic findings. *Yale J Biol Med* 1984; **57**(4): 685–696.
11. Burgdorfer W. et al. Erythema chronicum migrans - a tickborne spirochetosis. *Acta Trop* 1983; **40**(1): 79–83.
12. James A. M. et al. *Borrelia lonestari* Infection after a bite by an *Amblyomma americanum* Tick. *J Infect Dis* 2001; **183**(12): 1810–1814.
13. Gardner T. Chapter 11: Lyme disease. In: J. Remington, J. Klein (eds). *Infectious Diseases of the Fetus and Newborn Infant*. Philadelphia, PA: W.B. Saunders Company, 2001: 519–641.
14. Barbour A. G., Fish D. The biological and social phenomenon of Lyme disease. *Science* 1993; **260**(5114): 1610–1616.
15. Case definitions for infectious conditions under public health surveillance. Centers for Disease Control and Prevention. *MMWR Morb Mortal Wkly Rep* 1997; **46**(RR-10): 1–55.
16. Wharton M. et al. Case definitions for public health surveillance. *MMWR Morb Mortal Wkly Rep* 1990; **39**(RR-13): 1–43.
17. Lyme Disease. Internet web site ed: CDC Division of Vector-borne Infectious Diseases, 2001. [Cited 2001 Dec 6]. Available from URL: http//www.cdc.gov.ncidod/clvbid/lyme/index.htm.
18. Surveillance for Lyme Disease - United States, 1992–1998. *Morb Mortal Wkly Rep* 2000; **49**(SS03)): 1–11.
19. Billings A. N., Rawlings J. A., Walker D. H. Tick-borne diseases in Texas: a10-year retrospective examination of cases. *Tex Med* 1998; **94**(12): 66–76.
20. Chary-Valckenaere I. et al. Diagnosis of Lyme disease. Current difficulties and prospects. *Rev Rhum Engl Ed* 1995; **62**(4): 271–280.
21. Christen H. J. Lyme neuroborreliosis in children. *Ann Med* 1996; **28**(3): 235–240.
22. Cimmino M. et al. European Lyme borreliosis clinical spectrum. *Zentralbl Bakteriol* 1998; **287**(3): 248–252.
23. Hejka A. G. et al. The pathologist's view of Lyme disease. *Wis Med J* 1989; **88**(11): 17–20.
24. Hercogova J. et al. Early-stage lyme borreliosis during pregnancy: treatment in 15 women with erythema migrans. *Cesk Gynekol* 1993; **58**(5): 229–232.
25. Lesniak O. M., Belikov E. S. The classification of Lyme borreliosis (Lyme disease. *Ter Arkh* 1995; **67**(11): 49–51.
26. Malane M. S. et al. Diagnosis of Lyme disease based on dermatologic manifestations. *Ann Intern Med* 1991; **114**(6): 490–498.
27. Maraspin V. et al. Erythema migrans in pregnancy. *Wien Klin Wochenschr* 1999; **111**(22–23): 933–940.
28. Schmidt R. et al. Prevalence of erythema migrans borreliosis in blood donors. *Infusionstherapie* 1989; **16**(6): 248–251.
29. Baranton G. et al. Distinct levels of genetic diversity of *Borrelia burgdorferi* are associated with different aspects of pathogenicity. *Res Microbiol* 2001; **152**(2): 149–156.
30. Asbrink E., Brehmer-Andersson E., Hovmark A. Acrodermatitis chronica atrophicans - a spirochetosis. Clinical and histopathological picture based on 32 patients; course and relationship to erythema chronicum migrans Afzelius. *Am J Dermatopathol* 1986; **8**(3): 209–219.
31. Christian C. L. Management of asymptomatic *Borrelia burgdorferi* infection (see comments. *Arthritis Rheum* 1992; **35**(11): 1395.
32. Coyle P. K. et al. Detection of *Borrelia burgdorferi*-specific antigen in antibody-negative cerebrospinal fluid in neurologic Lyme disease. *Neurology* 1995; **45**(11): 2010–2015.
33. Coyle P. K. et al. *Borrelia burgdorferi* reactivity in patients with severe persistent fatigue who are from a region in which Lyme disease is endemic. *Clin Infect Dis* 1994; **18**(Suppl. 1): S24–S27.
34. Dournon E. Lyme disease: biological diagnosis and treatment. *Rev Prat* 1989; **39**(15): 1300–1303.
35. Fahrer H. et al. Prevalence of Lyme borreliosis in a Swiss population at risk. *Schweiz Med Wochenschr* 1988; **118**(2): 65–69.
36. Fahrer H. et al. Longterm survey (7 years) in a population at risk for Lyme borreliosis: what happens to the seropositive individuals? *Eur J Epidemiol* 1998; **14**(2): 117–123.
37. Fahrer H. et al. The prevalence and incidence of clinical and asymptomatic Lyme borreliosis in a population at risk. *J Infect Dis* 1991; **163**(2): 305–310.
38. Feder H. M., Jr et al. Prospective assessment of Lyme disease in a school-aged population in Connecticut. *J Infect Dis* 1995; **171**(5): 1371–1374.
39. Hanrahan J. P. et al. Incidence and cumulative frequency of endemic Lyme disease in a community. *J Infect Dis* 1984; **150**(4): 489–496.
40. Karch H. et al. Demonstration of *Borrelia burgdorferi* DNA in urine samples from healthy humans whose sera contain *B. burgdorferi*-specific antibodies. *J Clin Microbiol* 1994; **32**(9): 2312–2314.

41. Kubo N. et al. Questionnaire surveys of cases of tick bite and Lyme borreliosis in hunters in Hokkaido with reference to detection of anti-*Borrelia burgdorferi* antibody. *Intern Med* 1992; **31**(10): 1163–1168.
42. Kuiper H. et al. Evaluation of central nervous system involvement in Lyme borreliosis patients with a solitary erythema migrans lesion. *Eur J Clin Microbiol Infect Dis* 1994; **13**(5): 379–387.
43. MacDonald A. B., Berger B. W., Schwan T. G. Clinical implications of delayed growth of the Lyme borreliosis spirochete, *Borrelia burgdorferi*. *Acta Trop* 1990; **48**(2): 89–94.
44. Mautner V. F. et al. Epidemiology of *Borrelia burgdorferi* infection. Relation of the prevalence rate on determination by serologic procedures. *Nervenarzt* 1990; **61**(2): 94–97.
45. Nohlmans M. K. et al. Prevalence of Lyme borreliosis in The Netherlands. *Ned Tijdschr Geneeskd* 1991; **135**(48): 2288–2292.
46. Pfister H. W. et al. Latent Lyme neuroborreliosis: presence of *Borrelia burgdorferi* in the cerebrospinal fluid without concurrent inflammatory signs. *Neurology* 1989; **39**(8): 1118–1120.
47. Schmid G. P. et al. Failure to detect endotoxin in sera from patients with Lyme disease. *J Infect Dis* 1984; **150**(4): 616.
48. Schmutzhard E. et al. Infections following tickbites. Tick-borne encephalitis and Lyme borreliosis – a prospective epidemiological study from Tyrol. *Infection* 1988; **16**(5): 269–272.
49. Smith H. V., Gray J. S., McKenzie G. A Lyme borreliosis human serosurvey of asymptomatic adults in Ireland. *Zentralbl Bakteriol* 1991; **275**(3): 382–389.
50. Smith J. L., Israel C. W. Spirochetes in the aqueous humor in seronegative ocular syphilis. Persistence after penicillin therapy. *Arch Ophthalmol* 1967; **77**(4): 474–477.
51. Straubinger R. K. PCR-based quantification of *Borrelia burgdorferi* organisms in canine tissues over a 500-day postinfection period. *J Clin Microbiol* 2000; **38**(6): 2191–2199.
52. Straubinger R. K. et al. Status of *Borrelia burgdorferi* infection after antibiotic treatment and the effects of corticosteroids: an experimental study. *J Infect Dis* 2000; **181**(3): 1069–1081.
53. Weder B. et al. Chronic progressive neurological involvement in *Borrelia burgdorferi* infection. *J Neurol* 1987; **234**(1): 40–43.
54. Yoshinari N. H. et al. Outline of Lyme borreliosis in Brazil. *Rev Hosp Clin Fac Med Sao Paulo* 1997; **52**(2): 111–117.
55. Gylfe et al. Isolation of Lyme disease *Borrelia* from puffins (*Fratercula arctica*) and seabird ticks (*Ixodes uriae*) on the Faeroe Islands. *J Clin Microbiol* 1999; **37**(4): 890–896.
56. Lane R. S. et al. Risk factors for Lyme disease in a small rural community in northern California. *Am J Epidemiol* 1992; **136**(11): 1358–1368.
57. Steere A. C. et al. Longitudinal assessment of the clinical and epidemiological features of Lyme disease in a defined population. *J Infect Dis* 1986; **154**(2): 295–300.
58. Hoshinari N. H. et al. Epidemiological study of Lyme disease in Brazil. *Rev Hosp Clin Fac Med Sao Paulo* 1992; **47**(2): 71–75.
59. Baranton G. *Alphanumeric List of Borrelia burgdorferi* sensu Lato Strains. Paris, France: Pasteur Institute, Molecular Biology and Medicine Unit, 2001.
60. Straubinger R. et al. Two-lessons from the canine model of Lyme disease: migration of *Borrelia burgdorferi* in tissues and persistence after antibiotic treatment. *J Spirochetal Tick-Borne Dis* 1997; **4**(1/2).
61. Goebel K. M., Krause A., Neurath F. Acquired transient autoimmune reactions in Lyme arthritis: correlation between rheumatoid factor and disease activity. *Scand J Rheumatol* 1988; **75**(Suppl.): 314–317.
62. Albert S. et al. Lyme arthritis in a 12-year-old patient after a latency period of 5 years. *Infection* 1999; **27**(4–5): 286–288.
63. Bussen S., Steck T. Manifestation of Lyme arthritis in the puerperal period. *Z Geburtshilfe Perinatol* 1994; **198**(4): 150–152.
64. Flisiak R., Wiercinska-Drapalo A., Prokopowicz D. Immunologic reaction in patients with arthritis in the course of borreliosis with Lyme disease. *Przegl Epidemiol* 1996; **50**(3): 253–257.
65. Priem S. et al. Detection of *Borrelia burgdorferi* by polymerase chain reaction in synovial membrane, but not in synovial fluid from patients with persisting Lyme arthritis after antibiotic therapy. *Ann Rheum Dis* 1998; **57**(2): 118–121.
66. Sigal L. H. Musculoskeletal manifestations of Lyme arthritis. *Rheum Dis Clin North Am* 1998; **24**(2): 323–351.
67. Steere A. C., Hardin J. A., Malawista S. E. Erythema chronicum migrans and Lyme arthritis: cryoimmunoglobulins and clinical activity of skin and joints. *Science* 1977; **196**(4294): 1121–1122.
68. Steere A. C. Lyme arthritis: the joint lesions in Lyme borreliosis in the USA. *Ter Arkh* 1995; **67**(11): 43–45.
69. Weyand C. M., Goronzy J. J. Immune responses to *Borrelia burgdorferi* in patients with reactive arthritis. *Arthritis Rheum* 1989; **32**(9): 1057–1064.
70. Recommendations for test performance and interpretation from the Second National Conference on Serologic Diagnosis of Lyme Disease. *MMWR Morb Mortal Wkly Rep* 1995: 590–591.
71. Craft J. E. et al. Antigens of *Borrelia burgdorferi* recognized during Lyme disease. Appearance of a new immunoglobulin M response and expansion of the immunoglobulin G response late in the illness. *J Clin Invest* 1986; **78**(4): 934–939.
72. Ostrov B. E., Athreya B. H. Lyme disease. Difficulties in diagnosis and management. *Pediatr Clin North Am* 1991; **38**(3): 535–553.
73. Fung B. P. et al. Humoral immune response to outer surface protein C of *Borrelia burgdorferi* in Lyme disease: role of the immunoglobulin M response in the serodiagnosis of early infection. *Infect Immun* 1994; **62**(8): 3213–3221.
74. Padula S. J. et al. Use of recombinant OspC from *Borrelia burgdorferi* for serodiagnosis of early Lyme disease. *J Clin Microbiol* 1994; **32**(7): 1733–1738.
75. Petrovic M. et al. Lyme borreliosis – a review of the late stages and treatment of four cases. *Acta Clin Belg* 1998; **53**(3): 178–183.
76. Rahn D. W., Felz M. W. Lyme disease update. Current approach to early, disseminated, and late disease. *Postgrad Med* 1998; **103**(5): 51–54, , 57–9, 63–4 passim.
77. Schmid G. P. Epidemiology and clinical similarities of human spirochetal diseases. *Rev Infect Dis* 1989; **11**(Suppl. 6): S1460–S1469.

78. Zhong W., Oschmann P., Wellensiek H. J. Detection and preliminary characterization of circulating immune complexes in patients with Lyme disease. *Med Microbiol Immunol (Berl)* 1997; **186**(2–3): 153–158.
79. MacDonald A. B. Human fetal borreliosis, toxemia of pregnancy, and fetal death. *Zentralbl Bakteriol Mikrobiol Hyg [A]* 1986; **263**(1–2): 189–200.
80. Schlesinger P. A. et al. Maternal-fetal transmission of the Lyme disease spirochete, *Borrelia burgdorferi. Ann Intern Med* 1985; **103**(1): 67–68.
81. Gardner T. Chapter 11: Lyme disease. In: J. S. Remington, J. O. Klein (eds). *Infectious Diseases of the Fetus and Newborn Infant.* New York, NY: W.B. Saunders Company, 1995: 1373.
82. Lewis D. B., Wilson C. B. Chapter 2: Developmental immunology and role of host defenses in neonatal susceptibility to infection. In: J. S. Remington, J. O. Klein (eds). *Infectious Diseases of the Fetus and Newborn Infant.* New York, NY: W.B. Saunders Company, 1995: 1373.
83. Wormser G. P., Aguero-Rosenfeld M. E., Nadelman R. B. Lyme disease serology: problems and opportunities. *JAMA* 1999; **282**(1): 79–80.
84. Wilske B., Fingerle V. Diagnosis of Lyme borreliosis. How to corroborate suspected borreliosis. *MMW Fortschr Med* 2000; **142**(15): 28–31.
85. Kaiser R. False-negative serology in patients with neuroborreliosis and the value of employing of different borrelial strains in serological assays. *J Med Microbiol* 2000; **49**(10): 911–915.
86. Banyas G. T. Difficulties with Lyme serology. *J Am Optom Assoc* 1992; **63**(2): 135–139.
87. Guidelines for laboratory evaluation in the diagnosis of Lyme disease. American College of Physicians. *Ann Intern Med* 1997; **127**(12): 1106–1108.
88. Lawrence C. et al. Seronegative chronic relapsing neuroborreliosis (see comments). *Eur Neurol* 1995; **35**(2): 113–117.
89. Sigal L. H. Persisting complaints attributed to chronic Lyme disease: possible mechanisms and implications for management. *Am J Med* 1994; **96**(4): 365–374.
90. Preac-Mursic V. et al. Survival of *Borrelia burgdorferi* in antibiotically treated patients with Lyme borreliosis. *Infection* 1989; **17**(6): 355–359.
91. Nordstrand A., Barbour A. G., Bergstrom S. Borrelia pathogenesis research in the post-genomic and post-vaccine era. *Curr Opin Microbiol* 2000; **3**(1): 86–92.
92. Schutzer S. E. et al. Sequestration of antibody to *Borrelia burgdorferi* in immune complexes in seronegative Lyme disease. *Lancet* 1990; **335**(8685): 312–315.
93. Wang P. Hilton, Contribution of HLA alleles in the regulation of antibody production in Lyme disease. *Front Biosci* 2001; **6**: B10–B16.
94. Straubinger R. K. et al. Clinical manifestations, pathogenesis, and effect of antibiotic treatment on Lyme borreliosis in dogs. *Wien Klin Wochenschr* 1998; **110**(24): 874–881.
95. Burgess E. C., Windberg L. A. *Borrelia* sp. infection in coyotes, black-tailed jack rabbits and desert cottontails in southern Texas. *J Wildl Dis* 1989; **25**(1): 47–51.
96. Burgess E. C., Wachal M. D., Cleven T. D. *Borrelia burgdorferi* infection in dairy cows, rodents, and birds from four Wisconsin dairy farms. *Vet Microbiol* 1993; **35**(1–2): 61–77.
97. Burgess E. C. *Borrelia burgdorferi* infection in Wisconsin horses and cows. *Ann NY Acad Sci* 1988; **539**: 235–243.
98. Liebstein M. M., Khan M. I., Bushmich S. L. Evidence for in utero transmission of *Borrelia burgdorferi* from naturally infected cows. *J Spirochetal Tick-Borne Dis* 1998; **5**(4): 54–62.
99. Ghinsberg R. C., Nitzan Y. Is syphilis an incurable disease. *Med Hypotheses* 1992; **39**(1): 35–40.
100. Logigian E. L., Kaplan R. F., Steere A. C. Chronic neurologic manifestations of Lyme disease (see comments). *N Engl J Med* 1990; **323**(21): 1438–1444.
101. Jelic S., Filipovic-Ljeskovic I. Positive serology for Lyme disease borrelias in primary cutaneous B-cell lymphoma: a study in 22 patients; is it a fortuitous finding. *Hematol Oncol* 1999; **17**(3): 107–116.
102. Ma B. et al. Serodiagnosis of Lyme borreliosis by western immunoblot: reactivity of various significant antibodies against *Borrelia burgdorferi. J Clin Microbiol* 1992; **30**(2): 370–376.
103. Ma Y., Weis J. J. *Borrelia burgdorferi* outer surface lipoproteins OspA and OspB possess B-cell mitogenic and cytokine-stimulatory properties. *Infect Immun* 1993; **61**(9): 3843–3853.
104. Plorer A. et al. Effects of adequate versus inadequate treatment of cutaneous manifestations of Lyme borreliosis on the incidence of late complications and late serologic status. *J Invest Dermatol* 1993; **100**(2): 103–109.
105. Preac-Mursic V. et al. First isolation of *Borrelia burgdorferi* from an iris biopsy. *J Clin Neuroophthalmol* 1993; **13**(3): 155–161 (Discussion 162).
106. Sigal L. H. Lyme disease: a review of aspects of its immunology and immunopathogenesis. *Annu Rev Immunol* 1997; **15**: 63–92.
107. Honegr K. et al. In process citation. *Epidemiol Mikrobiol Immunol* 2001; **50**(1): 10–16.
108. Teltow G. J., Fournier P. V., Rawlings J. A. Isolation of *Borrelia burgdorferi* from arthropods collected in Texas. *Am J Trop Med Hyg* 1991; **44**(5): 469–474.
109. Hubalek Z., Halouzka J., Juricova Z. Investigation of haematophagous arthropods for borreliae - summarized data 1988–1996. *Folia Parasitol* 1998; **45**(1): 67–72.
110. Halouzka J. P. D., Hubalek Z. Isolation of the spirochete *Borrelia afzelii* from the mosquito *Aedes vexans* in the Czech Republic. *Med Vet Entomol* 1998; **12**(1): 103–105.
111. Magnarelli L. A., Anderson J. F. Ticks and biting insects infected with the etiologic agent of Lyme disease, *Borrelia burgdorferi. J Clin Microbiol* 1988; **26**(8): 1482–1486.
112. Hubalek Z., Halouzka J. Distribution of *Borrelia burgdorferi* sensu lato genomic groups in Europe, a review. *Eur J Epidemiol* 1997; **13**(8): 951–957.
113. Pokorny P. Incidence of the spirochete *Borrelia burgdorferi* in arthropods (Arthropoda) and antibodies in vertebrates (Vertebrata). *Cesk Epidemiol Mikrobiol Immunol* 1989; **38**(1): 52–60.
114. Badalian L. O. et al. The neurological syndromes in Lyme disease in children. *Zh Nevropatol Psikhiatr Im S S Korsakova* 1994; **94**(3): 3–6.
115. Gustafson J. M. et al. Intrauterine transmission of *Borrelia burgdorferi* in dogs. *Am J Vet Res* 1993; **54**(6): 882–890.
116. McFarlin B. L. et al. Epidemic syphilis: maternal factors associated with congenital infection. *Am J Obstet Gynecol* 1994; **170**(2): 535–540.

117. Hederstedt B. et al. IgM-antibodies against *T. pallidum* detected in sera from mothers of stillborn babies in Mozambique by the solid-phase haemadsorption assay (SPHA). *Int J STD AIDS* 1992; **3**(5): 347–349.
118. Schwartz D. A. et al. Pathology of the umbilical cord in congenital syphilis: analysis of 25 specimens using histochemistry and immunofluorescent antibody to *Treponema pallidum*. *Hum Pathol* 1995; **26**(7): 784–791.
119. Gerber M. A., Zalneraitis E. L. Childhood neurologic disorders and Lyme disease during pregnancy. *Pediatr Neurol* 1994; **11**(1): 41–43.
120. Nadal D. et al. Infants born to mothers with antibodies against *Borrelia burgdorferi* at delivery. *Eur J Pediatr* 1989; **148**(5): 426–427.
121. Strobino B. A. et al. Lyme disease and pregnancy outcome: a prospective study of two thousand prenatal patients. *Am J Obstet Gynecol* 1993; **169**(2 Pt 1): 367–374.
122. Strobino B., Abid S., Gewitz M. Maternal Lyme disease and congenital heart disease: a case-control study in an endemic area. *Am J Obstet Gynecol* 1999; **180**(3 Pt 1): 711–716.
123. Mather T. N., Telford S. R. d., Adler G. H. Absence of transplacental transmission of Lyme disease spirochetes from reservoir mice (*Peromyscus leucopus*) to their offspring. *J Infect Dis* 1991; **164**(3): 564–567.
124. Mather T. N., Fish D., Coughlin R. T. Competence of dogs as reservoirs for Lyme disease spirochetes (*Borrelia burgdorferi*). *J Am Vet Med Assoc* 1994; **205**(2): 186–188.
125. Moody K. D., Barthold S. W. Relative infectivity of *Borrelia burgdorferi* in Lewis rats by various routes of inoculation. *Am J Trop Med Hyg* 1991; **44**(2): 135–139.
126. Silver R. M. et al. Fetal outcome in murine Lyme disease. *Infect Immun* 1995; **63**(1): 66–72.
127. Klein J. O., Remington J. S. Chapter 1: Current Concepts of Infections of the Fetus and Newborn Infant. In J. S. a. K. Remington, J. O. (eds) *Infectious Diseases of the Fetus and Newborn Infant*. New York, NY: W.B. Saunders Company, 1995: 1373.
128. Kumi-Diaka J., Harris O. Viability of *Borrelia burgdorferi* in stored semen. *Br Vet J* 1995; **151**(2): 221–224.
129. Schmidt B. L. et al. Detection of *Borrelia burgdorferi* DNA by polymerase chain reaction in the urine and breast milk of patients with Lyme borreliosis. *Diagn Microbiol Infect Dis* 1995; **21**(3): 121–128.
130. MacDonald A. B. Gestational Lyme borreliosis. Implications for the fetus. *Rheum Dis Clin North Am* 1989; **15**(4): 657–677.
131. Bromberg K., Rawstron S., Tannis G. Diagnosis of congenital syphilis by combining *Treponema pallidum*-specific IgM detection with immunofluorescent antigen detection for *T. pallidum*. *J Infect Dis* 1993; **168**(1): 238–242.
132. Bayer M. E., Zhang L., Bayer M. H. *Borrelia burgdorferi* DNA in the urine of treated patients with chronic Lyme disease symptoms. A PCR study of 97 cases. *Infection* 1996; **24**(5): 347–353.
133. Dattwyler R. J., Halperin J. J. Failure of tetracycline therapy in early Lyme disease. *Arthritis Rheum* 1987; **30**(4): 448–450.
134. Nanagara R., Duray P. H., Schumacher H. R., Jr Ultrastructural demonstration of spirochetal antigens in synovial fluid and synovial membrane in chronic Lyme disease: possible factors contributing to persistence of organisms. *Hum Pathol* 1996; **27**(10): 1025–1034.
135. Steere A. C., Dwyer E., Winchester R. Association of chronic Lyme arthritis with HLA-DR4 and HLA-DR2 alleles. *N Engl J Med* 1990; **323**(4): 219–223.
136. Pachner A. R. Spirochetal diseases of the CNS. *Neurol Clin* 1986; **4**(1): 207–222.
137. Preac Mursic V. et al. Kill kinetics of *Borrelia burgdorferi* and bacterial findings in relation to the treatment of Lyme borreliosis (published erratum appears in Infection 1996 Mar–Apr; 24(2): 169). *Infection* 1996; **24**(1): 9–16.
138. Rittig M. G. et al. *Borrelia burgdorferi*-induced ultrastructural alterations in human phagocytes: a clue to pathogenicity? *J Pathol* 1994; **173**(3): 269–282.
139. Mursic V. P. et al. Formation and cultivation of *Borrelia burgdorferi* spheroplast-L-form variants (published erratum appears in Infection 1996 Jul–Aug; 24(4): 335). *Infection* 1996; **24**(3): 218–226.
140. Georgilis K., Steere A. C., Klempner M. S. Infectivity of *Borrelia burgdorferi* correlates with resistance to elimination by phagocytic cells. *J Infect Dis* 1991; **163**(1): 150–155.
141. Georgilis K., Peacocke M., Klempner M. S. Fibroblasts protect the Lyme disease spirochete, *Borrelia burgdorferi*, from ceftriaxone in vitro. *J Infect Dis* 1992; **166**(2): 440–444.
142. Pachner A. R. Neurologic manifestations of Lyme disease, the new 'great imitator". *Rev Infect Dis* 1989; **11**(Suppl. 6): S1482–S1486.
143. Gruntar I. et al. Conversion of *Borrelia garinii* cystic forms to motile spirochetes in vivo. *Apmis* 2001; **109**(5): 383–388.
144. Sell S. et al. Host response to *Treponema pallidum* in intradermally-infected rabbits: evidence for persistence of infection at local and distant sites. *J Invest Dermatol* 1980; **75**(6): 470–475.
145. Burmester G. R. et al. Immunology of reactive arthritides. *Annu Rev Immunol* 1995; **13**: 229–250.
146. Klempner M. S., Huber B. T. Is it thee or me? – autoimmunity in Lyme disease (news; comment). *Nat Med* 1999; **5**(12): 1346–1347.
147. Sigal L. H. Antibiotics for the treatment of rheumatologic syndromes. *Rheum Dis Clin North Am* 1999; **25**(4): 861–981, viii.
148. Sigal L. H., Williams S. A monoclonal antibody to *Borrelia burgdorferi* flagellin modifies neuroblastoma cell neuritogenesis in vitro: a possible role for autoimmunity in the neuropathy of Lyme disease. *Infect Immun* 1997; **65**(5): 1722–1728.
149. Asch E. S. et al. Lyme disease: an infectious and postinfectious syndrome. *J Rheumatol* 1994; **21**(3): 454–461.
150. Palacios R. et al. Positive IgG Western blot for *Borrelia burgdorferi* in Colombia. *Mem Inst Oswaldo Cruz* 1999; **94**(4): 499–503.
151. Baranton G., Marti Ras N., Postic D. *Borrelia burgdorferi*, taxonomy, pathogenicity and spread. *Ann Med Interne (Paris)* 1998; **149**(7): 455–458.
152. Brown R. N., Lane R. S. Lyme disease in California: a novel enzootic transmission cycle of *Borrelia burgdorferi*. *Science* 1992; **256**(5062): 1439–1442.

153. Cimmino M. A. et al. The epidemiology of Lyme borreliosis in Italy. *Microbiologica* 1992; **15**(4): 419–424.
154. Davidson M. M. et al. Isolation of *Borrelia burgdorferi* from ticks in the Highlands of Scotland. *J Med Microbiol* 1999; **48**(1): 59–65.
155. Fivaz B. H., Petney T. N. Lyme disease – a new disease in southern Africa? *J S Afr Vet Assoc* 1989; **60**(3): 155–158.
156. Fridriksdottir V., Nesse L. L., Gudding R. Seroepidemiological studies of *Borrelia burgdorferi* infection in sheep in Norway. *J Clin Microbiol* 1992; **30**(5): 1271–1277.
157. Gern L. et al. European reservoir hosts of *Borrelia burgdorferi* sensu lato. *Zentralbl Bakteriol* 1998; **287**(3): 196–204.
158. Gruver K. S., Guthrie J. W. Parasites and selected diseases of collared peccaries (*Tayassu tajacu*) in the trans-pecos region of Texas. *J Wildl Dis* 1996; **32**(3): 560–562.
159. Kim T. H. et al. Serologically diagnosed Lyme disease manifesting erythema migrans in Korea. *J Korean Med Sci* 1999; **14**(1): 85–88.
160. Lawrence R. H., Bradbury R., Cullen J. S. Lyme disease on the NSW central coast. *Med J Aust* 1986; **145**(7): 364.
161. Marguet C. et al. Lyme disease in Upper Normandy: report of a hospital survey. *Arch Pediatr* 2000; **7**(Suppl 3): 517s–522s.
162. Matuschka F. R. et al. Transmission of the agent of Lyme disease on a subtropical island. *Trop Med Parasitol* 1994; **45**(1): 39–44.
163. Matuschka F. R. et al. Characteristics of Lyme disease spirochetes in archived European ticks. *J Infect Dis* 1996; **174**(2): 424–426.
164. McCrossin I. Lyme disease on the NSW south coast. *Med J Aust* 1986; **144**(13): 724–725.
165. Mhalu F. S., Matre R. Serological evidence of Lyme borreliosis in Africa: results from studies in Dar es Salaam, Tanzania. *East Afr Med J* 1996; **73**(9): 583–585.
166. Neira O. et al. Lyme disease in Chile. Prevalence study in selected groups. *Rev Med Chil* 1996; **124**(5): 537–544.
167. Postic D. et al. Common ancestry of *Borrelia burgdorferi* sensu lato strains from North America and Europe. *J Clin Microbiol* 1999; **37**(9): 3010–3012.
168. Prukk T. et al. Seroprevalence of tick-borne Lyme borreliosis in a defined population in Estonia. *Scand J Infect Dis* 1999; **31**(4): 421–422.
169. Qiu W. G. et al. A population genetic study of *Borrelia burgdorferi sensu stricto* from eastern Long Island, New York, suggested frequency-dependent selection, gene flow and host adaptation. *Hereditas* 1997; **127**(3): 203–216.
170. Schmid G. The global distribution of Lyme Disease. *Rev Infect Dis* 1985; **7**(1): 41–50.
171. Stanek, G., Flamm H., Groh V., et al. Epidemiology of borrelia infections in Austria. *Zentralbl Bakteriol Mikrobiol Hyg [A]* 1987; **263**(3): 442–449.
172. Stanek G. et al. European Union concerted action on risk assessment in Lyme borreliosis: clinical case definitions for Lyme borreliosis. *Wien Klin Wochenschr* 1996; **108**(23): 741–747.
173. Smith R., O'Connell S., Palmer S. Lyme disease surveillance in England and Wales, 1986–1998. *Emerg Infect Dis* 2000; **6**(4): 404–407.
174. Shih C. M. et al. Lyme disease in Taiwan: first human patient with characteristic erythema chronicum migrans skin lesion. *J Clin Microbiol* 1998; **36**(3): 807–808.
175. Stefancikova A. et al. IgG antibodies to *Borrelia* in dogs in the area of Kosice. *Vet Med (Praha)* 1996; **41**(3): 83–86.
176. Strle F. Lyme borreliosis in Slovenia. *Zentralbl Bakteriol* 1999; **289**(5–7): 643–652.
177. Sugiyama Y., Minamoto N., Kinjo T. Serological surveillance of Lyme borreliosis in wild Japanese serows (*Capricornis crispus*). *J Vet Med Sci* 1998; **60**(6): 745–747.
178. Zhang Z. F., Wan K. L., Zhang J. S. Studies on epidemiology and etiology of Lyme disease in China. *Chung Hua Liu Hsing Ping Hsueh Tsa Chih* 1997; **18**(1): 8–11.
179. Zhioua E. et al. Longitudinal study of Lyme borreliosis in a high risk population in Switzerland. *Parasite* 1998; **5**(4): 383–386.
180. Marshall III W. F. et al. Detection of *Borrelia burgdorferi* DNA in museum specimens of *Peromyscus leucopus*. *J Infect Dis* 1994; **170**(4): 1027–1032.
181. Aberer E. et al. Heterogeneity of *Borrelia burgdorferi* in the skin. *Am J Dermatopathol* 1996; **18**(6): 571–579.
182. Duray P. H., Asbrink E., Weber K. The cutaneous manifestations of human Lyme disease: a widening spectrum. *Adv Dermatol* 1989; **4**: 255–275.
183. Houtman P. M., Tazelaar D. J. Joint and bone involvement in Dutch patients with Lyme borreliosis presenting with acrodermatitis chronica atrophicans. *Neth J Med* 1999; **54**(1): 5–9.
184. Kaufman L. D. et al. Late cutaneous Lyme disease: acrodermatitis chronica atrophicans. *Am J Med* 1989; **86**(6 Pt 2): 828–830.
185. Ohlenbusch A. et al. Etiology of the acrodermatitis chronica atrophicans lesion in Lyme disease. *J Infect Dis* 1996; **174**(2): 421–423.
186. Hinnebusch J., Barbour A. G. Linear plasmids of *Borrelia burgdorferi* have a telomeric structure and sequence similar to those of a eukaryotic virus. *J Bacteriol* 1991; **173**(22): 7233–7239.
187. Lewis B. A. Prehistoric juvenile rheumatoid arthritis in a precontact Louisiana native population reconsidered. *Am J Phys Anthropol* 1998; **106**(2): 229–248.
188. Lewis B. Treponematosis and Lyme borreliosis connections: explanation for Tchefuncte disease syndromes. *Am J Phys Anthropol* 1994; **93**(4): 455–475.
189. Baranton G., Marti Ras N., Postic D. Molecular epidemiology of the aetiological agents of Lyme borreliosis. *Wien Klin Wochenschr* 1998; **110**(24): 850–855.
190. Barskova V. G., Fedorov E. S., Ananieva L. P. The course of Lyme disease in different age groups. *Wien Klin Wochenschr* 1999; **111**(22–23): 978–980.
191. Hansen K., Lebech A. M. The clinical and epidemiological profile of Lyme neuroborreliosis in Denmark 1985–1990. A prospective study of 187 patients with *Borrelia burgdorferi* specific intrathecal antibody production. *Brain* 1992; **115**(Pt 2): 399–423.
192. Aaron L. A., Buchwald D. A review of the evidence for overlap among unexplained clinical conditions. *Ann Intern Med* 2001; **134**(9 Pt 2): 868–881.
193. Clauw D. J., Chrousos G. P. Chronic pain and fatigue syndromes: overlapping clinical and neuroendocrine features and potential pathogenic mechanisms. *Neuroimmunomodulation* 1997; **4**(3): 134–153.
194. Buchwald D., Garrity D. Comparison of patients with chronic fatigue syndrome, fibromyalgia, and multiple chemical sensitivities. *Arch Intern Med* 1994; **154**(18): 2049–2053.

195. Nicolson G. L., Bruton D. M., Jr, Nicolson N. L. Chronic fatigue illness and Operation Desert Storm. *J Occup Environ Med* 1996; **38**(1): 14–16.
196. Rowbottom D. G. et al. The haematological, biochemical and immunological profile of athletes suffering from the overtraining syndrome. *Eur J Appl Physiol Occup Physiol* 1995; **70**(6): 502–509.
197. Wessely S., Nimnuan C., Sharpe M. Functional somatic syndromes: one or many. *Lancet* 1999; **354**(9182): 936–939.
198. Pachner A. R., Steere A. C. The triad of neurologic manifestations of Lyme disease: meningitis, cranial neuritis, and radiculoneuritis. *Neurology* 1985; **35**(1): 47–53.
199. Brebner K. et al. Synergistic effects of interleukin-1β, interleukin-6, and tumor necrosis factor-α: central monoamine, corticosterone, and behavioral variations. *Neuropsychopharmacology* 2000; **22**(6): 566–580.
200. Coxon R. E. et al. The effect of antibody against TNF α on cytokine response in Jarisch-Herxheimer reactions of louse-borne relapsing fever. *Qjm* 1997; **90**(3): 213–221.
201. Erdile L. F., Guy B. OspA lipoprotein of *Borrelia burgdorferi* is a mucosal immunogen and adjuvant. *Vaccine* 1997; **15**(9): 988–996.
202. Giambartolomei G. H., Dennis V. A., Philipp M. T. *Borrelia burgdorferi* stimulates the production of interleukin-10 in peripheral blood mononuclear cells from uninfected humans and rhesus monkeys. *Infect Immun* 1998; **66**(6): 2691–2697.
203. Giambartolomei G. H. et al. Induction of pro- and anti-inflammatory cytokines by *Borrelia burgdorferi* lipoproteins in monocytes is mediated by CD14. *Infect Immun* 1999; **67**(1): 140–147.
204. Habicht G. S., Katona L. I., Benach J. L. Cytokines and the pathogenesis of neuroborreliosis: *Borrelia burgdorferi* induces glioma cells to secrete interleukin-6. *J Infect Dis* 1991; **164**(3): 568–574.
205. Hayashi F. et al. The innate immune response to bacterial flagellin is mediated by Toll-like receptor 5. *Nature* 2001; **410**(6832): 1099–1103.
206. Hurtenbach U. et al. Studies on early events of *Borrelia burgdorferi*-induced cytokine production in immunodeficient SCID mice by using a tissue chamber model for acute inflammation. *Int J Exp Pathol* 1995; **76**(2): 111–123.
207. Isogai E. et al. Cytokines in the serum and brain in mice infected with distinct species of Lyme disease *Borrelia*. *Microb Pathog* 1996; **21**(6): 413–419.
208. Isogai H. et al. Levels of endogenous interleukin-1, interleukin-6, and tumor necrosis factor in congenic mice infected with *Borrelia garinii*. *Microbiol Immunol* 1997; **41**(5): 427–430.
209. Miller L. C. et al. Live *Borrelia burgdorferi* preferentially activate interleukin-1 β gene expression and protein synthesis over the interleukin-1 receptor antagonist. *J Clin Invest* 1992; **90**(3): 906–912.
210. Moutschen M. et al. Pathogenic tracks in fatigue syndromes. *Acta Clin Belg* 1994; **49**(6): 274–289.
211. Porcella S. F., Schwan T. G. *Borrelia burgdorferi* and *Treponema pallidum*: a comparison of functional genomics, environmental adaptations, and pathogenic mechanisms. *J Clin Invest* 2001; **107**(6): 651–656.
212. Reichenberg A. et al. Cytokine-associated emotional and cognitive disturbances in humans. *Arch Gen Psychiatry* 2001; **58**(5): 445–452.
213. Straubinger R. K. et al. *Borrelia burgdorferi* induces the production and release of proinflammatory cytokines in canine synovial explant cultures. *Infect Immun* 1998; **66**(1): 247–258.
214. Talkington J., Nickell S. P. *Borrelia burgdorferi* spirochetes induce mast cell activation and cytokine release. *Infect Immun* 1999; **67**(3): 1107–1115.
215. Weis J. J. et al. Pathological manifestations in murine Lyme disease: association with tissue invasion and spirochete persistence. *Clin Infect Dis* 1997; **25**(Suppl. 1): S18–S24.
216. Wolfe F. Fibromyalgia. *Rheum Dis Clin North Am* 1990; **16**(3): 681–698.
217. Wolfe F. et al. The prevalence and characteristics of fibromyalgia in the general population. *Arthritis Rheum* 1995; **38**(1): 19–28.
218. Jason L. A. et al. A community-based study of chronic fatigue syndrome. *Arch Intern Med* 1999; **159**(18): 2129–2137.
219. Steele L. Prevalence and patterns of Gulf War illness in Kansas veterans: association of symptoms with characteristics of person, place, and time of military service. *Am J Epidemiol* 2000; **152**(10): 992–1002.
220. Proctor S. P. Chemical sensitivity and gulf war veterans' illnesses. *Occup Med* 2000; **15**(3): 587–599.
221. Masters E. J., Donnell H. D. Epidemiologic and diagnostic studies of patients with suspected early Lyme disease Missouri, 1990–1993 (letter; comment. *J Infect Dis* 1996; **173**(6): 1527–1528.
222. K. Frazier (ed). *The Hundredth Monkey*, 1st edn. Buffalo, NY: Promethius Books, 1991: 400.
223. Ruchlis H. In: *Clear Thinking: A Practical Introduction*, 1st edn. Buffalo, NY: Promethius Books, 1990: 271.
224. Kiple K., (ed.). *The Cambridge World History of Human Disease*, 1st edn. Vol. 1. New York, London, Melbourne: Cambridge University Press, 1993: 1176.

Attorney General forces Infectious Diseases Society of America to redo Lyme guidelines due to flawed development process

L Johnson,[1] R B Stricker[2]

[1] California Lyme Disease Association, Ukiah, California, USA; [2] International Lyme and Associated Diseases Society, Bethesda, Maryland, USA

Correspondence to: Dr R B Stricker, 450 Sutter Street, Suite 1504, San Francisco, California 94108, USA; rstricker@usmamed.com

Received 30 June 2008
Accepted 25 February 2009

ABSTRACT

Lyme disease is one of the most controversial illnesses in the history of medicine. In 2006 the Connecticut Attorney General launched an antitrust investigation into the Lyme guidelines development process of the Infectious Diseases Society of America (IDSA). In a recent settlement with IDSA, the Attorney General noted important commercial conflicts of interest and suppression of scientific evidence that had tainted the guidelines process. This paper explores two broad ethical themes that influenced the IDSA investigation. The first is the growing problem of conflicts of interest among guidelines developers, and the second is the increasing centralisation of medical decisions by insurance companies, which use treatment guidelines as a means of controlling the practices of individual doctors and denying treatment for patients. The implications of the first-ever antitrust investigation of medical guidelines and the proposed model to remediate the tainted IDSA guidelines process are also discussed.

The diagnosis and treatment of Lyme disease is highly controversial, and most patients are aware that obtaining a diagnosis and treatment for this tick-borne illness can be difficult. One group of doctors, the Infectious Diseases Society of America (IDSA), issued Lyme treatment guidelines in 2000 that promoted a narrow definition of the disease.[1] These guidelines excluded most Lyme patients and denied them treatment for their illness. The IDSA viewpoint has been adopted without question by government agencies, insurers, medical boards and hospitals. As a result, the diagnosis and treatment of Lyme disease has been suppressed, with profound healthcare implications for patients, their families and their communities. The level of disability of patients with Lyme disease is equal to that of patients with congestive heart failure and there are at least 21 studies documenting death in patients with this potentially devastating tick-borne illness.[1]

AN INVESTIGATION AGAINST THE IDSA

When the IDSA sought to revise its Lyme treatment guidelines in 2006, patients and their treating doctors tried to obtain a voice in the guidelines process. The IDSA denied their requests for participation and limited the guidelines panel to researchers known to have a bias against the diagnosis and treatment of Lyme disease. The IDSA panel then selectively ignored evidence of persistent infection or clinical improvement with antibiotic treatment in patients with persistent symptoms of the disease. From the perspective of antitrust law, the behaviour of IDSA drew attention to its monopoly power, the fact that its guidelines were treated as mandatory and that members of the guidelines panel had commercial conflicts of interest and intentionally excluded divergent viewpoints and evidence. These facts dovetailed with IDSA's power to control the playing field and enforce its guidelines by providing insurers with second opinions while instigating and testifying at unprofessional conduct actions against doctors who did not comply with the IDSA guidelines. In addition, the IDSA's ability to further suppress the debate through its role as the gatekeepers (on editorial boards and as peer reviewers) for medical journals, medical conferences and grand rounds supported the antitrust argument when patients started complaining that they were being denied care for their disease.

The California Lyme Disease Association (CALDA), the national Lyme Disease Association, Connecticut-based Time for Lyme and other groups affected by the guidelines approached the Connecticut Attorney General, Richard Blumenthal, and expressed their concerns about patients being denied care. In late 2006, the Attorney General launched an antitrust investigation into IDSA and its Lyme guidelines panel for misuse of monopoly power and exclusionary conduct in the development of the guidelines. The antitrust theory is that when a medical society has monopoly power such that its guidelines can take on the force of law, as the IDSA guidelines do, it has an obligation to ensure that the development process is fair, does not exclude competing points of view, and that its panel is not driven by commercial conflicts of interest. To our knowledge, this is the first-ever antitrust investigation into the development process for medical guidelines.

In May 2008, after an extensive investigation, the Attorney General announced a settlement of the antitrust investigation into the IDSA guidelines development process. The settlement stipulates that the IDSA must put together a new panel free from conflicts of interest, permit the introduction of evidence opposing its viewpoints, and hold a public hearing (aired live on the Internet) on controversial recommendations of the guidelines panel. While this is an important victory for the Lyme community, the settlement has broader implications for medical guidelines generally because it represents the first time that conflicts of interest in the guidelines development process have been addressed using antitrust theories.

There are two broad themes that set the stage for the investigation by the Attorney General. The first is the growing problem of conflicts of interest among guidelines developers, and the second is the increasing centralisation of medical decisions by insurance companies, who use treatment guidelines as a means of controlling the practices of individual doctors.

CONFLICTS OF INTEREST MEAN THAT THE QUALITY OF PATIENT CARE MAY TAKE A BACK SEAT TO OTHER COMMERCIAL INTERESTS HELD BY GUIDELINE PANEL MEMBERS

A survey of medical experts who write guidelines for treating conditions such as heart disease, depression and diabetes has found that nearly nine out of 10 have financial ties to the pharmaceutical industry, and the ties are almost never disclosed.[7] Drug companies foster relationships with key opinion leaders among academic researchers who can help develop, obtain Food and Drug Administration (FDA) approval and create a market for drugs, diagnostic tests or vaccines. Panel members may also have consulting relationships with insurers.

Before this case, there had been no effective remedy for guidelines developed by panels with conflicts of interest. While researchers argue that "all is well" provided conflicts are disclosed, other commentators have pointed out that disclosure is not a sufficient remedy when commercial interests drive the process (including selection and interpretation of evidence) and conclusions of a guidelines panel. Merrill Goozner, director of the Integrity in Science Project at the Center for Science in the Public Interest, testified before the Institute of Medicine[3]:

> "The system for reviewing the body of evidence in a field; deriving best practices through systematic reviews; writing clinical practice guidelines; conducting and evaluating comparative research; and, vitally important, evaluating evidence for regulatory purposes should be entirely free from conflicts of interest."

Goozner emphasises the need to maintain strong boundaries between those who determine how medicine is practised and researchers who conduct industry-funded research.

The most influential members of the IDSA guidelines panel had commercial interests related to Lyme vaccines, diagnostic tests, and insurance consulting (table 1 and appendix A). Some of the panellists had been involved in the development of the first Lyme vaccine and had run clinical trials for the vaccine, which was withdrawn from the market after patients reported serious arthritic and neurological side effects.[4] Several panellists had been sued as part of a class action lawsuit or served as expert witnesses for the vaccine manufacturer, and some are working on the second generation of Lyme vaccines, which are still under development. Some panellists acknowledged that they owned or had interests in Lyme diagnostic tests or consulted for insurers. The panel was composed of researchers who supported each other's work and who controlled enormous amounts of government funding for research. These conflicts are disclosed by key panel members themselves in their own publications or statements to the press (table 1 and appendix 1).

Commercial conflicts of interest on guidelines panels is a growing problem in healthcare because panellists may no longer hold the interests of the patient paramount, and the guidelines may determine the medical standard of care for patient treatment. When commercial interests drive the train, patient concerns take a backseat. The *New York Times* reported on a guidelines panel for blood pressure that reduced the threshold level at which patients should receive medication.[11] It turned out that many of the panellists on the hypertension panel had links to the drug companies that produced antihypertensive medications. These manufacturers stood to gain from disease definitions that expanded the size of their commercial market and increased sales. Many doctors believe that they can rise above commercial conflicts of interest, but common sense tells us otherwise. Put a little bit of money in the game and the nature of the debate simply changes.

The IDSA has said that it was not exclusionary in its panel selection and that it listened to competing points of view. This is not true. The association rejected out of hand requests for a seat at the table by patient groups, doctors' organisations and individual treating doctors—even those who were IDSA members. In its previous guidelines panel, IDSA summarily tossed off the panel one researcher who disagreed with the panel chair on the best approach for treatment of chronic Lyme disease.

Dr Gary Wormser, who chaired the Lyme guidelines panel, scoffs at the notion that commercial interests could have played a role in the development process[12]:

Table 1 Summary of disclosed conflicts of interest by five key guideline panel members

Author	Conflict	Source
G Wormser	Lyme diagnostic tests (Immunetics, Bio-Rad, Biopeptides, Diaspex, Abbott Laboratories)	Self-disclosure, IDSA Guidelines 2006[5] Self-disclosure, *New England Journal of Medicine* 2007[6]
	Lyme vaccines (Baxter, AstraZeneca, Biopeptides)	
	Expert witness for medical malpractice involving Lyme disease	
R Dattwyler	Lyme diagnostic tests (Biopeptides and Baxter)	Self-disclosure, IDSA Guidelines 2006
	Lyme vaccines (Baxter, Biopeptides)	Self-disclosure, *BMJ* Lyme Wars 2007[7]
	US patent 7008625 Recombinant Constructs of Bb	Self-disclosure, see individual patents listed in conflict column
	Provisional patent 60/812,595 on a live "bacterial vaccine", PCT/US2005/023106 "oral vaccine for Borrelia", a wildlife vaccine	Brook Technologies Release[8]
	Provisional patent 60/799,016, "Peptide Diagnostic Agent for Lyme"	
	Expert witness for medical malpractice involving Lyme disease	
E Shapiro	Vaccines: Sanofi-Aventis, NIH Grants K24RR022477, KL2RR024138, and UL1RR024139.	Self-disclosure, IDSA Guidelines 2006 Self-disclosure, *New England Journal of Medicine* 2007
	Expert testimony: medical malpractice and unprofessional conduct actions	Self-disclosure, American Academy of Neurology 2007[9]
	Insurance: reviews Lyme disease disability claims for Metropolitan Life Insurance	
A Steere	Lyme vaccines (Baxter, GlaxoSmithKline)	Self-disclosure, IDSA Guidelines 2006
	Lyme diagnostic tests (Viramed)	Self-disclosure, *Nature* 2006[10]
J Halperin	Vaccines: serves as an expert witness on behalf of Lymerix (GlaxoSmithKline) in litigation regarding adverse effects from first generation vaccines (ongoing)	Self-disclosure, IDSA Guidelines 2006

> "There's no potential financial gain for generic drugs that are recommended for short courses. It's inconceivable that anyone would think so. To me it seems disingenuous to make these allegations when they are so absurd."

In Wormser's view, because the panel members were not promoting drugs for treatment there could be no conflict of interest.

People are used to thinking about conflicts of interest in terms of drugs used for treatment, but the arena is much broader than that. There is tremendous financial gain in Lyme disease through vaccines, diagnostic tests and consulting with insurance companies. The IDSA guidelines restrict the definition of the disease and mandate laboratory testing. Guidelines that restrict the disease definition are favourable to vaccine manufacturers because they increase the effective rate for the vaccines so that fewer people taking the vaccine "get" the disease. Guidelines that mandate testing for disease diagnosis promote the interests of those who develop and manufacture diagnostic tests. Guidelines that deny treatment to patients are favourable to insurance companies and those who are paid to consult with them. The IDSA Lyme guidelines panel members had commercial interests in each of these areas.

CENTRALISED MEDICINE REDUCES CHOICE FOR PATIENTS AND LIMITS THE DOCTOR'S ABILITY TO USE CLINICAL JUDGEMENT

The increased concentration and centralisation of power in medicine was also an important factor leading up to the antitrust investigation. Twenty years ago, individual doctors had more autonomy than they do today in deciding whether to comply with medical guidelines. Medical malpractice and unprofessional conduct actions were always rooted in the standard of care, which was determined by the consensus of practising doctors, but guidelines became a vehicle for driving the standard of care. This transformed a very fluid environment where opinions in medical practice changed as individual doctors' viewpoints changed based on new information from the latest medical conference or grand rounds, the success or failure in treating patients or the latest study read by the doctors. The opinions of individual panel members on guidelines panels of powerful medical societies became a proxy for the opinions of doctors in the broader community. With "evidence-based" guidelines, someone other than the treating doctors selects, interprets and makes recommendations regarding treatment.

The problem arises when the ability of a doctor to select, interpret and exercise clinical judgement is replaced by an obligation to comply with guidelines that do not work or that are not appropriate for the individual patient. Population-based treatment approaches using average results leave individual patients who are not the "norm" out of the equation. This is why it is important to treat the patient rather than the disease, and why displacing the treating doctor's judgement is risky business. Commercial interests, particularly those of insurers and drug manufacturers, see guidelines as a means of controlling medical costs or furthering vaccines, drugs or diagnostic tests. As a result, guidelines became part of the "one-stop shopping" marketing strategy of pharmaceutical companies and part of the cost-containment strategy of insurers. In addition to the role of commercial interests and conflicts of interest discussed above, an equally important issue is the shift of guidelines from a "suggestion" to a "mandated standard of care" that is intended to displace doctors' autonomy with centralised medical decisions.

Guidelines permit insurers to shift the emphasis from clinical judgement to a centralised, largely administrative function, with an emphasis on actuarially predictable population-based care. Dr David Eddy, senior adviser to Kaiser Permanente, notes that "if the fight to control health care costs is to be successful, it will have to address [the decisions physicians make about treatments]."[13] Guidelines are the mechanism for doing this. Specialty societies embrace treatment guidelines because these official protocols expand their sphere of influence in an insurance-driven environment. Specialty societies such as the IDSA are extremely insurance-conscious because the livelihood of their members hinges on the acceptability of their guidelines and the role their members play as ambassadors and enforcers of second opinion of those guidelines.

According to Eddy, "[I]t would not be stretching things too far to say that whoever controls practice policies controls medicine."[14] What this means is that if one can control the development of treatment guidelines and can obtain compliance from doctors, one can effectively control the way doctors practise medicine and also control costs. This is why insurers are driven by guidelines. Insurers control doctors' practices through economic profiling that compels doctors within the insurer's network to conform to guidelines or cost parameters on threat of termination from the network. Insurers control out-of-network costs by refusing to reimburse claims for services that do not conform to guidelines. The government is the USA's largest insurer through Medicare and this fact, plus the drive towards universal healthcare, has placed more emphasis on cost control through guidelines.

The health insurance industry relies heavily on third party guidelines (such as the IDSA Lyme guidelines) to provide a shield against potential litigation as well as to control costs. Historically, health insurers have been held accountable for violations of the standard of care (just as doctors can be). However, when powerful third parties develop the guidelines, they can drive the standard of care. When large specialty societies drive the standard of care, no one is accountable for malpractice if these standards are "wrong". The specialty society does not have the individual physician–patient relationship that would create the duty of care necessary for malpractice, and the insurer is shielded because it is relying on an acceptable standard of care. In this case, the IDSA promulgates guidelines that the insurers rely on to justify denials of care, thereby reducing costs. When patients seek out a doctor who does not follow the IDSA guidelines, the insurers require a second opinion from an "infectious disease" expert, thereby creating a highly effective enforcement cycle for insurers using third party guideline developers. Guidelines by specialty societies provide a particularly effective means of controlling general medical practice.

The same control issues apply to appeals of insurance denials through the "independent medical review" process sanctioned by most states. This review process assists insurers by having a third party review their claims. Some insurers who are not required by law to use the review process nevertheless elect to use this approach because it is an inexpensive way of disposing of claims as a practical matter without litigation or arbitration. There are only a handful of "independent review organisations" (IROs) used by the states that have adopted independent review processes. These organisations represent insurers as their bread and butter work and perform independent reviews on the side. While the internal processes of IROs are a black box (there is no transparency in their procedures), the general concept is that these organisations also rely on guidelines by third parties, particularly the guidelines of a specialty society. As a result, specialty society guidelines have a large role in determining the care that may be provided, not only by members of their society but also by family doctors and internists. Insurers can also rely on these guidelines to police doctors within their networks, terminating the contracts of those who are not complying. Hospitals (which can operate like insurance providers these days) can use these guidelines to determine the care provided within the hospital and whether hospital privileges will be extended or revoked for doctors who do not follow the guidelines.

RESTRICTIVE GUIDELINES ARE VIEWED AS MANDATORY BY THE MEDICAL COMMUNITY

The guidelines published by the IDSA in November of 2006 were extremely restrictive and denied the use of clinical judgement in the diagnosis and treatment of Lyme disease. This is a critical point because when patients fail treatment under the IDSA guidelines (which restrict Lyme treatment to 30 days), they are given no alternative treatment. Doctors are essentially told to sit on their hands and let the patients experience a disability that is equivalent to that of congestive heart failure—with no treatment offered. Doctors are told that they must ignore their clinical experience and ignore the patient's history, course of treatment and past responsiveness to medication. It is the exclusion of treatment options and denial of the doctor's right to use clinical judgement that makes the guidelines so restrictive. Add the fact that IDSA is so powerful in the medical community and that its opinions are given the force of law by medical boards and insurers and one has all of the ingredients necessary to deny patients with chronic Lyme disease any treatment whatsoever. The IDSA's role in instigating and testifying at unprofessional conduct hearings and in supporting insurance denials of care makes compliance with its guidelines mandatory. This enforcement deters doctors who might otherwise treat patients with chronic Lyme disease from doing so.

THE ATTORNEY GENERAL'S INVESTIGATION

Findings of the investigation

The Attorney General found that the IDSA Lyme guidelines panel, which was hand-picked by Dr G Wormser, had important conflicts of interest, intentionally blocked the appointment of panel members with divergent viewpoints, and intentionally excluded evidence that was not in conformity with the bias of the panel[15]:

> "The IDSA's guideline panel improperly ignored or minimized consideration of alternative medical opinion and evidence regarding chronic Lyme disease, potentially raising serious questions about whether the recommendations reflected all relevant science".

Some of the specific findings were:

- Dr Wormser, the panel chair was selected inappropriately, "held a bias regarding the existence of chronic Lyme" and "handpick[ed] a likeminded panel without scrutiny by or formal approval of the IDSA's oversight committee".
- The IDSA panel members had financial interests—"in drug companies, Lyme disease diagnostic tests, patents and consulting arrangements with insurance companies" The IDSA failed to conduct a conflicts of interest review for any of the panellists, several of whom had conflicts of interests.
- The IDSA's 2000 and 2006 Lyme disease panels refused to accept or meaningfully consider information regarding the existence of chronic Lyme disease.
- The IDSA blocked appointment of scientists and doctors with divergent views on chronic Lyme who sought to serve on the 2006 guidelines panel by informing them that the panel was fully staffed, even though it was later expanded.
- The IDSA portrayed the American Association of Neurology copycat guidelines as corroborating its own when it knew that the two panels shared several authors, including the chairmen of both groups, and were working on guidelines at the same time.[16]

The settlement

The settlement is a process—essentially a reassessment of the guidelines by a panel free of conflicts—with safeguards to ensure that evidence and opinions are not suppressed

The Attorney General has always been clear that his role is not to make medical judgements or to trump science. Instead, his role is to make sure that the development process is fair, non-exclusionary, and not tainted by conflicts of interest. According to the Attorney General's findings,[15] the IDSA panel members had important conflicts:

> "The IDSA's 2006 Lyme disease guideline panel undercut its credibility by allowing individuals with financial interests—in drug companies, Lyme disease diagnostic tests, patents and consulting arrangements with insurance companies—to exclude divergent medical evidence and opinion."

The IDSA settlement establishes a model to redress these conflicts of interest and the consequent suppression of scientific evidence and patient treatment options.

The settlement requires the IDSA to reconvene a new Lyme treatment guidelines panel made up of conflict-free panellists under the auspices of an ethicist, to hold a public hearing and to review all recommendations of the guidelines. Panellists from the original guidelines panel are precluded from sitting on this new panel. The Attorney General's press release concerning the settlement highlights important findings of impropriety on the part of IDSA and forces the organisation to re-examine its guidelines in a public forum (aired live over the Internet) using an open scientific hearing that will consider evidence from a broad spectrum of science. All panelists will be screened for potential conflicts of interest by Dr Howard Brody, a medical ethicist specialising in such conflicts.

SETTLEMENT PROCESS PHASES

While no overall timetable is specified, it seems likely that the settlement process will take 6–12 months. The settlement has three phases:

- the selection of the chair and the panel;
- the internal collection of scientific evidence and call for submissions of scientific evidence from the public;
- the public hearing of the evidence, which will be aired live on the Internet.

The settlement stipulates that IDSA must set up a panel of 8–12 members (including the chair) "who, as a group, reflect a balanced variety of perspectives and experience across a broad range of relevant disciplines, ranging from clinical experience in treating patients with Lyme disease to experience in investigating the best methods to diagnose and treat Lyme disease or other infectious diseases" to review the recommendations in its guidelines.[15]

Selection of the chair

The chair of the panel is critically important because this person and the IDSA Standards and Practice Guidelines Committee will select the panel members from the pool of applicants. The chair will be selected in an open process—meaning any qualified individual can apply—by the IDSA Standards and Practice Guidelines Committee. The IDSA will post an announcement on its website encouraging qualified doctors or researchers to apply. Those who apply for the chair may also be considered for panel member positions. In addition to the requirements to be on the panel, the chair must:

- be trained in infectious disease;
- not have published a point of view on Lyme disease;
- be knowledgeable on Lyme disease but not necessarily an expert;
- have experience in the review and interpretation of the medical scientific literature;
- have known abilities to:
  - complete a task in a timely manner;
  - consider varying points of view;
  - bring groups of individuals to consensus.

Selection of the panel

The panel will be selected by the chair and the Standards and Practice Guidelines Committee. This too will be through an open process with IDSA posting an announcement on its website soliciting applicants. IDSA is required to give "fair consideration to all reasonable applicants". A prospective panel member cannot have previously served on a Lyme guidelines panel, must be free of conflicts of interest, must be a doctor or a researcher, and need not be a member of the IDSA. All panellists will be screened for potential conflicts of interest by Dr Brody, the independent medical ethicist. The panel members selected must as a group[15]:

> "reflect a balanced variety of perspectives and experience across a broad range of relevant disciplines, ranging from clinical experience in treating patients with Lyme disease to experience in investigating the best methods to diagnose and treat Lyme disease or other infectious diseases."

Evidence selection

The settlement agreement provides for an internal collection of evidence by the IDSA staff and provides a 60-day window for people who are not on the panel to submit scientific studies for review by the panel. The IDSA must post an announcement calling for submissions of evidence by individuals and organisations. The evidence submitted must be distributed to and considered by the guidelines panel.

Public presentations and hearing

Following the collection and review of scientific evidence, those who want to present evidence to the panel are invited to apply. Any stakeholder may apply to make a presentation, although preference will be given to researchers and doctors. The panel will work with the medical ethicist and the Connecticut Attorney General's office to finalise the list of presenters and must reserve time for divergent opinions. Presenters must disclose conflicts of interest, but the conflicts will not preclude the presenter from participating. Once the presenters have been selected, there will be a public hearing of the presentations that will be aired live over the Internet. The presenters will identify specific recommendations of the IDSA guidelines that they take issue with and will present the scientific evidence opposing the recommendation.

Panel determinations

The panel will make a determination whether each recommendation contested "is medically sound in light of all of the evidence and information provided".[15] Each determination will require a 75% supermajority vote of the panel members (9/12, if the panel comprises 12 members). So, if the recommendation that a tick bite not be treated is contested, for example, a supermajority of the panel would need to vote in favour of the original recommendation for it to stand. Once each of the contested recommendations has been reviewed, the panel will determine whether the guidelines need to be revised in whole, in part, or not at all. If the guidelines need to be revised, then the new treatment recommendations will also be subject to the 75% voting requirement. The notion here is that a "consensus" of the panel is 75%, and all determinations require a consensus.

THE ATTORNEY GENERAL INTENDS TO ENFORCE THE TERMS OF THE SETTLEMENT AGREEMENT

A number of comments by the IDSA president, Dr Donald Poretz, imply that the IDSA views its obligations under the Connecticut Attorney General's settlement agreement as being a process of merely "going through the motions" and that the guidelines will remain unchanged.[17] This type of dismissive attitude by the IDSA is shocking to patients. The Attorney General found important conflicts of interest for guidelines panel members, bias in the selection of participants, suppression of scientific evidence, blocking of divergent viewpoints and foreclosure of treatment options for patients. These are the types of findings that a responsible medical society would take seriously by launching an internal investigation into the guidelines panel. Restrictive guidelines constrain doctors from using clinical judgement and prevent them from using more effective treatments and individualised care. The notion of "going through the motions" on an issue of such enormous social, economic and medical importance is morally wrong. Moreover, it is likely to backfire politically. Attorney General Blumenthal has demonstrated that he is a man of courage, resolve and persistence—a man who intends to enforce the terms of the settlement agreement and expects the IDSA to comply with its terms.

Acknowledgements: The authors thank R Wolfram, K Newby, M Perez-Lizano and B Blossom for helpful discussion.

Competing interests: RBS serves without compensation on the medical advisory panel for QMedRx Inc. He has no financial ties to the company.

Provenance and peer review: Not commissioned; externally peer reviewed.

REFERENCES

1. **Johnson LB,** Stricker RB. Treatment of Lyme disease—a medicolegal assessment. *Expert Rev Anti-infect Ther* 2004;**2**:533–57.
2. **Stolberg S.** Study says clinical guides often hide ties of doctors. *New York Times*. 6 Feb 2002; National Desk. www.nytimes.com/2002/02/06/health/06DRUG.html (accessed 9 Mar 2009).
3. **Integrity in Science**. Integrity in Science Watch Week of 03/10/2008. IOM urged to recommend conflict-free zone for medicine. www.cspinet.org/integrity/watch/200803101.html (accessed 9 Mar 2009).
4. **Stricker RB.** Lymerix® risks revisited. *Microbe* 2008;**3**:1–2.
5. **Wormser GP,** Dattwyler RJ, Shapiro ED, *et al*. The clinical assessment, treatment, and prevention of Lyme disease, human granulocytic anaplasmosis, and babesiosis: Clinical Practice Guidelines by the Infectious Diseases Society of America. *Clin Infect Dis* 2006;**43**:1089–134. (See appendix A for details of competing interests.)
6. **Feder HM,** Johnson BJB, O'Connell S, *et al*, the Ad Hoc International Lyme Disease Group. A critical appraisal of "chronic Lyme disease". *N Engl J Med* 2007;**357**:1422–

Clinical ethics

30. Erratum in: *N Engl J Med* 2008;**358**:1084. (See appendix A for details of competing interests.)
7. **Porwancher RB,** Bockenstedt L, Dattwyler R, *et al*. Lyme Wars: Critique misses mark. *BMJ* rapid response 30 Nov 2007. www.bmj.com/cgi/eletters/335/7628/1008 (accessed 9 Mar 2009). (See appendix A for details of competing interests.)
8. **Center for Biotechnology**. Companies developed. Brook Biotechnologies. http://www.biotech.sunysb.edu/industDev/comp-dev.html (accessed 9 Mar 2009). (See appendix A for details of competing interests.)
9. **Halperin JJ,** Shapiro ED, Logigian E, *et al*. Practice parameter: treatment of nervous system Lyme disease (an evidence-based review): Report of the Quality Standards Subcommittee of the American Academy of Neurology, *Neurology* 2007;**69**:91–102. (See appendix A for details of competing interests.)
10. **Abbott A.** Uphill struggle. *Nature* 2006;**439**:524–5. (See appendix A for details of competing interests).
11. **Saul S.** Unease on industry's role in hypertension debate. *New York Times*. 20 May 2006. www.nytimes.com/2006/05/20/business/20hyper.html?ex=1148788800&en=c743a665286103ef&ei=5070&emc=eta1 (accessed 9 Mar 2009).
12. **Ferrette C.** Lyme disease expert defends research. *Journal News*. 6 May 2008. http://m.lohud.com/news.jsp?key=76504 (accessed 14 Mar 2009).
13. **Eddy DM.** Three battles to watch in the 1990s. *JAMA* 1993;**270**:520–6.
14. **Eddy DM.** Clinical decision making: from theory to practice, practice policies—what are they? *JAMA* 2000;**263**:877–8.
15. **Connecticut Attorney General's Office**. Attorney General's investigation reveals flawed Lyme disease guideline process, IDSA agrees to reassess guidelines, install independent arbiter. 1 May 2008. http://www.ct.gov/ag/cwp/view.asp?a=2795&q=414284 (accessed 9 Mar 2009).
16. **Stricker RB,** Johnson LB. Practice parameter: treatment of nervous system Lyme disease (an evidence-based review). *Neurology* 2008;**70**:1719.
17. **Landers SJ.** Lyme treatment accord ends antitrust probe. *American Medical News* 9 June 2008. http://www.ama-assn.org/amednews/2008/06/09/hlsa0609.htm (accessed 9 Mar 2009).

APPENDIX A

Conflicts of interests reported in references 5–10
Reference 5: IDSA Guidelines 2006. Potential conflicts of interest.

- G.P.W. has received consulting fees from Baxter and research support from Immunetics, and he is a founder of Diaspex, a company that does not offer products or services.
- R.J.D. has served as a speaker for Pfizer and is part owner of Biopeptides, a biotech company that develops vaccines and laboratory diagnostics, including products for Borrelia burgdorferi.
- J.J.H. has served as an expert witness on behalf of Lymerix (GlaxoSmithKline).
- A.C.S. has received consulting fees from Baxter.

Reference 6: Feder *et al, N Engl J Med* 2007

- Dr. Shapiro reports serving as an expert witness in medical-malpractice cases related to Lyme disease, reviewing claims of disability related to Lyme disease for Metropolitan Life Insurance Company, and receiving speaker's fees from Merck and Sanofi-Aventis.
- Dr. Steere reports receiving a research grant from Viramed and fees from Novartis.
- Dr. Wormser reports receiving research grants related to Lyme disease from Immunetics, Bio-Rad, and Biopeptides and education grants from Merck and AstraZeneca to New York Medical College for visiting lecturers for infectious-disease grand rounds, being part owner of Diaspex (a company that is now inactive with no products or services), owning equity in Abbott, serving as an expert witness in a medical-malpractice case, and being retained in other medical-malpractice cases involving Lyme disease. He may become a consultant to Biopeptides.

Reference 7: Porwancher *et al, BMJ* 2007

- Dr. Raymond Dattwyler reports that he is the principal owner of Biopeptides Corporation. He has a United States provisional patent 60/812,595 on a live "bacterial vaccine," an oral vaccine platform technology; PCT/US2005/023106 "oral vaccine for Borrelia," a wildlife vaccine; United States provisional patent 60/799,016, "Peptide Diagnostic Agent for Lyme." He has served as an expert witness in medical malpractice cases involving Lyme disease.
- Dr. John Halperin reports having served as an expert witness in malpractice cases involving Lyme disease. He was an expert witness for GlaxoSmithKline which made LYMErix.
- Dr. Robert B. Nadelman reports that he has been retained as an expert witness in medical malpractice cases related to Lyme disease.
- Dr. Eugene Shapiro reports having served as an expert witness in medical malpractice cases related to Lyme disease. He has reviewed claims of disability related to Lyme disease for Metropolitan Life Insurance Company.
- Dr. Gary P. Wormser reports that he has had research grants from Immunetics, Inc., BioRad, and may receive one from Biopeptides' He reports educational grants to NYMC to support ID grand rounds from Merck and AstraZeneca, and possibly Pfizer in the future. He has equity in Abbott and has been an expert witness in malpractice cases involving Lyme disease.

Reference 8

Brook Biotechnologies was created in 1994 to develop and commercialize the first FDA-approved diagnostic test kit for Lyme Disease. Brook Biotechnologies has recently ceased operations and the technology has been licensed to Baxter Diagnostics.

Reference 9: Halperin *et al, Neurology* 2007

- Dr. Halperin holds equity in Abbott, Bristol Myers Squibb, Johnson & Johnson, Schering Plough, and Vasogen. He has served as an expert witness in medical malpractice actions.
- Dr. Shapiro has received funds for reviewing disability claims from Metropolitan Life Insurance Company and has served as an expert witness in malpractice actions. He has also received honoraria from Merck, Inc. and Aventis for speaking engagements. Dr. Shapiro receives funding from NIH grants K24RR022477, KL2RR024138, and UL1RR024139.
- Dr. Wormser reports having received research grants related to Lyme disease from the Centers for Disease Control and Prevention, the National Institutes of Health, Immunetics, Inc., and BioRad. He was part owner of Diaspex, LLC, a company with no products or services. He has been an expert witness for the United States in a medical malpractice case and has been retained in other medical practice cases involving Lyme disease. Dr. Wormser has overseen educational grants to New York Medical College to support Infectious Diseases grand rounds from Merck and AstraZeneca, and one from Pfizer is expected in 2008.

Reference 10: Abbott, *Nature* 2006

- Steere, who has worked as a consultant for Baxter vaccines, says "There is no proof that autoimmunity ever developed in anyone, but it could be a very rare side effect."

CT Attorney General

Connecticut Attorney General's Office

Press Release

Attorney General's Investigation Reveals Flawed Lyme Disease Guideline Process, IDSA Agrees To Reassess Guidelines, Install Independent Arbiter

May 1, 2008

Attorney General Richard Blumenthal today announced that his antitrust investigation has uncovered serious flaws in the Infectious Diseases Society of America's (IDSA) process for writing its 2006 Lyme disease guidelines and the IDSA has agreed to reassess them with the assistance of an outside arbiter.

The IDSA guidelines have sweeping and significant impacts on Lyme disease medical care. They are commonly applied by insurance companies in restricting coverage for long-term antibiotic treatment or other medical care and also strongly influence physician treatment decisions.

Insurance companies have denied coverage for long-term antibiotic treatment relying on these guidelines as justification. The guidelines are also widely cited for conclusions that chronic Lyme disease is nonexistent.

"This agreement vindicates my investigation -- finding undisclosed financial interests and forcing a reassessment of IDSA guidelines," Blumenthal said. "My office uncovered undisclosed financial interests held by several of the most powerful IDSA panelists. The IDSA's guideline panel improperly ignored or minimized consideration of alternative medical opinion and evidence regarding chronic Lyme disease, potentially raising serious questions about whether the recommendations reflected all relevant science.

"The IDSA's Lyme guideline process lacked important procedural safeguards requiring complete reevaluation of the 2006 Lyme disease guidelines -- in effect a comprehensive reassessment through a new panel. The new panel will accept and analyze all evidence, including divergent opinion. An independent neutral ombudsman -- expert in medical ethics and conflicts of interest, selected by both the IDSA and my office -- will assess the new panel for conflicts of interests and ensure its integrity."

Blumenthal's findings include the following:

- The IDSA failed to conduct a conflicts of interest review for any of the panelists prior to their appointment to the 2006 Lyme disease guideline panel;
- Subsequent disclosures demonstrate that several of the 2006 Lyme disease panelists had conflicts of interest;
- The IDSA failed to follow its own procedures for appointing the 2006 panel chairman and members, enabling the chairman, who held a bias regarding the existence of chronic Lyme, to handpick a likeminded panel without scrutiny by or formal approval of the IDSA's oversight committee;
- The IDSA's 2000 and 2006 Lyme disease panels refused to accept or meaningfully consider information regarding the existence of chronic Lyme disease, once removing a panelist from the 2000 panel who dissented from the group's position on chronic Lyme

disease to achieve "consensus";

- The IDSA blocked appointment of scientists and physicians with divergent views on chronic Lyme who sought to serve on the 2006 guidelines panel by informing them that the panel was fully staffed, even though it was later expanded;
- The IDSA portrayed another medical association's Lyme disease guidelines as corroborating its own when it knew that the two panels shared several authors, including the chairmen of both groups, and were working on guidelines at the same time. In allowing its panelists to serve on both groups at the same time, IDSA violated its own conflicts of interest policy.

IDSA has reached an agreement with Blumenthal's office calling for creation of a review panel to thoroughly scrutinize the 2006 Lyme disease guidelines and update or revise them if necessary. The panel -- comprised of individuals without conflicts of interest -- will comprehensively review medical and scientific evidence and hold a scientific hearing to provide a forum for additional evidence. It will then determine whether each recommendation in the 2006 Lyme disease guidelines is justified by the evidence or needs revision or updating.

Blumenthal added, "The IDSA's 2006 Lyme disease guideline panel undercut its credibility by allowing individuals with financial interests -- in drug companies, Lyme disease diagnostic tests, patents and consulting arrangements with insurance companies -- to exclude divergent medical evidence and opinion. In today's healthcare system, clinical practice guidelines have tremendous influence on the marketing of medical services and products, insurance reimbursements and treatment decisions. As a result, medical societies that publish such guidelines have a legal and moral duty to use exacting safeguards and scientific standards.

"Our investigation was always about the IDSA's guidelines process -- not the science. IDSA should be recognized for its cooperation and agreement to address the serious concerns raised by my office. Our agreement with IDSA ensures that a new, conflicts-free panel will collect and review all pertinent information, reassess each recommendation and make necessary changes.

"This Action Plan -- incorporating a conflicts screen by an independent neutral expert and a public hearing to receive additional evidence -- can serve as a model for all medical organizations and societies that publish medical guidelines. This review should strengthen the public's confidence in such critical standards."

THE GUIDELINE REVIEW PROCESS

Under its agreement with the Attorney General's Office, the IDSA will create a review panel of eight to 12 members, none of whom served on the 2006 IDSA guideline panel. The IDSA must conduct an open application process and consider all applicants.

The agreement calls for the ombudsman selected by Blumenthal's office and the IDSA to ensure that the review panel and its chairperson are free of conflicts of interest.

Blumenthal and IDSA agreed to appoint Dr. Howard A. Brody as the ombudsman. Dr. Brody is a recognized expert and author on medical ethics and conflicts of interest and the director of the Institute for Medical Humanities at the University of Texas Medical Branch. Brody authored the book, "Hooked: Ethics, the Medical Profession and the Pharmaceutical Industry."

To assure that the review panel obtains divergent information, the panel will conduct an open scientific hearing at which it will hear scientific and medical presentations from interested parties. The agreement requires the hearing to be broadcast live to the public on the Internet via the IDSA's website. The Attorney General's Office, Dr. Brody and the review panel will together finalize the list of presenters at the hearing.

Once it has collected information from its review and open hearing, the panel will assess the information and determine whether the data and evidence supports each of the recommendations in the 2006 Lyme disease guidelines.

The panel will then vote on each recommendation in the IDSA's 2006 Lyme disease guidelines on whether it is supported by the scientific evidence. At least 75 percent of panel members must vote to sustain each recommendation or it will be revised.

Once the panel has acted on each recommendation, it will have three options: make no changes, modify the guidelines in part or replace them entirely.

The panel's final report will be published on the IDSA's website.

ADDITIONAL FINDINGS OF BLUMENTHAL'S INVESTIGATION

IDSA convened panels in 2000 and 2006 to research and publish guidelines for the diagnosis and treatment of Lyme disease. Blumenthal's office found that the IDSA disregarded a 2000 panel member who argued that chronic and persistent Lyme disease exists. The 2000 panel pressured the panelist to conform to the group consensus and removed him as an author when he refused.

IDSA sought to portray a second set of Lyme disease guidelines issued by the American Academy of Neurology (AAN) as independently corroborating its findings. In fact, IDSA knew that the two panels shared key members, including the respective panel chairmen and were working on both sets of guidelines a the same time -- a violation of IDSA's conflicts of interest policy.

The resulting IDSA and AAN guidelines not only reached the same conclusions regarding the non-existence of chronic Lyme disease, their reasoning at times used strikingly similar language. Both entities, for example, dubbed symptoms persisting after treatment "Post-Lyme Syndrome" and defined it the same way.

When IDSA learned of the improper links between its panel and the AAN's panel, instead of enforcing its conflict of interest policy, it aggressively sought the AAN's endorsement to "strengthen" its guidelines' impact. The AAN panel -- particularly members who also served on the IDSA panel -- worked equally hard to win AAN's backing of IDSA's conclusions.

The two entities sought to portray each other's guidelines as separate and independent when the facts call into question that contention.

The IDSA subsequently cited AAN's supposed independent corroboration of its findings as part of its attempts to defeat federal legislation to create a Lyme disease advisory committee and state legislation supporting antibiotic therapy for chronic Lyme disease.

In a step that the British Medical Journal deemed "unusual," the IDSA included in its Lyme guidelines a statement calling them "voluntary" with "the ultimate determination of their application to be made by the physician in light of each patient's individual circumstances." In fact, United Healthcare, Health Net, Blue Cross of California, Kaiser Foundation Health Plan and other insurers have used the guidelines as justification to deny reimbursement for long-term antibiotic treatment.

Blumenthal thanked members his office who worked on the investigation -- Assistant Attorney General Thomas Ryan, former Assistant Attorney General Steven Rutstein and Paralegal Lorraine Measer under the direction of Assistant Attorney General Michael Cole, Chief of the Attorney General's Antitrust Department.

FRANK R. WOLF
10TH DISTRICT, VIRGINIA

COMMITTEE ON APPROPRIATIONS
SUBCOMMITTEES:
RANKING MEMBER—STATE-FOREIGN OPERATIONS
TRANSPORTATION-HUD

CO-CHAIR—CONGRESSIONAL HUMAN RIGHTS CAUCUS

Congress of the United States
House of Representatives

241 CANNON HOUSE OFFICE BUILDING
WASHINGTON, DC 20515–4610
(202) 225–5136

13873 PARK CENTER ROAD
SUITE 130
HERNDON, VA 20171
(703) 709–5800
(800) 945–9653 (IN STATE)

110 NORTH CAMERON STREET
WINCHESTER, VA 22601
(540) 667–0990
(800) 850–3463 (IN STATE)

wolf.house.gov

September 4, 2008

Mr. Daniel R. Levinson
Inspector General
U.S. Department of Health and Human Services
Room 5250 Cohen Building
3330 Independence Ave SW
Washington DC 20201

Dear Mr. Levinson:

I write today to inquire about the Center for Disease Control and Prevention's (CDC) recognition of Lyme disease treatment guidelines set forth by the Infectious Disease Society of America (IDSA). I have become concerned about the integrity of these standards. I understand other members of Congress have asked for an investigation into this matter and want to join that request.

Last month I held a Lyme Disease Forum in my congressional district and nearly 300 people took time out of their summer schedule to attend. Many in attendance suffer from Bell's palsy, meningitis and other manifestations of Lyme Disease. I have seen firsthand the devastation of this disease. Between 1999 and 2007, the number of reported cases of Lyme Disease in Loudoun County, Virginia, increased from 29 to over 200 cases per year.

I am aware that earlier this year Connecticut Attorney General Richard Blumenthal reported that his antitrust investigation exposed conflicts of interests in the process used by IDSA to write 2006 Lyme disease guidelines. Mr. Blumenthal's findings of undisclosed financial interests held by several of the IDSA panelists and the panel's exclusion of divergent scientific evidence and opinion were shocking. How do you explain this injustice to my constituents and others who suffer from chronic Lyme?

CDC continues to link to the IDSA guidelines. While CDC maintains that the IDSA has "given rigorous peer review of the IDSA guidelines," numerous congressional requests for an explanation of how peer review requirements are met remain unanswered. Furthermore, why is it that another set of guidelines complied by another medical society, which have been published on the National Guidelines Clearing House, are not listed or taken into account by the CDC?

I request that the OIG investigate whether the CDC is justified in only using the IDSA Lyme guidelines given the host of questionable practices exposed during the IDSA approval process. There needs to be a concerted effort to ensure that clinicians working with Lyme disease patients and their families have all the tools necessary to treat this devastating disease.

I am committed to doing whatever I can to help address this issue and look forward to your response.

Best wishes.

Sincerely,

Frank R. Wolf
Member of Congress

Thank You

FRW:jp

This is very important.

DEPARTMENT OF HEALTH & HUMAN SERVICES

Office of Inspector General

Washington, D.C. 20201

OCT 2 0 2008

The Honorable Frank R. Wolf
House of Representatives
Washington, DC 20515

Dear Mr. Wolf:

I am writing in response to your letter dated September 4, 2008, in which you requested that the Office of Inspector General (OIG) determine whether the Centers for Disease Control and Prevention is justified in only using the Infectious Disease Society of America's (IDSA) Lyme disease guidelines given the host of questionable practices exposed during the IDSA approval process. Our Office of Investigations is currently reviewing the allegations identified in your letter. OIG will stay in touch with your staff as we determine appropriate action.

We appreciate your interest in the programs of the Department. If you have any questions regarding this matter, your staff may call Claire Barnard, Director of External Affairs, at (202) 205-9523.

Sincerely,

Timothy J. Menke
Deputy Inspector General
for Investigations

FRANK R. WOLF
10TH DISTRICT, VIRGINIA

COMMITTEE ON APPROPRIATIONS

SUBCOMMITTEES:

RANKING MEMBER—COMMERCE-JUSTICE-SCIENCE

TRANSPORTATION-HUD

CO-CHAIR—TOM LANTOS HUMAN RIGHTS COMMISSION

Congress of the United States
House of Representatives

241 CANNON HOUSE OFFICE BUILDING
WASHINGTON, DC 20515–4610
(202) 225–5136

13873 PARK CENTER ROAD
SUITE 130
HERNDON, VA 20171
(703) 709–5800
(800) 945–9653 (IN STATE)

110 NORTH CAMERON STREET
WINCHESTER, VA 22601
(540) 667–0990
(800) 850–3463 (IN STATE)

wolf.house.gov

January 26, 2010

Helke Ferrie
KOS Publishing Inc.
1997 Beechgrove Rd, Caledon, Ontario, Canada L7K 0N3

Dear Helke:

Thank you for your recent letter sharing your kind comments about my work on Lyme disease awareness on behalf of my constituent's in Virginia's 10th Congressional District. I appreciate having the benefit of your comments and understand that Lyme disease is also a growing public health concern in Canada.

As you know, in September of 2008 I wrote to the inspector general of the Department of Health and Human Services with regard to the Centers for Disease Control and Prevention's recognition of Lyme disease treatment guidelines set forth by the Infectious Disease Society of America. Since that letter, a funding bill which included an increase in the Centers for Disease Control and Prevention's budget for Lyme disease was signed into law. The House Appropriations Committee (July 17, 2009) and the Senate Appropriations Committee (July 30, 2009) both approved identical report language accompanying this Lyme disease research funding increase that included references to "chronic Lyme." I believe this reference to chronic Lyme, the merits of which the IDSA disputes, is a positive step for those suffering from this devastating disease.

For additional information about my work on Lyme disease, including bipartisan legislation I have proposed with co-chairs of the House Lyme Disease Caucus, please visit my Web site at www.wolf.house.gov/LYME.

Best wishes.

Sincerely,

Frank R. Wolf
Member of Congress

FRW:jp
enclosures

FY 2010: Labor-HHS-Education
S.Rept. 111-66: 7/30/09

Antimicrobial Resistance.—The Committee remains concerned by the emergence of life-threatening antimicrobial resistant pathogens in hospital and community settings. The Committee is pleased that CDC has set up a surveillance network similar to a sentinel surveillance system and encourages CDC to continue making such systems easy to use and compatible with the emergence of health information technology.

Lyme Disease.—The Committee encourages the CDC to expand its activities related to developing sensitive and more accurate diagnostic tools and tests for Lyme disease including the timely evaluation of emerging diagnostic methods and improving utilization of diagnostic testing to account for the multiple clinical manifestations of acute and chronic Lyme disease; to expand its epidemiological research activities on tick-borne diseases [TBDs] to include an objective to determine the long-term course of illness for Lyme disease; to improve surveillance and reporting of Lyme and other TBDs in order to produce more accurate data on the prevalence of the Lyme and other TBDs; to evaluate the feasibility of developing a national reporting system on Lyme including laboratory reporting; and to expand prevention of Lyme and TBDs through increased community-based public education and creating a physician education program that includes the full spectrum of scientific research on the diseases.

Syringe Re-use.—The Committee remains concerned about the re-use of syringes and other infection control errors. The Committee is pleased that the CDC Healthcare Infection Control Practices Advisory Committee is at work developing additional infection control guidance specifically for outpatient settings and that the CDC is planning to convene meetings with academia and industry to explore the development of "fail safe" systems and products. In addition, the Committee continues to support the CDC's education and outreach campaign. The Committee requests that the CDC report to the Committee on the progress of those efforts by April 15, 2010.

HIV, Viral Hepatitis, STD, and TB Prevention

The Committee has included $1,028,680,000 for the activities at this Center in fiscal year 2010. The fiscal year 2009 level was $1,006,375,000 and the 2010 budget request was $1,060,299,000. The Committee has included funding for the following activities at the following amounts:

[In thousands of dollars]

Activity	Fiscal year 2009 comparable	Fiscal year 2010 budget	Committee recommendation
HIV/AIDS	691,861	744,914	711,045
Viral Hepatitis	18,316	18,367	18,367
Tuberculosis	143,870	144,268	144,268

Hepatitis Testing.—The Committee encourages the CDC to expand testing and continue to validate interventions focused on the mother-child transmission issue and other efforts targeted on the prevention of the hepatitis B virus in the Asian-American community where currently 1 in 10 individuals are infected with the hepatitis B virus.

FY 2010: Labor-HHS-Education
H.Rept. 111-220: 7/17/09

Budget activity	FY 2010 Committee	FY 2010 Committee compared to—	
		FY 2009	FY 2010 Budget request
Vector-borne Diseases, including West Nile Virus	$26,717,000	+$418,000	$0
Lyme Disease	8,938,000	+3,668,000	+3,668,000
Food Safety	26,942,000	+4,422,000	0
Prion Disease	5,474,000	+86,000	0
Chronic Fatigue Syndrome	4,825,000	+75,000	0

Food Safety.—The Committee supports CDC's increased investment in food safety. Improving foodborne outbreak detection and response remains a critical priority for CDC, as well as the Federal, State, and local food safety regulatory agencies. CDC's proposed enhancement of PulseNet and other surveillance tools and capacities will help ensure continuing improvement in this area. The Committee also believes that an equally important priority for CDC is to invest in generating the epidemiological data and conducting the analyses that regulatory agencies and the food industry need to target to implement effective prevention strategies. The Committee expects CDC to focus an increasing share of its management attention and resources on such prevention-related activities and to work closely with the Food and Drug Administration and other key parties to help prevent foodborne illness.

Lyme Disease.—The Committee encourages CDC to expand its activities related to developing sensitive and more accurate diagnostic tools and tests for Lyme disease, including the evaluation of emerging diagnostic methods and improving utilization of diagnostic testing to account for the multiple clinical manifestations of acute and chronic Lyme disease; to expand its epidemiological research activities on tick-borne diseases to include an objective to determine the long-term course of illness for Lyme disease; to improve surveillance and reporting of Lyme and other tick-borne diseases in order to produce more accurate data on their prevalence; to evaluate the feasibility of developing a national reporting system on Lyme disease, including laboratory reporting; and to expand prevention of Lyme and tick-borne diseases through increased community-based public education and creating a physician education program that includes the full spectrum of scientific research on the diseases.

Preparedness, Detection, and Control of Infectious Diseases

The Committee provides $173,791,000 for Preparedness, Detection, and Control of Infectious Diseases, which is $16,365,000 more than the fiscal year 2009 funding level and $5,050,000 more than the budget request. In addition, the Recovery Act provided an additional $40,000,000 in the Prevention and Wellness Fund for States to develop and implement healthcare-associated infection reduction plans in fiscal years 2009 and 2010.

The National Center for Preparedness, Detection, and Control of Infectious Diseases provides focus on preparedness and response capacity for new and complex infectious disease outbreaks, and manages and coordinates emerging infectious diseases, integrates laboratory groups, and facilitates increased quality and capacity in clinical laboratories. The Center serves as a focal point for engaging outside agencies and partners in quality laboratory systems and improved healthcare settings.

MY LYME DISEASE RESEARCH JOURNEY

2

By John D. Scott

"A pessimist sees the difficulty in every opportunity; an optimist sees the opportunity in every difficulty."

—*Sir Winston Churchill*

"If I have seen farther than others, it is because I was standing on the shoulders of giants."

—*Sir Isaac Newton*

In September 1986, I stepped off the edge of the world with a perplexing, energy-draining disease. My local family physician initially diagnosed me with "mono," but I had experienced mononucleosis before and had recovered. He then referred me to a local internist who touted the same diagnosis. After more than 2½ years of illness, I had to quit work. I went to another local physician who specialized in chronic fatigue syndrome (CFS), and he diagnosed me with CFS with which he was familiar. Next, I went to an infectious disease specialist in Toronto, who diagnosed post infectious neuromyasthenia, and suggested that I was malingering. Then, my local physician referred me to a psychiatrist who concluded that my symptoms were those of an infectious agent. Finally, my wife put a 10-cm slab of foam in the back of our minivan, and I crawled in, and she drove me for 2 days to Ottawa to see a physician who specialized in CFS. He screened me for a myriad of medical causes, and initially diagnosed me with CFS. After 2 months, however, the Lyme disease test that he ordered came back positive. My local physician treated me with 2 weeks of tetracycline but the slight recovery did not last. After consulting other physicians, I finally found Dr. P.T. Williams (now deceased) in Ajax, Ontario, a Lyme-literate clinician, who confirmed that I had a classic case of Lyme neuroborreliosis (Lyme disease). Notably, over the years, I have tested positive for Lyme disease at 3 accredited laboratories.

After 4 years and 12 different doctors, I was pleased to have a definitive diagnosis of Lyme disease. Now, I could get on with serious and appropriate treatment and, gradually, I improved with ongoing antibiotic therapy. After 2 years my brain cleared, and it no longer showed evidence of white matter lesions on an MRI scan. Also, my spaced-out sensations improved. I was delighted because I did not want to lose my mind. In all, because of the long delay in diagnosis and treatment, I have endured chronic, persistent Lyme disease for over 20 years.

When diagnosed with Lyme, I started to ask many questions about this tick-borne zoonosis, and I was told by the teaching staff at the University of Guelph, as well as other medical professionals, that the only way I could contract Lyme disease was by visiting Long Point on the north shore of Lake Erie. They stated too that I had to have a bull's-eye rash, *erythema mygrans*. Frankly, I was baffled about the epidemiology of Lyme disease in Canada.

When I explained the dilemma about where I had contracted Lyme disease to Dr. Williams, he suggested that I get control of the ticks in Ontario. He encouraged me and my wife to start a support group for Lyme disease patients and caregivers. We launched the Lyme-Borreliosis Support Group on Ontario, now called the Lyme Disease Association of Ontario. We had the first meeting in October 1990, and for 17 years between 1990 and 2007, we held four meetings per year for patients and their families, and published a newsletter, *Lyme Alert*, 4 times a year. The group is ongoing today. As well, over the years, we talked to patients by phone, and did Lyme disease advocacy, and provided up-to-date information to anyone who requested it. We got hundreds of phone calls, which came from all over North America. Although medical peers labeled Dr. Williams a "renegade" and a "Lyme guru," he was a colourful man, and profoundly knowledgeable about internal medicine and ectoparasites as well as Lyme disease and associated tick-borne pathogens. We were grateful for his advice with the support group and his encouragement and interest in our tick research.

Since I have a science background and a dissecting microscope, I decided to do a tick study, and obtain ticks from veterinarians across Ontario. Initially, I tried to get the Public Health Branch (Ontario government), Health Canada (federal government), and the University of Guelph to help with research studies, but unfortunately I was turned down by all 3 institutions. One Health Canada microbiologist said he did not know what he would do if the deer ticks crossed the U.S.-Canada border. I told him that they were already here. In despair, I contacted Ms. Diane Kindree, West Vancouver, past President of the Vancouver, B.C. Lyme Borreliosis

Society, and she helped greatly by introducing me to Dr. Satyen N. Banerjee (now deceased), British Columbia Centre for Disease Control, Vancouver, B.C. Fortunately, he was willing to help by testing our ticks. What a breakthrough!

In May 1993, my wife and I met with our local federal member of parliament (M.P.) and a high-ranking government official in Ottawa, who insisted that one had to go to Long Point to get Lyme disease. However, my M.P. suggested that we apply for a National Research and Development Program (NHRDP) grant. We decided to apply, and got the guidelines and the protocol for the application forms. Drs. Satyen and Maya Banerjee helped us with the details. Our motto was: "Truth crushed to the ground will rise again."

Over the course of 3 years, we applied to 12 different grant sources for Lyme disease research funding including the federal government's NHRDP grant, corporate businesses, foundations, and institutional organizations. However, in all 12 applications we were turned down. In fact, one NHRDP rejection letter stated, "your proposal falls outside our terms of reference." Since I had worked for 3 months on this grant proposal with the profound fatigue of Chronic Lyme disease, I was furious! I decided there was no foreseeable way to cut through the stubbornness and backwardness of Canadian government officials and their research partners. We had to find another route to raise research money. Ironically, after 12 years, federal researchers called me in 2005, and wanted our blacklegged tick data. The nerve of this request was astounding. After much negotiation, we signed a contract, and sold part of our tick information. Of course, this money helped our support group to fund some of our research. Another federal researcher told me that, when he was hired, his job was to "put out fires." In other words, his mandate was to squelch anything that countered the federal government's Lyme disease philosophy. It became clearly evident that not only did we have to go out of the province for scientific expertise, we also had to go out of the country.

On May 13, 1991, I went out to a local farmer's meadow, and flagged for ticks, and got one tick. I was encouraged to continue searching for the natural vectors of Lyme disease spirochetes in Canada.

In 1993, we embarked on a 10-year, tick-host study during which we obtained ticks from veterinarians across Ontario. As the project progressed, I received up to 8 packages of ticks per day in the mail. Using taxonomic guides and scientific books, I identified these ticks, and sent their identification back to the veterinarians. In total, I spent over 10,000 hours working on this massive, decade-long tick project. In October 1994, we obtained the first live culture of *Borrelia burgdorferi,* the bacterium that causes Lyme disease, and confirmed its positivity using PCR testing; these motile spirochetes (helical-shaped) were cultured from a blacklegged tick, *Ixodes scapularis*, commonly called the deer tick. This engorged female was attached to a dog from Kenora, Ontario that had no history of travel. We were delighted to make this important discovery! Eventually, we got *B. burgdorferi*-infected adults (males, females) of *I. scapularis* from across Ontario including major urban centers; namely, Toronto, Hamilton, Windsor, Kingston, Ottawa, and Thunder Bay. This research was published in a 2006 issue of the *Journal of Medical Entomology*.

Now that we had observed this random distribution of *I. scapularis* ticks in Ontario, we wondered how they were covertly deposited in these scattered tick-friendly locations. We searched the scientific literature, and found that Drs. John F. Anderson and Louis Magnarelli of the Connecticut Agricultural Experiment Station, in New Haven, Connecticut had pioneered the initial studies of ticks on songbirds in North America during the early 1980s. These tick researchers mentioned that songbirds can disperse Lyme disease vector ticks over a long distance, and potentially start a new established population. From this research, we started our own research project whereby we got ticks from bird banders in eastern and central Canada.

In 1999, Dr. S. N. Banerjee and his staff cultured the first *B. burgdorferi* from an engorged *I. scapularis* nymph, which was collected from a Common Yellowthroat by bird banders in May 1999 on Bon Portage Island located off the south coast of Nova Scotia.

As our studies progressed, we received ticks from songbirds nationwide, which we had not previously encountered, and Dr. Lance A. Durden at Georgia Southern University, which houses the U.S. National Tick Collection, helped us with the identification. Some of these ticks were imported into Canada by neotropical passerines from South America, a distance of at least 5000 km. Over the past 12 years, Dr. Durden has helped us enormously to identify unusual tick species. Dr. Durden and I have found 18 different species of ticks (2 formally undescribed in the scientific literature) on songbirds in Canada. With the laboratory assistance of another U.S. researcher, we have been able to find 6 species of bird-feeding ticks harbouring the Lyme disease spirochetes. Using DNA sequence analysis, we have also found different strains of this bacterium in various locations. I was very pleased to have coordinated this bird-tick-pathogen research.

Thus, with the resilience and cooperation of these bird-tick-*Borrelia* researchers, we have unfolded the mystery of the wide dispersal of Lyme disease vector ticks countrywide. People and domestic animals do not have to go to an endemic area to contract Lyme disease. In fact, the 2007 Annual Report of the Ministry of Health and Long-Term Care states that 85% of patients, who acquired Lyme disease locally in Ontario between 2002 and 2006, had not been to an endemic area. Since 1995, we have published our research in 12 peer-reviewed articles in different scientific journals: *Journal of Vector Ecology*, *Journal of Parasitology*, *Journal of Medical Entomology*, *Canadian Medical Association Journal*, as well as the *North American Bird Bander*.

During our tick studies, we observed several tick patterns forming, especially along main songbird migration routes. Although the nymph of the blacklegged tick is reported as the principal vector of Lyme disease in the U.S., we did not obtain any *I. scapularis* nymphs from a dog, cat, horse, or person during our 10-year tick-host study from 1993 to 2002. Even though blacklegged tick females and males are larger and easier to see, no nymphs were submitted by the public and veterinarians. Coincidently, the infection rate of bird-associated, *I. scapularis* nymphs closely correlates with the infection rate of *I. scapularis* adults (males, females) on domestic animals and people. In essence, when fully engorged bird-feeding nymphs drop from songbirds, they molt to *I. scapularis* adults, which later attach to mammalian hosts (i.e., deer, dogs, cats, horses, and humans).

Therefore, songbirds are nature's way of dispersing Lyme disease vector ticks over a wide range in Canada. Blacklegged tick nymphs that are dispersed by songbirds during northward spring migration are ready to quest as adults for hosts in the fall. If these ticks do not find suitable hosts, they overwinter, and are ready for host-seeking activities in the spring. Any time that the ambient temperature is above freezing, and there is no snow cover, *I. scapularis* ticks can acquire *B. burgdorferi* from an infected host (i.e., mouse, shrew, chipmunk, songbird), and these blood-feeding ticks are infected for life. Obviously, ground-foraging songbirds play a major role in the natural enzootic cycle of *B. burgdorferi*, and the long- and short-range dispersal of Lyme disease vector ticks across Canada.

Epidemiologically, heavily tick-infested songbirds have the potential to start a new population of Lyme disease vector ticks in a new locale. Unquestionably, spring and fall migrating birds can transport larval and nymphal *Ixodes* species ticks well beyond the expected range. Of note, federal researchers estimated that spring migratory songbirds disperse between 50 million and 175 million immature blacklegged ticks Canada-wide annually. This is a lot of ticks! Our research clearly provides evidence that people can contract Lyme disease anywhere that an infected tick is dropped by a songbird. Any member of the medical profession who states that one has to go to Long Point to contract Lyme disease is at least 27 years out of date.

Since 1995, we have studied several populations of blacklegged ticks along the north shore of Lake Erie. These breeding colonies include Point Pelee National Park, Rondeau Provincial Park, Long Point (2 sites), and Turkey Point (2 sites including Turkey Point Provincial Park). Other Ontario-based populations of ticks are present at Wainfleet Bog, Presqu'ile Provincial Park, Prince Edward Point National Area, the St. Lawrence Island National Park area (at least 3 sites), and Charleston Lake Provincial Park. Different levels of *B. burgdorferi* infection have been detected at each of the above tick habitats; this infection rate will vary not only in the life stages of the tick, but it will also vary from year to year. Currently, we are aware of at least 23 established populations of blacklegged ticks from southeastern Manitoba to Nova Scotia.

Considering all the Lyme disease research that we have conducted, we are deeply troubled that the College of Physicians and Surgeons of Ontario (CPSO) are investigating Lyme-literate physicians in this province because they are treating their Lyme disease patients with long-term antibiotics. Currently, there is a tsunami of information on the persistence of the Lyme disease bacteria in the human body. This bacterium has many different morphological forms, such as spirochetes (spiral-shape), blebs (buds), granules (ultra-microscopic grains), and cysts (dormant, spore-shaped, no cell wall). These multiple forms undoubtedly add to the complexity of treating this stealth microorganism. As well, they sequester and hide in the brain, bone, eye, ligament and heart. When Chronic Lyme disease patients have treatment failures with short-term antibiotics, long-term antimicrobials as well as other remedial modalities, are a fact of life. The harassment of Lyme-literate physicians by CPSO is a travesty of justice, and a violation of human rights. Sadly, CPSO seems to have ignored our research and the wide distribution of Lyme disease-infected ticks across Canada.

Recent articles indicate that climate change is having a distinct effect on the northward spread of native ticks in Canada. This hypothesis is pure speculation because these studies are "inconclusive." This author analyzed the historical weather data for Winnipeg over the past 70 years, and found that the mean annual temperature has only increased by less than 0.5 degrees Celsius. In nature, ticks go down into the cool, moist leaf litter and topsoil humus to rehydrate during hot summer days. In the winter, blacklegged ticks, which have antifreeze-like compounds in their bodies, stay cozy under an insulating blanket of snow. Furthermore, studies show that blacklegged ticks on the East Coast, and western blacklegged ticks, *Ixodes pacificus*, on the West Coast can even withstand forest fires. Established populations of these tick species endure charcoal-burning heat during forest fires, and fully reestablish themselves again within a year or two. Ticks are great survivors!

Thankfully, over the past 20 years, there have been many people who have greatly supported our advocacy and research work. In the early 1990s, several resource people, including Dr. P. T. Williams, helped to give us our initial boost. Diane Kindree, West Vancouver, B.C. provided much encouragement and also her father, the late Laverne Kindree, M.D. of Squamish, B.C., who was awarded the Order of Canada in 2009. Dr. Kindree provided medical advice and shared first-hand information about field collections and in-house microbiological studies. Dr. John F. Anderson, Connecticut Agricultural Experiment Station, New Haven, CT, helped us test ticks for spirochetes. Drs. Satyen and Maya Banerjee, B.C.C.D.C., Vancouver, B.C., were very helpful for several years in testing ticks and providing all kinds of microbiological technical assistance. As we have progressed with our bird-tick studies, Dr. Lance A. Durden, Georgia Southern University, Statesboro, Georgia greatly helped us to identify ticks; he also helped us with manuscript submissions for scientific articles. Dr. Jesús Lizarraga of Valencia, Spain, and our friend for the past 17 years, has helped to keep me abreast of the Lyme borreliosis research and developments in Europe. We are also indebted to bird banders, wildlife rehabilitators, veterinarians, and the public for submitting ticks for our research. We are also grateful for numerous support group members who helped with tick studies and related group activities.

Our lifetime friends, John and Laura Taylor, Drumbo, Ontario, have always provided encouragement and support especially in the early years when we needed it the most. John and Laura always believed we were physically ill a belief not everyone in our life shared. They were the friends who walked in, when the rest of the world walked out! My wife, Catherine, has put up with a lot of in-house tick research, which likely should have been done in a Level 3 laboratory. Over the years, she has encouraged me to identify thousands of ticks, which we studied in our basement, and to keep going with the research when the going was tough for both of us. Her computer skills allowed us to keep constantly moving forward, and to communicate electronically with colleagues and the outside world. Due to limited physical energy, we have been very restricted with our social activities, which anyone with Lyme disease will understand.

Finally, we hope and believe that we have played a pivotal role as pioneers in the epidemiology and ecology of Lyme disease in Canada. We have shown that the Lyme disease vector ticks countrywide harbour many strains of the Lyme disease spirochete, and these ticks can parasitize and infect people and domestic animals. Also, our ongoing studies show that songbirds play a significant role in the dispersal of Lyme disease vector ticks to unexpected locations. Patients certainly do no have to go to an endemic area to contract Lyme disease.

John D. Scott
March 2010
Research Consultant, Lyme Disease Association of Ontario,
365 St. David St. South, Fergus, ON N1M 2L7

Research

Recherche

Research letter

Presence of spirochete causing Lyme disease, *Borrelia burgdorferi*, in the blacklegged tick, *Ixodes scapularis*, in southern Ontario

Satyendra N. Banerjee, Maya Banerjee, Keerthi Fernando, John D. Scott, Robert Mann, Muhammad G. Morshed

See related article page 1573

Lyme disease, the most common tick-borne disease in North America, is a multisystemic illness of humans and domestic animals caused by the spirochete *Borrelia burgdorferi sensu lato* ("in the broad sense").[1] Small mammals are the main reservoir hosts for this bacterium, and *Ixodes scapularis* (blacklegged tick; Fig. 1) and *Ixodes pacificus* (western blacklegged tick) found in British Columbia are the principal vectors in Canada.[2]

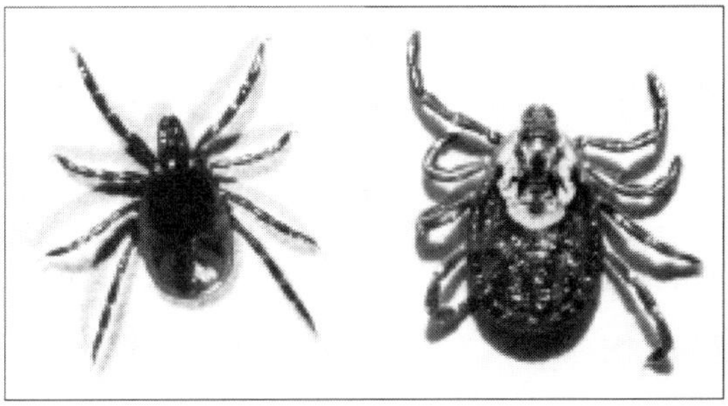

Fig. 1: Left: Blacklegged tick, *Ixodes scapularis,* unfed adult female. This tick is a competent vector for the spirochete causing Lyme disease, *Borrelia burgdorferi.* Total body length ranges from 2.0 to 3.5 mm; this specimen is 3.2 mm in length. Right: American dog tick, *Dermacentor variabilis,* unfed adult female. Total body length ranges from 3.0 to 5.0 mm; this specimen is 4.5 mm in length. This is the tick species most frequently submitted for identification in Ontario; it is not a competent vector for *B. burgdorferi.* Both ticks are found in southern Ontario.

As part of collaborative research between the Vector-borne Diseases Laboratory, BC Centre for Disease Control, and the Lyme Disease Association of Ontario, Ontario veterinarians submitted 139 *I. scapularis* ticks (collected from dogs in 1997 and 1998 in southern Ontario locations) to the laboratory to be tested for *B. burgdorferi.* For removal, a tick was held as close to the host's skin as possible with fine-pointed tweezers, and was removed from the skin with gentle but steady pressure. Each tick was stored in a small plastic vial with a moist paper towel for shipment to the laboratory for analysis.

The hosts of 121 (87%) of the ticks had no reported history of out-of-province travel. Two (1.6%) of these 121 ticks (1 from Mississauga and 1 from Etobicoke [part of Toronto]) produced motile spirochetes, which were subsequently identified as *B. burgdorferi* by monoclonal antibody and polymerase chain reaction tests (Table 1). In an additional 7 (5.8%) of the 121 ticks, *B. burgdorferi* was detected directly by polymerase chain reaction (Table 1). The first blood sample from host dogs was normally taken 4–6 weeks after tick removal. Subsequently, serum samples from all 9 dogs were tested by indirect immunofluorescence antibody assay and Western blot to identify specific antibodies against *B. burgdorferi*; such antibodies were observed in all samples. In a few cases the indirect immunofluorescence antibody titres were low (Table 1); however, all of the Western blots were reactive, with 5 or more bands needed for identification. Because most dogs with Lyme disease are asymptomatic, Western blot provides valuable diagnostic information about the presence of *B. burgdorferi* infection.

The wide distribution of *I. scapularis* ticks and the fact that some of them carry *B. burgdorferi* shows that the bacterium is present in southern Ontario. The fully engorged female ticks collected in Mississauga and Etobicoke not only produced live cultures of *B. burgdorferi*, but also laid eggs that hatched into larvae. The fact that these females had mated recently indicates that *I. scapularis* may be established in these locations, as well as at Long Point, Point Pelee National Park and Rondeau Provincial Park (on the north shore of Lake Erie), where the species is endemic. The Mississauga occurrence is the first report of a gravid *I. scapularis* female producing larvae in Ontario at a location other than Long Point. The other locations at which

Research letter

Table 1: Presence of *Borrelia burgdorferi* in engorged female *Ixodes scapularis* collected from dogs resident in southern Ontario with no history of out-of-province travel (1997 and 1998)

Collection site	Date of collection	Test results	IFA titre*	Comments
Mississauga	Apr. 24, 1997	PCR (c) positive Mab reactive	1:64	Antibiotic given same day tick was collected
Point Pelee	May 5, 1997	PCR positive	1:512	Antibiotic started 39 days after tick was collected
Ottawa	May 11, 1997	PCR positive	1:64	Antibiotic started 17 days after tick was collected
Bramalea	May 12, 1997	PCR positive	1:64	No antibiotic (dog had received Lyme vaccine 6 mo before tick was found)
Hamilton	May 13, 1997	PCR positive	1:256	Lyme vaccine given same day tick was collected
Scarborough	May 13, 1997	PCR positive	1:64	Antibiotic given after blood sample was drawn
Chatham	Apr. 9, 1998	PCR positive	1:128†	Antibiotic given after second blood sample was drawn
Etobicoke	Apr. 21, 1998	PCR(c) positive Mab reactive	1:256†	Antibiotic given after second blood sample was drawn
Westport	Nov. 1, 1998	PCR positive	1:256†	Antibiotic given after second blood sample was drawn

Note: PCR = polymerase chain reaction, (c) = live culture, Mab = monoclonal antibody test of live spirochete isolate, IFA = indirect fluorescence assay.
*All serum samples included in this table were tested by Western blot (MarDx Diagnostics, Inc., Carlsbad, Calif.) and were found to be reactive. A titre of 1:64 signifies a negative result, 1:128 an equivocal result and 1:256 a positive result.
†Two blood samples were tested by IFA, both with the same result.

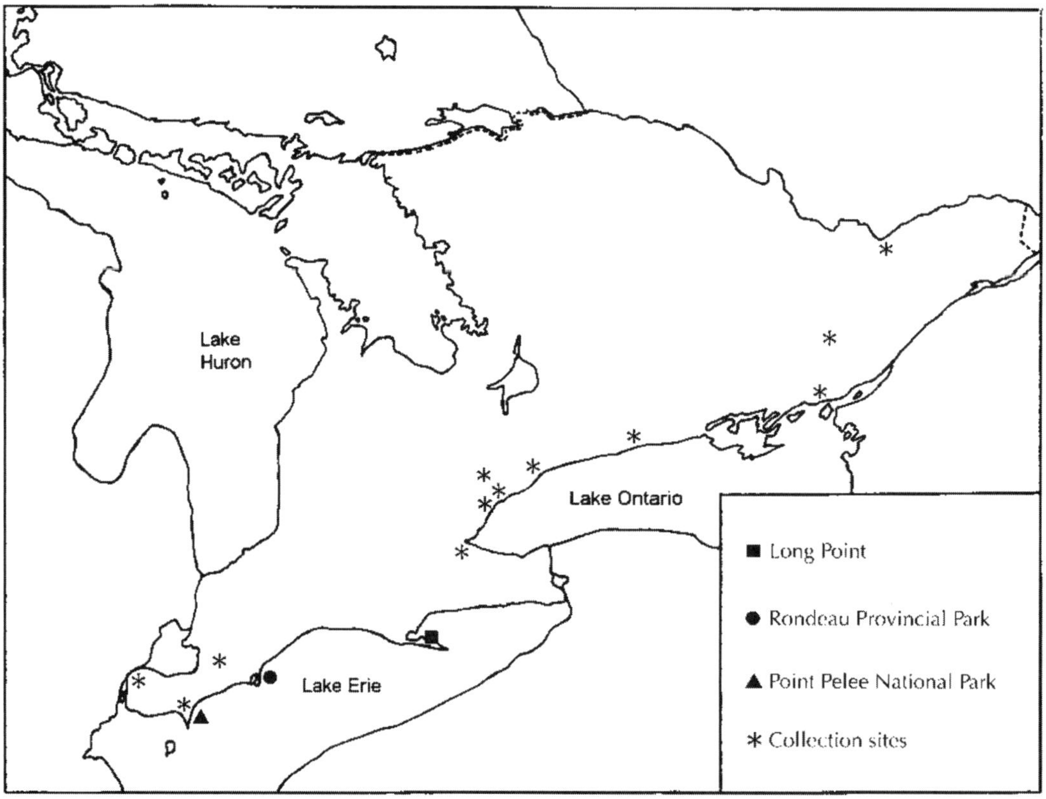

Fig. 2: Locations in southern Ontario (asterisks) where *Ixodes scapularis* ticks carrying *Borrelia burgdorferi* were collected, in 1997–1999, from dogs with no history of out-of-province travel. *Ixodes scapularis* ticks carrying *B. burgdorferi* are endemic at Long Point. At Rondeau Provincial Park *I. scapularis* ticks are established and *B. burgdorferi* is present.[3] *Ixodes scapularis* ticks are also established at Point Pelee National Park.

I. scapularis were positive for *B. burgdorferi* include Bramalea, Chatham, Hamilton, Ottawa, Point Pelee, Scarborough (part of Toronto) and Westport (Fig. 2).

On Apr. 28, 1997, a domestic cat from Aylmer, Que., was taken to an emergency veterinary clinic in nearby Ottawa where a fully engorged *I. scapularis* tick was removed; the tick later tested positive for *B. burgdorferi* (by polymerase chain reaction). Eight days before removal of the tick, the cat had been symptomatic (displaying anorexia and lethargy) and had been treated with antibiotics. This incident demonstrates that people and pets can bring *I. scapularis* ticks infected with *B. burgdorferi* into Ontario from bordering areas. Current evidence suggests that *I. scapularis* does not have an established population across southern Ontario. However, *I. scapularis* ticks are dropped haphazardly by birds during spring migration,[4] and in a recent study *B. burgdorferi* was isolated from an *I. scapularis* nymph retrieved from a common yellowthroat, *Geothlypis trichas*, in Nova Scotia during spring banding.[5]

A total of 280 cases of Lyme disease in humans were reported from 1981 to 1998 in Ontario. In 127 of these cases there was no history of out-of-province travel. In only 14 cases was there exposure at Long Point (Charles A. LeBer, Ontario Ministry of Health and Long-Term Care: personal communication, 1999). A recent study also reported co-infection by *B. burgdorferi* and *Babesia* spp. in a patient who had travelled to Nantucket, Mass.[6]

Across Canada, *B. burgdorferi* has been isolated in Prince Edward Island,[7] Nova Scotia,[5] New Brunswick, Quebec, Ontario,[8] Manitoba (unpublished data; isolate provided by Harvey Artsob, Laboratory Centre for Disease Control, Health Canada, Winnipeg, 1997), Alberta[9] and British Columbia.[10] Even though the risk of acquiring Lyme disease in Ontario is low, the possibility of *B. burgdorferi* infection should not be ignored.

The present study indicates that *I. scapularis* is widespread in southern Ontario and may act as a source of *B. burgdorferi* infection for humans, domestic animals and wildlife. Consequently, the medical community should be aware that people who frequent the outdoors may be exposed to *I. scapularis* ticks and are at risk of contracting Lyme disease.

Addendum

In 1999 isolates of *B. burgdorferi* were cultured in our laboratory from *I. scapularis* ticks collected in southern Ontario at Kingston, Cobourg and LaSalle. The ticks were removed on Oct. 25, Nov. 11, and Nov. 18 respectively, from dogs with no history of out-of-province travel.

We thank the veterinarians who submitted ticks and drew canine blood for serological testing. For designing the polymerase chain reaction (PCR) primers for this study, we thank Dr. Sean Byrne, British Columbia Centre for Disease Control. We also thank the Lyme Disease Association of Ontario for financial support and for providing information on the findings of *I. scapularis* in Ontario.

Dr. S.N. Banerjee, Mr. Fernando, Mr. Mann and Dr. Morshed are with the Vector-borne Diseases Laboratory, BC Centre for Disease Control, Vancouver, BC; Drs. S.N. Banerjee, M. Banerjee and M.G. Morshed are with the Department of Pathology and Laboratory Medicine, University of British Columbia, Vancouver, BC; and Mr. Scott is with the Lyme Disease Association of Ontario, Fergus, Ont.

This article has been peer reviewed.

Competing interests: None declared.

References

1. Dennis DT, Lance SE. Lyme borreliosis. In: Beran GW, editor. *Handbook of zoonoses. Section A: Bacterial, rickettsial, chlamydial and mycotic.* 2nd ed. Boca Raton (FL): CRC Press; 1994. p. 265-80.
2. Lane RS, Piesman J, Burgdorfer W. Lyme borreliosis: relation of its causative agent to its vectors and hosts in North America and Europe. *Ann Rev Entomol* 1991;36:587-609.
3. Morshed MG, Scott JD, Banerjee SN, Fernando K. Mann R, Isaac-Renton J. First isolation of Lyme disease spirochete, Borrelia Burgdorferi from black-legged tick, *Ixodes scapularis*, collected at Rondeau Provincial Park, Ontario. *Can Commun Dis Rep* 2000;26:42-4.
4. Klich M, Lankester MW, Wu KW. Spring migratory birds (Aves) extend the northern occurrence of blacklegged tick (Acari: Ixodidae). *J Med Entomol* 1996;33:581-5.
5. Morshed MG, Scott JD, Banerjee SN, Banerjee M, Fitzgerald T, Fernando K, et al. First isolation of Lyme disease spirochete, *Borrelia burgdorferi*, from blacklegged tick, *Ixodes scapularis*, removed from a bird in Nova Scotia, Canada. *Can Commun Dis Rep* 1999;25:153-5.
6. Dos Santos C, Kain K. Two tick-borne diseases in one: a case report of concurrent babesiosis and Lyme disease in Ontario. *CMAJ* 1999;160:1851-3. Available: www.cma.ca/cmaj/vol-160/issue-13/1851.htm
7. Artsob H, Garvie M, Cawthorn RJ, Horney B, Maloney R, Dick D, et al. Isolation of the Lyme disease spirochete, *Borrelia burgdorferi*, from *Ixodes dammini* (Acari: Ixodidae) collected on Prince Edward Island, Canada. *J Med Entomol* 1992;29:1063-6.
8. Banerjee S, Scott J, Lankester M, Kubinec J. Isolation of *Borrelia burgdorferi* — Thunder Bay District, Ontario. *Can Commun Dis Rep* 1996;22:138-40.
9. Banerjee SN, Banerjee M, Fernando K, Dong MY, Smith JA, Cook D. Isolation of *Borrelia burgdorferi*, the Lyme disease spirochete from rabbit ticks, *Haemaphysalis leporispalustris* from Alberta. *J Spirochetal Tick-borne Dis* 1995;2:23-4.
10. Banerjee S. Update on the status of Lyme borreliosis in British Columbia, Canada. *Clin Infect Dis* 1995;21:704.

Reprint requests to: *Dr. Muhammad G. Morshed, Department of Pathology and Laboratory Medicine, University of British Columbia, 655 W 12th Ave., Vancouver BC V5Z 4R4; fax 604 660-6073; mmorshed@interchange.ubc.ca*

Commentary

Lyme borreliosis in Ontario: determining the risks

Ian K. Barker, L. Robbin Lindsay

See related article page 1567

In this issue of *CMAJ* Satyendra Banerjee and colleagues highlight the possibility of exposure to Lyme borreliosis in Ontario.[1] What is the likelihood of encountering the blacklegged tick, *Ixodes scapularis*, the vector of Lyme borreliosis, in eastern Canada? Is this likelihood changing? And what are the implications?

Until recently, the only known Canadian population of *I. scapularis* was found at Long Point, on the north shore of Lake Erie.[2] However, many individual *I. scapularis* ticks have been found, on people and pets with no history of travel, throughout Saskatchewan, southern Manitoba, Ontario, Quebec and the Atlantic provinces.[3,4] Such ticks, found at sites where the species is not endemic, are "adventitious" (coming from without, accidental), having arrived as immature stages on birds migrating from tick-endemic areas to the south.[2,5,6]

Adventitious ticks may transmit *B. burgdorferi* if they have previously fed on an infected host.[6] Given that only 9 (6.5%) of the 139 adult ticks examined by Banerjee and colleagues carried *B. burgdorferi*, many probably originated in areas where few hosts were infected. However, in some localities up to about 20% of nymphs,[7] which seem most important in transmitting *B. burgdorferi* to people,[8] and more than 50% of adults[7] may be infected.

Despite their wide distribution, the density of adventitious ticks in the environment is very low; hence, indigenous Lyme borreliosis is uncommon in Ontario, accounting for 127 of 280 cases of the disease diagnosed in the province between 1981 and 1998 (Charles A. LeBer, Ontario Ministry of Health and Long-Term Care: personal communication, 1999). Passive surveillance underestimates incidence[9] but does permit comparisons of risk. From 1988 to 1998 the highest mean annual incidence of indigenous cases per 100 000 population in Ontario (0.4) was in the northwest, where an outdoor lifestyle may enhance exposure. In the region including Long Point, the annual incidence of indigenous cases for the same period was 0.2 per 100 000 population, whereas in the rest of the province it was 0.1 per 100 000 population. The overall mean annual incidence of Lyme borreliosis in Ontario, including cases acquired out of province, was 0.2 per 100 000 population (Charles A. LeBer: personal communication, 1999). These data are similar to the mean annual incidence per 100 000 over the period 1989 to 1998 in states such as Michigan (0.54 [0.18 in 1998]), Ohio (0.45 [0.42 in 1998]) and Illinois (0.25 [0.12 in 1998]),[10] where there are few established populations of *I. scapularis*. These rates are much lower than the annual incidence where vector populations are widespread and moderately high, such as Minnesota (3.83 [5.66 in 1998]) and Wisconsin (9.29 [12.83 in 1998]), and pale in comparison to data from New York (21.76 [25.51 in 1998]), Connecticut (55.62 [105 in 1998]) and Nantucket County, Massachusetts (more than 1200 in 1996),[11] where infected vectors are commonly encountered.

If enough adventitious immature ticks are introduced to an area, some may survive to find a mate and establish a local population. However, given that *B. burgdorferi* is not transmitted through the tick egg, subsequent generations of ticks will not pose a threat until an infected host, such as a migratory bird, introduces the spirochete into the host–vector cycle in that locality.

The range of *I. scapularis* in the United States is expanding.[12] Range expansion, and a concomitant local increase in the risk of Lyme borreliosis, is also occurring in Ontario. We have detected recently established populations of *I. scapularis* at Point Pelee National Park and Rondeau Provincial Park on the north shore of Lake Erie, as well as evidence for other populations at the eastern end of Lake Ontario, all on landfalls for spring migrant birds (unpublished data). Other such populations may remain undetected, as Banerjee and colleagues imply. Identification and communication of the location and extent of new areas of *I. scapularis* endemicity is required to inform public health education and to assist physicians in evaluating the risk of exposure.

I. scapularis can theoretically become established throughout Ontario south of North Bay, in the Kenora – Rainy River region of northwestern Ontario[3] and possibly in parts of southern Manitoba and Quebec. Climatic constraints on development of the various life stages will likely prevent establishment of populations in most of northern Ontario and possibly in the Maritimes and much of Manitoba and Quebec.

Physicians should recognize that exposure to *B. burgdorferi*, though uncommon, can occur in Canada. The low incidence complicates the diagnosis of an already problematic disease. Canadian primary care physicians can gain little experience with Lyme borreliosis. Unsuspected biting ticks may go unnoticed, and symptoms other than the characteristic erythema migrans rash, which occurs in about 90% of culture-confirmed cases, are nonspecific.[13] Because infection is uncommon, first-step serologic tests (indirect fluorescence assay, enzyme-linked immunosorbent assay and immunodot assay) are more likely to produce a false-positive result than a true-positive result.[14] The more specific second-step test, Western blotting, should be carried out as a sequel to a positive first-step test.[14] Such testing, which is required by the Central Public Health Laboratory in Ontario (Charles A. LeBer: personal communication, 1999), reduces the risk of misdiagnosis on the basis of serologic testing. To detect specific IgG antibodies, Western blotting must be carried out after a month of illness.[14,15] A diagnosis of Lyme borreliosis must be based on critical evaluation of all clinical and laboratory data,[13–15] including any history of exposure to ticks or travel to an area were *I. scapularis* is endemic.

I. scapularis also transmits *Babesia microti*, the agent of human granulocytic ehrlichiosis, and deer tick virus, which is closely related to Powassan virus but of unknown pathogenicity.[16] These agents, which may concurrently infect people with Lyme borreliosis and which do cause disease (although uncommonly) in the Unit ed States, have yet to be recognized in ticks in Canada. However, they may affect travellers.[17]

I. scapularis is not the most common tick on people and pets in Canada. The more common ticks do not transmit *B. burgdorferi*,[7,18] but they do serve as vectors for other zoonoses. *Dermacentor variabilis*, found east of central Saskatchewan, and *Dermacentor andersoni*, found further to the west, transmit Rocky Mountain spotted fever; *D. variabilis* also transmits Q fever and tularemia.[19] *Ixodes cookei* transmits Powassan virus.[20]

Simple measures can mitigate the risk of acquiring any tick-borne zoonoses. These include, at the societal level, publicizing areas where ticks are endemic, so that these areas may be avoided or greater vigilance taken by people who do visit them; and, at the individual level, tucking in pant cuffs and wearing long-sleeved shirts; applying DEET-based repellents to clothing and exposed skin; and carefully examining clothing and body for ticks after a day outdoors. The mouthparts of attached ticks should be grasped with forceps at skin level, and the tick slowly withdrawn. Early removal of ticks may diminish the probability of acquiring Lyme borreliosis and other zoonoses.

Current information on Lyme borreliosis, other than Canadian epidemiology, is readily accessible at the US Centers for Disease Control and Prevention Lyme disease Web site (www.cdc.gov/ncidod/dvbid/lymeinfo.htm).

Dr. Barker is with the Ontario Region, Canadian Cooperative Wildlife Health Centre and Department of Pathobiology, Ontario Veterinary College, University of Guelph, Guelph, Ont. Dr. Lindsay is with the Zoonotic Diseases Section, Health Canada, Canadian Science Centre for Human and Animal Health, Winnipeg, Man.

Competing interests: None declared.

References

1. Banerjee SN, Banerjee M, Fernando K, Scott JD, Mann R, Morshed MG. Presence of spirochete causing Lyme disease, *Borrelia burgdorferi*, in the blacklegged tick, *Ixodes scapularis*, in southern Ontario. *CMAJ* 2000; 162(11):1567-9.
2. Barker IK, Surgeoner GA, Artsob H, McEwen SA, Elliott LA, Campbell GD, et al. Distribution of the Lyme disease vector, *Ixodes dammini* (Acari: Ixodidae) and isolation of *Borrelia burgdorferi* in Ontario, Canada. *J Med Entomol* 1992; 29:1011-22.
3. Lindsay LR, Barker IK, Surgeoner GA, McEwen SA, Gillespie TJ, Robinson JT. Survival and development of *Ixodes scapularis* (Acari: Ixodidae) under various climatic conditions in Ontario, Canada. *J Med Entomol* 1995;32:143-52.
4. Lindsay R, Artsob H, Galloway T, Horsman G. Vector of Lyme borreliosis, *Ixodes scapularis*, identified in Saskatchewan. *Can Commun Dis Rep* 1999;25:81-3.
5. Klich M, Lankester MW, Wu KW. Spring migratory birds (Aves) extend the northern occurrence of blacklegged tick (Acari: Ixodidae). *J Med Entomol* 1996;33:581-5.
6. Morshed MG, Scott JD, Banerjee SN, Banerjee M, Fitzgerald T, Fernando K, et al. First isolation of Lyme disease spirochete, *Borrelia burgdorferi*, from blacklegged tick, *Ixodes scapularis*, removed from a bird in Nova Scotia, Canada. *Can Commun Dis Rep* 1999;25:153-5.
7. Lindsay LR, Barker IK, Surgeoner GA, McEwen SA, Elliott LA, Kolar J. Apparent incompetence of *Dermacentor variabilis* (Acari: Ixodidae) and fleas (Insecta: Siphonaptera) as vectors of *Borrelia burgdorferi* in an *Ixodes dammini* endemic area of Ontario, Canada. *J Med Entomol* 1991;28:750-3.
8. Falco RC, McKenna DF, Daniels TJ, Nadelman RB, Nowakowski J, Fish D, et al. Temporal relation between *Ixodes scapularis* abundance and risk for Lyme disease associated with erythema migrans. *Am J Epidemiol* 1999; 149:771-6.
9. Campbell GL, Fritz CL, Fish D, Nowakowski J, Nadelman RB, Wormser GP. Estimation of the incidence of Lyme disease. *Am J Epidemiol* 1998;148: 1018-26.
10. Division of Vector-Borne Infectious Diseases. Lyme disease: epidemiology [online publication]. Atlanta: US Centers for Disease Control and Prevention; updated 1999 Oct 8. Available: www.cdc.gov./ncidod/dvbid/lymeepi.htm (accessed 2000 Apr 6).
11. US Centers for Disease Control and Prevention. Lyme disease — United States, 1996. *MMWR* 1997;46:531-5.
12. Dennis DT, Nekomoto TS, Victor JC, Paul WS, Piesman J. Reported distribution of *Ixodes scapularis* and *Ixodes pacificus* (Acari: Ixodidae) in the United States. *J Med Entomol* 1998;35:629-38.
13. Nadelman RB, Wormser GP. Lyme borreliosis. *Lancet* 1998;352:557-65.
14. Brown SL, Hansen SL, Langone JJ. Role of serology in the diagnosis of Lyme disease. *JAMA* 1999;282:62-6.
15. Wormser GP, Aguero-Rosenfeld ME, Nadelman RB. Lyme disease serology: problems and opportunities. *JAMA* 1999;282:79-80.
16. Ebel GD, Foppa I, Spielman A, Telford SR 3rd. A focus of deer tick virus transmission in the northcentral United States. *Emerg Infect Dis* 1999;5(4):570-4 [serial online]. Available: www.cdc.gov/ncidod/EID/vol5no4 /ebel.htm (accessed 2000 Apr 6).
17. Dos Santos CC, Kain KC. Two tick-borne diseases in one: a case report of concurrent babesiosis and Lyme disease in Ontario. *CMAJ* 1999;160:1851-3. Available: www.cma.ca/cmaj/vol-160/issue-13/1851.htm
18. Barker IK, Lindsay LR, Campbell GD, Surgeoner GA, McEwen SA. The groundhog tick *Ixodes cookei* (Acari: Ixodidae): a poor potential vector of Lyme borreliosis. *J Wildl Dis* 1993;29:416-22.
19. Artsob H. Tick-transmitted human disease threats in Canada. *Germs Ideas* 1996;2:35-9.
20. Gholam BIA, Puksa S, Provias JP. Powassan encephalitis: a case report with neuropathology and literature review. *CMAJ* 1999;161:1419-22. Available: www.cma.ca/cmaj/vol-161/issue-11/1419.htm

Correspondence to: *Dr. Ian K. Barker, Ontario Region, Canadian Cooperative Wildlife Health Centre, Department of Pathobiology, Ontario Veterinary College, University of Guelph, Guelph ON N1G 2W1; ibarker@ovc.uoguelph.ca*

CMAJ REVIEW

The emergence of Lyme disease in Canada

Nicholas H. Ogden DPhil, L. Robbin Lindsay PhD, Muhammad Morshed PhD, Paul N. Sockett PhD, Harvey Artsob PhD

Lyme disease, caused by the bacterium *Borrelia burgdorferi* and transmitted by tick vectors, is the most commonly reported vector-borne disease in the temperate zone.[1] More than 20 000 cases are recorded annually in the United States.[2] In about 80% of cases, early Lyme disease is characterized by a skin lesion, erythema migrans, which expands to a diameter of more than 5 cm from the site of the tick bite.[3] If left untreated, the disease can progress to early disseminated Lyme disease with neurologic (facial palsy, meningitis and meningoradiculoneuritis, also known as Bannwarth syndrome) and cardiac (usually atrioventricular block, sometimes with myopericarditis) involvement, and then to late disseminated Lyme disease with neurologic manifestations (peripheral neuropathy or encephalomyelitis) and Lyme arthritis.[3,4]

B. burgdorferi is transmitted by ticks, which feed on wildlife reservoir hosts of the pathogen, particularly rodents and birds. *Ixodes scapularis*, the blacklegged tick (Figure 1), is the main vector in eastern and central North America. *Ixodes pacificus*, the western blacklegged tick, is the main vector west of the Rocky Mountains. Both tick species are indiscriminate in their choice of host and will feed on humans; as such, they can transmit pathogens from wildlife to humans.

Recent studies have suggested that the risk of exposure to Lyme disease is emerging in Canada because the range of *I. scapularis* is expanding, a process that is predicted to accelerate with climate change. Here we review the available and emerging surveillance information and discuss its relevance to the early diagnosis and prevention of Lyme disease. We based this review on a search of the MEDLINE database using the key words "Lyme," "*Ixodes*" and "Canada."

DOI:10.1503/cmaj.080148

Key points

- Expansion of the geographic range of the tick vector *Ixodes scapularis* in Canada is leading to increasing numbers of endemic areas for Lyme disease.
- Because the specificity of serologic tests for Lyme disease may not be high, epidemiologic findings about the likelihood of exposure to ticks that transmit Lyme disease inform the serologic diagnosis, rather than the other way around.
- Current passive surveillance for tick vectors has identified new endemic areas, but additional methods are needed to precisely identify where Lyme disease is emerging in Canada.
- Enhanced surveillance tools such as risk maps and risk algorithms help in identifying areas where *I. scapularis* ticks are becoming established
- Clinicians' vigilance for human cases, particularly in non-endemic areas, will greatly assist these surveillance efforts.

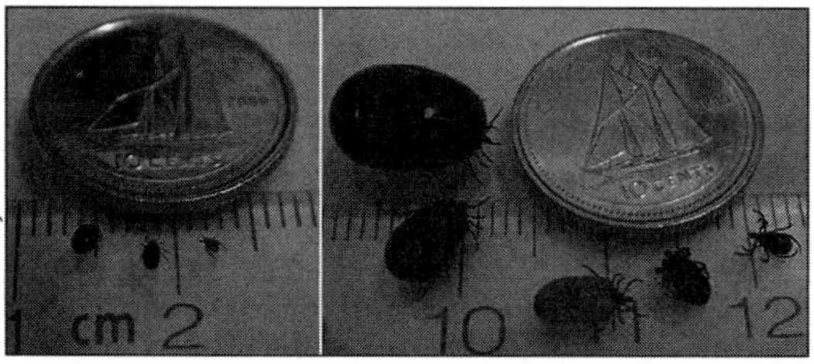

L. Robbin Lindsay

Figure 1: The life stages of the blacklegged tick, *Ixodes scapularis*, which transmits Lyme disease. Nymphs (left-hand photograph) and adult females (right-hand photograph) are shown in various stages of engorgement from unfed (at the right of each picture) to fully engorged (at the left of each picture). The western blacklegged tick, *Ixodes pacificus*, is morphologically very similar to *I. scapularis*.

Diagnosis of Lyme disease

Within several weeks after the tick bite and manifestation of the erythema migrans lesion, the lesion disappears and the bacterium disseminates hematogenously to other tissues, including additional skin sites (producing secondary erythema migrans lesions in some cases), the nervous system, the heart and the joints.[3] Bacterial culture or use of polymerase chain reaction to amplify target sequences in clinical material (such as blood, skin, synovial fluid or cerebrospinal fluid) are diagnostic methods with low to moderate sensitivity.[2,5] Public health laboratories in Canada,[6,7] the United States[2,8] and some European countries advocate a two-tiered serologic testing process, consisting of enzyme-linked immunosorbent assay followed by Western blot, to assist in diagnosis. Serologic testing is insensitive in very early Lyme disease, but the 2-tiered method is much more sensitive in detecting cases of disseminated Lyme disease.[2,5,7,9] When used alone, enzyme-linked immunosorbent assay has limited specificity, but the

From the Centre for Foodborne, Environmental and Zoonotic Infectious Diseases (Ogden), Public Health Agency of Canada, Saint-Hyacinthe, Que.; the Zoonoses and Special Pathogens Division (Lindsay, Artsob), National Microbiology Laboratory, Public Health Agency of Canada, Winnipeg, Man.; Zoonotic and Emerging Pathogens (Morshed), Laboratory Services, British Columbia Centre for Disease Control, Vancouver, BC; and First Nations and Inuit Health Branch (Sockett), Health Canada, Ottawa, Ont.

specificity is improved by Western blotting, provided that the bands are interpreted according to criteria for positivity set by the US Centers for Disease Control and Prevention.[8] Concerns about test specificity mean that interpretation of the 2-tiered test is informed by whether the patient has had contact with an endemic area, which is defined by ecological criteria.[10] The diagnosis should be guided by the patient's clinical situation, with the results of laboratory tests providing supportive evidence of infection.

Geographic distribution of risk and endemic areas

Endemic areas are localities where *B. burgdorferi* is demonstrably being transmitted by an established population of vector ticks.[6] The number of documented endemic areas in Canada has increased recently. In the early 1990s, only 1 geographically discrete population of *I. scapularis* was known, at Long Point on the Ontario shore of Lake Erie.[11] Since 1997, detection of human cases by vigilant clinicians and passive surveillance for ticks[12] has led to the identification of populations of *I. scapularis* in southern Ontario, Nova Scotia, southeastern Manitoba and New Brunswick (Figure 2).[13] In addition, active surveillance driven by risk maps (Box 1) has identified the possibility of additional emerging populations in southern Quebec, in the absence of a clear signal from passive surveillance.[14] Data on human cases from provinces where Lyme disease is reportable suggest a corresponding recent increase in the number of cases acquired by Canadians without any history of travel abroad (Figure 3).[15] Studies indicate that ambient temperature constrains the establishment of *I. scapularis* in Canada to the warmer regions of southeastern Manitoba, southern Ontario and Quebec and some regions of the Maritimes. As such, projected increases in temperature with climate change are expected to permit and accelerate the

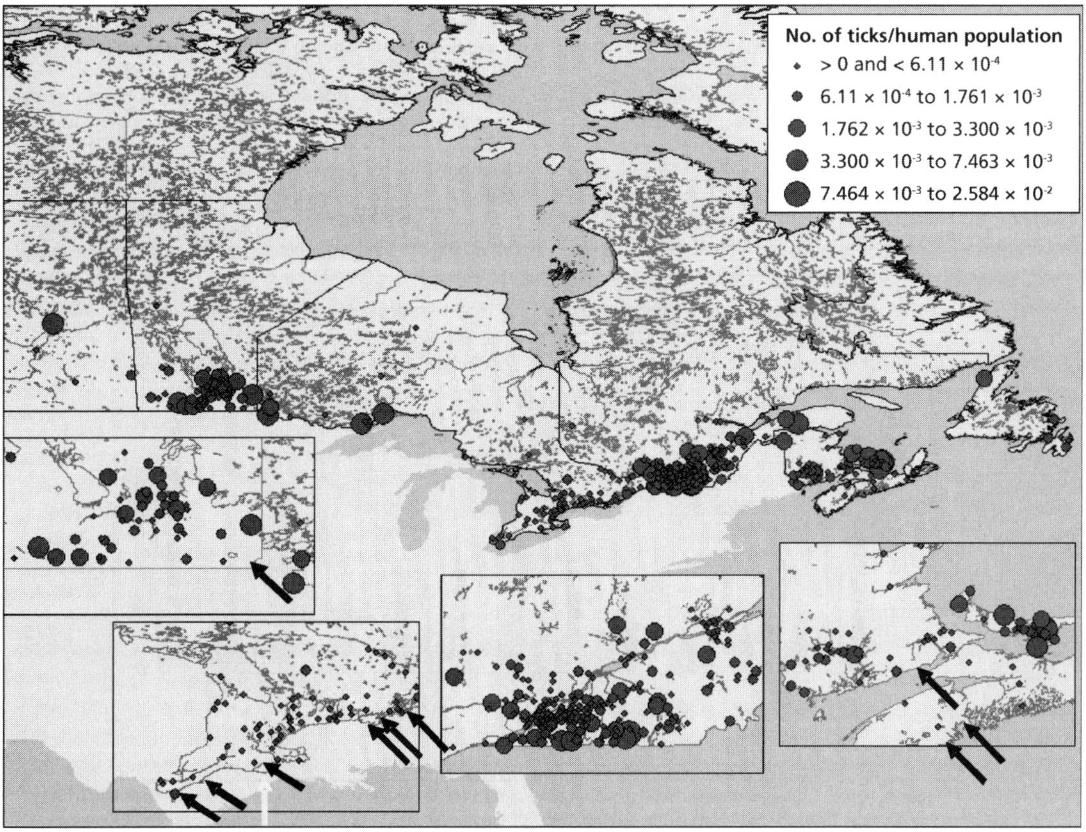

Figure 2: The distribution of *Ixodes scapularis*, reflecting information submitted to provincial and federal public health agencies from January 1990 to December 2003 and to the Lyme Disease Association of Ontario for 1993 to 1999 (red circles are centred on the centroid of the census subdivision from which the reports were submitted). Census subdivisions where resident populations of *I. scapularis* are currently known to occur are indicated by arrows, and the census subdivision containing the only *I. scapularis* population that was known in 1991 is indicated by the yellow arrow. Reproduced, with permission, from the Entomological Society of America.[12]

expansion of *I. scapularis* into Canada.[13,16]

Surveillance by the British Columbia Centre for Disease Control suggests that established populations of *I. pacificus* and areas where *B. burgdorferi* is endemic are widely distributed in southern British Columbia. The prevalence of *B. burgdorferi* infection in host-seeking *I. pacificus* ticks is usually lower (typically less than 10%[17,18]) than that in *I. scapularis* (typically greater than 25% in the northeastern United States and southeastern Canada[1,19]). Therefore, the risk of Lyme disease in endemic areas where *I. pacificus* is the vector is generally lower than where *I. scapularis* is the vector.

Overall, there is a low risk of exposure to Lyme disease from tick vectors in the nonendemic areas of all 10 provinces. This risk is due to ticks dispersed from endemic areas by migratory birds (Figure 2).[12,20,21] About 10% of these bird-transported ticks are infected with *B. burgdorferi*,[12] and small numbers of cases of human Lyme disease occur outside endemic areas.[22]

Box 1: Risk maps for the occurrence of the Lyme disease vector *Ixodes scapularis*

- The 2 most influential factors for the establishment of the tick in Canada are warmer temperatures and dispersion of the ticks on animal hosts.
- Risk maps employ a risk algorithm comprising these influential factors.
- The risk maps provide a model against which different surveillance methods can be compared and hypotheses on the likelihood of expanding geographic range tested.
- Initial field validation suggests that the risk algorithm is a useful tool to identify areas where *I. scalpularis* ticks are becoming established.

Conclusions and recommendations

The number of known endemic areas of Lyme disease in Canada is increasing because the range of *I. scapularis* is expanding in the eastern and central provinces. National surveillance must be able to identify this changing pattern. Lyme disease is potentially preventable if people wear appropriate clothing and use *N,N*-diethyl-*meta*-toluamide (DEET) repellents. Removal of infected ticks from a person within 24 hours of attachment usually prevents transmission of *B. burgdorferi*,[23] and early Lyme disease is usually easily treated with antibiotics.[4,24] However, prompt treatment requires recognition of vector ticks and erythema migrans lesions by affected members of the public and prompt diagnosis by clinicians.[24] If Lyme disease is not recognized during the early stages, patients may suffer seriously debilitating disease, which may be more difficult to treat.[4] Therefore, an important function of surveillance is to inform both the public and clinicians about the local risk level and the need for prudent administration of regimens appropriate for prevention and early diagnosis of Lyme disease.

As of 2009, physicians will be required to report clinically confirmed and suspected cases of Lyme disease to the national

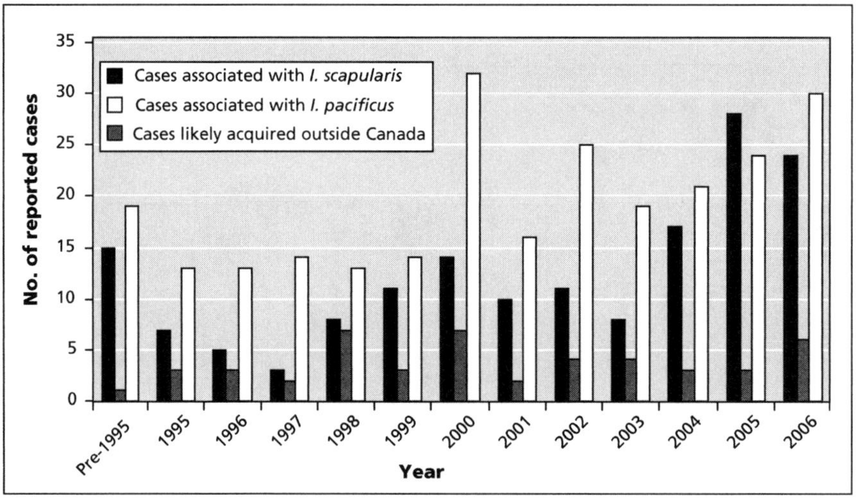

Figure 3: Annual number of cases of Lyme disease reported voluntarily by the provinces and territories since the late 1980s. Cases of Lyme disease in British Columbia were probably transmitted by *Ixodes pacificus*, whereas cases from all other provinces with cases that were potentially locally acquired (i.e., Manitoba, Ontario, Quebec, New Brunswick, Nova Scotia and Newfoundland and Labrador) were probably associated with *Ixodes scapularis*. Cases affecting patients with a history of travel to an endemic area outside Canada during the period when they likely acquired the infection are considered travel-related or nonendemic. Reproduced with permission from the Minister of Public Works and Government Services Canada, 2008.[15]

surveillance authority. Such reporting will assist in identifying the burden associated with this disease. We also advocate using environmental indicators of the risk of Lyme disease (i.e., the occurrence of ticks or environmental data for risk maps) for surveillance, to both support the diagnosis of the disease and to pre-empt its occurrence in humans. Researchers are now using the gold-standard surveillance method of intensive field study to validate risk maps for Lyme disease vectors[14] as public health tools, so that these maps can be used to identify new endemic areas (Box 1). These studies and the risk maps can then be used to evaluate, select and target surveillance methods, such as passive surveillance for tick vectors (already in use but with effort that varies geographically[12]) and surveillance for the presence of Lyme disease vectors on, and evidence of *B. burgdorferi* infection in, sentinel animals.[25,26] With these methods, it may be possible to predict and then confirm how ticks are spreading in Canada and how endemic areas are expanding, which should in turn allow the targeting of public and physician awareness programs to the areas of greatest risk, for maximum effect.

We conclude that Lyme disease is emerging in Canada, that effective, enhanced surveillance involving federal and provincial agencies needs to be instigated and that clinician awareness of Lyme disease will be crucial to minimizing its impact.

This article has been peer reviewed.

Competing interests: None declared.

Contributors: Dr. Ogden was the lead author and provided information on Lyme disease ecology and surveillance. Dr. Lindsay provided Figure 1, contributed to and critically assessed the article content, and provided information on surveillance and Lyme disease vectors in Canada. Dr. Morshed contributed to and critically assessed the article content and provided information on the ecology of Lyme disease in British Columbia. Dr. Sockett contributed to and critically assessed the article content and provided information on surveillance and public health policy. Dr. Artsob contributed to and critically assessed the article content and provided information on the laboratory diagnosis of Lyme disease. Each of the authors approved the final version submitted for publication.

REFERENCES

1. Kurtenbach K, Hanincova K, Tsao J, et al. Key processes in the evolutionary ecology of Lyme borreliosis. *Nat Rev Microbiol* 2006;4:660-9.
2. Centers for Disease Control and Prevention (CDC). Lyme disease — United States, 2003–2005. *MMWR Morb Mortal Wkly Rep* 2007;56:573-6.
3. Aguero-Rosenfeld ME, Wang G, Schwartz I, et al. Diagnosis of Lyme borreliosis. *Clin Microbiol Rev* 2005;18:484-509.
4. Wormser GP, Dattwyler RJ, Shapiro ED, et al. The clinical assessment, treatment, and prevention of Lyme disease, human granulocytic anaplasmosis, and babesiosis: clinical practice guidelines by the Infectious Diseases Society of America. *Clin Infect Dis* 2006;43:1089-134.
5. Nowakowski J, Schwartz I, Liveris D, et al. Laboratory diagnostic techniques for patients with early Lyme disease associated with erythema migrans: a comparison of different techniques. *Clin Infect Dis* 2001;33:2023-7.
6. Consensus conference on Lyme disease. *CMAJ* 1991;144:1627-32.
7. Canadian Public Health Laboratory Network. The laboratory diagnosis of Lyme borreliosis: guidelines from the Canadian Public Health Laboratory Network. *Can J Infect Dis Med Microbiol* 2007;18:145-8.
8. Centers for Disease Control and Prevention (CDC). Recommendations for test performance and interpretation from the Second National Conference on Serologic Diagnosis of Lyme Disease. *MMWR Morb Mortal Wkly Rep* 1995;44:590-1.
9. Dressler F, Whalen JA, Reinhardt BN, et al. Western blotting in the serodiagnosis of Lyme disease. *J Infect Dis* 1993;167:392-400.
10. Tugwell P, Dennis DT, Weinstein A, et al. Laboratory evaluation in the diagnosis of Lyme disease. *Ann Intern Med* 1997;127:1109-23.
11. Barker IK, Surgeoner GA, Artsob H, et al. Distribution of the Lyme disease vector, *Ixodes dammini* (Acari: Ixodidae) and isolation of *Borrelia burgdorferi* in Ontario, Canada. *J Med Entomol* 1992;29:1011-22.
12. Ogden NH, Trudel L, Artsob H, et al. *Ixodes scapularis* ticks collected by passive surveillance in Canada: analysis of geographic distribution and infection with the Lyme borreliosis agent *Borrelia burgdorferi* sensu lato. *J Med Entomol* 2006;43:600-9.
13. Ogden NH, Bigras-Poulin M, O'Callaghan CJ, et al. A dynamic population model to investigate effects of climate on geographic range and seasonality of the tick *Ixodes scapularis*. *Int J Parasitol* 2005;35:375-89.
14. Ogden NH, St-Onge L, Barker IK, et al. Risk maps for range expansion of the Lyme disease vector, *Ixodes scapularis*, in Canada now and with climate change. *Int J Health Geogr* 2008;7:24.
15. Ogden NH, Lindsay LR, Morshed M, et al. The rising challenge of Lyme borreliosis in Canada. *Can Commun Dis Rep* 2008;34:1-19. Available: www.phac-aspc.gc.ca/publicat/ccdr-rmtc/08vol34/dr-rm3401a-eng.php (accessed 2009 May 12).
16. Ogden NH, Maarouf A, Barker IK, et al. Climate change and the potential for range expansion of the Lyme disease vector *Ixodes scapularis* in Canada. *Int J Parasitol* 2006;36:63-70.
17. Holden K, Boothby JT, Kasten RW, et al. Co-detection of *Bartonella henselae*, *Borrelia burgdorferi*, and *Anaplasma phagocytophilum* in *Ixodes pacificus* ticks from California, USA. *Vector Borne Zoonotic Dis* 2006;6:99-102.
18. Lane RS, Foley JE, Eisen L, et al. Acarologic risk of exposure to emerging tick-borne bacterial pathogens in a semirural community in northern California. *Vector Borne Zoonotic Dis* 2001;1:197-210.
19. Lindsay LR, Barker IK, Surgeoner GA, et al. Duration of *Borrelia burgdorferi* infectivity in white-footed mice for the tick vector *Ixodes scapularis* under laboratory and field conditions in Ontario. *J Wildl Dis* 1997;33:766-75.
20. Ogden NH, Lindsay LR, Hanincová K, et al. Role of migratory birds in introduction and range expansion of *Ixodes scapularis* ticks, and *Borrelia burgdorferi* and *Anaplasma phagocytophilum* in Canada. *Appl Environ Microbiol* 2008;74:1780-90.
21. Morshed MG, Scott JD, Fernando K, et al. Migratory songbirds disperse ticks across Canada, and first isolation of the Lyme disease spirochete, *Borrelia burgdorferi*, from the avian tick, *Ixodes auritulus*. *J Parasitol* 2005;91:780-90.
22. Vrbova L, Middleton D. Descriptive epidemiology of Lyme disease in Ontario: 1999–2004. *Can Commun Dis Rep* 2006;32:247-57.
23. Schwan TG, Piesman J. Vector interactions and molecular adaptations of Lyme disease and relapsing fever spirochetes associated with transmission by ticks. *Emerg Infect Dis* 2002;8:115-21.
24. Wormser GP. Prevention of Lyme borreliosis. *Wien Klin Wochenschr* 2005;117:385-91.
25. Duncan AW, Correa MT, Levine JF, et al. The dog as a sentinel for human infection: prevalence of *Borrelia burgdorferi* C6 antibodies in dogs from southeastern and mid-Atlantic states. *Vector Borne Zoonotic Dis* 2004;4:221-9.
26. Johnson JL, Ginsberg HS, Zhioua E, et al. Passive tick surveillance, dog seropositivity, and incidence of human Lyme disease. *Vector Borne Zoonotic Dis* 2004;4:137-42.

Correspondence to: *Dr. Nicholas H. Ogden, Environmental Issues Division, Centre for Foodborne, Environmental and Zoonotic Infectious Diseases, Public Health Agency of Canada, 3200 rue Sicotte, CP 5000, Saint-Hyacinthe QC J2S 7C6; fax 450 778-8120; nicholas_ogden@phac-aspc.gc.ca*

First Isolation of Lyme Disease Spirochete, *Borrelia burgdorferi*, from Ticks Collected from Songbirds in Ontario, Canada

John D. Scott
Lyme Disease Association of Ontario
365 St. David St. South
Fergus, ON N1M 2L7
Email: jkscott@bserv.com

Lance A. Durden
Department of Biology
Georgia Southern University
Statesboro, GA 30460-8042
Email: ldurden@georgiasouthern.edu

ABSTRACT

This study documents the first isolation of the Lyme disease spirochete, Borrelia burgdorferi, *from ticks attached to songbirds in Ontario. Viable spirochetes were cultured from a nymph of the blacklegged tick,* Ixodes scapularis Say, *detached from a Hermit Thrush,* Catharus guttatus. *Similarly,* B. burgdorferi *isolates were obtained from* I. scapularis *nymphs collected from a House Wren,* Troglodytes aedon. *These* B. burgdorferi *isolates show divergent heterogeneity indicating that some strains originated from nearby locales and others from southern latitudes. Lyme disease vector ticks are transported by northward-migrating songbirds, and dispersed widely across southern Canada. Importantly,* B. burgdorferi-*infected* I. scapularis *ticks pose a public health risk to people and domestic animals wherever they are released.*

INTRODUCTION

The blacklegged tick, *Ixodes scapularis* Say (Acari: Ixodidae), the primary vector of the spirochete that causes Lyme disease, is distributed widely east of the Rocky Mountains by migratory songbirds (Anderson et al. 1990, Durden and Keirans 1996). Typically, *I. scapularis* immature stages (larvae, nymphs) parasitize ground- and shrub-frequenting passerine species. En route to breeding grounds, northward-migrating passerines make landfall at established populations of *I. scapularis*, which are scattered across northern United States (Steiner et al. 2008) and southern Canada, and some of these ticks are infected with the Lyme disease spirochete, *Borrelia burgdorferi* (Scott et al. 2001, Morshed et al. 2005, Ogden et al. 2008). At these stopovers, ground-foraging songbirds meander through grassy vegetation and arboreal leaf litter and are parasitized by bird-associated ticks. Fully engorged ticks later detach from these migrating songbirds farther afield in cool, humid, tick-friendly habitats where *I. scapularis* immature stages subsequently molt in 5-11 weeks to the next life stage. From mid-May to early June, northward migration of passerines overlaps directly with the peak questing activity of *I. scapularis* nymphs. Ogden et al. (2008) estimated 50 million to 175 million *I. scapularis* ticks are dispersed by birds annually across Canada.

Anderson and Magnarelli (1984) pioneered bird-tick-*Borrelia* studies in the Lyme, Connecticut area and cultured *B. burgdorferi* from the liver of a Veery, *Catharus fuscescens*, and *I. scapularis* larvae attached to it. In Canada, Scott et al. (2001) initially cultured *B. burgdorferi* from a live, fully engorged *I. scapularis* nymph, which was collected in May 1999 from a Common Yellowthroat, *Geothlypis trichas,* in Nova Scotia. Subsequently, *B. burgdorferi* was detected in Ontario in an ethanol-preserved *I. scapularis* nymph collected in May 2003 from a Common Yellowthroat, which was mist-netted at Long Point, Ontario (Morshed et al. 2005). More recently, *B. burgdorferi* has been detected in *I. scapularis* immature stages collected from songbirds in Ontario (Ogden et al. 2008, Scott et al., unpubl. data) because these ticks were dead specimens, spirochetes were mortal.

The aim of this study was to culture live *B. burgdorferi* from subadult *I. scapularis* collected from songbirds in Ontario, and to determine the viability and genetic variability of Lyme disease spirochetes in these bird-feeding ticks.

METHODS

Bird banders captured songbirds with mist nets, and ticks were removed using stainless steel tweezers (superfine tip). Ticks were inserted into self-sealing micro tubes, which contained slightly moistened, non-chlorinated filter paper. These ticks were sent by courier to Scott for identification, and ticks indigenous to southern latitudes were forwarded to Durden for confirmation of identification. In the molecular laboratory, individual live ticks were cultured in BSK-H media, and cultures were checked weekly by dark-field microscopy for four weeks.

PCR amplification was performed on the ribosomal *rrf* (5S)-*rrl* (23S) intergenic spacer gene and the linear plasmid *OspA* gene using the Stratagene Robocycler as described previously (Morshed et al. 2005). The *rrf-rrl* amplicons were sequenced with the ABI 3130 DNA sequencer and analyzed with DNAStar software.

The St. Williams Crown Forest reference isolate ON05FTP863 (GenBank accession no. FJ707480) cultured from an *I. scapularis* female is accessible via the GenBank website: http://www.ncbi.nlm.nih.gov/nuccore/224981432.

RESULTS

A partially engorged *I. scapularis* nymph (Fig. 1) was removed from a Hermit Thrush, *Catharus guttatus*, which was mist-netted at Long Point, Ontario (42.51N, 80.16W) on 13 May 2007. Likewise, six engorged *I. scapularis* subadults (five sent for identification) were collected from a House Wren, *Troglodytes aedon* on 14 May 2007. Motile spirochetes were observed by dark-field microscopy in cultures from a single nymph from the Hermit Thrush and two nymphs from the House Wren.

PCR amplification of the *rrf-rrl* intergenic spacer and *OspA* genes confirmed that the three isolates belong to the *B. burgdorferi sensu lato* complex. None of the three isolates had the same nucleotide sequences in the *rrf-rrl* region; they differed from

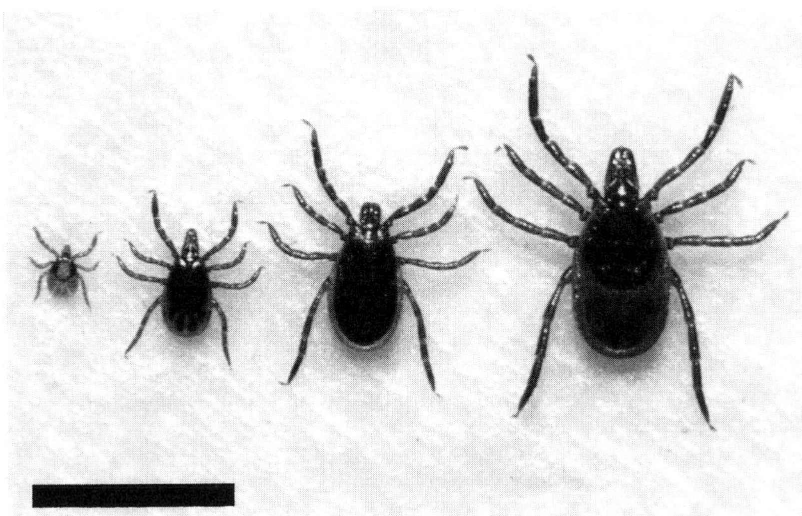

Fig. 1. Motile life stages of blacklegged tick, *Ixodes scapularis*: unfed larva, unfed nymph, male, unfed female. Bar, 3 mm. Photo by John D. Scott

Table 1. Isolates of *Borrelia burgdorferi* cultured from *I. scapularis* ticks collected from songbirds at Long Point, Ontario

Bird species	Tick stage, tick no.	Isolate	Amplicon size (bp)[b]	Genbank assession no.	Deviation[c] from strain B31	Website reference[a] http://www.ncbi.nlm.nih.
Hermit Thrush	nymph, 075A23	ON07FTP979	220	FJ707481	57	gov/nuccore/224981433
House Wren	nymph, 07-5A24C	ON07FTP981	218	FJ707482	3	gov/nuccore/224981434
	nymph, 07-5A24D	ON07FTP982	218	FJ707483	2	gov/nuccore/224981435

[a] The website prefix is provided in the subheading and the suffixes in the column below.
[b] bp, number of nucleotides sequenced in the *rrf* (5S)-*rrl* (23S) intergenic spacer amplicon.
[c] deviation within *rrf-rrl* region, in bp, from type strain B31.

each other by at least 3 base pairs (bp). The two isolates (ON07FTP981 [nymph 07-5A24C] and ON07FTP982 [nymph 07-5A24D]), which were collected from the House Wren (Table 1), had nucleotide sequence differences from the *B. burgdorferi sensu stricto* type strain B31consisting of 3 bp and 2 bp, respectively. In contrast, the isolate ON07FTP979 from the nymph (07-5A23), which was collected from the Hermit Thrush, had a 2-bp insertion plus 57-bp substitutions in the *rrf-rrl* region, compared to strain B31.

DISCUSSION

The present study shows that migratory songbirds disperse *I. scapularis* ticks in Ontario harboring *B. burgdorferi* with diverse heterogeneity. The *B. burgdorferi* isolate in the nymph attached to the Hermit Thrush, which winters as far south as Guatemala, had a marked difference (2-bp insertion, 57-bp substitutions) in the *rrf-rrl* 220-bp region. Researchers (Lin et al. 2004, Rudenko et al. 2009) report genetic diversity of *B. burgdorferi* in ticks and vertebrate hosts collected in the southern United States and, ultimately, these bird-associated ticks can be transported to Canada during spring migration. Because of the large number of nucleotide substitutions, it is likely that the isolate, which was cultured from the nymph attached to the Hermit Thrush, originated from southern United States.

The isolates from the two *I. scapularis* nymphs collected from the House Wren deviated from each other by three nucleotides in the *rrf-rrl* 218-bp amplicon. Even though certain songbirds, such as the American Robin, *Turdus migratorius*, may be competent reservoirs of *B. burgdorferi* (Richter et al. 2000), endogenous transmission of *B. burgdorferi* in our study via the House Wren was not evident during tick engorgement. One isolate (ON07FTP981) matched a Turkey Point Provincial Park isolate (ON06FTP933; Scott et al. 2008), and also it matched an isolate (ON05FTP863) cultured from an *I. scapularis* female collected at St. Williams Crown Forest at Turkey Point, Ontario. These isolates have been characterized as *B. burgdorferi* sensu stricto (Scott et al. 2008); this genospecies is common across North America, and causes Lyme disease in people and domestic animals. Genographically, the combination of these Lyme disease spirochetes reveals a direct genetic link between Turkey Point Provincial Park, St. Williams Crown Forest, and Long Point. The other isolate (ON07FTP982) cultured from the nymph on the House Wren had a 2-bp deviation from strain B31. In essence, at least one of the *B. burgdorferi* isolates was acquired by the House Wren in the Long Point region.

Bird-tick studies reveal evidence of *B. burgdorferi*-positive *I. scapularis* introduced by spring migrants across northern latitudes of central and eastern Canada. Ogden et al. (2008) reported that approximately 15% of the *I. scapularis* nymphs, which were collected from infested songbirds in eastern Canada, were positive for *B. burgdorferi*. During a 10-year tick-host study, Morshed et al. (2006) revealed an infection prevalence of 12.9% for *B. burgdorferi* in *I. scapularis* adults, which were collected from dogs, cats, horses, and humans as far north as the 50° N in Ontario. Similarly, Ogden et al. (2006) reported 12.5% of the *I. scapularis* (adults) collected from people, domestic and wildlife animals from Manitoba to Newfoundland and Labrador, to be infected with *B. burgdorferi*. The close correlation between bird-derived immature stages and mammalian-derived *I. scapularis* adults accentuates the fact that migratory passerines are dispersing agents of *B. burgdorferi*-infected blacklegged ticks in Ontario.

A heavily parasitized songbird, which drops ticks in one site, can start a new population of *I. scapularis*. Anderson and Magnarelli (1984) reported high infestations of *I. scapularis* (reported as *I. dammini*) on passerines in Connecticut: 21 *I. scapularis* larvae were removed from both a Gray Catbird, *Dumetella carolinensis* and a Swamp Sparrow, *Melospiza georgina* and, likewise, 19 *I. scapularis* nymphs from an American Robin. In the present study, six *I. scapularis* subadults were collected from the House Wren and, ultimately, provide the potential for *I. scapularis* and *B. burgdorferi* to become established in a new locale.

Recently, Stutchbury et al. (2009) used light-weight geolocators on passerines to track migratory routes, and found that certain songbirds fly 577 km/d or more during spring migration and, during a typical five-day engorgement period, can import bird-feeding *I. scapularis* nymphs from the southern United States into Canada. Aided by south winds and warm temperatures, southern temperate and Neotropical songbirds, including House Wrens and Hermit Thrushes, are able to import ticks into Ontario with a multitude of *B. burgdorferi* strains and other tick-associated pathogens.

Not only does the present study show viability of *B. burgdorferi* in bird-derived *I. scapularis*, it also reveals diverse heterogeneity of *B. burgdorferi*-infected ticks imported by migratory songbirds. Consistent with other studies (Morshed et al. 2006, Rudenko et al. 2009), our study shows that *B. burgdorferi* strains in Ontario are more heterogeneous than previously thought. Ultimately, this genetic diversity could substantially alter clinical manifestations and serological responses in Lyme disease patients and, as a result, may lead to a misdiagnosis. Ornithologists and medical practitioners need to be aware that outdoors people may encounter Lyme disease vector ticks that can result in diverse pathological symptoms.

In conclusion, songbirds act as hosts for bird-transported ticks and play an integral role in the enzootic cycle of Lyme disease. Not only do passerines act as transporting agents of *I. scapularis* harboring viable *B. burgdorferi*; but they may also act as reservoir-competent hosts. The heightened questing activity of *I. scapularis* nymphs in May and early June and the concurrent tick parasitism of passerine migrants during peak spring migration ostensively show that these avian hosts are long-range dispersing agents of Lyme disease vector ticks. Because migratory songbirds transport *B. burgdorferi*-infected *I. scapularis* anywhere in Ontario, people do not have to visit an endemic area to contract Lyme disease.

ACKNOWLEDGMENTS

We thank bird banders at Long Point Bird Observatory for collection of ticks from songbirds. Gratitude is extended to the Laboratory Services, British Columbia Centre for Disease Control for technical assistance in culturing and DNA sequence analysis. This study was supported in part by the Lyme Disease Association of Ontario.

LITERATURE CITED

Anderson, J.F. and L.A. Magnarelli. 1984. Avian and mammalian hosts for spirochete-infected ticks and insects in a Lyme disease focus in Connecticut. *Yale Journal of Biology and Medicine* 57:627-641.

Anderson, J.F., L.A. Magnarelli, and K.C. Stafford III. 1990. Bird-feeding ticks transstadially transmit *Borrelia burgdorferi* that infect Syrian hamsters. *Journal of Wildlife Diseases* 26:1-10.

Durden, L.A. and J.E. Keirans. 1996. Nymphs of the genus *Ixodes* (Acari: Ixodidae) of the United States: taxonomy, identification key, distribution, hosts, and medical/veterinary importance. Thomas Say Publications in Entomology. Entomological Society of America, Lanham, MD.

Lin, T., J.H. Oliver, Jr., and L. Gao. 2004. Molecular characterization of *Borrelia* isolates from ticks and mammals from the southern United States. *Journal of Parasitology* 90:1298-1307.

Morshed, M.G., J.D. Scott, K. Fernando, L. Beati, D.F. Mazerolle, G. Geddes, and L.A. Durden. 2005. Migratory songbirds disperse ticks across Canada, and first isolation of the Lyme disease spirochete, *Borrelia burgdorferi*, from the avian tick, *Ixodes auritulus*. *Journal of Parasitology* 91:780-790.

Morshed, M.G., J.D. Scott, K. Fernando, G. Geddes, A. McNabb, S. Mak, and L.A. Durden. 2006. Distribution and characterization of *Borrelia burgdorferi* isolates from *Ixodes scapularis* and presence in mammalian hosts in Ontario, Canada. *Journal of Medical Entomology* 43: 762-773.

Ogden, N.H., L. Trudel, H. Artsob, I.K. Barker, G. Beauchamp, D.F. Charron, M.A. Drebot, T.D. Galloway, R. O'Handley, R.A. Thompson, and L.R. Lindsay. 2006. *Ixodes scapularis* ticks collected by passive surveillance in Canada: analysis of geographic distribution and infection with Lyme borreliosis agent *Borrelia burgdorferi*. *Journal of Medical Entomology* 43:600-609.

Ogden, N.H., L.R. Lindsay, K. Hanincová, I.K. Barker, M. Bigras-Poulin, D.F. Charron, A. Heagy, C.M. Francis, C.J. O'Callaghan, I. Schwartz, and R.A. Thompson. 2008. Role of migratory birds in introduction and range expansion of *Ixodes scapularis* ticks and of *Borrelia burgdorferi* and *Anaplasma phagocytophilum* in Canada. *Applied and Environmental Microbiology* 74:1780-1790.

Richter, D., A. Spielman, N. Komar, and F.-R. Matuschka. 2000. Competence of American Robins as reservoir hosts for Lyme disease spirochetes. *Emerging Infectious Diseases* 6:133-138.

Rudenko, N., M. Golovchenko, L. Grubhoffer, and J.H. Oliver, Jr. 2009. *Borrelia carolinensis* sp. nov., a new (14th) member of the *Borrelia burgdorferi sensu lato* complex from the southeastern region of the United States. *Journal of Clinical Microbiology* 47:134-141.

Scott, J.D., K. Fernando, S.N. Banerjee, L.A. Durden, S.K. Byrne, M. Banerjee, R.B. Mann, and M.G. Morshed. 2001. Birds disperse ixodid (Acari: Ixodidae) and *Borrelia burgdorferi*-infected ticks in Canada. *Journal of Medical Entomology* 38:493-500.

Scott, J.D., M.-K. Lee, K. Fernando, D. R. Jorgensen, L.A. Durden, and M.G. Morshed. 2008. Rapid introduction of Lyme disease spirochete, *Borrelia burgdorferi sensu stricto*, in *Ixodes scapularis* (Acari: Ixodidae) established at Turkey Point Provincial Park, Ontario, Canada. *Journal of Vector Ecology* 33:64-69.

Steiner, F.E., R.R. Pinger, C.N. Vann, N. Grindle, D. Civitello, K. Clay, and C. Fuqua. 2008. Infection and co-infection rates of *Anaplasma phagocytophilum* variants, *Babesia* spp., *Borrelia burgdorferi*, and the rickettsial endosymbiont in *Ixodes scapularis* (Acari: Ixodidae) from sites in Indiana, Maine, Pennsylvania, and Wisconsin. *Journal of Medical Entomology* 45:289-297.

Stutchbury, B.J.M., S.A. Tarof, T. Done, E. Gow, P.M. Kramer, J. Tautin, J.W. Fox, and V. Afanasyev. 2009. Tracking long-distance songbird migration by using geolocators. *Science* 323:896.

LYME DISEASE CAN BE A DIAGNOSIS OF HOPE

3

By Felix Sperling PhD and
Janet Sperling MSc, Edmonton, Alberta

Lyme disease, or Lyme borreliosis as we prefer to call it, is a devilishly complicated disease. It has challenged many of our most firmly held preconceptions and turned our personal world upside down. In the darkest stages of Ed's story, the most honorable players have been psychiatrists, administrators, lawyers, and politicians—professions that we had previously viewed with suspicion. Our respect for the power of clinical diagnoses has multiplied in spite of their inherent subjectivity, while our regard for the kind of evidence-based medical diagnoses that focus on machine readouts has diminished in spite of their apparent objectivity. But our son's story has had a happy ending that underscores the power of reason and persistence.

The story has unfolded in four phases. First came our frantic search for answers, with dread clutching more tightly with every strange new development in our son's condition. Then came the growing realization that both the answer and a relatively simple solution lay in plain view, but the struggle to get Ed's primary physicians to see it that way would become a willful confrontation. This was followed by our son's slow, unsteady recovery, which continued to test everyone's resolve. Finally we entered a period in which Ed has moved on with his life but we as his parents have become increasingly more determined that no other Lyme sufferers should have to deal with a systemic failure that reflects as much about our medical system as it does about a bacterial assault on a Lyme patient. In the end this is not a narrative about one patient, one family, or one medical group, but about a deep, unresolved conflict at multiple biological and social levels.

July 2005: Desperately seeking answers.

The following is a lightly edited version of a description of Ed's symptoms that we wrote in late July 2005. We had hit a wall of intransigence and incomprehension among his doctors. As a desperate measure we sent this description to several colleagues and contacts that we hoped might be able to point us in a positive direction. Our audience was expected to be familiar with a variety of medical terms that might be obscure to more general readers.

Ed is a bright, personable youth with a delightful, gentle sense of humor. He retains that sense of humor in spite of his increasingly depressing circumstances. Currently 110 pounds and 5 feet 4 inches, he could be described as having a slight build. A year ago he would have seemed a bit chubby, with strong bones but short. He has always been exceptionally intelligent and energetic, and has read voraciously across a wide range of topics. He has ranked nationally in various math contests in recent years, and has easily maintained high grades in all his classes. He has an infectious enthusiasm for science and engineering, which is encouraged by numerous academics and engineers in his extended family and neighborhood in Edmonton, Alberta. His physical activities have included moderate levels of cross-country skiing and sailing, and he has consistently been a strong walker. He is the oldest of four boys (the youngest being 3 years old) in a stable family. Born one month premature, he has remained relatively small for his age but he has been healthy except for moderate asthma and a transient allergy to milk.

Ed's present alarming medical condition apparently started with a persistent but otherwise innocuous flu-like illness in late November 2004. His most noticeable symptoms were low energy levels and moderate congestion, periods of low fever and serious headache, a declining appetite, and eventually an apparent sinus infection. He had a period of dry, cracked lips in mid December. He seemed to be recovering later in December, and had no problem continuing with school until the winter holiday started on December 20th. In late November he weighed 135 lbs, a weight he had maintained through the previous year even though he grew almost 8 centimeters and become noticeably slimmer during this time.

Ed's first neurological symptoms were exhibited on the evening of December 25th, when we noticed that he was pacing around the house restlessly but pausing frequently to check the time on different clocks around the house. His explanation was that he kept losing track of time. This phase stopped after a couple of hours, after which he went back to sitting quietly on a sofa, which he had been doing more frequently during the preceding weeks. He had stopped eating and drinking freely a few days before this, needing to be prompted to finish his meals, and had commented on his mouth filling up with mucous at the same time, which we attributed to draining sinuses. Ed had previously been eating and drinking with gusto. He had been learning to cook, had no aversion to any foods and had an omnivorous diet, including occasional wild game in his early years.

December 26th was less eventful, though Ed remained lethargic. We took him to our regular health clinic on the first day it was open, December 27th, and the GP prescribed Biaxin antibiotic for what he considered to be a "terrible sinus infection."

A return visit on December 30th showed significant improvement, and we left that afternoon to visit Ed's grandparents four hours drive away, near Calgary.

On December 31st, after a modest amount of physical activity outside in snowy but dry conditions, he began to feel nauseous and went inside, but after an hour he began to vomit. This continued until he was taken to emergency at a Calgary hospital three hours later, where he was rapidly diagnosed with a small pneumothorax (presumably due to the vomiting). Most alarmingly, he had blood sodium levels of 166 mmol/L, though his potassium levels were in the normal range. He was transferred to Alberta Children's Hospital in Calgary for a week, with his sodium levels being gradually brought down to normal levels by the end of the week. No underlying cause was found for his electrolyte imbalance. He was admitted at about 100 lbs, but climbed to nearer 110 within a few days. He received three days of IV antibiotics. Near the end of this week, he began to show a slight twisting motion of his head when he tried to read; he did not ever read books on his own even though reading had previously been his favorite pastime. His discharge summary was that he had idiopathic hypernatraemia (unexplained unusual blood salt concentrations).

When Ed returned to Edmonton upon his release from hospital in Calgary on January 7th, his most noticeable symptom was fatigue, though he also had prominent, contracted neck muscles. He continued to have strong but intermittent headaches. He returned to school three days later, in response to medical advice that it was best to get him back into a stimulating environment. By the end of the week, however, it became clear that his ability to read and focus was continuing to decline. He was able to read very slowly, with continuous prompting, and invariably showed some twisting of his head at the same time. He described the problem as getting stuck on words, which was helped by using head motions to force his eyes to move forward on the line.

He was admitted to the local children's research hospital in Edmonton on January 14th. Neurological examination resulted in a diagnosis that he was suffering either from conversion syndrome (a controversial, purely psychological condition in which mental trauma is expressed physiologically) or from an autoimmune reaction, such as PANDAS, though no sign of a strep infection was later found. Consequently, he was given intravenous immunoglobulin, but almost immediately his blood pressure plummeted to 60/38. He hovered near that level for several hours even though the IV IG injection was stopped soon after his blood pressure initially declined. During this physiological crisis, we as Ed's parents were each, separately and sternly reprimanded by a resident for apparently creating his condition by being overanxious. The next day Ed was put on IV steroids for three days. He remained profoundly lethargic for most of that period.

During Ed's second hospital visit, we discovered that he had serious problems in doing any visual puzzles, and he appeared to have virtually no ability to read silently to himself. However when he was asked to read out loud he was able to do so fluently for multiple pages, though he eventually had to stop because of fatigue. He was released on January 19th. His discharge summary from hospital in Edmonton stated he had obsessive compulsive disorder and possible Tourette's. However, two visits to a psychiatrist shortly after his release produced a strong statement that his condition was not due to OCD or any other psychiatric illness.

Ed remained at home in the care of his mother and did not return to school during the ensuing 4 weeks. His ability to read seemed to decline through February to the point where he found it painfully difficult and exhausting to read out loud to the end of a paragraph. He read out several words at one time, and these were interspersed by a minute or so of circular motions with his hand (a motion that replaced his earlier head twisting). In early February, he took a battery of cognitive tests from a clinical psychologist, which showed that he had high intelligence but seriously diminished processing speed and ability to perform sequential operations. Throughout January and February, he experienced numerous periods of low blood pressure and low peripheral body temperature. However he was able to go on short walks (less than 1 km) and showed no balance problems even when walking in icy conditions. He needed to be spoon fed some of the time, but could dress himself slowly and go to the bathroom independently. He was kept stimulated by listening to the radio or books on tape, by regular visits with his grandparents at the end of the street, and by the normal household disruptions caused by his siblings. Throughout this period, Ed kept optimistically estimating that he would be largely recovered in about two weeks, which was in keeping with his generally positive and persistent nature.

Beginning in early March, his condition seemed to improve slightly. On the advice of doctors, he returned to school for one class per day, though he still had serious problems reading even a paragraph. On even days he attended a help session for a distance learning class in Social Studies. His lessons were read to him by a sympathetic teacher's aide and he was encouraged to read small sections for himself. On odd days he sat in on a lecture or discussion in the same Social Studies class that he would have taken with his original class cohort. Other students seemed to be uniformly sympathetic and supportive. During this period we discovered that he was able to write things out by hand fairly well, as long as he did not read what he was writing. We started to go on longer walks of 2–4 km every 2 or 3 days, during which Ed seemed to be sure footed, showed stamina (albeit with an oddly rapid pace at the start of each walk), and took pride in keeping ahead of his father. However, he remained completely indecisive whenever asked what direction he wanted to walk, and got lost easily.

In order to provide support as well as to respond to apparent pigeon-holing as OCD by hospital staff, Ed began visits with a private psychologist in early April. Visits continued on a monthly basis, after an initial 2 week interval. The psychologist was supportive, and unambiguously stated from the beginning that the underlying problem was neurological, not psychiatric.

In early April, Ed was able to compose short but lucid and grammatically correct essays of up to a page in length for his school work. At this time, all his symptoms started to improve more rapidly and in parallel. On about April 11th, he started to eat entire meals with only minor prompting at the start of the meal, instead of needing to be prompted for every mouthful. He also would usually go to the bathroom, or put on his clothes, and return without getting stalled. He no longer seemed to accumulate as much saliva in his mouth. By Friday April 22nd he seemed to have made a 70% recovery (estimate of parents) of his previously high energy levels, academic performance, and good humor.

On April 23rd, Ed was woken up complaining of fatigue and mental fogginess. Overnight, he had apparently reverted to the condition he had in February. There was no evident change in diet or stress levels. He seemed to have caught a cold virus, which some of his other siblings also came down with at that time, though his cold symptoms did not seem particularly pronounced. On the next Monday, his ability to read and to interact with his teacher's aide was also obviously greatly diminished. In the following weeks, his abilities continued to decline, which he found to be profoundly disheartening. He continued to be able to walk strongly during this period but, ominously, he started to occasionally exhibit sudden, transient halts in mid stride. When questioned about it, he had no explanation.

He was buoyed up briefly during May 16–19, during a previously scheduled period of day admission to the university hospital in order to facilitate his examination by a series of specialists in multiple medical disciplines. For one day in this time, he was able to partially feed himself without assistance. Nonetheless, in spite of an MRI, EEG, and examination by endocrinologists, neurologists, and specialists in infectious diseases and metabolic diseases, all tests returned results fully within the normal scale. One endocrinologist insisted that psychiatric problems were the most likely explanation, and the final discharge, by a neurologist, provided no summary statement or recommendations. Ed was particularly exhausted and demoralized when he returned home after the last day.

In late May, Ed lost the ability to open his school locker before going to class, even though he had had few difficulties with this task for the previous two months. Earlier in May, he started to consistently get disoriented as to what day it was and where to go in his school. This culminated with him getting caught up outside his locker on May 27th, unable to go forward or backward or even aware of the problem, while his teacher's aide waited upstairs for him for 80 minutes and eventually hundreds of students streamed by him in the hall during the break.

Now at the end of July, Ed still has periods of substantial declines in blood pressure and peripheral body temperature. These seem to have no clear correlation with any triggering conditions, although onset commonly occurs after he eats a meal. These symptoms appear to have declined over time, though it is hard to tell whether the improvement, compared to February, is due to substantially warmer summer weather conditions. Early in his illness, he had a strong mottled red flush on his cheeks, particularly back toward his ears but not below the eyes. This has declined gradually but remains noticeable.

Throughout his illness, Ed has remained verbally articulate, with no slurring of words, or syntax problems. He has some difficulty in finding words and his speech has slowed. Moreover he speaks only when spoken to, and most responses are monosyllabic, though he has no problem with complex answers or logically well-formulated responses when there is strong stimulation. From the beginning, he has expressed a strong aversion to eating or drinking, and says that he has no hunger at all. Apparently food has no appeal even when he has not eaten for extended periods, even though he claims that he has no problem in tasting differences.

He has been enrolled since early June in Pilates exercises and piano once per week. He seems to be learning chords well in the piano lessons though he tires rapidly. He continues to be competent in ping pong, with an instinctively fast reaction time, but cannot keep track of the score. Since late March, he has also visited once per week with an older friend who is a demonstrator in physics, while teaching labs are being set up. Ed's enthusiasm for this meeting has always been high, which is not surprising because this is the kind of thing in which he has taken the greatest pleasure ever since he was very young. However, he became much more passive in May and may be showing a slowly declining ability to keep up conceptually. His walks with family members became impractical in early June, when the frequency of his halt-walking increased to the point where it was happening every few steps. He has recently started to twist his head or upper body from side to side when he is standing for extended periods of time. He sometimes fidgets and taps his feet repetitively when he is left alone, although this is of less concern because he commonly did that before his illness.

In the year prior to Ed's health problems, he spent the first 8 months of 2004 in Canberra, Australia, with several weeks camping in numerous locations ranging from South Australia to Queensland. The only health issues noticed during this period were recurring sinus inflammation. Throughout his life, Ed spent a moderate amount of recreational time outdoors with his family, including Alberta (western Canada) during 1999-2004, California during 1994–1999, and Ontario or upstate New York during 1989-1994.

During the past 7 months, Ed has been examined by more than 30 medical specialists, mainly at the local university children's hospital. He has not been on any medication since his hospital stays in January, other than antibiotics for another sinus infection in February. Apparently his endocrine levels are normal, and he shows no signs of an elevated immune response. He had MRIs in January and May, and an EEG in May, which were deemed normal. He tested negative for Huntington's Disease, and did not have elevated copper levels (Wilson's disease). We are unclear what tests for pathogens have been performed; and the response to our repeated questions about the possibility of Lyme Disease or Western Equine Encephalitis was that the timing and nature of Ed's symptoms made these exceedingly unlikely. Prions (nvCJD) were considered a possibility, but no tests were performed and permission was never granted by the hospital for a tonsilar biopsy because of unspecified ethics concerns. One complicating factor in Ed's condition is that he is at his most alert when he is meeting people for the first time, such as at a medical examination, whereas he soon thereafter seems more exhausted and unresponsive than ever. However, by this time his condition is not visible to medical personnel.

No consensus has emerged, either for a diagnosis or a treatment plan. Medical opinions have varied from Ed's condition being primarily psychiatric (conversion syndrome, or obsessive compulsive disorder), an autoimmune reaction (PANDAS, ADEM, or Sydenham's Chorea), an unspecified mitochondrial metabolic disorder, or post-infection damage to the basal ganglia. Each opinion has had at least one other conflicting opinion, and it is notable that a psychiatrist and psychologist each expressed strong opinions that Ed's condition was primarily neurological and not psychiatric, whereas most neurologists have favored psychiatric diagnoses while others have reserved their opinions.

We are desperate to find something that might reverse our son's decline. Our wonderfully bright, considerate, and courageous boy is slipping away as his medical care goes around in circles. Is there a chance that his condition can be reversed, such as by treating a previously undetected pathogen with antibiotics? If we put him on a round of L-dopamine, as suggested by one doctor as an "exploratory" measure, would we be putting him on a one-way conveyor belt with a Russian roulette ending (as implied by Oliver Sacks' book *Awakenings*)?

Does anyone have ideas on how we can possibly help our son—please!?

December 2005: Increasing conflict while time runs out.

In response to our plea for diagnostic advice at the end of July 2005, friends and colleagues kept presenting Lyme disease as a possibility. When we started to pay more attention to this idea during the fall we were perplexed by the depth of resistance to it. We had been trained as researchers, albeit as entomologists who were more interested in the physiological and genetic diversity of insects than with humans. The following is how we perceived the situation when we provided a description of our son's case to a prominent law professor who was a leading scholar in the area of health law. By December 2005, Ed's condition had reached its lowest point, and our frustrations had peaked. We were desperately worried that we would lose our son, and we could not accept the consistently dismissive responses by medical specialists with whom we were trying to discuss Ed's condition.

Over the year prior to December, Edward's health had deteriorated to the point where he was in a zombie-like state and needed continuous assistance to perform even the most simple actions. Throughout this time, we had been dealing with doctors at the local children's hospital who seemed to have decided in the first week that his illness was either psychiatric or completely out of their realm and not worth treating. Meanwhile, we gathered supporting evidence that he had Lyme disease, and we tried desperately to get doctors to take this diagnosis seriously. We remained open to alternate diagnoses; however continued inaction was not an option while our son's condition continued to deteriorate. We were now seeking to either ensure appropriate treatment locally or to get access to sympathetic and knowledgeable medical treatment outside of Alberta.

Ed was now 16 years old and prior to this illness he had rarely had any kind of health problem. He had always been very bright and mentally stable. When he first got sick with a serious sinus infection late in 2004, it seemed quite unremarkable for him to be treated with antibiotics by our family doctor. After his physiological crisis with low sodium, we had returned to Edmonton with instructions to see a particular pediatrician at the local children's hospital within a week if we had any further concerns. We phoned this doctor repeatedly because we feared potential brain damage since Ed couldn't read without moving his head. He had strange writhing and jerking movements and was drooling. But we were told by the pediatrician to go to the nearest shopping mall to see an optometrist. As surprising as this response was, it became clear over the following months that it indicated a widespread attitude by the doctors at this hospital.

Eventually (January 14, 2005) we were able to see a different doctor, who admitted Edward for investigation. When he suffered a drastic drop in his blood pressure after being given intravenous immunoglobulin, he was given steroids to depress his immune system. At discharge, Edward was diagnosed as having an unspecified tic disorder (a reference to nervous tics, not arthropod ticks) by a specialist trained in infectious diseases and another trained in neurology. A week later, a psychiatrist disagreed strongly with this diagnosis and sent us back for further investigation. Another neurologist then diagnosed conversion syndrome and sent Ed back to the psychiatrist who again disagreed. For the next 6 months Ed was batted back and forth between the physiological and mental health doctors. During this time we asked a private psychologist to examine Ed, and he was emphatic that Ed was suffering from a neurological rather than a psychiatric condition.

During February, Edward was given oral antibiotics for three weeks to treat an apparent resumption of his serious sinus problems. This was the only medical treatment that any doctors would give him between mid January and November 2005. During late March and throughout the month of April, Ed's condition slowly improved to the point where he was able to read laboriously and to feed himself. However in the last few days of April his condition declined precipitously again over a period of just a few days and then gradually worsened so that in a few weeks he was as bad as he had been in late January. Ed was examined again by a series of doctors at the local children's hospital in mid May, but was discharged without a treatment plan and with only a vague diagnosis of neurological degeneration. No doctors seemed willing or able to help, though there was no shortage of opinions that implied that the situation was either psychological (Edward or his parents) or too mysterious to fathom. To our horror, more than one doctor suggested that the mystery would be cleared up upon autopsy.

After seven months of getting passed from one doctor to another, with numerous contradicting opinions, the original psychiatrist admitted Edward to another hospital for three weeks in August in order to more definitively evaluate potential psychiatric diagnoses. At the end of this period, he stated that he did not believe that Ed's medical problems were psychiatric in origin.

Throughout Ed's illness, we repeatedly asked his doctors whether it might be possible that he had an infectious disease like West Nile Virus, Western Equine Encephalitis, and especially Lyme disease. We were repeatedly told that it was not worth following up on those potential diagnoses, even though we had just returned from eight months in Australia, and had also lived in areas like California where we had removed potentially infected ticks from Ed when we were camping. Eventually, we became more insistent that Lyme disease should be taken more seriously. It became clear that all the doctors at the local children's hospital were part of a camp that believes that Lyme disease does not exist in Alberta or perhaps even Canada. We were also told that he must have contracted his illness in Alberta since there had been too long a period between a possible exposure to Lyme or any other diseases outside of Alberta and the time that Ed fell ill.

Nonetheless, we insisted that the possibility should be considered, and Edward saw a specialist in infectious diseases at the local children's hospital on August 30th. She stated that she was willing to request an ELISA and Western Blot for Lyme disease although she was certain that this was not Lyme disease. We did not receive any further communication from her until November 3.

Eventually, a pediatrician at a third hospital checked the Western Blots on the computer system and discovered that they were negative. Knowing that the Lyme ELISA is notoriously inaccurate, we flew to Victoria, B.C., on October 22 to meet with Dr. E. Murakami, who had treated many cases of Lyme disease. He believed that Edward had Lyme disease based on his clinical experience. He ordered tests for co-infections with Lyme disease and was surprised to receive a phone call a few days later from the Alberta provincial lab saying that the *Babesia* test (a co-infection) was suspicious. We then received a phone call from the infectious diseases doctor to discuss Edward's case, since she had heard from a colleague who was also one of our neighbors that we had taken Ed to Dr. Murakami. She said her receptionist had been asked to book a follow up appointment but had not gotten around to it. Her opinion was that *Babesia* only caused a mild and self limiting disease and there was no evidence of anything else, after which our discussion over the phone deteriorated. On November 8th, one day after our frustrating conversation with this infectious diseases doctor, we got a requisition from a sympathetic family doctor for blood to be drawn from Ed. We had it sent at our own expense to a highly rated lab, IGeneX, which tests for Lyme and associated diseases in California.

After it became clear that the specialist in infectious diseases who had seen him on August 30th would not grant Ed another appointment, a different infectious diseases doctor agreed to see Edward on November 14th, The second ID specialist reluctantly allowed a trial of doxycycline with the comment that it was equivalent to giving a teenager antibiotics for acne. She stated that she was sure that Ed's condition was not Lyme disease, even though we cited research studies that had found low doxycycline doses to be ineffective for treating Chronic Lyme disease (which Ed's condition would have become due to the lack of treatment for at least a year). We agreed to this treatment because we hoped that it would at least halt his continued deterioration.

Four days after starting doxycycline in mid November, Ed became very ill and suffered extremely low blood pressure much like he experienced in late December and early January. Although it was quite worrisome, this condition was nonetheless consistent with a reaction known to be typical in antibiotic treatment of Lyme borrelioses, called a Jarisch-Herxheimer reaction, which is considered by many Lyme-literate doctors to be strong evidence for the existence of Lyme disease. When we told the doctor about Edward's reaction to the doxycycline, she did not consider it to be medically significant, implying that she was dubious that Herxheimer reactions even occur in Lyme disease.

On November 29th we found that IGeneX had returned to our family physician a positive Lyme disease result for IgM on a Western Blot and a borderline positive on the IgG component. However, a second *Babesia* test that was ordered in Alberta by the ID specialist was delayed many weeks and came back as negative.

Consequently, by December we believed that Ed suffered from a *Borrelia* (= Lyme disease) infection which he acquired either in North America or Australia. This was supported by 1) Ed's symptoms, 2) Dr. Murakami's clinical diagnosis, 3) the Herxheimer reaction, and 4) IGeneX test results. He may also have had *Babesia* (a common co-infection with *Borrelia*) which he could have acquired in Australia, with the *Babesia* testing weakly positive because only North American strains were tested.

We anticipated continued recalcitrance on the part of the local children's hospital doctors in spite of the positive test result from IGeneX, and so we contacted an Edmonton MLA, to help us be taken more seriously. His people contacted a senior administrator at the children's hospital who interceded on our behalf. Very reluctantly, the second ID doctor agreed to put Ed on a two week round of IV antibiotics, which he started on December 12th. But we were aware of published research that showed that two weeks of IV antibiotics often was not nearly enough to cure Chronic

Lyme disease. The crux of the problem was that if Edward really had Lyme disease, then he probably needed several months of antibiotics, not just two weeks. In retrospect, it was likely that his brief period of partial recovery in March and April was due to the antibiotics he got in February, and that the *Borrelia* that cause Lyme resurged at the end of April. However the infectious diseases doctor treating Ed in early December 2008 was at most willing to extend the IV treatment from two weeks to 28 days, but was very clear in saying that she would not extend it beyond that.

We tried for a full year to work with the doctors at the local children's hospital but by the end of 2005 our frustrations overwhelmed us. We had come full circle back to one of the doctors who made the original psychiatric diagnoses that colored the opinions of subsequent doctors. This infectious diseases doctor was resistant to our interpretation of Ed's behaviour as well as to considering any objective data such as blood pressure readings. For example she neglected to order blood tests before, during, or after Ed started taking doxycycline. The antibiotics that Ed did get were viewed as a palliative measure in response to strong parental and administrative pressure, not a serious medical intervention.

We didn't understand why the doctors at the local children's hospital were so resistant to a diagnosis of Lyme disease. No one offered any positive treatment plans, and we had been the only ones to come up with a plausible explanation for Edward's completely disabling condition. In numerous interactions with doctors, we were told to "relax," "let nature take its course," or "be glad you have other children," leaving us with the overwhelming implication that these doctors expected him to die. They didn't really know what the medical problem was, but they seemed to want to keep some connection with his case in the eventuality that an interesting autopsy result came out of it and they could write up a research paper. They were clearly not considering the circumstances from the stance of trying to maximize Edward's chances of recovery. The risk of adverse effects from antibiotic treatment were minor compared to the disabling condition that Edward now suffered, but all the doctors we dealt with were reluctant to give him the kind of treatment that would maximize the chances of his recovery as recommended by Lyme experts. Instead it appeared that the doctors at the local children's hospital were more interested in upholding each other's psychiatric diagnoses than reading up on Lyme disease. When we asked for clarification, the only response was that they were following minimal CDC guidelines for a disease that they didn't believe Edward had.

This left us with a plea to a prominent health lawyer for any way that he could help us through this complicated mess so that we could continue to get appropriate medical treatment for our son. Was our main alternative to go deeply in debt and split up our family by moving Ed to a place where there were Lyme-literate doctors?

2006 and 2007: A slow return to health

Upon meeting with us, the law professor's immediate and generous response was to write a formal letter informing the pertinent hospital that he was taking on our case. Privately, he told us that he appreciated being able to make a constructive contribution to a legal case before a tragedy had run its course, while there still was some opportunity to truly help the patient.

The response by the local children's hospital was to assign us to a senior administrator. With her mediation, Edward's care was transferred to another pediatrician. A temporary IV line was installed in Ed's arm, and for three agonizing months, with us making a new case for continued treatment every couple of weeks, Ed's condition slowly started to improve.

We took hope from knowing about a case in British Columbia where a Lyme patient received IV antibiotics for three months before her condition made a more dramatic improvement. More fundamentally, we took refuge in the simple logic that, of all the dire diagnoses that Ed had been offered, including MS, Parkinson's, and a variety of immunological and genetic meltdowns like ALS and Huntington's, only Lyme borreliosis truly offered hope of a sustained recovery. Between the certainty of death and a very small chance of success, it was only reasonable to treat for the disease where the treatment would make a difference rather than to assume that the condition was due to alternatives that provide no hope.

Instead we were offered a variety of counter arguments. The first and most persistently proffered was that "excessive" use of antibiotics would breed antibiotic resistance. It is a fine argument if the main consideration is to reduce costs due to long term antibiotics. But it requires that we as a society accept that some proportion of patients will die for the sake of the extending the useful life of a particular antibiotic, even though that antibiotic might have saved the patient. In practice even animal breeders have not followed this advice, instead releasing tonnes of antibiotics into the environment in animal feed, meat products, or farm effluent. The real test is whether the doctors concerned would deny their own children antibiotics under the same conditions, and we never got a straight answer when we posed the question that way.

The second objection was that Lyme borreliosis is very rare in Alberta and really not worth investing energy into pursuing. It is a valid approach when a disease first presents—a reasonable doctor will start by investigating the most prevalent diagnoses that will explain the symptoms. But it is not reasonable after the most likely prior explanations have been eliminated, since under these conditions a rare illness becomes increasingly more likely as the more common illnesses are removed as explanations. As Sir Arthur Conan Doyle had Sherlock Holmes say, once you have eliminated the impossible, whatever remains, however improbable, must be true. But we were amazed that more than one medical specialist clung to a repetition of the statement that Lyme borreliosis was vanishingly rare in Alberta and the diagnosis therefore could not apply.

A third objection was that none of the accepted tick vectors were known to be established in Alberta, or that an onset of illness in late November implied too long an incubation period for it to have been tick-borne. Here we were on firm ground, as entomologists, but that didn't seem to give us much credibility. We knew that *Ixodes* ticks belonging to undoubtedly competent vector species had occasionally been found in Alberta, both on birds and on humans. It is also quite normal for ticks to bite in late September or October, and that initial symptoms like the characteristic bulls-eye rash may be missed or simply not manifested. All of this assumed that Ed contracted his illness in Alberta, but we had been in tropical Australia in late August. There is also ample evidence that Lyme and many other bacterial infections can have a relatively latent period of months or even years, and so our residency in Lyme endemic areas of the US was relevant. But all this was deemed too far-fetched to be worth considering, with vague psychiatric diagnoses made by non-psychiatrists being the main alternatives that were offered.

A fourth objection to the possibility of Lyme, held up as irrefutable by various specialists, was that the Canadian tests had definitively shown that Ed did not have Lyme. The problem there was that we were able to find a great deal of peer-reviewed research literature that demonstrated a dismal rate of false negatives for those tests even when they were performed at fully accredited institutions. Other studies documented a substantial amount of genetic diversity in *Borrelia* genotypes across North America. These studies carried the logical corollary that genetic diversity in disease causing organisms can be expected to lead to variation in diagnostic effectiveness if, as is the case for Lyme, the accredited diagnostic tests were standardized on the basis of a single strain from the eastern USA. An additional wild card was the suite of other kinds of bacteria or even viruses that routinely are co-transmitted with *Borrelia* when a tick bites. Pathogens such as *Babesia*, *Bartonella* and *Ehrlichia* can have synergistic effects with *Borrelia* but may need to be treated with completely different antibiotics. However when we made these counterarguments, fully supported by research literature, we were usually summarily written off. Most doctors simply don't have the time or the training to think about diseases that don't fit predefined boxes. Holistic diagnoses that require an integrated understanding of statistical probability and biological diversity are more conveniently referred to a "soft" specialty like psychiatry.

Meanwhile, as spring 2006 spread its warmth in Edmonton, a miracle started to unfold. Ed's IV antibiotics were stopped, with our agreement, in mid March, but he continued on oral antibiotics both for *Borrelia* and *Babesia,* under the care of a supportive psychiatrist. In early May, Ed's rate of improvement accelerated, but his involuntary halting continued into June, with a brief but alarming reversal in early July. Problems with jerky coordination continued through to the end of 2006, though he was able to start school again full time in September.

A strange set of stretch marks appeared in July 2006, spreading over large parts of Ed's back and shoulders in the ensuing months. Only when we stumbled across images of *Bartonella*-infected patients with red stripes almost identical to those on Ed, did we have any clue what the cause might be. Within two weeks of starting antibiotics for *Bartonella* in mid December, Ed's brothers were remarking how much "less flippy" his motions seemed, and he continued to improve incrementally during the next year, 2007, although his stretch marks took much longer to fade. It seems too incredible to be true, and yet it is well established that a single tick can contain two or three or even more kinds of pathogens. Nor did Ed necessarily get everything that made him sick from one tick or even during one narrow period of time. The fact is that, when he was eventually treated as if he had Lyme borreliosis, he got better in a manner that was consistent with him having been infected by *Borrelia*. When he was subsequently treated as if he had also acquired other tick-borne bacterial infections, his health improved even more. Eventually, it took until the end of 2007 before the cloud seemed to fully lift from Ed's brow.

In addition to a few beleaguered health professionals who stood by Ed within the medical system (most of whom prefer not to have attention drawn to their courageous, peer-disapproved actions), he received excellent support from a devoted teacher's aide (Rita Fraser) within a supportive Edmonton public school system, an innovative exercise facility for disabled patients (the Steadward Center at the University of Alberta), a patient music teacher, a substantial extended family, a full time mother, and a father's medical benefits plan that absorbed most of the financial costs. But it took all of these, along with his own natural resilience, to pull through. Not many other Lyme sufferers have had the same advantages, and have ended up losing their homes, their families, and eventually most remnants of a normal life.

Wouldn't it be so much more humane—and cost effective—if our medical establishment were to take Lyme borreliosis seriously in the first place?

2008 and onward: Can we fix the machine?

In June 2008, Ed finished high school, having lost only a year because he had support during his illness and was able to catch up once his health returned. During the summer, he went off to French language school in Quebec for five weeks with his next younger brother. He returned happy, healthy, and ready to plunge into the rigors of first year engineering, which he passed a year later with a solid array of A's and B's. Understandably, he became increasingly more reluctant to be identified as "that kid who had Lyme," preferring to immerse himself in designing and building racing cars as part of an engineering club.

For us as Ed's parents, however, there was a sense of unfinished business. During the period of Ed's recovery, Dr. Murakami was forced into retirement through the stress of continued investigations by the B.C. College of Physicians and Surgeons. One of the most public medical advocates of Lyme patients in Canada had been removed. We had been fortunate to be able to get support from Dr. Murakami and a few other sympathetic medical people, most of whom were limited in what they could do because infectious diseases were not their specialty. We were also able to use our own research training, our contacts, and our knowledge of the system to help our son recover in spite of a medical system that was divided against itself. But adherents to the dominant medical opinion were willing, for various ideological reasons, to let patients like Ed perish. What could rural patients or First Nations people do to help themselves if they were suffering from Lyme? After all they are far more likely to be exposed to ticks than city dwellers would be. How could we even know if dozens of people have not already died of Lyme borreliosis in Alberta? Between flawed tests and a severe reluctance to even consider the diagnosis, we may never know how many ALS, MS, or Parkinson's deaths might really have had a preventable bacterial origin. It simply didn't seem fair.

The need to help shift the balance of this profoundly wrong situation has offered a kind of therapy for us that has helped us to cope with some horrific memories. Janet began to get increasingly more involved with the Canadian Lyme Disease Foundation, a group that advocates for greater investment in Lyme disease research in Canada. She has participated in rallies in Ottawa, met several times with the

Deputy Minister of Health and Wellness in Manitoba, organized a Lyme Wall of Hope in Edmonton, successfully elicited a private member's statement on Lyme Disease in the Alberta Legislature (K. Taft, November 20, 2008), and written briefs to health authorities across Canada (e.g. Appendix 1 and 2). The two of us have coauthored a peer-reviewed overview of Lyme borreliosis in Canada from the viewpoint of entomologists. Felix has shifted the focus of his lab to include the population genetics and evolution of ticks in Alberta. Much work is left before our understanding of Lyme borreliosis is on a solid footing in Canada.

Much of that unfinished work lies in translating research results into policy that allows effective diagnoses and treatment of a complex disease like Lyme in spite of a variety of constraining factors like institutional inertia and incomplete medical certainty. To illustrate this point, Appendix 1 and 2 below are emails sent by Janet Sperling to British Columbia public health authorities to support more flexible consideration of clinical diagnoses of Lyme disease. In spite of a polite acknowledgement of receipt, accompanied by the statement that a reply would be forthcoming shortly, no response or refutation has ever been received. The same brief has also been submitted by Lyme patient advocates to the Federal Public Health Agency, again without anything more than an acknowledgement of receipt.

Conclusion

So we end on an optimistic note, even though the saga remains unfinished. Considering the alternatives, Lyme really is a diagnosis of hope when it is the most treatable disease among grim alternatives. After a period of panic and confusion, we were able to concentrate on doing whatever it took to provide our son Ed with treatment that ultimately had few differences from the long term antibiotic regimes widely accepted for bacterial diseases like tuberculosis. When he was properly treated for Lyme borreliosis, he got better as if he had had the disease. After that, it didn't really matter whether he actually had the particular strains or even species that current Lyme immunological diagnostics are narrowly focused on.

We strongly believe that patient and doctor education can make a positive difference. But effective support and protection are needed for medical practitioners who are willing to try to treat Lyme patients on the basis of flexible clinical judgment. Continued research into the diversity of Lyme, Lyme-like and associated bacteria is sure to pay dividends. In a fundamentally important sense, Lyme disease is also a metaphor for our trying times, as we struggle to simultaneously manage diversity, complexity and change.

Appendix 1: Lyme diagnosis

E-mail letter to British Columbia Deputy Provincial Health Officer, August 2008. I am a member of CanLyme with an interest in peer-reviewed literature on Lyme disease. I am also an entomologist by training and the mother of a now-recovered Lyme victim. My understanding is that you are particularly interested in Lyme research concerning diagnosis and treatment. Here I will deal with the diagnosis of Lyme disease. In my second email, I will cover its treatment.

British Columbia uses a two tier testing protocol that starts with an ELISA. If that is positive then the sample is further tested with a Western Blot before the patient is considered to have tested positive for Lyme disease. If the ELISA is negative, a Western Blot is rarely attempted. The rigid interpretation of these tests is what we are challenging.

The ELISA is a first step that is generally considered more sensitive than the Western Blot; however numerous reports contradict this (Cordoliani et al 1997, Evans et al 2005, Harrer et al 2007, Mantovani et al 2007). An ELISA is a more economical test to run and is more easily automated than a Western Blot, which presumably explains the use of an ELISA as an initial screening test.

The CDC criteria (MMWR 1995 44: 590–591) for interpreting Lyme disease Western Blots are used in British Columbia as well as by the CDC in Washington. The problem is that the criteria are both too specific and not specific enough.

The criteria for interpretation of the Western Blot are based on two serotypes of *Borrelia*, strain G39/40 (Dressler et al 1993) and strain 297 (Engstrom et al 1995), which do not reflect the extensive and well documented diversity of strains found in North America (Bunikis et al 2004). The choice of strains G39/40 and 297 is especially perplexing since they are considered to be non-infectious strains (Coburn et al 1994) and G39/40 is rarely referenced in later work. These criteria, established at a conference in 1994, were designed to produce a statistically relevant pattern of banding. Yet they specifically exclude both Osp A and Osp B (Dressler et al 1993) even though these bands are highly informative, so much so that Osp A was chosen as a target for vaccine development (Bergstrom et al 2002). Since the criteria include cross reacting proteins such as flagellin, but exclude more strain specific proteins such as Osp A and Osp B, it is possible in British Columbia to have a banding pattern that includes Osp A, Osp B, and flagellin proteins and still be considered negative for Lyme disease. Flagellin proteins may cross-react with other spirochetes but I am not aware of cross reacting proteins for either Osp A or Osp B.

Current commercial test kits generally rely on strain B31, a strain that is highly associated with the arthritis form of Lyme and not neuroborreliosis (Assous et al 1993). In Table 4 of Aguero-Rosenfeld et al (2005) they indisputably demonstrate that circular logic is involved in Lyme Disease diagnosis using the two-tier approach. Their Table 4 shows only 38% sensitivity (early EM) to 87% (early neuroborreliosis) to 97% with Lyme arthritis. Thus the two-tier approach is skewed to favor a restricted view of Lyme disease. It is circular logic to state that Lyme arthritis can be detected in 97% of cases and that therefore Lyme arthritis is the main manifestation of Lyme disease, since the test was designed using the arthritic form of Lyme in the first place. This doesn't help people with early Lyme or those with neuroborreliosis, and these are the people who come to CanLyme desperate for help because their ELISA did not pick up 13% or more of these real Lyme cases.

In Europe, where multiple strains of Lyme disease are acknowledged, Western Blots are interpreted differently. A positive result can be based on the presence of 2 or 3 bands for a specific series of proteins for *Borrelia burgdorferi*. At no point are 5 bands required for a positive result (Robertson et al 2000).

In Brazil a positive Western Blot is defined as 4 bands for IgG, 2 for IgM or 2 IgG associated with one IgM. Significant positive clinical response to antibiotics has been documented for patients who exhibit the reduced number of bands (Mantovani et al 2007). Their condition is termed a 'Lyme Disease-like syndrome' because of the fewer number of Western Blot bands than the strict CDC definition for Lyme. Consequently, in Brazil, the diagnosis of Lyme Disease is made based on the clinical picture and serology is only used as supporting evidence.

Another recent article that shows that the best diagnosis of Lyme disease is clinical is Pavan (2002) who concludes that the diagnosis of LB is mainly clinical, while laboratory testing is a valid help but insufficient to make a diagnosis (and listing 9 references to support his statement).

On the other hand, some authors of the Infectious Diseases Society of America's guidelines for the treatment of Lyme disease represent an extremely restrictive view of Lyme Disease and state that neuroborreliosis is self-limited in most patients even without antibiotic treatment (Wormser and Halperin 2008). This stance trivializes the suffering of our members, and is only weakly supported by two older references from 1983 and 1990. This view is not supported by any peer reviewed treatment guidelines. Antibiotic treatment to differing degrees is recommended in all peer reviewed guidelines as I will demonstrate in my next email. The attitude of these vocal and influential IDSA practitioners has resulted in considerable suffering from undiagnosed and untreated Lyme disease in British Columbia.

We at CanLyme believe that many desperately ill British Columbians are suffering from a treatable illness. The peer reviewed literature, when examined from the perspective of empirical success when a clinical diagnosis is given, clearly shows that the use of serology to diagnose Lyme disease is an inexact art. The use of negative serology to deny a Lyme disease diagnosis, the current standard in British Columbia, is highly inappropriate. We are dealing with many serologically and genetically distinct strains of a putatively single disease that has correspondingly diverse manifestations ranging from mild to severe.

In short, the current tests for Lyme disease are inadequate. We strongly advocate diagnosis on the basis of clinical symptoms, supported but not limited by testing that takes into account the serological diversity of *Borrelia*, as well as any associated diseases.

References

Aguero-Rosenfeld ME, Wang G, Schwartz I, Wormser GP. 2005. Diagnosis of Lyme Borreliosis. *Clinical Microbiology Reviews* 18: 484-509.

Assous MV, Postic D, Paul G, Nevot P, Baranton G. 1993. Western Blot Analysis of Sera from Lyme Borreliosis Patients According to the Genomic Species of the *Borrelia* Strains Used as Antigens. *European Journal of Clinical Microbiology and Infectious Disease.* 12: 261-268.

Bergstrom S, Noppa L, Gylfe A, Ostberg,Y. 2002. Molecular and Cellular Biology of Borrelia burgdorferi sensu lato. Chapter 3 pages 47–90 in *Lyme Borreliosis: Biology, Epidemiology and Control* (eds J Gray, O Kahl,R Lane and G. Stanek)

Bunikis J, Garpmo U, Tsao J, Berglund J, Fish D, Barbour AG. 2004. Sequence typing reveals extensive strain diversity of the Lyme borreliosis agents *Borrelia burgdorferi* in North America and *Borrelia afzelii* in Europe. *Microbiology* 150: 1741–1755.

Coburn J, Barthold SW, Leong JM. 1994. Diverse Lyme disease spirochetes bind integrin alpha IIb beta 3 on human platelets. *Infection and Immunity* 62: 5559–5567.

Cordoliani F, Vignon-Pennamen MD, Assous, MV, Vabres P, Dronne P, Rybojad M, Morel P. 1997. Atypical Lyme borreliosis in an HIV-infected man. *British Journal of Dermatology* 37: 437-439.

Dressler F, Whalen JA, Reinhardt BN, Steere AC. 1993. Western blotting in the serodiagnosis of Lyme disease. *The Journal of Infectious Diseases* 167: 392–400.

Engstrom SM, Shoop E, Johnson RC. 1995. Immunoblot interpretation criteria for serodiagnosis of early Lyme disease. *Journal of Clinical Microbiology* 33: 419-27.

Evans R, Mavin S, Ho-Yin D. 2005. Audit of the laboratory diagnosis of Lyme disease in Scotland. *Journal of Medical Microbiology* 54: 1139-41.

Harrer T, Geißdörfer W, Schoerner C, Lang E, Helm G. 2007. Seronegative Lyme neuroborreliosis in a patient on treatment for chronic lymphatic leukemia, *Infection* 35: 110–113.

Heikkilä T, Seppälä I, Saxén H, Panelius J, Peltomaa M, Julin T, Carlsson SA, Lahdenne P. 2002. Recombinant BBK32 protein in serodiagnosis of early and late Lyme borreliosis. *Journal of Clinical Microbiology* 40: 1174–1180.

Mantovani E, Costa IP, Gauditano G, Bonoldi VL, Higuchi, ML, Yoshinari NH. 2007. Description of Lyme disease-like syndrome in Brazil. Is it a new tick-borne disease or Lyme disease variation? *Brazilian Journal of Medical and Biological Research* 40: 443-56.

Oksi J, Nikoskelainen J, Hiekkanen H, Lauhio A, Peltomaa M, Pitkäranta A, Nyman D, Granlund H, Carlsson S-H, Seppälä I, Valtonen V, Viljanen M. 2007. Duration of antibiotic treatment in disseminated Lyme borreliosis: a double-blind, randomized, placebo-controlled, multicenter clinical study. *European Journal of Clinical Microbiology and Infectious Diseases* 26: 571–581

Pavan, WO. 2002. Need of interdisciplinary competence and the role of the Department of Health in the struggle against Lyme borreliosis *ACTA Dermatovenerologica* 11 (1) http://ibmi.mf.uni-lj.si/acta-apa/acta-apa-02-1/pavan.html

Robertson J, Guy E, Andrews N, Wilske B, Anda P, Granstrom M, Hauser U, Moosmann Y, Sambri V, Schellekens J, Stanek G, Gray J. 2000. A European multicenter study of immunoblotting in serodiagnosis of Lyme borreliosis. *Journal of Clinical Microbiology* 38: 2097–2102.

Wormser GP and Halperin JJ. 2008. Oral doxycycline for neuroborreliosis. *The Lancet Neurology* 7: 665-666.

Appendix 2: Lyme disease treatment

Email letter to a BC Deputy Provincial Health Officer, August 2008.

This is the second of two emails describing Lyme disease from the perspective of an entomologist whose son has now made a complete recovery from Lyme disease. My purpose is to demonstrate, based on peer reviewed research publications, that the current treatment of Lyme disease based on IDSA guidelines is inadequate and that a sincere investment in further research is crucial, owing to many unresolved issues relating to long term persistence and co-infections.

Lyme is most successfully treated early in the course of the disease (Cameron et al 2004, Diterich et al 2001, Evison et al 2006, Exner 2004, Vanousova and Hercogova 2008). Conversely, any delay in diagnosis causes increasing challenges in achieving successful treatment. While doctors are understandably reluctant to make a clinical diagnosis for a disease that they have rarely confronted, diagnosis remains problematic throughout the course of the disease (as described in my email on Lyme diagnosis). The fundamental fact remains that early diagnosis and treatment of Lyme can save lives. Our daily newspapers are chronicling the consequences of neglect of the same principle for Listeria.

Dissemination to distant tissues and long term persistence are pathogenic processes found for all major human spirochetal infections (Wormser 2006). Yet in the IDSA Guidelines authored by Wormser et al (2006), only 14–30 days of antibiotic are recommended. Other treatment recommendations for later stages of Lyme range from no antibiotics (Steere et al 1983) to 12 weeks of Ceftriaxone and open ended antibiotics (Harvey and Martz 2007). The most contentious issue in peer reviewed literature is not the early treatment but the endpoint. Acceptance of long term disability is the basis of the current IDSA Guidelines which include a category of 'Post-Lyme Disease Syndromes', an ill defined and progressively disabling constellation of symptoms.

The practice parameter review for neurologists produced by Halperin et al (2007) is instructive. They have chosen to interpret as 'excellent' a response to treatment in which 63% of patients improved, 22% improved but relapsed, and 15% remained unchanged. This left 37% of patients unsatisfied with the outcome of their treatment. A further study used by Halperin et al (2007) to support their point of view states that at post-treatment follow-up, half the patients reported headache and concentration problems. A third study states that 25% of patients assessed 5 years after treatment reported persistent "neurologic" difficulties. Thus a large body of research shows that many patients are not returning to their previous good health, a remarkable result considering that Halperin (2008) claims that the medical establishment has reached consensus over short term treatment of Lyme disease. The clear message for a substantial proportion of Lyme patients is that it is the accepted medical norm to give up on them.

In our experience, many Canadian doctors (Johnston and Conly 2005, Bowie 2007), cite Klempner et al (2001) as the basis to deny treatment of Lyme disease. Yet Cameron's 2006 analysis has unambiguously demonstrated numerous flaws in that study. The Klempner study enrolled the subset of patients who were the most difficult to treat—those who had been ill for several years and had previously failed treatment. Then the trial was halted when no significant difference in health-related quality of life was experienced by patients who received 30 days IV plus 60 days oral antibiotic compared to those receiving a placebo, even though those patients represented a group preselected for their lack of prior response to treatment. No consideration was given to the tautology in the study or the possibility that incomplete prior treatment may have selected for bacterial strains that exhibited resistance to subsequent antibiotic treatments.

Study designs, like Klempner et al (2001), that presuppose a particular narrow definition of Lyme disease and then draw conclusions based on a preselected subset of patients are the norm. In contrast, a study by Oksi et al (2007) enrolled patients with both definite and possible Lyme borreliosis. As with other studies, they reported good or excellent response to extended antibiotic in only 79% of cases, with three weeks of IV followed by 100 days oral penicillin being insufficient to improve the health of 21% of the patients. However, this study not only confirmed the refractory nature of a substantial proportion of Lyme cases, but it demonstrated the existence of seronegative Lyme, a finding that was made possible by enrolling a less restricted subset of patients. Thus it is clear that the results of any study are contingent on the prior definition of Lyme that is used to admit patients into a study, a practice that may increase the chances of confirming a prior hypothesis but one that is not conducive to allowing better treatment or understanding of Lyme disease.

In an even more recent study, Fallon et al (2008) showed that 10 weeks of IV antibiotics resulted in short term cognitive improvement, reduced pain and increased physical functioning. However, the cognitive improvements observed upon cessation of antibiotics were not maintained 24 weeks after commencement of the antibiotic, although improvement in pain and physical functioning was sustained. The fact that 10 weeks of IV did not result in long term cognitive improvement in patients who had previously received IV therapy was taken to suggest that IV therapy did not eradicate the motile form of Lyme in sequestered or immune privileged sites (Fallon et al 2008), and may also be explained by persistence of a cystic form of Lyme disease (Alban et al 2000, Brorson and Brorson 2004, Murgia and Cinco 2006, Brorson and Brorson 2007).

Hodzic et al (2008) used xenodiagnosis in mice to unambiguously demonstrate that *Borrelia burgdorferi* (specifically the N40 strain also known for its virulence in humans) is able to survive and retain its infectivity after three months of antibiotics, especially when treatment was started after the infection was advanced. Hodzic et al (2008) thus convincingly showed that infectious spirochetes are able to survive treatment that was previously assumed to eradicate the motile form of *Borrelia*. Infective spirochetes persisted in various tissues as well as collagen, with collagen being a major niche for both spirochete survival and possibly immune evasion.

In a contrasting interpretation of similar results, Ljøstad et al (2008) compared results of oral doxycycline and IV ceftriaxone in patients who were serologically positive for *B. afzelii,* one of the European variants of Lyme disease. They followed patients for 4 months and reported that 59% of patients had residual symptoms. These results coincided with two other studies that showed that two to five years after treatment 25–59% of patients reported residual symptoms (Berglund et al 2002, Vrethem et al 2002). However, Ljøstad et al (2008) discounted the possibility of bacterial survival and did not back up their interpretation with evidence or references, despite older studies that contradict this stance (Alban et al 2000, Brorson and Brorson 2004, Murgia and Cinco 2006, Brorson and Brorson 2007). This interpretation is further undermined by a recent Hodzic et al (2008) study which shows that *Borrelia* can survive antibiotic levels in excess of those used in any of these studies.

Borrelia are not alone in their ability to survive long term antibiotics. For example, lifelong prophylaxis is recommended for severe rheumatic fever (World Health Organization 2001). Rheumatic fever is similar to Lyme disease in that erythema marginatum, infective arthritis and Sydenham's chorea are major manifestations. The World Health Organization report states: "It is evident from the preceding discussion that the pathogenesis of RF and RHD is a complex maze of events that are immunologically intricate, pathologically significant, and clinically devastating for the patients. It is ironic that a rather innocuous "sore throat" should extract such a high price from the host. As scientific research evolves, it is hoped that the gaps in our understanding will be filled, and better strategies for prophylaxis and treatment will become available." The same can certainly be said for Lyme disease. Other diseases for which long term antibiotic treatment is the accepted norm include, but are certainly not limited to, latent TB (9 months antibiotic—Inge and Wilson 2008), leprosy (12 months of multidrug therapy—World Health Organization 1997) and actinomycosis (IV for 2–6 weeks and 6–12 months of oral antibiotic—Russo 2008). This raises an obvious question: if long term antibiotic treatment is freely accepted for numerous other bacterial diseases, why is it so vigorously opposed by the IDSA for Lyme disease?

In addition to the simple persistence of *Borrelia*, whatever the life form, another complication that can cause Lyme disease to remain refractory to treatment is the presence of co-infections by other bacteria. The fact that late Lyme disease is sometimes associated with treatment failure (Bratton et al 2008, Ogden et al 2008) has resulted in differing approaches to treatment. For example, a Czech treatment protocol for Lyme disease emphasizes the importance of considering co-infections, especially when treatment results in a worsening of symptoms (Vanousova and Hercogova 2008). This principle is also emphasized in the ILADS treatment protocol described in Cameron et al (2004).

A suite of several diseases is commonly associated with borreliosis, and these are often reported simultaneously in the tick vectors (Alekseev and Dubinina 2003, Belongia 2002, Hamer et al 2007, Pichon et al 2006). For example, Eskow et al (2001) have recommended that patients with incomplete resolution of their symptoms should be routinely assessed for evidence of *Bartonella* as a co-infection. Co-infection of *Borrelia* and *Babesia* results in increased severity of arthritis in dogs (Moro 2006). In fact, Harvey and Martz (2007) have postulated that co-infection of *Borrelia* and *Babesia* may cause antibiotic responsive ALS, a disease that is normally considered a death sentence and for which the disadvantages of antibiotics cannot reasonably be considered sufficiently important to deny treatment for the individual. As a further complication, multiple co-infections may result in confusing laboratory results (Walid et al 2007). Consequently, the complexity of Lyme disease and its treatment has led Owen (2006) to suggest that Lyme disease is actually a polymicrobial disease.

Interestingly, the existence of co-infections is much less contentious than is the view that such simultaneous infections may have any influence on each other. For example, although Wormser et al (2006) acknowledge that concurrent infection by *Babesia*, *Anaplasma* and *Borrelia* is possible, they see each disease as a single independent entity. As with Lyme disease, they discount the possibility that testing for co-infections may result in a false negative result or that the infections may be synergistic, especially at the level of the individual patient. In contrast, Diterich et al (2001 and 2003) maintain that the host immune response is modulated by *Borrelia* infection. *Babesia* infections, especially *Babesia microti* are also capable of transient immune suppression (Allred 2003). Telfer et al (2008) have written an excellent review of the impact of co-infecting bacterial or even viral species and elegantly describe an interaction network for a field vole, a potential reservoir host for *Borrelia burgdorferi* and its co-infections (Brisson et al 2008). In light of the strong evidence for the importance of co-infections in animal models, the neglect of these same processes by the IDSA guidelines (Wormser et al 2006) seems perversely retrograde for humans.

Co-infections are not the only factors that necessitate variable and flexible treatment for Lyme disease. The recent spread of a high-virulence strain of *Borrelia burgdorferi* in North America has now been established (Qiu et al 2008), and these authors suggest that this pathogenic strain may also be successful in infecting a broad range of host as well as vector species. Furthermore, the ranges of the accepted tick vectors of Lyme disease, *Ixodes scapularis* and *I. pacificus*, may be expanding due to global climate change (Ogden et al 2008). Thus the current practice of treating Lyme disease only in geographical areas where *I. scapularis* or *I. pacificus* is known to be endemic, as has been recommended in Canada by Barker and Lindsay (2000), is likely to unnecessarily limit the effective treatment of individuals.

As further demonstration of the lack of consensus on the treatment of Lyme disease (in contrast to the non-independent claims made by the joint authors of both the IDSA and neurology guidelines), some other respected medical bodies have refrained from issuing similar statements. For example, the Cochrane Collaboration is a highly respected global network of volunteers who review medical interventions, publish their results in a library of evidence based medicine, and are considered free from conflicted funding. They have not yet published an accepted protocol for Lyme treatment. A proposal for a Cochrane study (Cadavid et al 2008) specifically excludes 'post Lyme syndrome' an action that implies that there remains considerable difference of opinion on treatment of late Lyme disease and they consider its treatment to not yet be at the stage of consensus.

Based on the peer reviewed literature summarized above, it should be abundantly clear that the treatment of Lyme disease requires an open-minded, flexible approach tailored to each individual patient. The medical adage 'treat the patient, not the disease' is especially appropriate in light of co-infections and other complications that mean that Lyme borreliosis is not a simple, single entity. Unfortunately, the experience of CanLyme members demonstrates that, in our technologically driven medical system that often emphasizes machine readouts over clinical diagnoses, few patients are fortunate enough to receive meaningful treatment at any stage of infection.

In recognition of the lack of real consensus on the treatment of Lyme disease, I consider it important to emphasize that CanLyme members are supportive of any treatment protocol that results in improved quality of life for its members, from those with a recent tick bite and spreading rash to those with late Lyme disease. If you are aware of any double-blind study that shows that the ILADS treatment protocol, with its emphasis on treating co-infections and extended antibiotics, does not result in improved quality of life, I would appreciate the reference. In every study that I have read, the limitations of viewing Lyme as 'easy to diagnose and easy to treat' are tragically clear and the shortcomings of the IDSA treatment guidelines can only ultimately be explained by a lack of appreciation of the suffering of our members.

I sincerely hope to be able to continue our discussion and to thereby contribute to resolving the current impasse in the treatment of Lyme disease. Numerous patients continue to suffer from both Lyme disease as well as a serious misinterpretation of their symptoms. If you, in your position as deputy medical officer of health, could foster a climate that encourages real flexibility and research on Lyme disease as it exists in British Columbia, this would surely make a huge difference in alleviating the suffering of Lyme patients and their families.

References

Alban PS, Johnson PW, and Nelson DR. 2000. Serum starvation induced changes in protein synthesis and morphology of *Borrelia burgdorferi*. *Microbiology* 146: 119–127.

Alekseev AN and Dubinina HV. 2003. Multiple infections of tick-borne pathogens in *Ixodes* spp. (Acarina, Ixodidae). *Acta Zoologica Lituanica* 13: 311-321.

Allred DR. 2003. Babesiosis: persistence in the face of adversity. *Trends in Parasitology* 19: 51-5.

Barker IK and Lindsay LR. 2000. *Canadian Medical Association Journal* 162: 1573-4.

Belongia EA, 2002 Epidemiology and impact of coinfections acquired from *Ixodes* ticks. *Vector-Borne and Zoonotic Diseases* 2: 265-273.

Berglund J, Stjernberg L, Ornstein K, Tykesson-Joelsson K, Walter H. 2002. 5-y follow-up study of patients with neuroborreliosis. *Scandinavian Journal of Infectious Diseases* 34: 421–25.

Bowie WR. 2007. Guidelines for the management of Lyme Disease. The controversy and the quandary. *Drugs* 67: 2661-6.

Bratton RL, Whiteside JW, Hovan MJ, Engle RL, Edwards FD. 2008. Diagnosis and treatment of Lyme disease. *Mayo Clinic Proceedings* 83: 566-571.

Brisson, D, Dykhuizen DE, Ostfeld RS. 2008. Conspicuous impacts of inconspicuous hosts on the Lyme disease epidemic. *Proceedings of the Royal Society, Biological Sciences* 275: 227-35.

Brorson Ø and Brorson S-H. 2004. An in vitro study of the susceptibility of mobile and cystic forms of *Borrelia burgdorferi* to tinidazole. *International Microbiology* 7: 139–142.

Brorson Ø and Brorson S-H. 2007. Grapefruit seed extract is a powerful in vitro agent against motile and cystic forms of *Borrelia burgdorferi* sensu lato. Infection 35: 206-8.

Cadavid D, Auwaerter P, Aucott J, Rumbaugh J. 2008. Treatment for the neurological complications of Lyme disease. (Protocol) *Cochrane Database of Systematic Reviews* 2008, Issue 1. CD006978.

Cameron D. 2006. Generalizability in two clinical trials of Lyme disease. *Epidemiologic Perspectives and Innovations* 3: 12 doi:10.1186/1742-5573-3-12.

Cameron, DJ. Gaito, A, Harris, N, Bach, G, Bellovin, S, Bock, S, Burrascano, J, Dickey, C, Horowitz, R, Phillips, S, Meer-Sheerer, L, Raxlen, B, Sherr, V, Smith, H, Smith, P, and Stricker, R. 2004. *Evidence-based guidelines for the management of Lyme disease. Expert Review of Anti-infective Therapy*, 2: S1-13.

Diterich I, Harter L, Hassler D, Wendel A, Hartung T. 2001. Modulation of cytokine release in ex vivo-stimulated blood from borreliosis patients. *Infection and Immunity* 69: 687-694.

Diterich I, Rauter C, Kirschning CJ, Hartung T. 2003. *Borrelia burgdorferi*-induced tolerance as a model of persistence via immunosuppression. *Infection and Immunity* 71: 3979-3987.

Eskow E, Rao R-V, Mordechai E. 2001. Concurrent infection of the central nervous system by *Borrelia burgdorferi* and *Bartonella henselae*: evidence for a novel tick-borne disease complex. *Archives of Neurology* 58: 1357-1363.

Evison, J, Aebi C, Francioli P, Péter, O, Bassetti, S, Gervaix A, Zimmerli S, Weber, R. 2006. Borréliose de Lyme 2e partie: Clinique et traitement. *Revue Medicale Suisse* No 60 http://revue.medhyg.ch/article.php3?sid=31227

Exner M. 2004. *Borrelia* spp., *Encyclopedia of Medical Genomics and Proteomics*, 1:1, 146 -9.

Fallon, B.A., Keilp, J.G., Corbera, K.M., Petkova, E., Britton, C.B., Dwyer, E., Slavov, I., Cheng, J., Dobkin, J., Nelson, D.R., and Sackeim, H.A. 2008. A randomized, placebo-controlled trial of repeated IV antibiotic therapy for Lyme encephalopathy. *Neurology* 70: 992-1003.

Halperin JJ, Shapiro ED, Logigian E, Belman, AL, Dotevall, L, Wormser, GP, Krupp, L, Gronseth, G, Bever, CT. 2007. Practice parameter: treatment of nervous system Lyme disease (an evidence-based review): report of the Quality Standards Subcommittee of the American Academy of Neurology. *Neurology* 69: 91–102.

Halperin JJ. 2008. Prolonged Lyme disease treatment. Enough is enough. *Neurobiology* 70: 986-987.

Hamer SA, Roy PL Hickling GJ, Walker ED, Foster ES, Barber CC, Tsao JI. 2007. Zoonotic pathogens in *Ixodes scapularis*, *Michigan Emerging Infectious Diseases* 13: 1131-3.

Harvey WT, Martz D. 2007. Motor neuron disease recovery associated with IV ceftriaxone and anti-Babesia therapy. *Acta Neurologica Scandinavica* 115: 129–131.

Hodzic E, Feng S, Holden K, Freet, KJ, Barthold, SW. 2008. Persistence of *Borrelia burdorferi* following antibiotic treatment in mice. *Antimicrobial Agents and Chemotherapy* 52: 1728-36.

Inge LD and Wilson JW. 2008. Update on the treatment of tuberculosis. *American Family Physician* 78: 457-465, 469-470.

Johnston BL and Conly JM. 2005. Lyme Disease: Is it or is it not? *Canadian Journal of Infectious Diseases and Medical Microbiology* 16: 325-328.

Klempner M, Hu L, Evans J, Schmid, CH, Johnson, GM, Trevino, RP, Norton, D, Levy, L, Wall, D, McCall, J, Kosinski, M, Weinstein, A. 2001, Two controlled trials of antibiotic treatment in patients with persistent symptoms and a history of Lyme disease. *New England Journal of Medicine* 345: 85–92.

Ljøstad U, Skogvoll E, Eikeland R, Midgard R, Skarpaas T, Berg A, Mygland A. 2008. Oral doxycycline versus intravenous ceftriaxone for European Lyme neuroborreliosis: a multicentre, non-inferiority, double-blind, randomised trial. *Lancet Neurology* 7: 690–95.

Moro MH, Zegarra-Moro, OL, Persing DH. 2006. *Babesia microti* and *Borrelia burgdorferi* coinfection associated with increased severity of arthritis. *The Journal of Infectious Diseases* 194: 716-716.

Murgia R and Cinco M. 2004. Induction of cystic forms by different stress conditions in *Borrelia burgdorferi*. APMIS 112: 57–62.

Ogden NH, St-Onge L, Barker IK, Brazeau S, Bigras-Poulin M, Charron DF, Francis CM, Heagy A, Lindsay LR, Maarouf A, Michel P, Milord F, O'Callaghan CJ, Trudel L, Thompson RA. 2008. Risk maps for range expansion of the Lyme disease vector, *Ixodes scapularis*, in Canada now and with climate change. *International Journal of Health Geographics* 22: 24 http://www.ij-healthgeographics.com /content/pdf/1476-072X-7-24.pdf

Oksi J, Nikoskelainen J, Hiekkanen H, Lauhio, A, Peltomaa, M, Pitkaranta, Nyman, D, Granlund, H, Carlsson, S-A, Seppala, I, Valtonen, V, Viljanen, M. 2007. Duration of antibiotic treatment in disseminated Lyme borreliosis: a double-blind, randomized, placebo-controlled, multicenter clinical study. *European Journal of Clinical Microbiology and Infectious Diseases* 26: 571–581.

Owen D, 2006. Is Lyme disease always poly microbial?—The jigsaw hypothesis. *Medical Hypotheses* 67, 860–864.

Pichon B, Kahl O, Hammer B, Gray JS. 2006. Pathogens and host DNA in *Ixodes ricinus* nymphal ticks from a German forest. Vector-Borne and Zoonotic Diseases 6: 382–387.

Qiu W-G, Bruno JF, McCaig WD, Xu Y,Livey I, Schriefer MM, Luft BJ. 2008. Wide distribution of a high-virulence *Borrelia burgdorferi* clone in Europe and North America. *Emerging Infectious Diseases* 14: 1097–1104.

Russo T. 2008. part 7 section 7 Actinomycosis in Harrison's principles of internal medicine 17th edition (editors Fauci et al) New York: McGraw-Hill Medical.

Steere AC, Pachner AR, Malawista SE. 1983. Neurologic abnormalities of Lyme disease: successful treatment with high-dose intravenous penicillin. *Annals of Internal Medicine* 99: 767–72.

Telfer S, Birtles R, Bennet M, Lambin X, Paterson S, Begon M. 2008. Parasite interactions in natural populations: insights from longitudinal data. *Parasitology* 135: 767-781.

Vanousova D and Hercogova J. 2008. Lyme borreliosis treatment. *Dermatologic Therapy* 21: 101–109.

Vrethem M, Hellblom L, Widlund M, Ahl, M, Danielsson, O, Ernerudh, J, Forsberg, P. 2002 Chronic symptoms are common in patients with neuroborreliosis—a questionnaire follow-up study. *Acta Neurologica Scandinavica* 106: 205–08.

Walid, M S, Ajjan M, Patel N. 2007. Borreliosis and human granulocytic anaplasmosis coinfection with positive rheumatoid factor and monospot test: case-report. *The Internet Journal of Infectious Diseases*. Volume 6 Number 1. http://www.ispub.com/journal/the_internet_journal_of_infectious_diseases/volume_6_number_1_14/article_printable/borreliosis_and_human_granulocytic_anaplasmosis_coinfection_with_positive_rheumatoid_factor_and_monospot_test_case_report.html

WHO Expert Consultation on Rheumatic Fever and Rheumatic Heart Disease (2001: Geneva, Switzerland) Rheumatic fever and rheumatic heart disease: report of a WHO Expert Consultation, Geneva, 29 October–1 November 2001. (WHO technical report series; 923)

WHO Expert Committee on Leprosy (1997: Geneva Switzerland) Expert Committee on Leprosy seventh report (WHO technical report series; 874)

Wormser GP. 2006. Dissemination and persistence are pathogenic events common to all of the major human spirochetal infections. *Molecular Biology of Spirochetes*, F.C. Cabello et al Eds IOS Press.

Wormser GP, Dattwyler RJ, Shapiro, ED, Halperin, JJ, Steere AC, Klempner MS, Krause PJ,Bakken JS, Strle F. Stanek G, Bockenstedt L, Fish D, Dumler JS, Nadelman RB. 2006. The clinical assessment, treatment, and prevention of Lyme disease, human granulocytic anaplasmosis, and babesiosis. *Clinical Infectious Diseases* 43: 1089–134.

521

C.P. Alexander review / Revue C.P. Alexander[1]

Lyme borreliosis in Canada: biological diversity and diagnostic complexity from an entomological perspective

Janet L.H. Sperling, Felix A.H. Sperling[2]

Department of Biological Sciences, University of Alberta, Edmonton, Alberta, Canada T6G 2E9

Abstract—Lyme borreliosis (LB), also known as Lyme disease, is emerging as a serious tick-borne illness across Canada. More than three decades of research on LB in North America and Europe have provided a large, complex body of research involving well-documented difficulties at several levels. However, entomologists are well situated to contribute to resolving some of these challenges. The central pathogen in LB, the spirochete *Borrelia burgdorferi* Johnson *et al.*, includes numerous genospecies and strains that are associated with different disease symptoms and distributions. The primary vectors of LB are ticks of various *Ixodes* Latreille species (Acari: Ixodida: Ixodidae), but questions linger concerning the status of a number of other arthropods that may be infected with *B. burgdorferi* but do not transmit it biologically. A variety of vertebrates may serve as reservoirs for LB, but differences in their ability to transmit LB are not well understood at the community level. Persistent cystic forms of and immune-system evasion by *B. burgdorferi* contribute to extraordinary challenges in diagnosing LB. Multiple trade-offs constrain the effectiveness of assays like ELISA, Western blot, polymerase chain reaction, and microscopic visualization of the spirochetes. Consequently, opportunities abound for entomologists to contribute to documenting the diversity of the players and their interactions in this devilishly complex disease.

Résumé—La borréliose de Lyme (LB), connue aussi sous le nom de maladie de Lyme, est en train de devenir une importante maladie transmise par les tiques dans l'ensemble du Canada. Les recherches au cours de plus de trois décennies sur LB en Amérique du Nord et en Europe ont fourni un ensemble considérable et complexe de travaux qui comporte des problèmes bien identifiés à différents niveaux. Les entomologistes sont, cependant, bien placés pour contribuer à solutionner certains de ces défis. Le pathogène principal de LB, le spirochète *Borrelia burgdorferi* Johnson *et al.*, englobe plusieurs espèces génétiques et souches qui sont associées à des symptômes et des répartitions différentes de la maladie. Les vecteurs principaux de LB sont des tiques de différentes espèces d'*Ixodes* Latreille (Acari: Ixodida: Ixodidae), mais il reste des questions concernant le statut de plusieurs autres arthropodes qui peuvent être infectés par *B. burgdorferi*, mais qui ne le transmettent pas biologiquement. Divers vertébrés peuvent servir de réservoirs pour LB, mais les différences relatives dans leur capacité à transmettre LB ne sont

Received 26 March 2009. Accepted 26 June 2009.

[1]This series is supported by a fund established in memory of the late Charles P. Alexander. The Entomological Society of Canada uses the fund to support the publication of invited articles or reviews on topics that broaden the scope of *The Canadian Entomologist* and (or) are of current significance to entomology.
Cette série est financée par un fond établi à la mémoire de feu Charles P. Alexander. La Société d'entomologie du Canada utilise les fonds afin de supporter la publication d'articles ou de revues sur invitation portant sur des sujets qui élargissent le champ de *The Canadian Entomologist* et (ou) sont présentement pertinents en entomologie.

[2]Corresponding author (e-mail: felix.sperling@ualberta.ca).
doi: 10.4039/n08-CPA04

pas bien comprises au niveau de la communauté. Les formes kystiques persistantes et l'évasion du système immunitaire chez *B. burgdorferi* rendent le diagnostic de LB extraordinairement compliqué. De nombreux compromis limitent l'efficacité de tests biologiques, tels que la méthode ELISA, le buvardage western, l'amplification en chaîne par polymérase et la visualisation des spirochètes au microscope. En conséquence, il existe de multiples occasions pour les entomologistes de contribuer à l'étude de la diversité des intervenants et de leurs interactions dans cette maladie diablement complexe.

[Traduit par la Rédaction]

Introduction

Lyme borreliosis (LB) is a potentially debilitating illness that is typically vectored by ixodid ticks (Acari: Ixodida: Ixodidae) and caused by infection by the spirochete *Borrelia burgdorferi* Johnson *et al.* or other closely related species of *Borrelia* Swellengrebel. While the disease is also known as Lyme disease, the term Lyme borreliosis is becoming increasingly prominent internationally, to emphasize the causative organism (Gray *et al.* 2002). It has become the most common disease vectored by arthropods in the United States of America (USA), with the majority of cases occurring in the northeastern and north-central regions. In 2005, a total of 12 914 cases were reported among the 56 million inhabitants of the 10 states that border eastern and central Canadian provinces, and the incidence of LB has more than doubled since it became nationally notifiable in the USA in 1991 (Centers for Disease Control and Prevention (CDC) 2007). In contrast, although most of the 32 million inhabitants of Canada lived within 150 km of the United States border in 2005, fewer than 50 cases of LB per year were diagnosed in humans by Canadian laboratories and approximately half of these were associated with travel to areas outside Canada (Charron and Sockett 2005).

In Canada, accurate LB statistics have been difficult to obtain because the disease is not yet nationally notifiable (Ogden *et al.* 2008*a*; Canadian Paediatric Society Infectious Diseases and Immunization Committee (CPS) 2009). Nonetheless, *B. burgdorferi* has now been recognized in every province (Table 1). Recent passive surveillance from Manitoba eastward has shown that 12.5% of sampled specimens of the tick vector *Ixodes scapularis* Say were infected with *B. burgdorferi*, including 10% of those collected on humans (Ogden *et al.* 2006). Infected ticks are not a new phenomenon in Canada; soon after the original description of *B. burgdorferi*, Lindsay *et al.* (1991) reported a 58% prevalence of *B. burgdorferi* in adult *Ixodes* Latreille at Long Point, Ontario.

LB has been recognized by the Public Health Agency of Canada as becoming increasingly important for Canadians (Ogden *et al.* 2008*a*, 2008*d*). Even so, some infectious-diseases specialists disagree, noting that the disease is rare and reports of endemic cases have not increased in Canada during the past two decades (CPS 2009). In the USA, controversy over the diagnosis and treatment of LB has resulted in an increasing polarization of views, with some doctors interpreting it as a serious illness with long-term sequelae (*e.g.*, Fallon *et al.* 2008; Stricker and Johnson 2008; Cameron 2009) and others viewing it as a faddish ailment used by patients to displace the less socially palatable medical explanation of psychiatric difficulties (Sigal and Hassett 2002; Hassett *et al.* 2008). Ballantyne (2008) concluded that such controversies can only be resolved with further research. Limitations in the sensitivity and specificity of blood tests across the genetic diversity of *Borrelia* species, an incomplete understanding of their immune-system evasion and persistence, variation in the degree of human immunity, and complications due to co-infections by other disease-causing microorganisms all contribute to the complexity of the interactions between the spirochetes, their vectors, and their vertebrate hosts. Even in Connecticut, where LB was first described and incidence is still very high, treatment has been sufficiently controversial that the Connecticut General Assembly recently passed legislation protecting doctors from disciplinary action for prescribing long-term treatment with antibiotics (Connecticut General Assembly 2009).

Table 1. Reports of Lyme borreliosis (LB) and *Ixodes* ticks in Canada.

	First report of human LB in *Canada Diseases Weekly Report*	First report of *I. scapularis* or *I. pacificus*	PCR (or IFA) positive for *Borrelia burgdorferi* in ticks	Positive cases for dogs in 2007[1]
Nova Scotia	—	1984[2]	1999[3]	34
New Brunswick	1987[4]	1990[2]	1996[5] (IFA)	11
Newfoundland	1989[4]	1994[6]	2001[7] (*B. burgdorferi*); 2006[8] (*B. garinii*)	n/a
Prince Edward Island	—	1989[2]	1991[9] (IFA)	1
Quebec	1984[10]	1989[2]	1996[11]	65
Ontario	1977[10]	1904[12]	1988[13] (IFA), 1993[14]	395
Manitoba	1988[4]	1989[2]	2002[15]	229
Saskatchewan	1999[16]	1998[16]	—	3
Alberta	1989[4]	1998[3]; 2002[15]	1994[17]	5
British Columbia	1988[4]	1910[18]	1993[19]	4

Note: Sources are as follows: 1, IDEXX Laboratories, Inc. (2008); 2, Costero (1990); 3, Scott *et al.* (2001); 4, Mackenzie (1990); 5, Bjerkelund (1997); 6, Artsob *et al.* (2000); 7, Whitney (2005); 8, Smith *et al.* (2006); 9, Artsob *et al.* (1992); 10, Bollegraaf (1988); 11, Louise Trudel, Laboratoire de santé publique du Québec, Institut national de santé publique du Québec, Sainte-Anne-de-Bellevue, personal communication, 26 March 2009; 12, Nuttall and Warburton (1911); 13, Barker *et al.* (1988); 14, Banerjee *et al.* (1995*b*); 15, Morshed *et al.* (2005); 16, Lindsay et al. (1999*c*); 17, Banerjee *et al.* (1995*a*); 18, Gregson (1956); 19, Banerjee (1993).

Entomologists are no strangers to the complexity that accompanies diversity, and are well positioned to make positive contributions to resolving some of the controversies that surround LB. In fact, entomologists have a vested interest in LB because many are potentially exposed to infection during fieldwork (Piacentino and Schwartz 2002; Vázquez *et al.* 2008) and yet are also aware of the potential for entomophobic hysteria. Furthermore, entomologists in Canada have an opportunity to make a fresh start, taking advantage of the currently low profile of the disease in Canada but building on the large volume of recent scientific studies from the USA and Europe. The purpose of this review is to explore the scientific, peer-reviewed research on LB that is relevant to Canada, with particular focus on biological and diagnostic factors that contribute to making this disease so challenging.

The natural history and ecology of LB

Diversity of *Borrelia* species and delimitation of *B. burgdorferi*

After investigating bacteria in ticks that were implicated in a cluster of juvenile arthritis cases from Old Lyme, Connecticut (41°19′N, 72°20′W), Burgdorfer *et al.* (1982) proposed that a spirochete was the etiologic agent of this illness. European researchers isolated a morphologically and immunologically similar spirochete from the skin and cerebrospinal fluid of a patient suffering from Bannwarth's syndrome (Pfister *et al.* 1984). The spirochete was formally named *B. burgdorferi* by Johnson *et al.* (1984) and later shown to include three distinct phyletic groups (Welsh *et al.* 1992). These three groups of strains, referred to as *B. burgdorferi sensu stricto* (s.s.), *B. garinii* Baranton *et al.*, and *B. afzelii* Canica *et al.*, were associated with differences in clinical symptoms within a broad definition of LB (Lebech *et al.* 1994). *Borrelia burgdorferi* tends to produce arthritic symptoms, *B. garinii* tends to infect neural tissue, and *B. afzelii* may persist in the skin (Terekhova *et al.* 2006; Tilly *et al.* 2008; Craig-Mylius *et al.* 2009; Hildenbrand *et al.* 2009; Kudryashev *et al.* 2009).

Rudenko *et al.* (2009) have now described *Borrelia carolinensis* from the southeastern USA as the 14th species of the *B. burgdorferi sensu lato* (s.l.) complex. The members of this species complex vary in host/vector associations, pathogenicity, and distribution, and have now been recorded in many areas where they were not previously thought to occur (Rudenko *et al.* 2009). In North America, Lyme-like borreliosis may also be caused by *B. lonestari* Armstrong *et al.* (Stromdahl *et al.* 2003) and *B. bissettii* Postic *et al.* (Schneider *et al.* 2008), both of which occur widely on the continent. A Colorado isolate of *B. bissettii* has been shown to be pathogenic to mice, but an isolate from British Columbia was not (Schneider *et al.* 2008). Another species, *B. californiensis* Postic *et al.*, is of unknown pathogenicity and has so far only been documented from California, where it is primarily associated with the California kangaroo rat, *Dipodomys californicus* Merriam (Postic *et al.* 2007).

Outside the *B. burgdorferi* s.l. complex, other *Borrelia* species can cause relapsing fever, with *B. hermsii* (Davis) vectored by argasid ticks (Ixodida: Argasidae) and occurring in British Columbia, Montana, and south through the Rocky Mountains (Schwan *et al.* 2007), and *B. recurrentis* (Lebert) vectored by the human body louse, *Pediculus humanus* L. (Anoplura: Pediculidae), in several widely separated Third World countries (Cutler *et al.* 1997). *Borrelia recurrentis* infection may occur either by crushing infected lice into broken skin or by contact with infected louse feces (Houhamdi and Raoult 2005). Difficulties in diagnosing *Borrelia* spp. have been reviewed by Exner (2004).

Unexpectedly large genetic diversity has also been found within *B. burgdorferi* s.s. For example, nine distinct clonal lineages were found at one field site in the northeastern USA (Bunikis *et al.* 2004). Differences in fitness between two of these genotypes, one isolated from blood and the other from skin, were studied in mice by Hanincová *et al.* (2008). The blood isolate retained its infectivity to xenodiagnostic ticks, whereas the skin isolate did not, suggesting partial diversification into more specialized subtypes in North America. Additional research in North America and Europe has shown further diversity in *B. burgdorferi* s.s.; at least 12 distinct sequence types defined by DNA sequence differences in outer-surface protein C (OspC) coexist in the northeastern USA and at least 17 OspC types are found across the USA and Europe (Qiu *et al.* 2008). *OspC-A* genotypes are associated with a highly virulent clonal group that has a wide distribution, suggesting recent migration of *OspC-A* genes into North America from Europe within the past few hundred years (Qiu *et al.* 2008). Interestingly, the *OspC-A* sequence at the *OspC* locus characterizes isolate B31, which was explicitly identified as the "type strain" in the original description of *B. burgdorferi* (Johnson *et al.* 1984). Most of the genome of B31 has subsequently been sequenced by Casjens *et al.* (2000).

Based on multilocus sequences for several slow-evolving housekeeping genes (MLSTs), Margos *et al.* (2008) agreed with Qiu *et al.* (2008) about the European origin of *B. burgdorferi*; however, they contended that *B. burgdorferi* has existed in North American refugia for much longer, in the order of millions of years. Although Margos *et al.* (2008) documented substantial discordance in topology as well as evolutionary processes between their concatenated MLST markers compared with the *OspC* locus, they did not consider whether recent introgression and hybridization of genes introduced from Europe may have contributed to the virulence of LB *via* hybridization. In other words, differences between MLSTs and OspC topology may reflect legitimately distinct biological processes in which housekeeping genes characterize a portion of the genome that has remained geographically stable, whereas *OspC* genes show signs of strong selection and recent trans-Atlantic gene flow. If so, this would mean that MLSTs may not unambiguously genotype *B. burgdorferi* samples or establish their evolutionary relationships and population structure at different levels, as was maintained by Margos *et al.* (2008).

Although intellectually fascinating, the complexity of *B. burgdorferi* s.l. has provoked spirited disagreement. Even the delimitation of LB is contentious. One school of thought is represented by the Infectious Diseases Society of America (Wormser *et al.* 2006, 2007) and relies on narrowly focused serology that is commonly applied in Canada using commercial diagnostic kits such as MarDx (Canadian Public Health Laboratory Network (CPHLN) 2007), which were developed using the B31 strain of *B. burgdorferi* s.s. In contrast, the International Lyme and Associated Diseases Society defines LB more broadly as infection with *B. burgdorferi* s.l., which may be confounded with associated co-infections (Cameron *et al.* 2004). A small minority of practitioners even prefer to describe LB as a disease that is primarily a polymicrobial infection, emphasizing synergies of co-infections and host factors rather than the diversity of *Borrelia* spp. to explain the complex and notoriously variable clinical presentations of LB (Owen 2006). In common with other spirochetal diseases, LB has a wide spectrum of clinical symptoms that usually occur in successive stages (Miklossy 2008; Hildenbrand *et al.* 2009), and this diversity of symptoms, whether they are concurrent or successive, certainly contribute to the challenge of determining which of these symptoms are due to *B. burgdorferi.*

Vector incidence and distribution

Borrelia burgdorferi is almost exclusively vectored by *Ixodes* ticks throughout its temperate Northern Hemisphere distribution (Eisen and Lane 2002). In British Columbia the primary vector is *I. pacificus* Cooley and Kohls, whereas across central and eastern Canada it is *I. scapularis*; together these two tick species are believed to be responsible for almost all human LB infections in Canada (Ogden *et al.* 2008*d*).

There are various methods of sampling ticks for study. Probably the most common is flagging (or dragging), which usually involves dragging a flannel sheet about 1 m^2 in area lightly against vegetation for a specific amount of time before inspecting it visually for adhering ticks (*e.g.*, Faulde and Robbins 2008; Ogden *et al.* 2008*d*; Scott *et al.* 2008). Alternatively, humans wearing protective clothing may be inspected for attached ticks (Lane *et al.* 2004; Faulde and Robbins 2008). These techniques suffer from the disadvantages that sampling takes place over a relatively short time period and is subject to weather conditions (Gray 1985).

Longer term sampling may be accomplished using caged sentinel animals (Burkot *et al.* 2001) or carbon dioxide traps (Gray 1985) but is problematic because *I. scapularis* has very limited horizontal movement (Falco and Fish 1991). Livetrapped animals can be inspected visually for ticks (Ogden *et al.*, 2008*c*; Salkeld *et al.* 2008) or their cages can be suspended over water into which the ticks fall (Ginsberg *et al.* 2005). Lane and Loye (1991) reported that visual inspection detected as few as 45% of the number of *I. pacificus* that were found using drop-off collection. Birds can be a source of ticks during banding (Scott *et al.* 2001; Morshed *et al.* 2005; Smith *et al.* 2006), as can deer killed by hunters (Lindsay *et al.* 1999*b*; Shariat *et al.* 2007). Passive surveillance may involve taking advantage of ticks removed in medical or veterinary clinics (Ogden *et al.* 2006, 2008*d*). A flaw of passive sampling is that the nymph is the tick life stage most likely to transmit disease to humans (Mather *et al.* 1996), but most ticks submitted as a result of passive surveillance are adult females, which are more easily detected (Morshed *et al.* 2006; Ogden *et al.* 2006).

The basic phenology of *Ixodes* ticks in Canada can be described relatively simply (Fig. 1) but there is substantial variation in the basic pattern within and between regions. An established population at Long Point in southern Ontario has received the best documentation to date (Lindsay *et al.* 1999*a*, 1999*b*). Larval activity in this area was lengthy, with weak peaks in mid to late June and mid-August (Lindsay *et al.* 1999*a*). On the other hand, nymphs were most abundant during a narrower time range, in June and July (Lindsay *et al.* 1999*a*), and adult activity was distinctly bimodal, with peaks in April and October (Lindsay *et al.* 1999*b*). The bimodal questing activity of adult *I. scapularis* in Ontario has been confirmed by Morshed *et al.* (2006), and in Manitoba, peak activity of adult *I. scapularis* occurs between September and November, with a second peak from April to June (Galloway 2002). Elsewhere in Canada the phenology of *Ixodes* may vary depending on local conditions; however, detailed studies are not generally available. In California, adult *I. pacificus* have a bimodal activity pattern, with peak

Fig. 1. Typical life cycle of the blacklegged tick, *Ixodes scapularis*, and associated infection by *Borrelia burgdorferi* in Canada, showing the succession of immunological and environmental challenges to spirochetes (broken lines and "wiggles") as they cope with tick searches for hosts, successive tick life stages, variation in blood-meal sources, and transmission to and from vertebrate hosts. Phenology is largely taken from Lindsay *et al.* (1999*a*, 1999*b*) and Galloway (2002), although the cycle may be extended for 1 or more years if ticks are unable to find food in any given year.

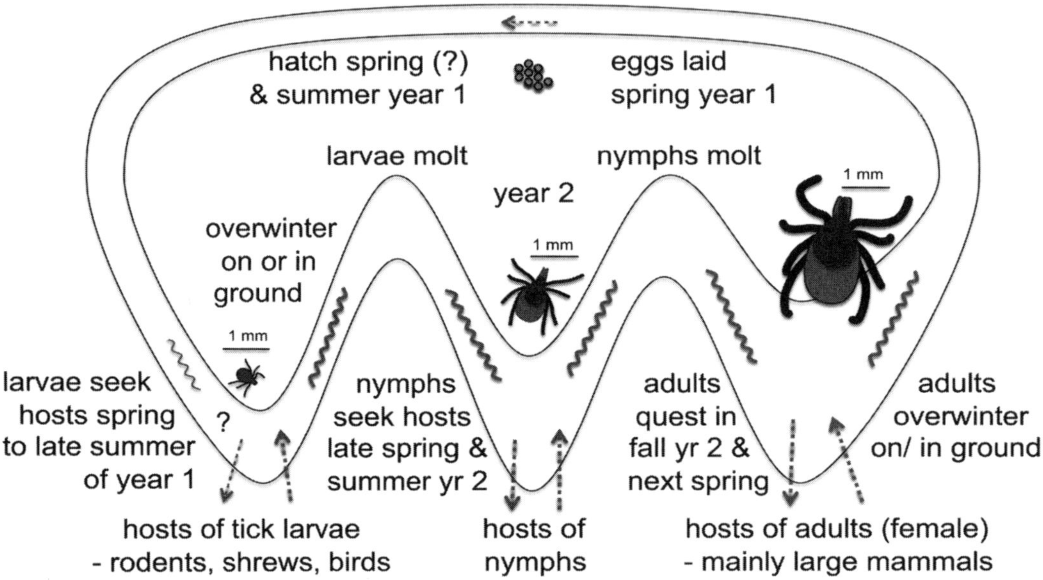

activity in both March and December and nymphs occurring between April and August (Clover and Lane 1995).

In agreement with Lindsay *et al.*'s (1999*b*) findings for southern Ontario, long duration and weak bimodality are also evident in the activity of larval *I. scapularis* from both the northeast and Upper Midwest of the USA (Gatewood *et al.* 2009), although the authors chose to fit a unimodal curve to their larval-occurrence data. In contrast, the seasonal activity of nymphs was explicitly recognized as bimodal, and the variation in size of the two nymphal-activity peaks was interpreted as the result of variation in the number of larvae that hatch in midsummer and then may or may not be able to feed before overwintering (Gatewood *et al.* 2009). However, it is plausible that adult phenology also contributes to the biomodality of both larval and nymphal activity. Extended larval activity may be due to the overlap of two cohorts: larvae hatching from eggs laid early in spring by females that had fed in the fall and overwintered, and those resulting from females that fed in spring and laid eggs somewhat later. As Killilea *et al.* (2008) have emphasized, there is a strong need for standardized sampling of all life stages of ticks across broad geographic regions.

Primary tick identification guides that are likely to be useful in Canada include Gregson (1956), Keirans and Clifford (1978), Furman and Loomis (1984), Durden and Keirans (1996), and Web sites such as *Ticks of Canada* (Canadian Lyme Disease Foundation 2009) and Anderson and Harrington (2009). Lindquist *et al.* (1999) produced couplets that augment the keys of Gregson (1956), Keirans and Clifford (1978), and Durden and Keirans (1996).

Established populations of *I. scapularis* have been well documented in localized areas of Nova Scotia, Ontario, and Manitoba

(Ogden *et al.* 2008*d*). Populations of *I. pacificus* have been established for at least a century in southern British Columbia (Gregson 1956). The dispersal and population structure of *I. pacificus* are still poorly understood, but work based on both allozymes and mtDNA has shown patterns of high local genetic diversity and locus-specific isolation or selection in localities ranging from West Vancouver, British Columbia, to southern California and Utah (Kain *et al.* 1997, 1999). *Ixodes* vectors can be spread by migratory birds across most of Canada (Scott *et al.* 2001; Morshed *et al.* 2005; Ogden *et al.* 2008*c*), which means that sporadic cases of LB can occur throughout Canada and transient populations of *Ixodes* ticks could establish in suitable localized habitats. Because *I. scapularis* and *I. pacificus* commonly feed on deer and other vertebrates that live in woodlands, increases in tick numbers can result from restoration of woodlands, especially in semi-urban areas, where hunting of deer is discouraged (Killilea *et al.* 2008). Changes in the distribution of ticks as a result of climate change are predicted to be disproportionately serious in Canada, with consequent increases in cases of LB (Ogden *et al.* 2006, 2008*a*, 2008*c*, 2008*d*).

Other confirmed vectors of *B. burgdorferi* that are known to range into Canada include *Ixodes angustus* Neumann, *I. dentatus* Marx, *I. jellisoni* Cooley and Kohls, *I. muris* Bishopp and Smith, and *I. spinipalpis* Hadwen and Nuttall (Gregson 1956; Eisen and Lane 2002). Older literature that lists *I. dammini* Spielman *et al.* as a vector of *B. burdorferi* (*e.g.*, Lindsay *et al.* 1991) refers to *I. scapularis*; these two species are now considered conspecific (Wesson *et al.* 1993). *Ixodes cookei* Packard is not considered to be a competent vector of *B. burgdorferi* (Barker *et al.* 1993), although *B. burgdorferi* is documented from a specimen of *I. cookei* and its dog host in central Alberta (Fernando *et al.* 2008). *Borrelia garinii,* the most neurotropic of the European forms of LB, has been found in *I. uriae* White on seabirds in Newfoundland (Smith *et al.* 2006). In general, most *Ixodes* ticks in Canada appear to be competent, although not necessarily efficient, vectors of *B. burgdorferi* (Eisen and Lane 2002). *Ixodes gregsoni* has been newly described from mustelids in Canada Lindquist *et al.* (1999), but is unlikely to have much of an effect on transmission of *B. burgdorferi* because mustelids are poor reservoirs (LoGiudice *et al.* 2003). A number of ticks can acquire *B. burgdorferi* infections but are considered incompetent because they are unable to pass the infection on to the next host; these include *Amblyomma americanum* (L.), *Haemaphysalis leporispalustris* Packard, all species of *Dermacentor* C.L. Koch, and a few species of *Ixodes* (Eisen and Lane 2002). Vector competence is defined as the ability to (*i*) acquire spirochetes when feeding on an infected host, then (*ii*) pass them between tick life stages, and subsequently (*iii*) pass the infection to a susceptible host while feeding (Eisen and Lane 2002). Transmission of *Borrelia* from younger to older tick life stages is well established and such trans-stadial transmission is important because ticks generally feed on only one individual host per tick life stage (Oliver 1989). Less is known about the prevalence and importance of infection passed to larvae from adult females *via* the egg stage (Eisen and Lane 2002), although such transovarial infection may be important in Europe (Kurtenbach *et al.* 1995). For all forms of transmission, however, it is difficult to distinguish experimentally between complete incompetence and rare vectoring because of low tick infectivity (Kahl *et al.* 2002). The *B. burgdorferi*-vectoring competence of ticks is distinguished from mechanical transmission, where pathogens are not passed *via* the normal tick salivary secretions but are introduced past broken skin by a mechanism such as pathogens clinging to the mouthparts (an unlikely scenario considering the sensitivity of *Borrelia* to oxygen; Barbour and Hayes 1986) or, more plausibly, crushing a tick into a wound in the course of attempted removal. For a tick-borne proteobacterium, *Anaplasma* Theiler, in cattle, mechanical vectoring *via* the mouthparts of biting flies is approximately two orders of magnitude less efficient than biological vectoring (Scoles *et al.* 2005). However, the efficiency of mechanical vectoring of *Borrelia* and its role in human illness are not known. Until recently, autoinoculation by crushing lice into wounds was thought to be the only way that *B. recurrentis* was transmitted (Houhamdi and Raoult 2005).

In addition to tick species, mosquitoes (Diptera: Culicidae), tabanid flies (Diptera: Tabanidae), and fleas (Siphonaptera) are known to harbor *B. burgdorferi*
but none has been shown to be competent as defined by Eisen and Lane (2002). In mosquitoes, for example, 7%–8% of adult female *Aedes* Meigen in Connecticut (Magnarelli *et al.* 1986) and 1.7% of *Culex pipiens* (L.) in Poland carried *B. burgdorferi* (Kosik-Bogacka *et al.* 2007). Furthermore, transmission between mosquito life stages is suggested by the occurrence of *Borrelia* in 1.6% of larval *Culex* L. in the Czech Republic (Zákovská *et al.* 2002) and 3.2% of larval and 1.6% of pupal *C. pipiens* in Poland (Kosik-Bogacka *et al.* 2007). Mites may also contain *B. burgdorferi* (Zakovska *et al.* 2008), but no surveyed spiders have been found to harbor *Borrelia* (Suffridge *et al.* 1999).

There are anecdotal reports of LB transmitted by vectors other than ticks in Canada (Doby *et al.* 1987) and the USA (*e.g.*, Luger 1990). These are unsupported by any of the evidence normally required to demonstrate competence or even mechanical vectoring. Nonetheless, although statements such as "fleas, flies, and mosquitoes are not vectors for Lyme disease" (Bratton *et al.* 2008) are common in the medical literature, it is conceivable that the detailed documentation of transmission by tick vectors has overshadowed occasional mechanical transmission by secondary vectors. Eisen and Lane (2002) state, "Although insects may prove incompetent to serve as vectors for *B. burgdorferi s.l.*, the possibility of occasional mechanical transmission should not be discounted". Further study is clearly needed.

Diversity and dynamics of reservoir hosts

The primary reservoir host of LB in North America has long been assumed to be white-footed mice (Levine *et al.* 1985), although recent research in the northeastern USA shows that two shrew species are each at least as likely as white-footed mice to be a potential source of infection for humans in some locations (Brisson *et al.* 2008). On the west coast of North America, infection rates demonstrate that squirrels are highly competent reservoirs and their infection rates correlate closely with rates of human infection (Salkeld *et al.* 2008). Major described hosts of *B. burgdorferi* that interact with humans include white-footed mice, chipmunks, squirrels, wood rats, and shrews (Killilea *et al.* 2008).

Some animals that act as common hosts for tick vectors, most notably deer in Europe and North America (Kurtenbach *et al.* 1998; Ullmann *et al.* 2003) and lizards in California (Lane 1990; Giery and Ostfeld 2007), are able to clear infection by *B. burgdorferi* and thereby may actively contribute to reducing rates of infection with *B. burgdorferi*. Thus, high deer densities could have both a positive and a negative influence on the zoonotic cycle of LB by allowing tick populations to be high while reducing rates of *Borrelia* infection in ticks if deer are the primary intermediate host between rodents, such as shrews, and humans. However, a recent report from Tennessee shows that 33% of winter ticks, *Dermacentor albipictus* (Packard), collected from white-tailed deer were positive for *B. burgdorferi* or *B. lonestari* (Shariat *et al.* 2007). The observation that *Borrelia* was not cleared from ticks feeding on these deer suggests that in some areas deer may still be significant reservoir hosts. The report by Shariat *et al.* (2007), however, is anomalous and it remains to be shown that *D. albipictus* could vector *Borrelia*. Lizards are also variable in their ability to clear *B. burgdorferi* infection (Clark *et al.* 2005) and are not universal in their incompetence as reservoir hosts (Giery and Ostfeld 2007).

Since birds, including migratory song birds that nest in urban habitats, are important for long-distance dispersal of ticks (Morshed *et al.* 2005; Ogden *et al.* 2008*c*; Scott *et al.* 2001) and some are important reservoirs for *B. burgdorferi* (Ginsberg *et al.* 2005), they can play an important role in peridomestic exposure to LB (Ginsberg *et al.* 2005).

In addition to variation in the strains of *Borrelia* that they tend to carry, reservoir animals exhibit differing symptoms of infection. For example, mice, commonly used as models for human infection, do not develop the characteristic bull's-eye rash or exhibit clear neurological manifestations of LB, although they are excellent models for the arthritis form of LB (Yrjänäinen *et al.* 2007). This may explain the greater attention paid to the arthritis form of LB, for which an excellent animal model exists, than to the neurological form, where animal models are more problematic (Nardelli *et al.* 2008; Rupprecht *et al.* 2008).

Rates of infection of *I. pacificus* by *B. burgdorferi* are considered low in British Columbia (Ogden *et al.* 2008*d*) and reported as being less than 1% across the province (British Columbia Ministry of Health 2008). Charron and Sockett (2005) have speculated that this is due to the preference for lizard hosts shown by *I. pacificus* in the nymphal stage, presumably based on the borreliacidal properties of lizard blood demonstrated in California (Lane 1990; Slowik and Lane 2009). However the significance of such an interaction remains to be demonstrated in British Columbia, where lizards, being at the extreme northern edge of their ranges, are at much lower density. In British Columbia, the effect of climate change and the importance of patchiness in the distribution of *B. burgdorferi* and infected hosts are currently unpredictable (Ogden *et al.* 2008*d*).

Risk of human exposure to LB

The risk of human exposure to LB is related to numerous factors, such as the identity of ticks, the particular *Borrelia* strain, previous hosts, local ecological interactions, or human behavior (Horobik *et al.* 2006). Human behaviors that bring people into contact with ticks include sitting on logs, gathering wood, leaning against trees, walking in natural areas, and stirring or sitting on leaf litter (Lane *et al.* 2004). Even when considerable personal protection measures are taken by highly motivated entomologists, potentially infected ticks have been removed up to 2 days later, demonstrating that the risk of exposure to LB is still significant (Lane *et al.* 2004; Vázquez *et al.* 2008). Forest fragmentation may increase the risk of LB through loss of predators from smaller patches and a consequent increase in the abundance of small rodents, leading to higher densities of infected nymphal ticks (Allan *et al.* 2003). Also, highly diverse communities of vertebrates are less likely to bring infected nymphs into contact with humans, owing to "dilution effects" (LoGiudice *et al.* 2003). The dilution effect hypothesis states that when there are multiple vertebrate hosts for ticks, and these hosts differ in how well they clear infection but do not differ in resistance to ticks, then *B. burgdorferi* will no longer be transmitted as efficiently as when only the most susceptible hosts are infected. A number of other factors are also likely to influence the distribution and infection rates of ticks and there is a clear need for tick occurrence to be documented in a more standardized manner at multiple spatial and temporal scales (Killilea *et al.* 2008).

In the USA, the number of infected nymphs of *I. scapularis* and *I. pacificus* correlates with reported human disease more than does the incidence of adult ticks, and therefore nymphs are the life stage most commonly associated with disease transmission (Clover and Lane 1995; Mather *et al.* 1996; CDC 2007). The small size of *Ixodes* tick nymphs and their rapid feeding rate compared with that of adults are considered to be factors in increasing spirochete transmission to humans by nymphs (Clover and Lane 1995). Moreover, if nymphs are more likely than larvae to feed on hosts with borreliacidal blood, such as lizards or potentially even deer, this may also contribute to reducing rates of disease transmission by adult ticks relative to earlier life stages. Regardless of the underlying mechanism, it is important to survey nymphal ticks as well as adults to accurately assess disease incidence.

In regions of Canada where ticks are not endemic, however, the role of adults in vectoring should be clarified because, in such regions, a relatively high proportion of adults may have fed on migratory birds rather than on mammals when they were in the nymphal stage (Morshed *et al.* 2006). Birds from near Long Island, New York, have been demonstrated to be competent reservoirs for *Borrelia*, with wild-caught robins infecting 16% of larval ticks placed on them, whereas robins that were previously infected by nymphal ticks in the laboratory passed that infection on to 82% of larvae that subsequently fed on them (Ginsberg *et al.* 2005). Although it is unclear whether similar infection rates apply to adult ticks that fed on birds as nymphs, it remains to be seen whether the adult stage of ticks may have greater importance in disease transmission in regions of Canada where *Ixodes* spp. are primarily derived from birds.

Physiological processes

Gene regulation and transmission dynamics

For *B. burgdorferi* to be transmitted from a cold-blooded tick vector to a warm-blooded host, it must regulate its gene expression in a complex and as yet incompletely understood manner. Models of gene regulation range from simple ones based solely on temperature and pH (Schwan *et al.* 1995) to a new paradigm suggested by Stevenson *et al.* (2006), who cautioned that the effects of temperature and pH may not predict the *in vivo* expression of genes. The synthesis of each of five different lipoproteins is controlled in a distinct manner, in some cases opposite to that predicted from temperature and pH effects *in vitro* (Stevenson *et al.* 2006).

Studies of the transmission dynamics of *B. burgdorferi* in *I. scapularis* indicate that the risk of transmission of strain B31 by a single bite from an infected tick is about 2% and that the risk increases with the length of time that the tick is attached (Hojgaard *et al.* 2008). When a tick first attaches, spirochetes are still found in the midgut and are producing outer-surface protein A (OspA), which helps spirochetes adhere to a midgut protein, TROPSA. When feeding begins, the spirochetes are exposed to warm mammalian blood and lowered pH, and OspA is downregulated while OspC is upregulated. Spirochetes then migrate from the midgut to the salivary gland and transmission to the vertebrate host can be achieved (*e.g.*, Hojgaard *et al.* 2008). This delay in transmission explains why transmission is reduced when ticks are removed within 24 h of attachment (Hojgaard *et al.* 2008). In Europe, transmission of *B. burgdorferi* s.s. and *B. afzelii* by *I. ricinus* occurs in less than 24 h, but the risk of transmission still increases over time (Kahl *et al.* 1998; Crippa *et al.* 2002). In a further complication of the host–tick–pathogen interaction, *B. burgdorferi* s.l. is able to increase expression of an *Ixodes* salivary protein, Salp15, to protect against complement-mediated killing of *Borrelia* by the host's innate immune system (Ramamoorthi *et al.* 2005). This protective effect was greater when the vector was *I. ricinus* rather than *I. scapularis* (Schuijt *et al.* 2008). The early expression of *osp*C appears to be essential for *B. burgdorferi* to escape innate immunity and disseminate in the host (Gilbert *et al.* 2007), and yet persistent infection of the host is only possible when *osp*C is downregulated after infection because acquired antibodies to OspC allow the spirochetes to be cleared (Tilly *et al.* 2007). Current understanding of the interactions of tick saliva and *B. burgdorferi* is discussed in Anderson and Valenzuela (2007).

Even though vectoring by ticks is the most likely way to contract LB (and gene regulation of outer-surface proteins on *Borrelia* as well as increased expression of Salp15 in the tick vector will increase the probability of infection of the vertebrate host), there is nonetheless some evidence that contact transmission of *B. burgdorferi* can also occur without a vector. Burgess and Patrican (1987) have shown that deer mice can be infected orally by ingesting saline containing *B. burgdorferi* and that these mice can in turn infect ticks that feed on them. Despite an explicit search of the LB literature, it is not apparent that any studies have addressed whether *Borrelia* can be transmitted to vertebrate hosts that eat infected ticks or, for that matter, by contact between hosts *via* body fluids such as urine or sperm. However, Kurtenbach *et al.* (1994) have demonstrated differences in the antibody responses of various mouse species infected by needle inoculation *versus* tick bites. Tick-infected mice did not express antibodies to OspA or outer-surface protein B (OspB) early in the infection, whereas intradermally injected mice did (Kurtenbach *et al.* 1994). However, infection proceeded in both groups; in fact, intradermal inoculation is commonly used to ensure that a controlled quantity of pathogen is transferred in studies of LB (*e.g.*, Hodzic *et al.* 2008). Recent research has shown that both OspA and OspB are involved in binding to the tick gut, so the results of Kurtenbach *et al.*'s (1994) study are counter to what would be expected. OspB-deficient *B. burgdorferi* is infectious and pathogenic in mice but is unable to survive in *Ixodes* (Neelakanta *et al.* 2007).

Careful and prompt removal of attached ticks is nonetheless important in reducing the probability of transmission of *B. burgdorferi* (Hojgaard *et al.* 2008). The preferred method is to grasp the mouthparts firmly with fine-pointed forceps and pull them straight out in a single action without twisting. This should reduce the risk of regurgitation of gut contents (Gammons and Salam 2002). An alternative method for removing attached ticks is the "straw and knot method" of Murakami (2009): a drinking straw is used to guide a thread to the base of the mouthparts, allowing the tick be pulled out in a single motion. Any remaining mouthparts should be excised and the area cleaned with antiseptic solution. Removal of the cement plug attaching the mouthparts to the wound may be important because *B. burgdorferi* can be present in it (Alekseev *et al.* 1995).

Persistent infection

Borrelia spp. are capable of persistent infection, and such persistence is the norm in mice, rats, hamsters, dogs, and monkeys (Barthold 2000; Straubinger 2000; Summers *et al.* 2005; Hodzic *et al.* 2008). Persistence in reservoir hosts can be interpreted as an evolutionarily shaped survival strategy linked to the asynchronous phenology of the tick vectors (Kurtenbach *et al.* 2006). Although natural infections are less controlled and defined, there is strong evidence that they persist in humans also (Oksi *et al.* 1999; Breier *et al.* 2001; Miklossy *et al.* 2004, 2008; Hunfeld *et al.* 2005). Immune evasion has been extensively documented in *Borrelia* (Liang *et al.* 2002; Bankhead and Chaconas 2007; Rupprecht *et al.* 2008; Xu *et al.* 2008*a*; Yang *et al.* 2009). Although *B. burgdorferi* is generally considered to be an extracellular pathogen, localization has been demonstrated within endothelial cells (Ma *et al.* 1991; Thomas *et al.* 1994), synovial cells (Girschick *et al.* 1996), and neuronal and glial cells (Livengood and Gilmore 2006; Miklossy *et al.* 2006). Infiltration of blood vessels, cardiac myocytes, and collagen tissues has also been demonstrated (Pachner *et al.* 1995), and adherence and escape of *Borrelia* from vasculature has recently been visualized directly by Moriarty *et al.* (2008). Sequestration and physical protection from the immune system in the extracellular matrix have been reviewed by Cabello *et al.* (2007) and Rupprecht *et al.* (2008).

When exposed to unfavorable conditions such as osmotic and heat shock, *B. burgdorferi* produces atypical forms (*e.g.*, Brorson and Brorson 1998, 2004; Singh and Girschick 2004; Miklossy *et al.* 2008; Margulis *et al.* 2009). The extracellular and intracellular presence of these atypical forms has been demonstrated in brain tissue of humans with confirmed neuroborreliosis, and atypical forms can exist in the absence of spirochetal forms (Miklossy *et al.* 2008). A thickened external membrane, observed by Miklossy *et al.* (2008) to surround cystic forms, was reactive to anti-OspA antibody and a full characterization of other immunogenic proteins was not attempted. Thus, a full understanding of the serology of LB must include the atypical forms as well as the typical spiral forms (Miklossy *et al.* 2008).

***Borrelia* has a unique, flexible genome**

Borrelia burgdorferi contains both circular and linear DNA molecules in roughly equal numbers (Rosa *et al.* 2005). Most replicons are linear molecules that are terminated by hairpin turns, which are unusual in bacteria and of much interest to molecular biologists (Chaconas 2005; Tourand *et al.* 2009). In addition to one large linear chromosome, *B. burgdorferi* has over 20 plasmids, the largest number so far described in any living organism (Chaconas 2005; Rosa *et al.* 2005) . Some of these plasmids carry crucial information for survival in tick vectors or mammalian hosts. The linear plasmid Ip28–1 is required for persistent infection with *B. burgdorferi* and the presence of the *vls* locus on this plasmid appears to be an absolute requirement for persisting infection. Antigenic variation at *vlsE* by recombination of cassette fragments allows a large number of antigenically distinct variants to be produced, thus facilitating avoidance of the host's immune system (Bankhead and Chaconas 2007). The genetics of *B. burgdorferi* has been reviewed by Rosa *et al.* (2005) and Tilly *et al.* (2008). Furthermore, *Borrelia* spp. are unusual in having evaded the usual limiting factor of iron availability in the host cells by using manganese for electron transport (Posey and Gherardini 2000; Ouyang *et al.* 2009). Typically, at the onset of infection, humans secrete lactoferrin to limit available iron and inhibit bacterial growth (Arnold *et al.* 1982). *Borrelia burgdorferi* has eliminated most of the genes that encode proteins that require iron as a cofactor, and a manganese transporter is required for virulence in *B. burgdorferi* (Posey and Gherardini 2000; Ouyang *et al.* 2009).

Immune-system selection

Antigenic variation is a common mechanism whereby pathogenic bacteria can evade the immune system. *Borrelia* species are the subject of intense study that has revealed at least two different ways in which they achieve such antigenic variation. For *B. hermsii*, recombination of *vlp* and *vsp* sequences is responsible for antigenic variation, whereas in *B. burgdorferi*, recombination occurs at *vlsE* (Norris 2006). Furthermore, variation in VlsE of *B. burgdorferi* is not, by itself, sufficient to achieve resistance to reinfection, and is only part of a complex system that may confine the adaptive response of the host (Bankhead and Chaconas 2007).

Immune-system selection on *B. burgdorferi* has received extensive study and host specialization is thought to result from negative selection mediated by the complement system of the host's innate immune system (Schroeder *et al.* 2009). Spirochetes that are susceptible to destruction by the complement system of a given species are lysed early in the midgut of the tick (Kurtenbach *et al.* 2002*a*). This has led to the hypothesis that the host range of a spirochete strain is restricted by the genes that encode ligands that bind to complement inhibitors (Kurtenbach *et al.* 2002*b*).

The second main component of the mammalian immune system is the adaptive immune system, which introduces nonlinear frequency-dependent fitness, leading to fluctuations in the abundance of spirochete genotypes. Balancing selection by the adaptive immune system on the *ospC* gene maintains spirochete diversity within local tick populations (Schroeder *et al.* 2009), with persistent *B. burgdorferi* strains being favored over "boom and bust" ones (Kurtenbach *et al.* 2006). In a further refinement by Gatewood *et al.* (2009), persistent *B. burgdorferi* strains were interpreted as being favored when tick seasonality is asynchronous because of climatic conditions such as the relatively small difference between summer- and winter-temperature extremes in the northeastern USA. In the Upper Midwest of the USA, in contrast, less-persistent strains are favored because greater seasonal temperature disparities are associated with more overlap in the durations of larval and nymphal activity, allowing easier transmission of *B. burgdorferi* strains from infected nymphs to uninfected larvae (Gatewood *et al.* 2009). Modeling of tick phenology has been expanded to include synchronicity with reservoir hosts and photoperiod (Ogden *et al.* 2006, 2008*b*), and it is clear that further complexity remains to be modeled.

Diagnosis and serology of LB

Initial diagnostic steps

Although all evidence indicates that ticks are necessary for infection with *B. burgdorferi*, the ticks themselves are often not noticed. Steere (1989) reported that only 50%–70% of people report a tick bite before being diagnosed with LB. Tick saliva is well documented as containing an anaesthetic that reduces the probability of tick detection (Ribeiro and Francischetti 2003) and, considering their small size, immature ticks are likely to have an even lower rate of detection than adults.

On the other hand, knowledge of the presence of *Ixodes* ticks in an area can contribute to a diagnosis of LB. For example, an erythema migrans (EM) rash is considered sufficient by itself for a diagnosis of LB, but only in geographic areas where *I. scapularis* or

I. pacificus is established (CPS 2009). The presence of an EM rash, with its characteristic bull's-eye appearance, is not enough to justify treatment in areas of Canada where these *Ixodes* species are not believed to be endemic; in such cases confirmatory serology is advised before the diagnosis is given (CPS 2009). Variability in the presence and appearance of the EM rash has been extensively documented (Tibbles and Edlow 2007; Egberts *et al.* 2008). About 80% of confirmed LB patients are reported to show the rash (Aguero-Rosenfeld *et al.* 2005; Bratton *et al.* 2008), and American researchers often explicitly require the EM rash to be present for a patient to be considered for enrollment in a study (*e.g.*, Wormser *et al.* 2008). Of 95 children presenting with facial palsy in an area of the USA where LB is endemic who later received serological confirmation of LB, only 35 reported the rash (Nigrovic *et al.* 2008). In Europe, only 18% of Swedish children with confirmed neuroborreliosis reported the rash (Skogman *et al.* 2008).

For a serological diagnosis of LB worldwide, either an enzyme-linked immunosorbent assay (ELISA) or an immunofluorescent assay (IFA) is expected to constitute the first step of a two-step diagnosis (Aguero-Rosenfeld *et al.* 2005). If the ELISA or IFA is positive, the second step is a Western blot immunoassay. Both the ELISA and the IFA are designed to detect serum antibodies produced by the host against proteins of *B. burgdorferi*. In Canada, only a positive or equivocal ELISA is currently accepted before a Western blot, which is more specific but more expensive, can be requested (CPHLN 2007). In the USA and Europe, either an ELISA or an IFA will fulfill the first step (CDC 1995; Brouqui *et al.* 2004). Like an ELISA, an IFA can use antibodies to whole-cell lysates or purified antigens such as flagellin, OspC, or P39. However, interpretation of an IFA requires well-trained personnel, whereas the more frequently used ELISA is more easily automated (Aguero-Rosenfeld *et al.* 2005). In Canada, the sensitivity of ELISA is considered to be close to 100% for tests performed 4 weeks post tick bite (Barker and Lindsay 2000; Forward 2005; Zaretsky 2006; CPHLN 2007; CPS 2009). This contrasts with Aguero-Rosenfeld *et al.* (2005), whose Table 4 reports that ELISA sensitivity is always less than 50% in the acute phase of an EM rash and only about 80% in the convalescent phase after antimicrobial treatment for an EM rash or a diagnosis of LB has been obtained because of neurological involvement. Only the arthritis form of LB was associated with higher ELISA sensitivity. There is considerable debate over the sensitivity of ELISA, especially in late stages of the disease (*e.g.*, Donta 2007; Wilson 2007; Stricker and Johnson 2008).

In laboratory diagnoses, sensitivity is defined as the percentage of people truly suffering from a disease who are identified as positive by means of an assay (Saah and Hoover 1997). This is not the same as the more commonly understood use of the term sensitivity for analyses, which refers to an assay's ability to detect a low concentration or signal in a sample (*e.g.*, the ability of an ELISA to detect low quantities of antibodies to *B. burgdorferi*). Diagnostic specificity, on the other hand, is defined as the percentage of people who do not have a disease and who are identified as negative by means of an assay (Saah and Hoover 1997). High diagnostic sensitivity means that an assay produces a high rate of true positives and a low rate of false negatives. Furthermore, high diagnostic specificity means a high rate of true negatives and a low rate of false positives. Laboratory diagnosis of LB has tended to emphasize diagnostic specificity and the need to eliminate false positives, rather than high sensitivity and the elimination of false negatives (CPHLN 2007; CPS 2009). Thus, a patient may eventually be diagnosed as having LB on the basis of PCR tests, observations of spirochetes in tissue, or clinical symptoms, in spite of an earlier ELISA test that returned a negative result. Clinicians, however, are often not aware of the potential for such false negatives, especially in late disease (Donta 2002, 2003, 2007; Wilson 2007).

Because ELISA is used as a screening method in Canada (CPHLN 2007), a negative ELISA may be taken as evidence that there is no infection with *Borrelia*. This interpretation of ELISA has resulted in the claim that there is no valid support for the idea that LB is underdiagnosed in Canada (CPS 2009). This viewpoint contrasts with Ogden *et al.* (2008*d*), who stated that underreporting is more biologically plausible. The documented genetic diversity and biological complexity of *B. burgdorferi* s.l. cannot help but contribute to difficulties in detecting *Borrelia* with both high sensitivity and high specificity, especially when the spirochetes enter tissues, such as collagen, to which the host's immune system has limited access (Cabello *et al.* 2007; Miklossy *et al.* 2008).

Effectiveness of specific ELISA tests

Commercial ELISA kits can be based on whole-cell sonicates or more specific antigens like flagellin and C6 peptide. Currently, whole-cell sonicates of strain B31 are used in Canada for humans (CPHLN 2007), whereas C6 peptide kits (IDEXX Laboratories, Inc. 2008) are favored for dogs. The C6 peptide ELISA relies on a single peptide from the VlsE protein, a lipoprotein with an invariable region, C6, which is highly antigenic. Because the assay based on C6 peptide is different from the standard ELISA used for the same organisms, dogs may serve as sentinels for some *B. burgdorferi* s.l. strains that are not detected using the whole cell sonicate ELISA kits used for humans.

The use of dogs as sentinels for LB is controversial and has recently been reviewed by Fritz (2009). The C6 peptide assay is considered to allow greater specificity than earlier assays, since it is only expressed in actively infected animals (Liang *et al.* 1999, 2002). Although treatment of seropositive dogs is discouraged unless clinical signs are present, the use of domestic dogs to demonstrate the presence of *B. burgdorferi* in areas where ticks are localized may lead to an underestimate rather than an overestimate of the presence of *B. burgdorferi* (Fritz 2009).

Some researchers use an in-house sonicate derived from strain B31 (*e.g.*, Steere *et al.* 2008), whereas others use whole-cell sonicates of N40 (*e.g.*, Pachner *et al.* 2002). Wormser *et al.* (2008) maintained that the diversity of LB strains is unlikely to be relevant to the diagnosis of human disease provided a whole-cell sonicate is used in the ELISA. However, use of whole-cell sonicates produces a high level of background absorbance, necessitating correction for false positives and potentially reducing the detection of true positives (Lawrenz *et al.* 1999; Donta 2002). It has been suggested that this effect explains the low sensitivity in a serological survey of deer in Ontario (Gallivan *et al.* 1998). Wilske *et al.* (2007) recommend that because of the heterogeneity of causative agents of LB in Europe, ELISAs should be based on OspC as well as DbpA, VlsE, or C6 peptide to improve sensitivity.

Commercial ELISA kits licensed for use in the USA vary substantially in sensitivity. Aguero-Rosenfeld *et al.* (2005) reported ranges from 33% (EM rash) to 79% (neuroborreliosis) and 100% (Lyme arthritis). Such an ascertainment bias in favor of the arthritis form of LB may account for statements that Lyme arthritis, the original name of the disease, is the most common form of late LB in North America (Wormser *et al.* 2006, 2007). Furthermore, the B31 strain has been shown to cause arthritic symptoms disproportionately relative to other members of *B. burgdorferi* s.l. (Terekhova *et al.* 2006; Tilly *et al.* 2008; Craig-Mylius *et al.* 2009; Hildenbrand *et al.* 2009; Kudryashev *et al.* 2009), so it is not unexpected that serological testing based on B31 is particularly effective in detecting the arthritis form of LB.

Western blots

Western blots, also called immunoblots, use gel electrophoresis to separate proteins by size or shape, after which they are visualized by staining with antibodies specific to the target proteins and scored for presence and intensity of the banding pattern. They are generally more expensive to run than an ELISA because they are more labor-intensive and require highly trained personnel to interpret the banding patterns (Bjerrum and Heegaard 2001).

A Western blot of patient serum antibodies to LB antigens is required as the second step in a serological diagnosis of LB. In Canada, the Western blot must have at least 2 of 3 bands for immunoglobulin M (IgM) as well as at least 5 of 10 bands for immunoglobulin G

(IgG) (CPHLN 2007). These criteria were established for active or previous infection and were designed to identify a banding pattern that gave high statistical specificity. Bands for IgM antibodies to both OspA and OspB and for IgG antibodies to OspB were explicitly excluded (Dressler *et al.* 1993), even though these bands are highly diagnostic. Because these proteins were intended as candidates for vaccine development (Fikrig *et al.* 1992), assays based on these bands would have been unable to distinguish between active LB and vaccination. An OspA vaccine was eventually released but withdrawn in 2002, ostensibly for economic reasons but there were suggestions that it had autoimmune effects (Rosé *et al.* 2001; Nigrovic and Thompson 2007; Nardelli *et al.* 2008).

It is generally accepted that OspC is the immunodominant protein involved in the IgM response, while decorin-binding protein A (DbpA) is the immunodominant protein in the IgG response (Jovicić *et al.* 2003; Wilske *et al.* 2007). However, Fingerle *et al.* (1998) demonstrated that 31% of *B. burgdorferi* from ticks that had been feeding on humans in southern Germany expressed OspA rather than OspC and that these *B. burgdorferi* were capable of causing disease in humans. Some current Western blot kits used in Canada, such as MarDx (CPHLN 2007), are based on a sonicate of strain B31. False-negative serology is considered a significant risk in neuroborreliosis unless multiple *Borrelia* strains are tested for (Kaiser 2000; Jovicić *et al.* 2003). In Europe, multiple *Borrelia* species are acknowledged and Western blots are interpreted differently than in North America, where *B. burgdorferi* s.s. is often assumed to be responsible for all human LB (CDC 1995; Robertson *et al.* 2000; Wormser *et al.* 2006, 2007; Vanousová and Hercogová 2008).

To confirm a LB diagnosis, it may be considered necessary to document conversion from IgM to IgG about 4 weeks or more after infection (Aguero-Rosenfeld *et al.* 2005; Wormser *et al.* 2006, 2007). In some people, however, seronegativity with only a cell-mediated immune response is possible (Singh and Girschick 2004). In addition, detection of antibodies that are tied up in complexes would be missed by standard tests that rely on free antibodies (Singh and Girschick 2004; Holl-Wieden *et al.* 2007).

Antigenic variation

Preferential expression of proteins by *B. burgdorferi* in both the tick vector and the mammalian host results in differential expression of antibodies that can be detected by immunoblots. For example, OspA/B is expressed in ticks (Neelakanta *et al.* 2007), whereas dmpA/B and bmpA/B are expressed in the mammalian host (Pal *et al.* 2008; Shi *et al.* 2008). The serological response in early LB would be expected to include proteins that may be downgraded in later disease while the antibody response to later disease would be expected to show different proteins. As with vlsE, antigenic variation within a single immunogenic protein allows *B. burgdorferi* to evade the host response and so immunblots would be expected to allow only variable detection of some proteins. Fortunately, multiple immunogenic proteins have been described and in recent work a genome-wide proteome array and protein microassay have been used to expand the number of diagnostic antigenic proteins that are useful in serological diagnosis (Barbour *et al.* 2008; Xu *et al.* 2008*b*).

PCR assays

North American practitioners have been reluctant to accept PCR tests as the primary basis for a diagnosis of LB (*e.g.*, Halperin and Wormser 2001). Such tests can show a large variation in specificity among studies, tissue categories, and geographic regions. Meta-analysis of PCR assays carried out in North America and Europe generally show moderate median sensitivity for skin biopsy (69%) and synovial fluid (78%) but low median sensitivity for cerebrospinal fluid (38%) and blood/plasma/serum (14%) (Aguero-Rosenfeld *et al.* 2005). The ranges of these values were at least 50% among individual studies, and when the studies were grouped by continent the difference in median sensitivity between North

America and Europe ranged from 8% (blood/plasma/serum) to 50% (cerebrospinal fluid). However, specificity rates for these categories are much higher, usually 100%, with the lowest being 93% (Aguero-Rosenfeld *et al.* 2005), which means that there are very few false positives. Thus, in spite of extensive documented variation in specificity and high rates of false negatives, PCR tests can be useful for confirming clinical diagnoses in individual cases. For example, a case of seronegative Lyme arthritis has been described where PCR-positive synovial fluid allowed a diagnosis to be made in the absence of a serological response (Holl-Wieden *et al.* 2007).

Although PCR-based diagnosis of LB in humans is problematic, presumably because spirochetes can be sequestered in tissues that were not tested, this is not such an impediment to the detection of *Borrelia* in ticks. Numerous studies have consistently demonstrated that whole or partial ticks can be homogenized to give sufficient DNA for identifying a substantial variety of bacterial symbionts (*e.g.*, van Overbeek *et al.* 2008). Furthermore, DNA-based identification of the ticks themselves is feasible *via* DNA barcoding or other DNA-based techniques (Sperling and Roe 2009), which should be especially useful for identifying immature stages, where diagnostic characters visible in their morphology are limited.

Future directions

Human cases of LB in Canada can be devastating to affected individuals, not only because of increasingly debilitating health effects over time, but because of the psychologically draining process of obtaining a formal diagnosis that allows treatment *via* the Canadian health system. It is easy to understand why a diagnosis of LB can be difficult to obtain in the face of its ecological complexity, genetic diversity, and immunological heterogeneity. With so much specialized information to assimilate and comprehend, it can be equally difficult to know where efforts to improve the situation can make a significant difference. Fortunately, it is likely that entomologists can contribute in a number of ways to a positive resolution of the challenges presented by LB.

First, there is a strong need for better means of identifying tick species and for detailed documentation of their distributions across Canada. Morphology-based keys that require only the use of a good microscope have been available for many decades, but relatively little new work on publicly accessible identification guides for ticks in Canada has been done since Gregson (1956). However, a handbook to the ticks of Canada is nearing completion (T. Galloway, University of Manitoba, Winnipeg, personal communication) and should fill an urgent need. Furthermore, there is good potential for DNA-based identification and delimitation of tick species (Sperling and Roe 2009), and internet-accessible guides can supplement these efforts. Such efforts should facilitate localized surveys of tick distributions, which are essential to more effective modeling and prediction of changes in tick and LB distributions in the context of climate change (Ogden *et al.* 2008*a*, 2008*c*, 2008*d*). The patchy distributions of *B. burgdorferi*-infected hosts and ticks means that using average numbers of infected ticks across a large area may underestimate the prevalence of LB. Efforts to identify patches should focus on areas where exposure of humans or their companion animals has been reported, because large-scale inventories of ticks are unlikely to pick up infrequent patches. The dispersal and population structure of ticks can be studied using molecular markers such as microsatellites, and the field is ripe for further work of this kind (*e.g.*, Kain *et al.* 1999).

The second way in which entomologists can contribute, in conjunction with microbiologists, is through more effective identification of *Borrelia* species and other symbionts in ticks. This will allow more effective study of the factors that regulate the behavior and interaction of ticks with their vertebrate hosts and bacterial symbionts. PCR-based diagnostics of *Borrelia* species and surveys of the diversity of bacterial strains in ticks are now commonplace. These should enable more comprehensive documentation of the distribution and evolution of these symbionts in spite of the challenges of growing them in culture (Aguero-Rosenfeld *et al.* 2005). Furthermore, new techniques for *in vivo* visualization of *Borrelia* are providing insights into the behavior of spirochetes (Moriarty *et al.* 2008). Round bodies of *B. burgdorferi* have also been visualized post mortem in confirmed cases of LB (Miklossy *et al.* 2008); this method may therefore assist in confirming previously inconclusive cases.

Consistent identification of *Borrelia* cannot help but increase our understanding of the transmission dynamics of these bacteria in specific ecological or behavioral circumstances. For example, Faulde and Robbins (2008) recently demonstrated that fewer infected ticks were picked up by dragging for the main European vector of LB, *I. ricinus*, than by collecting from exposed human volunteers, which suggests that *Borrelia burgdorferi* s.l. may increase the host-finding efficacy of female *I. ricinus* under natural conditions. Such an effect may explain why some of the low numbers of ticks collected in Canada by dragging or flagging test positive. It also supports the use of passive surveillance, because a higher percentage of positive ticks would be expected from ticks collected on hosts. Furthermore, *Borrelia* incidence and vector competence should be addressed more comprehensively in tick species other than those of *Ixodes*. An example is the competence of deer and other ungulates as reservoirs for *B. burgdorferi*. Even for *Ixodes* ticks, little is published that gives deer infection rates in Canada beyond the studies done in Ontario by Gallivan *et al.* (1998). Although the finding obviously needs to be confirmed, the Tennessee study by Shariat *et al.* (2007) opens up the possibility that deer are effective reservoir species in some areas, and *Dermacentor* ticks may even be involved as vectors.

A third major research gap in Canada is the synergistic effect of co-infections in vectors or alternative reservoirs, which opens up opportunities for entomological collaboration with public health researchers as well as with microbiologists. The diversity of species and strains of *Borrelia* is still incompletely understood and the most important combinations involved in these co-infections are largely unknown. Simultaneous infection by *B. burgdorferi* and *Babesia microti* Franca increases the severity of arthritis in mice (Moro *et al.* 2002). Human infection with both *B. burgdorferi* and *Babesia microti* was described in Ontario in 1997, with the recognition that more serious disease symptoms are associated with co-infection (dosSantos and Kain 1998). More severe symptoms continue to be reported for LB cases with co-infections (Rawling *et al.* 2009). For vectors, Zhong *et al.* (2007) have demonstrated that in *Amblyomma* C.L. Koch ticks treated with antibiotics, reproductive fitness is reduced. In their study system, *Coxiella* sp. Philip was the identified endosymbiont. Because *I. scapularis* also has an endosymbiont, a *Rickettsia*-like bacterium (Noda *et al.* 1997), this information may have relevance to the LB system. Not only would treating the ticks with antibiotics potentially reduce the incidence of *B. burgdorferi*, it might also reduce the population of the tick vector. The effectiveness of antibiotic-baited traps that target mice (Dolan *et al.* 2008) may have further advantages for integrated pest management strategies for controlling LB by lowering populations of *Ixodes* in subsequent years.

Practitioners of integrated pest management and other aspects of economic entomology will recognize a fourth research need: a long-term and broad-scale analysis of the costs and challenges of LB to humans, which is essential to a more effective deployment of resources to combat this disease. Recognizing that human cases are possible across the geographic expanse of Canada is vital to reducing the burden on the public health care system. Furthermore, recognizing and monitoring the changing effects of LB over time will pay dividends on a human scale. In Scotland the cost of treating a case of early LB is estimated to be one-third that of treating late LB (Joss *et al.* 2003), and early and effective treatment is viewed as a cost-saving measure. In Scotland, regular audits of the interpretation of Western blots that are tailored to local areas has been emphasized. This has resulted in improved management of patients, and it is now recognized that the 58-kilodalton protein is a highly specific indicator of infection by *B. burgdorferi*

(Evans *et al.* 2005). A revised antigen for IgG Western blotting has been produced and has increased sensitivity for Scottish patients (Mavin *et al.* 2009). Canadians might do well to follow this example and conduct an audit of the proteins used to establish a positive Western blot. The various ELISA tests are also in need of renewed scrutiny.

Variability and recurrence of symptoms are hallmarks of LB (Cameron *et al.* 2004; Holl-Wieden *et al.* 2007; Nardelli *et al.* 2008). Establishment of the initial infection, its dissemination, and the development of pathology are all stages in this complex disease. Debate is ongoing concerning the severity of symptoms and the role of persistent infection and immunological dysfunction in continued symptoms. The ecology of LB is challenging: at every spatial scale studied so far, the risk is unevenly distributed (Killilea *et al.* 2008). A coordinated, multidisciplinary, and flexible approach to understanding LB is needed to reduce the burden of this disease in Canada and abroad. Entomologists are in an ideal position to achieve rapprochement between the highly divergent groups of people concerned with LB and to contribute to a better understanding of its practical and intellectual challenges.

Acknowlegements

We thank Reuben Kaufman, Kathy Magor, Judith Miklossy, George Chaconas, and two anonymous reviewers for comments on an earlier draft of the manuscript, as well as Harvey Artsob, Saswati Das, Terry Galloway, Robbin Lindsay, and Louise Trudel for providing useful information. F.A.H.S. gratefully acknowledges support from a Discovery Grant from the Natural Sciences and Engineering Research Council of Canada and funding from Genome Alberta / Genome British Columbia.

References

Aguero-Rosenfeld, M.E., Wang, G., Schwartz, I., and Wormser, G.P. 2005. Diagnosis of lyme borreliosis. Clinical Microbiology Reviews, **18**(3): 484–509. PMID:16020686 doi:10.1128/CMR.18.3.484-509.2005.

Alekseev, A.N., Arumova, E.A., and Vasilieva, I.S. 1995. *Borrelia burgdorferi* sensu lato in female cement plug of *Ixodes persulcatus* ticks (Acari, Ixodidae). Experimental and Applied Acarology, **19**(9): 519–522. PMID:8575271 doi:10.1007/BF00052920.

Allan, B.F., Keesing, F., and Ostfeld, R. 2003. Effect of forest fragmentation on Lyme disease risk. Conservation Biology, **17**(1): 267–272. doi:10.1046/j.1523-1739.2003.01260.x.

Anderson, J.M., and Valenzuela, J.G. 2007. Spit-acular entry: *Borrelia* gets help from a tick salivary protein to move from the mammalian host to the arthropod vector. Cell Host and Microbe, **2**(1): 3–4. PMID:18005711 doi:10.1016/j.chom.2007.06.007.

Anderson, R.R., and Harrington, L.C. 2009. Tick biology for the home owner [on-line]. Available from http://www.entomology.cornell.edu/MedEnt/TickBioFS/TickBioFS.html [accessed 31 May 2009].

Arnold, R.R., Russell, J.E., Champion, W.J., Brewer, M., and Gauthier, J.J. 1982. Bactericidal activity of human lactoferrin: differentiation from the stasis of iron deprivation. Infection and Immunity, **35**(3): 792–799 PMID:6802759.

Artsob, H., Garvie, M., Cawthorn, R.J., Horney, B., Maloney, R., Dick, D., and McBurney, S. 1992. Isolation of the Lyme disease spirochete, *Borrelia burgdorferi*, from *Ixodes dammini* (Acari: Ixodidae) collected on Prince Edward Island, Canada. Journal of Medical Entomology, **29**(6): 1063–1066 PMID:1460625.

Artsob, H., Maloney, R., Conboy, G., and Horney, B. 2000. Identification of *Ixodes scapularis* in Newfoundland, Canada. Canada Communicable Disease Report, **26**(16): 133–134.

Ballantyne, C. 2008. The chronic debate over Lyme disease. Nature Medicine, **14**(11): 1135–1139. PMID:18989271 doi:10.1038/nm1108-1135.

Banerjee, S. 1993. Isolation of *Borrelia burgdorferi* in British Columbia. Canada Diseases Weekly Report No. 19-24. pp. 204–205.

Banerjee, S.N., Banerjee, M., Fernando, K., Dong, M.Y., Smith, J.A., and Cook, D. 1995a. Isolation of *Borrelia burgdorferi*, the Lyme disease spirochete from rabbit ticks, *Haemaphysalis leporispalustris* from Alberta. Journal of Spirochetal and Tick-Borne Diseases, **2**: 23–24.

Banerjee, S.N., Christensen, C.I., and Scott, J.D. 1995b. Lyme disease in Canada. Canada Communicable Disease Report **21**(10). PMID:7881380.

Bankhead, T., and Chaconas, G. 2007. The role of VlsE antigenic variation in the Lyme disease spirochete: persistence through a mechanism that differs from other pathogens. Molecular Microbiology, **65**(6): 1547–1558. PMID:17714442 doi:10.1111/j.1365-2958.2007.05895.x.

Barbour, A.G., and Hayes, S.F. 1986. Biology of *Borrelia* species. Microbiological Reviews, **50**(4): 381–400 PMID:3540570.

Barbour, A.G., Jasinskas, A., Kayala, M.A., Davies, D.H., Steere, A.C., Baldi, P., and Felgner, P.L. 2008. A genome-wide proteome array reveals a limited set of immunogens in natural infections of humans and white-footed mice with *Borrelia burgdorferi*. Infection and Immunity, **76**(8): 3374–3389. PMID:18474646 doi:10.1128/IAI.00048-08.

Barker, I.K., and Lindsay, L.R. 2000. Lyme borreliosis in Ontario: determining the risks. Canadian Medical Association Journal, **162**(11): 1573–1574 PMID:10862232.

Barker, I.K., Surgeoner, G.A., McEwen, S.A., and Artsob, H. 1988. *Borrelia burgdorferi*, the agent of Lyme disease, in tick vectors and wildlife reservoirs in southern Ontario. Ontario Disease Surveillance Report No. 9. pp. 151–154.

Barker, I.K., Lindsay, L.R., Campbell, G.D., Surgeoner, G.A., and McEwen, S.A. 1993. The groundhog tick *Ixodes cookei* (Acari: Ixodidae): a poor potential vector of Lyme borreliosis. Journal of Wildlife Diseases, **29**: 416–422.

Barthold, S. 2000. Lyme borreliosis. *In* Persistent bacterial infections. *Edited by* J.P. Nataro, M.J. Blaser, and S. Cunningham-Rundles. ASM Press, Washington, D.C. pp. 281–304.

Bjerkelund, J. 1997. New Brunswick Veterinary Medical Association Newsletter June 1997, Saint John, New Brunswick. pp. 15–16.

Bjerrum, O.J., and Heegaard, N.H.H. 2001. Western blotting. *In* Encyclopedia of life sciences. John Wiley and Sons, London. pp. 1–6.

Bollegraaf, E. 1988. Lyme disease in Canada. Canada Diseases Weekly Report No. 14-22. pp. 95–97.

Bratton, R.L., Whiteside, J.W., Hovan, M.J., Engle, R.L., and Edwards, F.D. 2008. Diagnosis and treatment of Lyme disease. Mayo Clinic Proceedings, **83**(5): 566–571. PMID:18452688 doi:10.4065/83.5.566.

Breier, F., Khanakah, G., Stanek, G., Kunz, G., Aberer, E., Schmidt, B., and Tappeiner, G. 2001. Isolation and polymerase chain reaction typing of *Borrelia afzelii* from a skin lesion in a seronegative patient with generalized ulcerating bullous lichen sclerosus et atrophicus. The British Journal of Dermatology, **144**(2): 387–392. PMID:11251580 doi:10.1046/j.1365-2133.2001.04034.x.

Brisson, D., Dykhuizen, D.E., and Ostfeld, R.S. 2008. Conspicuous impacts of inconspicuous hosts on the Lyme disease epidemic. Proceedings of the Royal Society, Biological Sciences, **275**: 227–235.

British Columbia Ministry of Health. 2008. Press release: Lyme disease in B.C., February 29 2008 [on-line]. Available from http://www.health.gov.bc.ca/cpa/mediasite/pdf/fr_Lyme_disease_Feb29_2008.pdf [accessed 21 February 2009].

Brorson, Ø., Brorson, S.H. 1998. In vitro conversion of *Borrelia burgdorferi* to cystic forms in spinal fluid, and transformation to mobile spirochetes by incubation in BSK-H medium. Infection, **26**(3): 144–150. PMID:9646104 doi:10.1007/BF02771839.

Brorson, Ø., Brorson, S.H. 2004. An in vitro study of the susceptibility of mobile and cystic forms of *Borrelia burgdorferi* to tinidazole. International Microbiology, **7**(2): 139–142 PMID:15248163.

Brouqui, P., Bacellar, F., Baranton, G., Birtles, R.J., Bjoërsdorff, A., Blanco, J.R., *et al.* 2004. Guidelines for the diagnosis of tick-borne bacterial diseases in Europe. Clinical Microbiology and Infection, **10**(12): 1108–1132. PMID:15606643 doi:10.1111/j.1469-0691.2004.01019.x.

Bunikis, J., Garpmo, U., Tsao, J., Berglund, J., Fish, D., and Barbour, A.G. 2004. Sequence typing reveals extensive strain diversity of the Lyme borreliosis agents *Borrelia burgdorferi* in North America and *Borrelia afzelii* in Europe. Microbiology, 150(**6**): 1741–1755. PMID:1518 4561 doi:10.1099/mic.0.26944-0.

Burgdorfer, W., Barbour, A.G., Hayes, S.F., Benach, J.L., Grunwaldt, E., and Davis, J.P. 1982. Lyme disease — a tick-borne spirochetosis? Science (Washington, D.C.), **216**(4552): 1317–1319. PMID:7043737 doi:10.1126/science.7043737.

Burgess, E.C., and Patrican, L.A. 1987. Oral infection of *Peromyscus maniculatus* with *Borrelia burgdorferi* and subsequent transmission by *Ixodes dammini.* The American Journal of Tropical Medicine and Hygiene, **36**(2): 402–407 PMID:3826500.

Burkot, T.R., Maupin, G.O., Schneider, B.S., Denatale, C., Happ, C.M., Rutherford, J.S., and Zeidner, N.S. 2001. Use of a sentinel host system to study the questing behavior of *Ixodes spinipalpis* and its role in the transmission of *Borrelia bissettii*, human granulocytic ehrlichiosis, and *Babesia microti.* The American Journal of Tropical Medicine and Hygiene, **65**(4): 293–299 PMID:11693872.

Cabello, F.C., Godfrey, H.P., and Newman, S.A. 2007. Hidden in plain sight: *Borrelia burgdorferi* and the extracellular matrix. Trends in Microbiology, **15**(8): 350–354. PMID:17600717 doi:10.1016/j.tim.2007.06.003.

Cameron, D.J. 2009. Clinical trials validate the severity of persistent Lyme disease symptoms. Medical Hypotheses, **72**(2): 153–156. PMID:19013025 doi:10.1016/j.mehy.2008.09.030.

Cameron, D.J., Gaito, A., Harris, N., Bach, G., Bellovin, S., Bock, K., *et al.* 2004. Evidence-based guidelines for the management of Lyme disease. Expert Review of Anti-Infective Therapy, **2**(1 Suppl): S1–S13. PMID:15581390 doi:10.1586/14789072.2.1.S1.

Canadian Lyme Disease Foundation. 2009. Ticks of Canada [online]. Available from http://www.canlyme.com/tickscanada.html [accessed 25 March 2009].

Canadian Paediatric Society (CPS). 2009. Lyme disease in Canada: Q and A for paediatricians. Paediatrics and Child Health (Oxford), **14**: 103–105.

Canadian Public Health Laboratory Network (CPHLN). 2007. The laboratory diagnosis of Lyme borreliosis: guidelines from the Canadian Public Health Laboratory Network. The Canadian Journal of Infectious Diseases and Medical Microbiology. **18**(2): 145–148 PMID:18923770.

Casjens, S., Palmer, N., van Vugt, R., Huang, W.M., Stevenson, B., Rosa, P., *et al.* 2000. A bacterial genome in flux: the twelve linear and nine circular extrachromosomal DNAs in an infectious isolate of the Lyme disease spirochete *Borrelia burgdorferi.* Molecular Microbiology, **35**(3): 490–516. PMID:10672174 doi:10.1046/j.1365-2958.2000.01698.x.

Centers for Disease Control and Prevention (CDC). 1995. Recommendations for test performance and interpretation. *In* Proceedings of the Second National Conference on Serologic Diagnosis of Lyme Disease. Morbidity and Mortality Weekly Report, **44**: 590–591.

Centers for Disease Control and Prevention (CDC). 2007. Lyme disease — United States, 2003−2005. Morbidity and Mortality Weekly Report, **56**(23): 573–576 PMID:17568368.

Chaconas, G. 2005. Hairpin telomeres and genome plasticity in *Borrelia*: all mixed up in the end. Molecular Microbiology, **58**(3): 625–635. PMID: 16238614 doi:10.1111/j.1365-2958.2005.04872.x.

Charron, D., and Sockett, P. 2005. Signs of change, signs of trouble: finding the evidence in climate change: preparing for the health impacts. Health Policy Research Bulletin, **11**: 27–30.

Clark, K., Hendricks, A., and Burge, D. 2005. Molecular identification and analysis of *Borrelia burgdorferi sensu lato* in lizards in the southeastern United States. Applied and Environmental Microbiology, **71**(5): 2616–2625. PMID:15870353 doi:10.1128/AEM.71.5.2616-2625.2005.

Clover, J.R., and Lane, R.S. 1995. Evidence implicating nymphal *Ixodes pacificus* (Acari: Ixodidae) in the epidemiology of Lyme disease in California. The American Journal of Tropical Medicine and Hygiene, **53**(3): 237–240 PMID:7573703.

Connecticut General Assembly. 2009. An act concerning the use of long-term antibiotics for the treatment of Lyme disease [online]. Available from http://www.cga.ct.gov/asp/cgabillstatus/cgabillstatus.asp?selBillType=Bill&bill_num=HB-6200 [accessed 30 May 2009].

Costero, A. 1990. Identification of the Lyme disease vector in Canada. Canada Diseases Weekly Report No. 16-30. pp. 142–147.

Craig-Mylius, K.A., Lee, M., Jones, K.L., and Glickstein, L.J. 2009. Arthritogenicity of *Borrelia burgdorferi* and *Borrelia garinii*: comparison of infection in mice. The American Journal of Tropical Medicine and Hygiene, **80**(2): 252–258 PMID:19190223.

Crippa, M., Rais, O., and Gern, L. 2002. Investigations on the mode and dynamics of transmission and infectivity of *Borrelia burgdorferi* sensu stricto and *Borrelia afzelii* in *Ixodes ricinus* ticks. Vector Borne and Zoonotic Diseases (Larchmont, N.Y.), **2**(1): 3–9. PMID:12656125 doi:10.1089/153036602760260724.

Cutler, S.J., Moss, J., Fukunaga, M., Wright, D.J.M., Fekade, D., and Warrell, D. 1997. *Borrelia recurrentis* characterization and comparison with relapsing-fever, Lyme-associated, and other *Borrelia* spp. International Journal of Systematic Bacteriology, **47**(4): 958–968 PMID:9336893.

Doby, J.M., Anderson, J.F., Couatarmanac'h, A., Magnarelli, L.A., and Martin, A. 1987. Lyme disease in Canada with possible transmission by an insect. Zentralblatt für Bakteriologie, Mikrobiologie und Hygiene Series A, **263**: 488–490.

Dolan, M.C., Zeidner, N.S., Gabitzsch, E., Dietrich, G., Borchert, J.N., Poché, R.M., and Piesman, J. 2008. A doxycycline hyclate rodent bait formulation for prophylaxis and treatment of tick-transmitted *Borrelia burgdorferi.* The American Journal of Tropical Medicine and Hygiene, **78**(5): 803–805 PMID:18458316.

Donta, S.T. 2002. Late and chronic Lyme disease. The Medical Clinics of North America, **86**(2): 341–349., vii PMID:11982305 doi:10.1016/S0025-7125(03)00090-7.

Donta, S.T. 2003. Macrolide therapy of chronic Lyme disease. Medical Science Monitor, **9**: 136–142.

Donta, S.T. 2007. Lyme disease guidelines — it's time to move forward. Clinical Infectious Diseases, **44**(8): 1134–1135, author reply 1137–1139. PMID:17366465 doi:10.1086/51297.

dosSantos, C., and Kain, K. 1998. Concurrent babesiosis and Lyme disease diagnosed in Ontario. Canada Communicable Disease Report No. 24-12. pp. 1–3.

Dressler, F., Whalen, J.A., Reinhardt, B.N., and Steere, A.C. 1993. Western blotting in the serodiagnosis of Lyme disease. The Journal of Infectious Diseases, **167**(2): 392–400 PMID:8380611.

Durden, L.A., and Keirans, J.E. 1996. Nymphs of the genus *Ixodes* (Acari Ixodidae) of the United States:taxonomy, identification key, distribution, hosts, and medical/veterinary importance. Entomological Society of America, Lanham, Maryland, pp. 1–95.

Egberts, F., Moller, M., Proksch, E., and Schwarz, T. 2008. Multiple erythema migrans — manifestation of systemic cutaneous borreliosis.

Journal of the German Society of Dermatology, **6**: 350–353.

Eisen, L., and Lane, R.S. 2002. Vectors of *Borrelia burgdorferi* sensu lato. *In* Lyme borreliosis: biology, epidemiology and control. *Edited by* J. Gray, O. Kahl, R.S. Lane, and G. Stanek. CABI Publishing, New York.

Evans, R., Mavin, S., and Ho-Yen, D.O. 2005. Audit of the laboratory diagnosis of Lyme disease in Scotland. Journal of Medical Microbiology, **54**(12): 1139–1141. PMID:16278426 doi:10.1099/jmm.0.46003-0.

Exner, M. 2004. *Borrelia* spp. *In* Encyclopedia of medical genomics and proteomics. Volume 1. Part 1. pp. 146–149.

Falco, R.C., and Fish, D. 1991. Horizontal movement of adult *Ixodes dammini* (Acari: Ixodidae) attracted to CO_2-baited traps. Journal of Medical Entomology, **28**(5): 726–729 PMID:1941943.

Fallon, B.A., Keilp, J.G., Corbera, K.M., Petkova, E., Britton, C.B., Dwyer, E., *et al.* 2008. A randomized, placebo-controlled trial of repeated IV antibiotic therapy for Lyme encephalopathy. Neurology, **70**(13): 992–1003. PMID: 17928580 doi:10.1212/01.WNL.0000284604.61160.2d.

Faulde, M.K., and Robbins, R.G. 2008. Tick infestation risk and *Borrelia burgdorferi* s.l. infection-induced increase in host-finding efficacy of female *Ixodes ricinus* under natural conditions. Experimental and Applied Acarology, **44**: 127–145.

Fernando, K., Lee, M.-K., Wong, Q., Burgess, K., Durden, L., and Morshed, M. 2008. First Isolation of *Borrelia burgdorferi* from *Ixodes cookei* removed from a dog in Alberta. The Canadian Journal of Infectious Diseases and Medical Microbiology, **19**: 130.

Fikrig, E., Barthold, S.W., Marcantonio, N., Deponte, K., Kantor, F.S., and Flavell, R.A. 1992. Roles of OspA, OspB, and flagellin in protective immunity to Lyme borreliosis in laboratory mice. Infection and Immunity, **60**(2): 657–661 PMID:1730500.

Fingerle, V., Liegl, G., Munderloh, U., and Wilske, B. 1998. Expression of outer surface proteins A and C of *Borrelia burgdorferi* in *Ixodes ricinus* ticks removed from humans. Medical Microbiology and Immunology, **187**(2): 121–126. PMID:9832327 doi:10.1007/s004300050083.

Forward, K.R. 2005. Lyme Disease: dispelling the myth. The Canadian Journal of Continuing Medical Education, **17**: 73–75.

Fritz, C.L. 2009. Emerging tick-borne diseases. The Veterinary Clinics of North America, Small Animal Practice, **39**(2): 265–278. PMID: 19185193 doi:10.1016/j.cvsm.2008.10.019.

Furman, D.P., and Loomis, E.C. 1984. the ticks of California. Bulletin of the California Insect Survey, **25**.

Gallivan, G.J., Barker, I.K., Artsob, H., Magnarelli, L.A., Robinson, J.T., and Voigt, D.R. 1998. Serologic survey for antibodies to *Borrelia burgdorferi* in white-tailed deer in Ontario. Journal of Wildlife Diseases, **34**(2): 411–414 PMID:9577798.

Galloway, T.D. 2002. Getting to know your ticks. Blue Jay, **60**: 107–112.

Gammons, M., and Salam, G. 2002. Tick removal. American Family Physician, **66**(4): 643–645 PMID:12201558.

Gatewood, A.G., Liebman, K.A., Vourc'h, G., Bunikis, J., Hamer, S.A., Cortinas, R., *et al.* 2009. Climate and tick seasonality are predictors of *Borrelia burgdorferi* genotype distribution. Applied and Environmental Microbiology, **75**(8): 2476–2483. PMID:19251900 doi:10.1128/AEM.02633-08.

Giery, S.T., and Ostfeld, R.S. 2007. The role of lizards in the ecology of Lyme disease in two endemic zones of the northeastern United States. The Journal of Parasitology, **93**(3): 511–517. PMID:17626342 doi:10.1645/GE-1053R1.1.

Gilbert, M.A., Morton, E.A., Bundle, S.F., and Samuels, D.S. 2007. Artificial regulation of ospC expression in *Borrelia burgdorferi.* Molecular Microbiology, **63**(4): 1259–1273. PMID: 17257307 doi:10.1111/j.1365-2958.2007.05593.x.

Ginsberg, H.S., Buckley, P.A., Balmforth, M.G., Zhioua, E., Mitra, S., and Buckley, F.G. 2005. Reservoir competence of native North American birds for the Lyme disease spirochete, *Borrelia burgdorfieri.* Journal of Medical Entomology, **42**(3): 445–449. PMID:15962798 doi:10.1603/0022-2585(2005)042[0445:RCONNA]2.0.CO;2.

Girschick, H.J., Huppertz, H.I., Rüssmann, H., Krenn, V., and Karch, H. 1996. Intracellular persistence of *Borrelia burgdorferi* in human synovial cells. Rheumatology International, **16**(3): 125–132 PMID:8893378 doi:10.1007/BF01409985.

Gray, J.S. 1985. A carbon dioxide trap for prolonged sampling of *Ixodes ricinus* L. populations. Experimental and Applied Acarology, **1**(1): 35–44. PMID:3939717 doi:10.1007/BF01262198.

Gray, J.S., Kahl, O., Lane, R.S., and Stanek, G. (Editors). 2002. Lyme borreliosis: biology, epidemiology and control. CABI Publishing, New York.

Gregson, J.D. 1956. The Ixodidae of Canada. Publication 930, Canada Department of Agriculture, Ottawa, Ontario.

Halperin, J.J., and Wormser, G.P. 2001. Of fleas and ticks on cats and mice.... Archives of Neurology, **58**(9): 1345–1347. PMID:11559304 doi:10.1001/archneur.58.9.1345.

Hanincová, K., Ogden, N.H., Diuk-Wasser, M., Pappas, C.J., Iyer, R., Fish, D., Schwartz, I., and Kurtenbach, K. 2008. Fitness variation of *Borrelia burgdorferi* sensu stricto strains in mice.

Applied and Environmental Microbiology, **74**(1): 153–157. PMID:17981941 doi:10.1128/AEM.01567-07.

Hassett, A.L., Radvanski, D.C., Buyske, S., Savage, S.V., Gara, M., Escobar, J.I., and Sigal, L.H. 2008. Role of psychiatric comorbidity in chronic Lyme disease. Arthritis and Rheumatism, **59**(12): 1742–1749. PMID:19035409 doi:10.1002/art.24314.

Hildenbrand, P., Craven, D.E., Jones, R., and Nemeskal, P. 2009. Lyme neuroborreliosis: manifestations of a rapidly emerging zoonosis. American Journal of Neuroradiology, **30**(6): 1079–1087. PMID:19346313 doi:10.3174/ajnr.A1579.

Hodzic, E., Feng, S., Holden, K., Freet, K.J., and Barthold, S.W. 2008. Persistence of *Borrelia burgdorferi* following antibiotic treatment in mice. Antimicrobial Agents and Chemotherapy, **52**(5): 1728–1736. PMID:18316520 doi:10.1128/AAC.01050-07.

Hojgaard, A., Eisen, R.J., and Piesman, J. 2008. Transmission dynamics of *Borrelia burgdorferi* s.s. during the key third day of feeding by nymphal *Ixodes scapularis* (Acari: Ixodidae). Journal of Medical Entomology, **45**(4): 732–736. PMID:18714875 doi:10.1603/0022-2585(2008)45[732:TDOBBS]2.0.CO;2.

Holl-Wieden, A., Suerbaum, S., and Girschick, H.J. 2007. Seronegative Lyme arthritis. Rheumatology International, **27**(11): 1091–1093. doi:10.1007/s00296-007-0333-6.

Horobik, V., Keesing, F., and Ostfeld, R.S. 2006. Abundance and *Borrelia burgdorferi*-infection prevalence of nymphal *Ixodes scapularis* ticks along forest–field edges. EcoHealth, **3**(4): 262–268. doi:10.1007/s10393-006-0065-1.

Houhamdi, L., and Raoult, D. 2005. Excretion of living *Borrelia recurrentis* in feces of infected human body lice. The Journal of Infectious Diseases, **191**(11): 1898–1906. PMID:15871124 doi:10.1086/429920.

Hunfeld, K.P., Ruzic-Sabljic, E., Norris, D.E., Kraiczy, P., and Strle, F. 2005. In vitro susceptibility testing of *Borrelia burgdorferi* sensu lato isolates cultured from patients with erythema migrans before and after antimicrobial chemotherapy. Antimicrobial Agents and Chemotherapy, **49**(4): 1294–1301. PMID:15793100 doi:10.1128/AAC.49.4.1294-1301.2005.

IDEXX Laboratories, Inc. 2008. Incidence of heartworm, *Ehrlichia canis*, Lyme disease, and anplasmosis in dogs across Canada as determined by the IDEXX SNAP® 3Dx® and 4Dx® tests. 2007 national incidence study results. IDEXX Laboratories, Inc., Markham, Ontario. pp. 1–13.

Johnson, R.C., Schmid, G.P., Hyde, F.W., Steigerwalt, A.G., and Brenner, D.J. 1984. *Borrelia burgdorferi* sp. nov.: etiologic agent of Lyme disease. International Journal of Systematic Bacteriology, **34**: 496–497.

Joss, A.W.L., Davidson, M.M., Ho-Yen, D.O., and Ludbrook, A. 2003. Lyme disease — what is the cost for Scotland? Public Health, **117**(4): 264–273 PMID:12966749 doi:10.1016/S0033-3506(03)00067-2.

Jovicić, V.Lj., Grego, E.M., Lako, B.L., Ristović, B.M., Lepsanović, Z.A., and Stajković, N.T. 2003. Improved serodiagnosis of early Lyme borreliosis: immunoblot with local *Borrelia afzelii* strain. Acta Pathologica, Microbiologica et Immunologica, **111**(11): 1053–1059. PMID:14629271 doi:10.1111/j.1600-0463.2003.apm1111107.x.

Kahl, O., Janetzki-Mittmann, C., Gray, J.S., Jonas, R., Stein, J., and de Boer, R. 1998. Risk of infection with *Borrelia burgdorferi* sensu lato for a host in relation to the duration of nymphal *Ixodes ricinus* feeding and the method of tick removal. Zentralblatt für Bakteriologie, **287**(1–2): 41–52 PMID:9532263.

Kahl, O., Gern, L., Eisen, L., and Lane, R.S. 2002. Ecological research on *Borrelia burgdorferi* sensu lato: terminology and some methodological pitfalls. *In* Lyme borreliosis: biology, epidemiology and control. *Edited by* J. Gray, O. Kahl, R.S. Lane, and G. Stanek. CABI Publishing, New York.

Kain, D.E., Sperling, F.A.H., and Lane, R.S. 1997. Population genetic structure of *Ixodes pacificus* (Acari: Ixodidae) using allozymes. Journal of Medical Entomology, **34**(4): 441–450 PMID:9220679.

Kain, D.E., Sperling, F.A.H., Daly, H.V., and Lane, R.S. 1999. Mitochondrial DNA sequence variation in *Ixodes pacificus* (Acari: Ixodidae). Heredity, **83**(4): 378–386. PMID:10583539 doi:10.1038/sj.hdy.6886110.

Kaiser, R. 2000. False-negative serology in patients with neuroborreliosis and the value of employing of different borrelial strains in serological assays. Journal of Medical Microbiology, **49**(10): 911–915 PMID:11023188.

Keirans, J.E., and Clifford, C.M. 1978. The genus *Ixodes* in the United States: a scanning electron microscope study and key to the adults. Journal of Medical Entomology. Supplement 2.

Killilea, M.E., Swei, A., Lane, R.S., Briggs, C.J., and Ostfeld, R.S. 2008. Spatial dynamics of Lyme disease: a review. EcoHealth, **5**(2): 167–195. PMID:18787920 doi:10.1007/s10393-008-0171-3.

Kosik-Bogacka, D.I., Kuźna-Grygiel, W., and Jaborowska, M. 2007. Ticks and mosquitoes as vectors of *Borrelia burgdorferi* s. l. in the forested areas of Szczecin. Folia Biologica, **55**(3-4): 143–146. PMID:18274258 doi:10.3409/173491607781492542.

Kudryashev, M., Cyrklaff, M., Baumeister, W., Simon, M.M., Wallich, R., and Frischknecht, F.

2009. Comparative cryo-electron tomography of pathogenic Lyme disease spirochetes. Molecular Microbiology, **71**(6): 1415–1434. PMID:19210619 doi:10.1111/j.1365-2958.2009.06613.x.

Kurtenbach, K., Dizij, A., Seitz, H.M., Margos, G., Moter, S.E., Kramer, M.D., *et al.* 1994. Differential immune responses to *Borrelia burgdorferi* in European wild rodent species influence spirochete transmission to *Ixodes ricinus* L. (Acari: Ixodidae). Infection and Immunity, **62**(12): 5344–5352 PMID:7960113.

Kurtenbach, K., Kampen, H., Dizij, A., Arndt, S., Seitz, H.M., Schaible, U.E., and Simon, M.M. 1995. Infestation of rodents with larval *Ixodes ricinus* (Acari: Ixodidae) is an important factor in the transmission cycle of *Borrelia burgdorferi* s.l. in German woodlands. Journal of Medical Entomology, **32**(6): 807–817 PMID: 8551503.

Kurtenbach, K., Sewell, H.-S., Ogden, N.H., Randolph, S.E., and Nuttall, P.A. 1998. Serum complement sensitivity as a key factor in Lyme disease ecology. Infection and Immunity, **66**(3): 1248–1251 PMID:9488421.

Kurtenbach, K., De Michelis, S., Etti, S., Schäfer, S.M., Sewell, H.-S., Brade, V., and Kraiczy, P. 2002a. Host association of *Borrelia burgdorferi* sensu lato — the key role of host complement. Trends in Microbiology, **10**(2): 74–79 PMID: 11827808 doi:10.1016/S0966-842X(01)02298-3.

Kurtenbach, K., Schäfer, S.M., Sewell, H.-S., Peacey, M., Hoodless, A., Nuttall, P.A., and Randolph, S.E. 2002b. Differential survival of Lyme borreliosis spirochetes in ticks that feed on birds. Infection and Immunity, **70**(10): 5893–5895. PMID:12228325 doi:10.1128/IAI.70.10.5893-5895.2002.

Kurtenbach, K., Hanincová, K., Tsao, J.I., Margos, G., Fish, D., and Ogden, N.H. 2006. Fundamental processes in the evolutionary ecology of Lyme borreliosis. Nature Reviews Microbiology, **4**(9): 660–669. PMID:16894341 doi:10.1038/nrmicro1475.

Lane, R.S. 1990. Susceptibility of the western fence lizard (*Sceloporus occidentalis*) to the Lyme borreliosis spirochete (*Borrelia burgdorferi*). The American Journal of Tropical Medicine and Hygiene, **42**(1): 75–82 PMID:2301709.

Lane, R.S., and Loye, J.E. 1991. Lyme disease in California: interrelationship of ixodid ticks (Acari), rodents, and *Borrelia burgdorferi.* Journal of Medical Entomology, **28**(5): 719–725 PMID:1941942.

Lane, R.S., Steinlein, D.B., and Mun, J. 2004. Human behaviors elevating exposure to *Ixodes pacificus* (Acari: Ixodidae) nymphs and their associated bacterial zoonotic agents in a hardwood forest. Journal of Medical Entomology, **41**(2): 239–248 PMID:15061284.

Lawrenz, M.B., Hardham, J.M., Owens, R.T., Nowakowski, J., Steere, A.C., Wormser, G.P., and Norris, S.J. 1999. Human antibody responses to VlsE antigenic variation protein of *Borrelia burgdorferi.* Journal of Clinical Microbiology, **37**(12): 3997–4004 PMID:10565921.

Lebech, A.M., Hansen, K., Wilske, B., and Theisen, M. 1994. Taxonomic classification of 29 *Borrelia burgdorferi* strains isolated from patients with Lyme borreliosis: a comparison of five different phenotypic and genotypic typing schemes. Medical Microbiology and Immunology, **183**(6): 325–341. PMID:7541107 doi:10.1007/BF00196683.

Levine, J.F., Wilson, M.L., and Spielman, A. 1985. Mice as reservoirs of the Lyme disease spirochete. The American Journal of Tropical Medicine and Hygiene, **34**(2): 355–360 PMID:3985277.

Liang, F.T., Steere, A.C., Marques, A.R., Johnson, B.J.B., Miller, J.N., and Philipp, M.T. 1999. Sensitive and specific serodiagnosis of Lyme disease by enzyme-linked immunosorbent assay with a peptide based on an immunodominant conserved region of *Borrelia burgdorferi* VlsE. Journal of Clinical Microbiology, **37**: 3990–3996 PMID:10565920.

Liang, F.T., Jacobs, M.B., Bowers, L.C., and Philipp, M.T. 2002. An immune evasion mechanism for spirochetal persistence in Lyme borreliosis. The Journal of Experimental Medicine, **195**(4): 415–422. PMID:11854355 doi:10.1084/jem.20011870.

Lindquist, E.E., Wu, K.W., and Redner, J.H. 1999. A new species of the tick genus *Ixodes* (Acari: Ixodidae) parasitic on mustelids (Mammalia: Carnivora in Canada. The Canadian Entomologist, **131**: 151–170.

Lindsay, L.R., Barker, I.K., Surgeoner, G.A., McEwen, S.A., Elliott, L.A., and Kolar, J. 1991. Apparent incompetence of *Dermacentor variabilis* (Acari: Ixodidae) and fleas (Insecta: Siphonaptera) as vectors of *Borrelia burgdorferi* in an *Ixodes dammini* endemic area of Ontario, Canada. Journal of Medical Entomology, **28**(5): 750–753 PMID:1941949.

Lindsay, L.R., Mathison, S.W., Barker, I.K., McEwen, S.A., Gillespie, T.J., and Surgeoner, G.A. 1999*a*. Microclimate and habitat in relation to *Ixodes scapularis* (Acari: Ixodidae) populations on Long Point, Ontario, Canada. Journal of Medical Entomology, **36**(3): 255–262 PMID:10337093.

Lindsay, L.R., Mathison, S.W., Barker, I.K., McEwen, S.A., and Surgeoner, G.A. 1999*b*. Abundance of *Ixodes scapularis* (Acari: Ixodidae) larvae and nymphs in relation to host density and habitat on Long Point, Ontario. Journal of Medical Entomology, **36**(3): 243–254 PMID:10337092.

Lindsay, R., Artsob, H., Galloway, T., and Horsman, G. 1999*c*. Vector of Lyme borreliosis, *Ixodes scapularis*, identified in Saskatchewan.

Canada Communicable Disease Report, 25(9). pp. 81–83 PMID:10079579.

Livengood, J.A., and Gilmore, R.D., Jr. 2006. Invasion of human neuronal and glial cells by an infectious strain of *Borrelia burgdorferi*. Microbes and Infection, **8**(14–15): 2832–2840. PMID: 17045505 doi:10.1016/j.micinf.2006.08.014.

LoGiudice, K., Ostfeld, R.S., Schmidt, K.A., and Keesing, F. 2003. The ecology of infectious disease: effects of host diversity and community composition on Lyme disease risk. Proceedings of the National Academy of Sciences of the United States of America, **100**(2): 567–571. PMID:12525705 doi:10.1073/pnas.0233733100.

Luger, S.W. 1990. Lyme disease transmitted by a biting fly. The New England Journal of Medicine, **322**(24): 1752. PMID:2342543.

Ma, Y., Sturrock, A., and Weis, J.J. 1991. Intracellular localization of *Borrelia burgdorferi* within human endothelial cells. Infection and Immunity, **59**(2): 671–678 PMID:1987083.

Mackenzie, S.G. 1990. Lyme disease in Canada. Canada Diseases Weekly Report No. 16-30. pp. 141–142.

Magnarelli, L.A., Anderson, J.F., and Barbour, A.G. 1986. The etiologic agent of Lyme disease in deer flies, horse flies, and mosquitoes. The Journal of Infectious Diseases, **154**(2): 355–358 PMID:2873190.

Margos, G., Gatewood, A.G., Aanensen, D.M., Hanincová, K., Terekhova, D., Vollmer, S.A., *et al.* 2008. MLST of housekeeping genes captures geographic population structure and suggests a European origin of *Borrelia burgdorferi*. Proceedings of the National Academy of Sciences of the United States of America, **105**(25): 8730–8735. PMID:18574151 doi:10.1073/pnas.0800323105.

Margulis, L., Maniotis, A., MacAllister, J., Scythes, J., Brorson, O., Hall, J., Krumbein, W.E., and Chapman, M.J. 2009. Spirochete round bodies. Syphilis, Lyme disease and AIDS: resurgence of "the great imitator"? Symbiosis, **47**: 51–58.

Mather, T.N., Nicholson, M.C., Donnelly, E.F., and Matyas, B.T. 1996. Entomologic index for human risk of Lyme disease. American Journal of Epidemiology, **144**(11): 1066–1069 PMID: 8942438.

Mavin, S., Evans, R., Milner, R.M., Chatterton, J.M.W., and Ho-Yen, D.O. 2009. Local *Borrelia burgdorferi* sensu stricto and *Borrelia afzelii* strains in a single mixed antigen improves western blot sensitivity. Journal of Clinical Pathology, **62**(6): 552–554. PMID:19240047 doi:10.1136/jcp.2008.063461.

Miklossy, J. 2008. Biology and neuropathology of dementia in syphilis and Lyme disease. *In* Handbook of clinical neurology; dementias. Volume 89. *Edited by* C. Duyckaerts and I. Litvan. Elsevier, Amsterdam; New York.

Miklossy, J., Khalili, K., Gern, L., Ericson, R.L., Darekar, P., Bolle, L., Hurlimann, J., and Paster, B.J. 2004. *Borrelia burgdorferi* persists in the brain in chronic Lyme neuroborreliosis and may be associated with Alzheimer disease. Journal of Alzheimer's Disease, **6**: 639–649.

Miklossy, J., Kis, A., Radenovic, A., Miller, L., Forro, L., Martins, R., *et al.* 2006. Beta-amyloid deposition and Alzheimer's type changes induced by *Borrelia* spirochetes. Neurobiology of Aging, **27**(2): 228–236. PMID:15894409 doi:10.1016/j.neurobiolaging.2005.01.018.

Miklossy, J., Kasas, S., Zurn, A.D., McCall, S., Yu, S., and McGeer, P.L. 2008. Persisting atypical and cystic forms of *Borrelia burgdorferi* and local inflammation in Lyme neuroborreliosis. Journal of Neuroinflammation, **5**(1): 40. doi:10.1186/1742-2094-5-40 PMID:18817547.

Moriarty, T.J., Norman, M.U., Colarusso, P., Bankhead, T., Kubes, P., Chaconas, G., and Coburn, J. 2008. Real-time high resolution 3D imaging of the Lyme disease spirochete adhering to and escaping from the vasculature of a living host. PLoS Pathogens, **4**(6): e1000090. doi: 10.1371/journal.ppat.1000090 PMID:18566656.

Moro, M.H., Zegarra-Moro, O.L., Bjornsson, J., Hofmeister, E.K., Bruinsma, E., Germer, J.J., and Persing, D.H. 2002. Increased arthritis severity in mice coinfected with *Borrelia burgdorferi* and *Babesia microti*. The Journal of Infectious Diseases, **186**(3): 428–431. PMID: 12134242 doi:10.1086/341452.

Morshed, M.G., Scott, J.D., Fernando, K., Beati, L., Mazerolle, D.F., Geddes, G., and Durden, L.A. 2005. Migratory songbirds disperse ticks across Canada, and first isolation of the Lyme disease spirochete, *Borrelia burgdorferi*, from the avian tick, *Ixodes auritulus*. The Journal of Parasitology, **91**(4): 780–790. PMID:17089744 doi:10.1645/GE-3437.1.

Morshed, M.G., Scott, J.D., Fernando, K., Geddes, G., McNabb, A., Mak, S., and Durden, L.A. 2006. Distribution and characterization of *Borrelia burgdorferi* isolates from *Ixodes scapularis* and presence in mammalian hosts in Ontario, Canada. Journal of Medical Entomology, **43**(4): 762–773. PMID:16892637 doi:10.1603/0022-2585(2006)43[762:DACOBB]2.0.CO;2.

Murakami, E. 2009. Tick removal: blister and straw and knot methods [online]. Available from http://www.youtube.com/watch?v=x9dsmFVPDqs [accessed 31 May 2009].

Nardelli, D.T., Callister, S.M., and Schell, R.F. 2008. Lyme arthritis: current concepts and a change in paradigm. Clinical and Vaccine Immunology; CVI, **15**(1): 21–34. PMID:18003815 doi:10.1128/CVI.00330-07.

Neelakanta, G., Li, X., Pal, U., Liu, X., Beck, D.S., DePonte, K., *et al.* 2007. Outer surface protein B is critical for *Borrelia burgdorferi* adherence and survival within *Ixodes* ticks. PLoS Pathogens,

3(3): e33. doi:10.1371/journal.ppat.0030033 PMID:17352535.

Nigrovic, L.E., and Thompson, K.M. 2007. The Lyme vaccine: a cautionary tale. Epidemiology and Infection, **135**(1): 1–8. PMID:16893489 doi:10.1017/S0950268806007096.

Nigrovic, L.E., Thompson, A.D., Fine, A.M., and Kimia, A. 2008. Clinical predictors of Lyme disease among children with a peripheral facial palsy at an emergency department in a Lyme disease-endemic area. Pediatrics, **122**(5): e1080–e1085. doi:10.1542/peds.2008-1273 PMID:18931 349.

Noda, H., Munderloh, U.G., and Kurtti, T.J. 1997. Endosymbionts of ticks and their relationship to *Wolbachia* spp. and tick-borne pathogens of humans and animals. Applied and Environmental Microbiology, **63**(10): 3926–3932 PMID:9327557.

Norris, S.J. 2006. Antigenic variation with a twist — the *Borrelia* story. Molecular Microbiology, **60**(6): 1319–1322 PMID:16796669 doi:10.1111/j.1365-2958.2006.05204.x.

Nuttall, G.H.F., and Warburton, C. 1911. Ixodidae. Section II. The genus *Ixodes*. *In* Ticks. A monograph of the Ixodoidea. Part II. *Edited by* G.H.F. Nuttall, C. Warburton, W. F. Cooper, and L.E. Robinson. Cambridge University Press, London, United Kingdom. pp. 133–293.

Ogden, N.H., Trudel, L., Artsob, H., Barker, I.K., Beauchamp, G., Charron, D.F., *et al.* 2006. *Ixodes scapularis* ticks collected by passive surveillance in Canada: analysis of geographic distribution and infection with Lyme borreliosis agent *Borrelia burgdorferi*. Journal of Medical Entomology, **43**(3): 600–609. PMID:16739422 doi:10.1603/0022-2585(2006)43[600:ISTCBP]2.0.CO;2.

Ogden, N.H., Artsob, H., Lindsay, L.R., and Sockett, P.N. 2008*a*. Lyme disease: a zoonotic disease of increasing importance to Canadians. Canadian Family Physician, **54**(10): 1381–1384 PMID:18854461.

Ogden, N.H., Bigras-Poulin, M., Hanincová, K., Maarouf, A., O'Callaghan, C.J., and Kurtenbach, K. 2008*b*. Projected effects of climate change on tick phenology and fitness of pathogens transmitted by the North American tick *Ixodes scapularis*. Journal of Theoretical Biology, **254**(3): 621–632. PMID:18634803 doi:10.1016/j.jtbi.2008.06.020.

Ogden, N.H., Lindsay, L.R., Hanincová, K., Barker, I.K., Bigras-Poulin, M., Charron, D.F., *et al.* 2008*c*. Role of migratory birds in introduction and range expansion of *Ixodes scapularis* ticks and of *Borrelia burgdorferi* and *Anaplasma phagocytophilum* in Canada. Applied and Environmental Microbiology, **74**(6): 1780–1790. PMID:18245258 doi:10.1128/AEM.01982-07.

Ogden, N.H., Lindsay, L.R., Morshed, M., Sockett, P.N., and Artsob, H. 2008*d*. The rising challenge of Lyme borreliosis in Canada. Canada Communicable Disease Report, **34**(1): 1–19. PMID:18290267–19.

Oksi, J., Marjamäki, M., Nikoskelainen, J., and Viljanen, M.K. 1999. *Borrelia burgdorferi* detected by culture and PCR in clinical relapse of disseminated Lyme borreliosis. Annals of Medicine, **31**(3): 225–232. PMID:10442678 doi:10.3109/07853899909115982.

Oliver, J.H., Jr. 1989. Biology and systematics of ticks (Acari: Ixodida). Annual Review of Ecology and Systematics, **20**(1): 397–430. doi:10.1146/annurev.es.20.110189.002145.

Ouyang, Z., He, M., Oman, T., Yang, X.F., and Norgard, M.V. 2009. A manganese transporter, BB0219 (BmtA), is required for virulence by the Lyme disease spirochete, *Borrelia burgdorferi*. Proceedings of the National Academy of Sciences of the United States of America, **106**(9): 3449–3454. doi:10.1073/pnas.0812999106 PMID:19218460.

Owen, D.C. 2006. Is Lyme disease always poly microbial? — The jigsaw hypothesis. Medical Hypotheses, **67**(4): 860–864 PMID:16814477 doi:10.1016/j.mehy.2006.03.046.

Pachner, A.R., Basta, J., Delaney, E., and Hulinska, D. 1995. Localization of *Borrelia burgdorferi* in murine Lyme borreliosis by electron microscopy. The American Journal of Tropical Medicine and Hygiene, **52**(2): 128–133 PMID:7872439.

Pachner, A.R., Dail, D., Li, L., Gurey, L., Feng, S., Hodzic, E., and Barthold, S. 2002. Humoral immune response associated with Lyme borreliosis in nonhuman primates: analysis by immunoblotting and enzyme-linked immunosorbent assay with sonicates or recombinant proteins. Clinical and Diagnostic Laboratory Immunology, **9**(6): 1348–1355 PMID:12414773.

Pal, U., Wang, P., Bao, F., Yang, X., Samanta, S., Schoen, R., *et al.* 2008. *Borrelia burgdorferi* basic membrane proteins A and B participate in the genesis of Lyme arthritis. The Journal of Experimental Medicine, **205**(1): 133–141. PMID:18166 585 doi:10.1084/jem.20070962.

Pfister, H.W., Einhäupl, K., Preac-Mursic, V., Wilske, B., and Schierz, G. 1984. The spirochetal etiology of lymphocytic meningoradiculitis of Bannwarth (Bannwarth's syndrome). Journal of Neurology, **231**(3): 141–144 PMID:6481420 doi:10.1007/BF00313682.

Piacentino, J.D., and Schwartz, B.S. 2002. Occupational risk of Lyme disease: an epidemiological review. Occupational and Environmental Medicine, **59**(2): 75–84. PMID:11850549 doi:10.1136/oem.59.2.75.

Posey, J.E., and Gherardini, F.C. 2000. Lack of a role for iron in the Lyme disease pathogen. Science (Washington, D.C.), **288**(5471): 1651–1653. PMID:10834845 doi:10.1126/science.288.5471.1651.

Postic, D., Garnier, M., and Baranton, G. 2007. Multilocus sequence analysis of atypical *Borrelia burgdorferi* sensu lato isolates — description of *Borrelia californiensis* sp. nov., and genomospecies 1 and 2. International Journal of Medical Microbiology, **297**(4): 263–271 PMID:17374507 doi:10.1016/j.ijmm.2007.01.006.

Qiu, W.G., Bruno, J.F., McCaig, W.D., Xu, Y., Livey, I., Schriefer, M.E., and Luft, B.J. 2008. Wide distribution of a high-virulence *Borrelia burgdorferi* clone in Europe and North America. Emerging Infectious Diseases, **14**(7): 1097–1104. PMID:18598631 doi:10.3201/eid1407.070880.

Ramamoorthi, N., Narasimhan, S., Pal, U., Bao, F., Yang, X.F., Fish, D., *et al.* 2005. The Lyme disease agent exploits a tick protein to infect the mammalian host. Nature (London), **436**(7050): 573–577. PMID:16049492 doi:10.1038/nature 03812.

Rawling, R.A., Strouse, K., and Granato, P.A. 2009. *Borrelia burgdorferi* and *Babesia microti* coinfection in a 79-year-old camper. Clinical Microbiology Newsletter, **31**(5): 37–39. doi:10.1016/j.clinmicnews.2009.02.002.

Ribeiro, J.M.C., and Francischetti, I.M.B. 2003. Role of arthropod saliva in blood feeding: sialome and post-sialome perspectives. Annual Review of Entomology, **48**(1): 73–88. PMID:12194906 doi:10.1146/annurev.ento.48.060402.102812.

Robertson, J., Guy, E., Andrews, N., Wilske, B., Anda, P., Granström, M., *et al.* 2000. A European multicenter study of immunoblotting in serodiagnosis of Lyme borreliosis. Journal of Clinical Microbiology, **38**(6): 2097–2102 PMID: 10834959.

Rosa, P.A., Tilly, K., and Stewart, P.E. 2005. The burgeoning molecular genetics of the Lyme disease spirochaete. Nature Reviews Microbiology, **3**(2): 129–143. PMID:15685224 doi:10.1038/nrmicro1086.

Rosé, C.D., Fawcett, P.T., and Gibney, K.M. 2001. Arthritis following recombinant outer surface protein A vaccination for Lyme disease. The Journal of Rheumatology, **28**(11): 2555–2557 PMID:11708435.

Rudenko, N., Golovchenko, M., Grubhoffer, L., and Oliver, J.H., Jr. 2009. *Borrelia carolinensis* sp. nov., a new (14th) member of the *Borrelia burgdorferi* sensu lato complex from the southeastern region of the United States. Journal of Clinical Microbiology, **47**(1): 134–141. PMID:19020062 doi:10.1128/JCM.0118 3-08.

Rupprecht, T.A., Koedel, U., Fingerle, V., and Pfister, H.-W. 2008. The pathogenesis of Lyme neuroborreliosis: from infection to inflammation. Molecular Medicine (Cambridge, Mass.), **14**(3-4): 205–212 PMID:18097481.

Saah, A.J., and Hoover, D.R. 1997. "Sensitivity" and "specificity" reconsidered: the meaning of these terms in analytical and diagnostic settings. Annals of Internal Medicine, **126**(1): 91–94 PMID:8992938.

Salkeld, D.J., Leonhard, S., Girard, Y.A., Hahn, N., Mun, J., Padgett, K.A., and Lane, R.S. 2008. Identifying the reservoir hosts of the Lyme disease spirochete *Borrelia burgdorferi* in California: the role of the western gray squirrel (*Sciurus griseus*). The American Journal of Tropical Medicine and Hygiene, **79**(4): 535–540 PMID:18840740.

Schneider, B.S., Schriefer, M.E., Dietrich, G., Dolan, M.C., Morshed, M.G., and Zeidner, N.S. 2008. *Borrelia bissettii* isolates induce pathology in a murine model of disease. Vector-Borne and Zoonotic Diseases (Larchmont, N.Y.), **8**(5): 623–633. PMID:18454594 doi:10.1089/vbz.2007.0251.

Schroeder, H., Skelly, P.J., Zipfel, P.F., Losson, B., and Vanderplasschen, A. 2009. Subversion of complement by hematophagous parasites. Developmental and Comparative Immunology, **33**(1): 5–13. PMID:18762211 doi:10.1016/j.dci.2008. 07.010.

Schuijt, T.J., Hovius, J.W.R., van Burgel, N.D., Ramamoorthi, N., Fikrig, E., and van Dam, A.P. 2008. The tick salivary protein Salp15 inhibits the killing of serum-sensitive *Borrelia burgdorferi* sensu lato isolates. Infection and Immunity, **76**(7): 2888–2894. PMID:18426890 doi:10.1128/IAI.00232-08.

Schwan, T.G., Piesman, J., Golde, W.T., Dolan, M.C., and Rosa, P.A. 1995. Induction of an outer surface protein on *Borrelia burgdorferi* during tick feeding. Proceedings of the National Academy of Sciences of the United States of America, **92**(7): 2909–2913. PMID:7708747 doi:10.1073/pnas.92.7.2909.

Schwan, T.G., Raffel, S.J., Schrumpf, M.E., and Porcella, S.F. 2007. Diversity and distribution of *Borrelia hermsii*. Emerging Infectious Diseases, **13**(3): 436–442 PMID:17552097.

Scoles, G.A., Broce, A.B., Lysyk, T.J., and Palmer, G.H. 2005. Relative efficiency of biological transmission of *Anaplasma marginale* (Rickettsiales: Anaplasmataceae) by *Dermacentor andersoni* (Acari: Ixodidae) compared with mechanical transmission by *Stomoxys calcitrans* (Diptera: Muscidae). Journal of Medical Entomology, **42**(4): 668–675. PMID:16119558 doi:10.1603/0022-2585(2005)042[0668:REOBTO] 2.0.CO;2.

Scott, J.D., Fernando, K., Banerjee, S.N., Durden, L.A., Byrne, S.K., Banerjee, M., Mann, R.B., and Morshed, M.G. 2001. Birds disperse ixodid (Acari: Ixodidae) and *Borrelia burgdorferi*-infected ticks in Canada. Journal of Medical Entomology, **38**(4): 493–500 PMID: 11476328.

Scott, J.D., Lee, M.-K., Fernando, K., Jorgensen, D.R., Durden, L.A., and Morshed, M.G. 2008. Rapid introduction of Lyme disease spirochete,

Borrelia burgdorferi sensu stricto, in *Ixodes scapularis* (Acari: Ixodidae) established at Turkey Point Provincial Park, Ontario, Canada. Journal of Vector Ecology, **33**(1): 64–69. PMID:18697308 doi:10.3376/1081-1710(2008)33[64:RIOLDS]2.0.CO;2.

Shariat, B.M., Freimund, J.A., Wright, S.M., Murphree, C.S., and Thomas, J.T. 2007. *Borrelia* infection rates in winter ticks (*Dermacentor albipictus*) removed from white-tailed deer (*Odocoileus virginianus*) in Cheatham County, Tennessee. Journal of the Tennessee Academy of Science, **82**: 57–61.

Shi, Y., Xu, Q., McShan, K., and Liang, F.T. 2008. Both decorin-binding proteins A and B are critical for the overall virulence of *Borrelia burgdorferi*. Infection and Immunity, **76**(3): 1239–1246. PMID:18195034 doi:10.1128/IAI.00897-07.

Sigal, L.H., and Hassett, A.L. 2002. Contributions of societal and geographical environments to "chronic Lyme disease": the psychopathogenesis and aporology of a new "medically unexplained symptoms" syndrome. Environmental Health Perspectives, **110**(Supplement 4): 607–611 PMID:12194894.

Singh, S.K., and Girschick, H.J. 2004. Lyme borreliosis: from infection to autoimmunity. Clinical Microbiology and Infection, **10**(7): 598–614. PMID:15214872 doi:10.1111/j.1469-0691.2004.00895.x.

Skogman, B.H., Croner, S., Nordwall, M., Eknefelt, M., Ernerudh, J., and Forsberg, P. 2008. Lyme neuroborreliosis in children: a prospective study of clinical features, prognosis, and outcome. The Pediatric Infectious Disease Journal, **27**(12): 1089–1094. PMID:19008771 doi:10.1097/INF.0b013e31817fd423.

Slowik, T.J., and Lane, R.S. 2009. Feeding preferences of the immature stages of three western North American ixodid ticks (Acari) for avian, reptilian, or rodent hosts. Journal of Medical Entomology, **46**(1): 115–122. PMID:19198525 doi:10.1603/033.046.0115.

Smith, R.P., Jr., Muzaffar, S.B., Lavers, J., Lacombe, E.H., Cahill, B.K., Lubelczyk, C.B., *et al.* 2006. *Borrelia garinii* in seabird ticks (*Ixodes uriae*), Atlantic coast, North America. Emerging Infectious Diseases, **12**(12): 1909–1912 PMID:17326943.

Sperling, F.A.H., and Roe, A.M. 2009. Molecular dimensions of insect taxonomy. *In* Insect biodiversity: science and society. *Edited by* R.G. Foottit and P.H. Adler. Blackwell Publishing, Oxford, United Kingdom.

Steere, A.C. 1989. Lyme disease. The New England Journal of Medicine, **321**(9): 586–596 PMID:2668764.

Steere, A.C., McHugh, G., Damle, N., and Sikand, V.K. 2008. Prospective study of serologic tests for Lyme disease. Clinical Infectious Diseases, **47**(2): 188–195. PMID:18532885 doi:10.1086/589242.

Stevenson, B., von Lackum, K., Riley, S.P., Cooley, A.E., Woodman, M.E., and Bykowski, T. 2006. Evolving models of Lyme disease spirochete gene regulation. Wiener Klinische Wochenschrift, **118**(21-22): 643–652. PMID:17160602 doi:10.1007/s00508-006-0690-2.

Straubinger, R.K. 2000. Lyme borreliosis in dogs. *In* Recent advances in canine infectious diseases. *Edited by* L.E. Carmichael. International Veterinary Information Service, Ithaca, New York.

Stricker, R.B., and Johnson, L. 2008. Serologic tests for Lyme disease: more smoke and mirrors. Clinical Infectious Diseases, **47**(8): 1111–1112, author's reply 1112–1113. PMID:18800935 doi:10.1086/592121.

Stromdahl, E.Y., Williamson, P.C., Kollars, T.M., JrEvans, S.R., Barry, R.K., Vince, M.A., and Dobbs, N.A. 2003. Evidence of *Borrelia lonestari* DNA in *Amblyomma americanum* (Acari: Ixodidae) removed from humans. Journal of Clinical Microbiology, **41**(12): 5557–5562. PMID:14662940 doi:10.1128/JCM.41.12.5557-5562.2003.

Suffridge, P.J., Smoller, B.R., and Carrington, P.R. 1999. Spiders and *Borrelia burgdorferi*: no evidence of reservoir occurrence in central Arkansas. International Journal of Dermatology, **38**(4): 296–297. PMID:10321947 doi:10.1046/j.1365-4362.1999.00602.x.

Summers, B.A., Straubinger, A.F., Jacobson, R.H., Chang, Y.F., Appel, M.J., and Straubinger, R.K. 2005. Histopathological studies of experimental Lyme disease in the dog. Journal of Comparative Pathology, **133**(1): 1–13. PMID:15904927 doi:10.1016/j.jcpa.2004.11.006.

Terekhova, D., Iyer, R., Wormser, G.P., and Schwartz, I. 2006. Comparative genome hybridization reveals substantial variation among clinical isolates of *Borrelia burgdorferi* sensu stricto with different pathogenic properties. Journal of Bacteriology, **188**(17): 6124–6134. PMID:16923879 doi:10.1128/JB.00459-06.

Thomas, D.D., Cadavid, D., and Barbour, A.G. 1994. Differential association of *Borrelia* species with cultured neural cells. The Journal of Infectious Diseases, **169**(2): 445–448 PMID:8106781.

Tibbles, C.D., and Edlow, J.A. 2007. Does this patient have erythema migrans? Journal of the American Medical Association, **297**(23): 2617–2627. doi:10.1001/jama.297.23.2617.

Tilly, K., Bestor, A., Jewett, M.W., and Rosa, P. 2007. Rapid clearance of Lyme disease spirochetes lacking OspC from skin. Infection and Immunity, **75**(3): 1517–1519. PMID:17158906 doi:10.1128/IAI.01725-06.

Tilly, K., Rosa, P.A., and Stewart, P.E. 2008. Biology of infection with *Borrelia burgdorferi*. Infectious Disease Clinics of North America,

22(2): 217–234., v PMID:18452798 doi:10.1016/j.idc.2007.12.013.

Tourand, Y., Deneke, J., Moriarty, T.J., and Chaconas, G. 2009. Characterization and in vitro reaction properties of 19 unique hairpin telomeres from the linear plasmids of the Lyme disease spirochete. The Journal of Biological Chemistry, **284**(11): 7264–7272. PMID:19122193 doi:10.1074/jbc.M808918200.

Ullmann, A.J., Lane, R.S., Kurtenbach, K., Miller, M., Schriefer, M.E., Zeldner, N., and Piesman, J. 2003. Bacteriolytic activity of selected vertebrate sera for *Borrelia burgdorferi* sensu stricto and *Borrelia bissettii*. Journal of Parasitology, **89**(6): 1256–1257. PMID:14740924 doi:10.1645/Ge-3081RN.

Vanousová, D., and Hercogová, J. 2008. Lyme borreliosis treatment. Dermatologic Therapy, **21**(2): 101–109. PMID:18394084 doi:10.1111/j.1529-8019.2008.00177.x.

van Overbeek, L., Gassner, F., van der Plas, C.L., Kastelein, P., Nunes-da Rocha, U., and Takken, W. 2008. Diversity of *Ixodes ricinus* tick-associated bacterial communities from different forests. FEMS Microbiology Ecology, **66**(1): 72–84. PMID:18355299 doi:10.1111/j.1574-6941.2008.00468.x.

Vázquez, M., Muehlenbein, C., Cartter, M., Hayes, E.B., Ertel, S., and Shapiro, E.D. 2008. Effectiveness of personal protective measures to prevent Lyme disease. Emerging Infectious Diseases, **14**(2): 210–216. PMID:18258112 doi:10.3201/eid1402.070725.

Welsh, J., Pretzman, C., Postic, D., Saint Girons, I., Baranton, G., and McClelland, M. 1992. Genomic fingerprinting by arbitrarily primed polymerase chain reaction resolves *Borrelia burgdorferi* into three distinct phyletic groups. International Journal of Systematic Bacteriology, **42**(3): 370–377 PMID:1503971.

Wesson, D.M., McLain, D.K., Oliver, J.H., Piesman, J., and Collins, F.H. 1993. Investigation of the validity of species status of *Ixodes dammini* (Acari: Ixodidae) using rDNA. Proceedings of the National Academy of Sciences of the United States of America, **90**(21): 10221–10225. PMID:8234280 doi:10.1073/pnas.90.21.10221.

Whitney, H. 2005. Lyme Disease in Newfoundland. Animal Health Fact Sheet AP053, Newfoundland and Labrador Department of Agriculture, St. John's, Newfoundland.

Wilske, B., Fingerle, V., and Schulte-Spechtel, U. 2007. Microbiological and serological diagnosis of Lyme borreliosis. FEMS Immunology and Medical Microbiology, **49**(1): 13–21. PMID:17266710 doi:10.1111/j.1574-695X.2006.00139.x.

Wilson, J.M. 2007. Concerns regarding the Infectious Diseases Society of America Lyme disease clinical practice guidelines. Clinical Infectious Diseases, **44**(8): 1135–1137., author's reply 1137–1139. PMID:17366466 doi:10.1086/513030.

Wormser, G.P., Dattwyler, R.J., Shapiro, E.D., Halperin, J.J., Steere, A.C., Klempner, M.S., *et al.* 2006. The clinical assessment, treatment, and prevention of Lyme disease, human granulocytic anaplasmosis, and babesiosis: clinical practice guidelines by the Infectious Diseases Society of America. Clinical Infectious Disease. Clinical Infactious Disease, **45**: 1089–1134.

Wormser, G.P., Dattwyler, R.J., Shapiro, E.D., Halperin, J.J., Steere, A.C., Klempner, M.S. *et al.* 2007. Erratum: The clinical assessment, treatment, and prevention of Lyme disease, human granulocytic anaplasmosis, and babesiosis: clinical practice guidelines by the Infectious Diseases Society of America. Clinical Infactious Disease, **45**: 941.

Wormser, G.P., Liveris, D., Hanincová, K., Brisson, D., Ludin, S., Stracuzzi, V.J., *et al.* 2008. Effect of *Borrelia burgdorferi* genotype on the sensitivity of C6 and 2-tier testing in North American patients with culture-confirmed Lyme disease. Clinical Infectious Diseases, **47**(7): 910–914. PMID:18724824 doi:10.1086/591529.

Xu, Q., McShan, K., and Liang, F.T. 2008a. Modification of *Borrelia burgdorferi* to overproduce OspA or VlsE alters its infectious behaviour. Microbiology, **154**(Pt 11): 3420–3429. PMID:18957595 doi:10.1099/mic.0.2008/019737-0.

Xu, Y., Bruno, J.F., and Luft, B.J. 2008b. Profiling the humoral immune response to *Borrelia burgdorferi* infection with protein microarrays. Microbial Pathogenesis, **45**(5–6): 403–407. PMID:18976702 doi:10.1016/j.micpath.2008.09.006.

Yang, X., Coleman, A.S., Anguita, J., Pal, U., and Coburn, J. 2009. A chromosomally encoded virulence factor protects the Lyme disease pathogen against host-adaptive immunity. PLoS Pathogens, **5**(3): e1000326. doi:10.1371/journal.ppat.1000326 PMID:19266024.

Yrjänäinen, H., Hytönen, J., Song, X.Y., Oksi, J., Hartiala, K., and Viljanen, M.-K. 2007. Anti-tumor necrosis factor-alpha treatment activates *Borrelia burgdorferi* spirochetes 4 weeks after ceftriaxone treatment in C3H/He mice. The Journal of Infectious Diseases, **195**(10): 1489–1496. PMID:17436229 doi:10.1086/513873.

Žákovská, A., Nejedla, P., Holíková, A., and Dendis. 2002. Positive findings of *Borrelia burgdorferi* in *Culex* (*Culex*) *pipiens pipiens* larvae in the surrounding of Brno city determined by the PCR method. Annals of Agricultural and Environmental Medicine, **9**(2): 257–259 PMID:12498597.

Žakovska, A., Janouškovcová, E., Pejchalová, K., Halouzka, J., and Dendis, M. 2008. Identification and characterization of 31 isolates of *Borrelia burgdorferi* (Spirochaetales, Spirochaetaceae) obtained from various hosts and vectors using PCR-RFLP and SDS-PAGE analysis. Acta Parasitologica, **53**(2): 186–192. doi:10.2478/s11686-008-0028-5.

Zaretsky, L. 2006. Lyme disease in Canada. Canadian Pharmacists Journal, **139**(4): 29–32.

Zhong, J., Jasinskas, A., Barbour, A.G., and Romesberg, F. 2007. Antibiotic treatment of the tick vector *Amblyomma americanum* reduced reproductive fitness. PLoS ONE, **2**(5): e405. doi:10.1371/journal.pone.0000405 PMID:17476327.

4

CANADA'S BLOOD SUPPLY ENDANGERED—AGAIN?

By Karin Klouman & Helke Ferrie

"The safety of the blood supply is paramount—the principle of safety must transcend other principles and policies.... If harm can occur, then it should be assumed that it will occur. If there are no measures that will entirely prevent the harm, measures that may only partially prevent transmission should be taken..."

—Justice Horace Krever
From the *Krever Commission Report, 1999*

One Awful Déjà Vu

The following information on what has so far transpired between the Lyme Action Group (LAG) and the Canadian Blood Services (CBS) may give the reader the feeling of an eerie déjà vu. While déjà vu is a psychological phenomenon, this one is not a question of subjective perception—Canadians actually *have* been here before. And here we go again.

When LAG was formed in the fall of 2008, by mostly victims of Chronic Lyme disease, the four areas of concern that were unanimously agreed upon were

1. the appalling and obsolete state of medical testing in Canada;
2. the lack of even the most basic knowledge about this disease among most of Canada's doctors, who are kept ignorant due to a pervasive systemic bias in public health and medical education and by government-mandated obsolete testing protocols that block adequate investigation;
3. the hostility with which those few doctors, who have become Lyme-literate, are met by their licensing authorities; and
4. the apparent lack of concern about the integrity of Canada's blood supply, with respect to the Lyme disease pathogens and their known co-infections because they are linked to inappropriate testing protocols.

Though Lyme disease is universally acknowledged as the most common vector-borne infectious disease for most of the world, Canada met this rising epidemic, and its certain danger to the blood supply, with an attitude of see no evil, hear no evil, speak no evil. Almost everybody in this entire chain of command, from Health Canada down to the local Public Health office, has bought into that appalling nonsense, supported by no evidence whatsoever, about Lyme disease being "hard to catch and easy to treat"—as the now discredited 2006 Guidelines produced by the Infectious Disease Society of America (IDSA) so emphatically maintain.

Starting with a press conference held on Nov 7, 2008, in Ontario's Legislative Building's media studio, LAG began to bring attention to the great human suffering caused by the ignored and unrecognized fact of Lyme disease in Canada, especially in Ontario which is the most populated province.

The specter of another blood scandal was always most important in LAG's publicly voiced concerns. Anyone who has ever had the chronic form of this infectious disease will be utterly horrified imagining others becoming infected, simply because no effort was made to prevent it; indeed, Canadians are misled into trusting the system, when actually not even the most basic cautionary information is provided.

Lorraine Johnson, a member for the California Lyme Disease Association and legal advisor to it as well as to the International Lyme and Associated Diseases Society (ILADS), had this to say at the National Lyme Disease meeting convened in March of 2006 by the Public Health Agency of Canada: *"The failure to provide objective and unbiased health care information violates the right of the individual to make autonomous decisions. Misleading information erodes public confidence in government, forecloses democratic debate about health care values, suppresses market place autonomy and research, and may empower some stakeholders at the expense of others... Misleading information can constitute a form of coercion when the distortion provokes fear or anxiety. Autonomy is the principle most violated by deceptive communications. Individuals should make their own decisions based on unbiased information ... omissions in health care information are forms of paternalism."**

Johnson's observations—that catalogue of potential failures of responsibility resulting in harm to real human beings—has actually come true and is in evidence in Canada's federal and provincial government policies, the public health services of the country, the medical schools, and the regulatory authorities controlling our doctors. The blood supply is just one, albeit an extremely important, component of our healthcare system.

*Although this National Lyme Disease Meeting was convened by the Public Health Agency of Canada in 2006, gathering federal and provincial representatives and Lyme experts from both sides of the border, instead of acting on their advice, the wholly inadequate and scientifically insupportable Canadian Public Health Laboratory Network guidelines on Lyme disease were published *after* this meeting in 2007, as if it had never even taken place.

Since 2006 a great deal has happened in the field of Lyme disease with regard to increasingly alarming and well-documented information, but no policy changes have happened in Canada whatsoever. Not even one of the recommendations from the National Lyme Disease Meeting (published two years later!) has been implemented, and by now most of that report is already obsolete, in the light of the cascade of new information and policy developments in the US. Far more radical action is needed now than was proposed in 2006. For the blood supply, being of the greatest importance to the day-to-day work of medicine, which absolutely relies on the blood supply's integrity, Lyme spirochetes and the co-infections that usually appear with them, are a ticking time bomb.

On January 14, 2009, LAG then made a formal written presentation, supported by relevant scientific publications and other related material, to Ontario's Premier (Dalton McGuinty), Minister of Health (then David Caplan), and the Attorney General (Chris Bentley); all members of the Legislative Assembly received copies. The Premier responded on March 16, 2009, informing LAG that the matter was to be handled by the appropriate Minister; he did *"appreciate [LAG's] concern about the safety of blood products and recognize[d] its vital importance to our citizens."* Subsequently, the Hon. David Caplan, arranged for a meeting for LAG with his Senior Policy Advisor, Shabnum Durrani, who clearly understood that the central problem was with the testing policy. Yet, the letters that from then on came from that Minister's office as well as later on from his successor, the Hon. D. Matthews, did not address—in fact ignored—this central issue totally and told LAG what we already know, and seriously object to and want changed, that Ontario's testing policy is in accord with current knowledge and the US CDC policy.

Governments excel at producing those well-crafted "hot potato" letters, which invariably suggest somebody else should be contacted and insist that overall, the system is doing everything it can.

For the patient suffering from Chronic Lyme disease and trying to cope on a daily basis with its debilitating symptoms, the nation's blood supply may not at first appear to be the most pressing issue. In fact, however, the policies and personal suffering are intimately linked.

The correspondence with the Canadian Blood Services (CBS) began even before Premier McGuinty's letter: the Lyme Action Group wrote to CBS for the first time on December 16, 2008. Addressing Dr. Verna M. Skanes, the Chair of the CBS, Karin Klouman wrote for LAG as follows:*

* For her own story about 9 years with Chronic Lyme disease, see Chapter 8

"I am writing this letter on behalf of the Lyme Action Group to draw your attention to the Canadian Blood Services' lack of policy in regards to the growing threat of Lyme Disease in Canada. There is currently no screening process in place to guard against the Canadian blood supply becoming infected with the causative agent for Lyme disease, this being the bacterium Borrelia burgdorferi.

There are several peer-reviewed published studies that alert to the findings of various strains of Borrelia surviving in collected and treated blood products for up to 48 days.

Other tick-borne and co-infectious agents, which often occur in conjunction with the Borrelia burgdorferi bacterium (such as Babesia microti), have furthermore been shown to be transmitted through blood transfusions. There are many medical and scientific reports on full-blown tick-borne infections in the recipients of such transfusions.

In our experience it is, unfortunately, common practice for the various local branches of your agency to repeatedly ask ***diagnosed*** Lyme Disease patients to still continue to donate blood, since Lyme is not one of the infections listed as being of concern to the Canadian Blood Services. This occurs even after such patients have informed the blood service centres that they consider themselves no longer eligible for donating blood because of their Lyme diagnosis.

Lyme is recognized as an emerging epidemic in North America. Most other blood service organizations, such as the American Red Cross, have developed specific policies to prevent the transmission of Lyme disease through blood transfusions, yet our Canadian Blood Services still remains inactive in regards to this issue. It could become a serious legal matter if Canadian Blood Services do not follow the lead of the other blood service agencies in North America.

Ignoring the possible Lyme contamination of our blood supply is, in our opinion, a completely unacceptable position for the Canadian Blood Service Agency to take. It is our sincere hope that once you have considered all the evidence, you will review and reconsider your practice."

The CBS replied on January 12, 2009; the letter was signed by Dr. Graham D. Sher, the CBS's Chief Executive Officer. It was a clear statement of the "all is well" variety. The problem with that response was three-fold: the supporting evidence referred to was significantly outdated; the fact that there appears to be no specific screening process for tick-borne diseases for blood donors in Canada (as is the case in many other countries) was not addressed; and the phrase "theoretical risk" was used as the *excuse* for CBS inaction. This phrase is loaded historically, as discussed below.

Karin Klouman replied for the Lyme Action Group on February 26, 2009, and addressed these three main issues, all of which required—and still require—immediate attention. The ignored, up-to-date scientific literature was once again cited. The first point she addressed concerned the outdated information and the importance of a new federal law, which the CBS was also ignoring:

> " ... the CBS continues to rely on ***outdated research material*** from the 1990s to conclude that 'Lyme disease is not judged to be an emerging threat to the blood supply.' We find it totally unacceptable that your current policy on Lyme disease is based on a CDC and FDA workshop that was held as far back as 1999.
>
> In the last decade, Lyme has become ***an emerging epidemic*** in parts of this continent. Lyme disease is now widespread across Canada. Furthermore, the new *Safety and Security Act of Canada* [passed into law later in 2009] with respect to human pathogens and toxins" (C-11) recognizes Borrelia burgdorferi as a serious infectious agent in Canada that the public needs to be protected against.
>
> The Lyme Action Group, therefore, considers it imperative that you ***immediately review*** your position on Lyme and that you base this on ***recent scientific findings*** in the blood transfusion literature.
>
> Since it is an established fact, that the Lyme spirochete survives in treated and stored blood products, it is our concern that the spread of tick-borne organisms can be occurring throughout our blood supply, especially ***since no steps have been taken*** to screen donors for any ***clinical signs of Lyme disease*** or other Tick-Borne Diseases (TBDs).
>
> Other tick-borne organisms, such as Babesia microti and Anaplasma phagocytophilum, are also considered to be a current risk to the blood supply. Babesios and Human Anaplasmosis have been well documented to ***transmit through blood transfusions.*** These other TBD organisms also often occur as co-infections in individuals that are infected by Borrelia burgdorferi. A screening process of donors that considers ***all tick-borne infections*** as a risk to the blood supply will, therefore, likely eliminate many that have not yet been diagnosed with a Borrelia infection, but have still tested positive for other tick-borne organisms.
>
> Canadian Blood Services, furthermore, obviously recognizes the danger of syphilis, another spirochetal disease being spread through the blood supply and has a clearly established protocol to prevent this from happening. It therefore ***defies all logic*** that no such screening process is in place to stop the contamination of our blood supply by the equally dangerous spirochete bacterium Borrelia burgdorferi. ***Lyme disease and syphilis bear many similarities***: Both diseases are caused by a spirochete and are difficult to diagnose, both are called "the great

imitator," both will eventually cause a multisystem collapse and both can manifest as severe neurological impairment.

a. There is no specific question about Lyme disease on your health assessment questionnaire.

b. Your health assessment form addresses general questions of acute ill health, such as "Are you feeling well today?" but you do not red-flag signs of Lyme disease (such as recurring flu-like symptoms). You ask, "Have you been under a doctor's care in the past 6 months?" but you do not screen for Chronic Lyme disease symptoms.

c. Your staff erroneously believes that TBDs cannot be spread through the blood supply. We have personal testimony from diagnosed Lyme patients who have been asked to continue to donate blood.

The finding of Lyme disease in any individual remains ***primarily a clinical diagnosis***, supported only in part by blood tests. In Canada, however, the official blood test recommended (ELISA) is considered by most in the treatment field to be deeply flawed, as it will miss the vast majority of Lyme disease sufferers. Many Lyme patients have furthermore had this disease for several years before diagnosis because our doctors are not receiving adequate training to consider Lyme as a possible underlying cause for a wide variety of medical complaints.

As a result of these factors many Lyme patients will continue to donate blood in good faith, having no idea that their vague recurring flu-like symptoms, their neurological issues and/or their poly-arthritic complaints etc. might be an indicator of Lyme disease.

The Lyme Action Group considers it outrageous that your staff is so unaware of the threat of Lyme disease that they are encouraging those with a Lyme disease diagnosis to still donate blood. However, given the unreliability of the current Canadian blood tests for Lyme disease, your staff needs not only to ask about a Lyme diagnosis, but must also be better trained to ask ***the right clinical questions*** in a health assessment interview. If the simple measure of a revised Health Questionnaire was implemented, then we would reduce the risk of contamination of our blood supply by any TBD organisms."

Karin Klouman then pointed out that all is most definitely not well with the Canadian Blood Services because

"There are some ***significant differences*** between CBS policy on Lyme disease and that of several other international blood service industries. The American Red Cross has a deferral policy on Lyme and one of ***permanent deferral*** in the case of Babesiosis, while the Centers for Disease Control in Atlanta recommends that

> affected Lyme patients do not donate in the US. Furthermore, European/Scandinavian blood bank industries have deferral guidelines in regards to Lyme disease. The AABB advisory board is currently considering appropriate official new guidelines in regards to screening for Babesiosis and other TBDs.
>
> The fact that various international blood service industries have developed (or are developing) policies on Lyme disease, while Canada lags substantially behind, could put the Canadian Blood Services in a difficult legal situation as well as possibly on the cusp of another "tainted blood" scandal.
>
> The complete inaction of the CBS in regards to Lyme disease and other TBDs is hard to understand, especially when considering the explosive increase in Lyme disease in Canada. Many Canadians also travel to ***endemic areas in the U.S, Asia and Europe***, returning to Canada unaware that they are infected by tick-borne organisms. They might, therefore, still donate blood, unless informed otherwise by an urgently needed and vastly improved Canadian Blood Services' screening process.
>
> It is the position of the Lyme Action Group that the time has come to act on this urgent matter. We, therefore, ***strongly urge you to immediately establish new guidelines on Lyme disease***. It is our opinion that you can no longer willfully ignore the growing threat of a possible contamination of our blood supply by the various tick-borne organisms."

The CBS replied on April 7 again, this time in a conciliatory tone, ending with the provision of a phone number and the suggestion of the Lyme Action Group meeting with representatives of the CBS. Special attention should be paid again to the use of the word "theoretical" in that April 7, 2009, letter. In it the Chief Executive Officer Dr. Graham Sher, states; *"Although we must remain vigilant regarding transmissibility of this agent [the spirochetal bacterium that causes Lyme disease, Borrelia borgdorferi], to date this risk remains* ***theoretical.****"* [Emphasis added.] We need to examine the use of the term "theoretical" more closely.

For readers too young to remember that infamous Canadian Blood Scandal, it needs to be briefly mentioned that during the 1970s and 1980s the Canadian Red Cross, then in charge of the nation's blood supply, took no precautions against contamination of donated blood when the threats HIV and hepatitis C emerged. At the same time, other countries' blood services were rapidly responding to that emerging threat. On many occasions members of the public tried to raise the alarm to the Canadian authorities, yet nothing was done. At that time, the sole focus had been on maintaining the maximum number of donations. Following a nation-wide investigation with hundreds of public hearings, Justice Horace Krever released a report in 1997 confirming that, due to extreme negligence, *"arguably the largest public health catastrophe in this country's history"* took place—as the *Canadian Medical Association Journal* observed on the 10th anniversary of the issuing of that report. *"About 1,000 individuals who received blood transfusions between the late 1970s and 1980s were infected with HIV, and another 30,000 were infected with hepatitis C."* In addition, the fact emerged after the Krever Commission's report was issued, that *all* Canadians with hemophilia, living during that time period, were infected and most died.

Justice Krever is quoted in that CMAJ article as follows:

> "The slowness in taking appropriate measures to prevent the contamination of the blood supply was in large measure the result of the rejection, or at least the non-acceptance, of an important tenet in the philosophy of public health: ***action to reduce risk should not await scientific certainty***. [Emphasis added.] When there was reasonable evidence that serious infectious disease could be transmitted by blood, the principal actors in the blood supply system in Canada refrained from taking essential preventive measures until causation had been proved with scientific certainty. The result was a national public health disaster."

The author of that CMAJ article feels: *"In retrospect, the findings of the Krever Commission could perhaps be considered the most influential report on public health in Canadian history."*

While it is true, that subsequently preventive measures were taken by CBS with regard to Creutzfeldt Jacob disease (a.k.a. Mad Cow Disease, caused by prions), SARS, and West Nile virus, when it comes to this newly emerging Lyme disease epidemic, the blood service hides behind semantics by interpreting "theoretical risk" ***in exactly the opposite way*** from what it was intended to mean; for Justice Krever this word was of central importance to the fifty recommendations he made in 1997.

Because all medical activity requires informed consent as a legal imperative, Justice Krever recommended that when learning of a *potential* risk to the safety of the blood supply, CBS should *"cause the recipients to be informed"* because we are "entitled" to be informed of any potential risk *"even in circumstances where the risk is* ***theoretical*** *and no treatment is currently available."* (Emphasis added.) In the words of bioethics lawyer Pamela Jones of Bennett Jones of Toronto, this emphasis on even a theoretical risk "***established a non-negotiable safety threshold***."

Significantly, she cites the Ontario case of *Pittman vs Bain* where the court ruled that upon learning that a blood product *may* have been contaminated, a blood bank or service is under the obligation to advise the patient of this fact and to do so in a timely manner.

Well, it is this book—not the Canadian Blood Services—that informs those Canadians who happen to read it, that our blood supply must be assumed to be contaminated with one of the most virulent and most difficult-to-treat infectious disease agents known to medicine. It is also likely to be contaminated by various other tick-borne disease pathogens about many of which it is known, with certainty, that they are transmissible through donated blood. Once again, a warning is now given to the current blood services of Canada—again by patient groups, namely LAG and CanLyme. In the past, the process of developing policies and technical ways of protecting recipients of donated blood had to be developed for hepatitis C and HIV; similarly this must happen now for tick-borne diseases. To do so is mandatory.

The numbers of people who contracted HIV and Hepatitis C infections, the last time the blood supply was contaminated in Canada, caused some 30,000 human disasters over the period of a decade.

In the US, the number of new, reported cases of Lyme disease *per year,* as Congressman Frank R. Wolf states in his March 11, 2009, letter to Congressman Frank Pallone Jr. (chairman of the US Energy and Commerce Subcommittee on Health) was 27,444 new ***confirmed*** Lyme cases for the year 2007. Wolf also states, that the CDC assumes under-reporting, due to various factors known to be standard for data gathering on infectious diseases and that, therefore, in 2007 alone, actually 270,000 Americans must have become infected with Lyme disease. According to the American Red Cross, which administers the blood supply in the US, some of those are assumed to have contracted the disease, or passed it on, through blood transfusions—hence their mandatory, exhaustive intake questionnaire and their policy to see known co-infections as red flags for Lyme.

Given that pathogen reduction techniques are still evolving in transfusion research, the US blood service explicitly tries to prevent the possibility of Lyme being transmitted through blood products by using this very detailed questionnaire that helps donors to identify the possibility of this infection in themselves. Canada does not ask any such questions from potential donors. Is this for the same obvious reasons that came to haunt the blood supply back in the '70s and '80s, namely that such screening through updated questionnaires would reduce the available blood supply? It undoubtedly would.

Lyme, like many other tick-borne or mosquito-transmitted diseases, are *relapsing fevers*; the intervals between fever events are unpredictable in duration and occurrence. People who regularly donate blood may mistake a first fever event as the flu, upon the cessation of that fever they may then donate blood, and only after several such fever events develop the classic symptoms of Lyme disease. By that time, other people may have been infected with Lyme spirochetes themselves and/or the commonly known co- infections. Both donors and recipients are, of course, clueless about this process.

Furthermore, the Lyme-causing spirochete appears in a person's blood stream at not well-understood intervals, then disappears in deep tissues and reappears in bodily fluids, often accompanied by other pathogens. Lyme being a bacterial spirochete, like syphilis (transmissible through blood and other bodily fluids) must be viewed with very high suspicion; our blood supply is protected from contamination with syphilis going back to the 1970s, but not from the Lyme-causing spirochete *Borrelia burgdorferi*. Ignoring an infectious disease agent of such extreme morbidity is unacceptable.

As Karin Klouman had pointed out to the CBS, the "theoretical risk" of acquiring Lyme disease through a blood transfusion was signaled in 1989 by the American Red Cross Blood Services in the journal *Transfusion* when reporting the results of their experiment with *B.burgdorferi*. Testing for the spirochetes survival in donated, stored blood, they found that it stayed alive for up to 45 days. The CBS acknowledged knowing about this study in the above-cited correspondence. A quick Google search in November 2009—twenty years later—revealed that there are more than 1,400 articles on PubMed (a major internet gateway to medical journals) on just transfusion-related reports on Lyme and associated tick-borne diseases; some of those reports are found in the *Canadian Medical Association Journal*. Clearly, a lot of knowledgeable people are concerned with this issue.

Cognitive Dissonance Canadian Style

The cognitive dissonance between facts ignored and complacency maintained has now become once again a national issue of concern. The CBS assure Lyme patients that we don't have to worry about a "theoretical threat" to the blood supply. Now, it so happens that scientists informing the federal government on the recently passed Bill C-11 (*An Act to promote security with respect to human pathogens and toxins)* don't share that complacent view. That federal Act explicitly focuses on a long list of specific bacteria, viruses, prions, and other disease-causing agents against which the Canadian public must be protected—because we now know, beyond any doubt, just how nasty those can be. *Borrelia burgdorferi*, the Lyme-causing pathogen as well as most of its co-infections are listed in that bill, which is now law. The websites of Canada's major teaching hospitals explicitly refer to this new Act and inform of policy changes with respect to many of the listed pathogens.

But this is not all—it gets even stranger! Denial was taken to another level absurdity and irresponsibility in May of 2009. Given this tremendous *increase* of interest around the world in the contamination of donated blood with new and emerging pathogens, something totally incomprehensible occurred on the website of the Public Health Agency of Canada's Transfusion Transmitted Diseases section. There the medical profession and patients go to find the list of diseases known to be transmitted by blood transfusions, or carrying a risk of doing so. Canada's doctors are now misled if consulting this Health Canada website. For years, Lyme disease and its co-infections were included as a "theoretical risk" with regard to some of them, and a known risk respecting others; the appropriate supporting citations from the medical literature were also appended—***until May 26, 2009***. On that date, the website was inexplicably modified and the Lyme spirochete disappeared.

Around that same time, the federal Bill C-11 was moving its way into law. The right hand certainly was clueless as to whatever the left hand was doing. Whoever was told clean up that Health Canada website by taking Lyme disease off the list of potentially transfusion-transmissible diseases was, apparently, not told to also wipe off his or her fingerprints when leaving the website—all the literature citations, which refer to Lyme disease as a potential risk to the safety of the blood supply, are still on there! Those citations include one of the most important research reports on Lyme disease in Canada, published on May 30, 2000, in the *Canadian Medical Association Journal* (reproduced in Chapter 2). It was co-authored and initiated by John Scott, author of that chapter.

It appears, that the Canadian Blood Service takes the concept of "theoretical risk" to mean that removing Lyme spirochetes out of sight and potential discussion meets the requirement of safety—which was not what Justice Krever ordered at all.

The CBS has not made it clear so far, and maybe does not know the answer either, by what authority safety and risk may be interpreted in this idiosyncratic manner. Most importantly, there is no new publication anywhere that suddenly proved, beyond a reasonable doubt, that the Lyme spirochete and its co-infections no longer pose a risk of transmissibility through blood products. It is utterly amazing that this action was taken *after* the US Centers for Disease Control declared Lyme an epidemic in 2008; since then, most other blood services have increased their vigilance with regard to tick-borne diseases. Canada, instead of acting on this alarming and wholly verifiable news from the world's largest surveillance centers, the CDC, goes to sleep—once again.

On May 24, 2009, Karin Klouman replied to the CBS again, two days before Lyme disease so mysteriously disappeared from that Health Canada website. By now the references she appended were becoming as long as the text of the letter. (As an aside to any would-be activists, the following caution might be helpful: when dealing with authorities or governments, always assume that you may be better informed than they are.) She wrote:

> "We appreciate your invitation for a meeting with the Canadian Blood Services (CBS) and are currently in the process of putting together a delegation to do so. Despite your insistence that no change is currently warranted in the CBS' screening policy for blood donors, in our opinion there are many areas of concern that need your immediate attention. We are particularly concerned about the following issues:
>
> 1. The necessity of considering the co-infectious agents in Lyme disease:
>
>   We find it disappointing that despite the fact that we have clearly voiced our concern over the possibility that *several tick-borne organisms* could be spreading through our blood supply, in your reply to us you have still chosen to focus exclusively on Borrelia burgdorferi (Bb), as if this organism is the only pathogen of interest.
>
>   Bb, in the vast majority of cases, occurs as a co-infection with *other* tick-borne organisms, such as *Babesia microti* and *Anaplasma phagocytophilum*, which have already been well documented to transmit through blood transfusions, *sometimes with fatal results*. If you implemented a deferral-policy for Babesiosis alone, then you would be taking a step towards also ruling out a good portion of the people with Lyme disease.
>
>   In our opinion it is unacceptable that there is no attention paid to *any* Tick-Borne Disease (TBD) as part of the CBS screening process, despite the American Association of Blood Banks' (AABB's) position that it "requires that all donors **be asked** if they have a history of Babesiosis. Those individuals with a history of the disease are permanently deferred from donating blood."
>
> 2. The CBS position on TBDs, in view of international blood service policies
>
>   Despite your insistence that you are fully aligned with other international blood agencies in regard to TBDs, the evidence is clearly to the contrary. The AABB recommends that a diagnosis of *Babesiosis* must cause a permanent deferral. The CBS does not mention such a necessary deferral on its website. The AABB furthermore state that "Donors with a history of Lyme disease can donate, provided they have undergone a full course of antibiotic treatment and no longer have symptoms." There are many published policies of deferral for Lyme

and associated TBDs by the American and international blood service industries, as illustrated by the following few examples:

The American Red Cross Blood Services, New York-Penn Region: Lyme disease "If this is a chronic condition you cannot donate. If treated with antibiotics and completely recovered, you can donate 12 months after last dose of antibiotics was taken" (4a)

The New York Blood Center: "*Babesiosis*: Permanent deferral. *Ehrlichiosis*: Accept if asymptomatic and treatment is complete. If signs or symptoms; defer for six months after completion of treatment. *Lyme Disease*: If no current signs: Defer until treatment is completed. If symptoms are present, defer for six months and asymptomatic."

The American Red Cross of Northern New Jersey. Jan. 14th/09 press release: "Among the conditions that would temporarily limit donor eligibility are travel to certain foreign countries and medical issues such as... a one-year deferral for Lyme disease. "

The UK Blood Transfusion Services: "Lyme disease: Must not donate while infected... *Babesiosis*: Must not donate."

The Australian Red Cross blood service: "Lyme disease: I have had Lyme disease. Can I donate?... You are eligible to donate 2 weeks after you have recovered fully and you are certified fit by your doctor."

The Norwegian Red Cross: "if bitten by a tick with no occurrence of symptoms there is a deferral for 4 weeks. If borelliosis occurs then there is a minimum of a 6 month deferral, after treatment has been completed."

For the CBS to use a recent AABB's subcommittee report on Borrelia burgdorferi as the reason for not implementing a screening process ... is an illogical position to take, especially since the AABB's official position is still to warn that Lyme disease patients can only donate after successful treatment has been completed ... The CBS also clearly do not follow the AABB recommendations in screening for Babesiosis. It will be a difficult legal position to defend that Canada continues to insist upon inaction in this matter, while so many international blood service industries have developed well-defined policies for Lyme disease and other TBDs.

3. The CBS' position on screening for Lyme disease, in view of Canadian Law

The new "Safety and Security Act of Canada," with respect to human pathogens and toxins (*C-11*) has named Borrelia burgdorferi as a dangerous pathogen that the public must be protected against. We fully expect that this 'protection of the public' extends to our blood supply. Therefore; the fact that the CBS do not look for tick-borne infections is bound to shortly come under close scrutiny. It is our position that if your current donor screening protocol does not immediately change to include looking for TBD, then the CBS will find itself in contempt of the law. In view of C-11, we believe that you have no choice but to implement a vastly improved health interview to substantially reduce the risk that Bb and other tick-borne organisms could be infecting our blood supply.

4. The importance of the clinical screening interview

According to experts in the treatment field a thorough ***clinical evaluation*** is the only way to arrive at a diagnosis of Lyme disease. A battery of blood tests is only helpful in that this can support such a diagnosis, once it has been made.

We therefore suggest that the primary approach to screening for TBDs must be a detailed clinical interview. Due to the general lack of education regarding the signs of Lyme disease, many donors with Lyme (and associated diseases) will have no idea that they may have contracted tick-borne infections. These people will, as it currently stands, be accepted by the CBS, as long as they are not showing any acute signs of febrile illness. Inexplicably your staff at local branches also actively encourages continued blood donation from those ***that have already informed the blood services*** that they have been diagnosed with Lyme. To alert you to this alarming trend we have referred to personal testimony from identified Lyme patients that have been blood donors ***in all our correspondence*** with you to date.

The causative agent for Lyme disease in North America; *Borrelia burgdorferi*, has been proven to survive in stored blood products and therefore ***must*** be considered a risk to our blood-supply. In North America, however, the Borrelia blood tests are only aimed at screening for ***Bb***, while any person traveling outside of North America is likely to pick up other strains of this pathogen. In Europe and Asia the more prevalent strains are Borrelia garinii and Borrelia afzelii, while in Africa the most common organism is Borrelia lusitaniae. Since blood tests for Borrelia have been shown to be notoriously unreliable and testing is only done for Bb (and none of the other subspecies) the simplest way to substantially reduce the risk of borreliosis in blood donors has to be a carefully developed questionnaire, which truly acknowledges the real danger that all the various Borrelia pathogens pose.

For the CBS to claim that your current health questionnaire already rules out any TBD-infected blood-donors is frankly absurd. You ask none of the questions that would be relevant in screening for any of the known TBDs, most of which are relapsing illnesses. Especially early on in the progression of Lyme disease a person can have a full-blown infection, yet still have periods of feeling relatively well. Under your present screening procedure, during times of 'apparent good health' such a person will be welcomed as a blood donor, despite the fact

> that he/she is a carrier of TBD. However, if an urgently needed revised Health Questionnaire was implemented, then we would substantively reduce the risk of any tick-borne organisms contaminating our blood supply.
>
> **In conclusion:** There is an agreement that Lyme disease is an emerging epidemic in North America and that there has been an explosive increase in Canada in the past decade. Furthermore, there are many patients in Canada who do not remember ever having had a tick bite, but yet they have full blown Lyme disease. Some of these patients have been the recipients of blood transfusions in the past and are now wondering whether they could have become infected through the blood supply. Other Lyme patients know that they have donated blood in good faith, having been unaware of the fact that they were infected by TBD. Others again are deeply disturbed by phone calls from the CBS, asking them ***to continue to donate blood***, despite being diagnosed with Lyme disease.
>
> There is a growing outrage among Lyme patients in Canada directed at the CBS' lack of action in protecting our blood supply. We would like to meet with you in the near future, in order to discuss in more detail these aforementioned serious issues in regard to your donor screening policies."

Two days after this letter went to Ottawa, Lyme disappeared from that website of the Public Health Agency of Canada's Transfusion Transmitted Diseases section. Coincidence? Maybe.

For the Canadian Blood Services *B. burgdorferi* and its co-pathogens are certainly very inconvenient. This was what in the past the Canadian Red Cross had found HIV and hepatitis C to be; and back then, too, other countries understood more rapidly their danger, while Canada denied and ignored them. This denial with all its attending potential for largely avoidable human suffering, is borne by the Canadian public—once again. Undoubtedly, Lyme disease, as a high-risk contaminant in blood products, will hit the fan in due course; it is inevitable.

What is especially poignant in this new development is the fact that it follows almost immediately upon the death of one of CBS's most renowned board members, the health activist James Kreppner. The chair of the CBS board, Verna Skanes, is quoted in the May 16, 2009, *Globe & Mail* obituary that Kreppner *"in many ways was the conscience of our board. He [a hemophiliac who contracted AIDS from a transfusion] was a pretty eloquent reminder of what we are all there for ... and to remind us of Justice Krever's recommendations."* The obituary quoted his partner Antonia Swann who said that Kreppner *"was passionate about protecting the blood system ... because he was fearful of future and as yet unknown pathogens. He wanted us to put safety above all else."*

Lyme Action Group and Canadian Blood Services Meeting

Between May and December 2009 this correspondence took place. In June LAG took up the invitation from CBS to meet personally. The CBS were even willing to fly from Ottawa to Toronto just for that purpose, to which LAG replied that doing so would be an unnecessary waste of tax-payers' money and suggested the meeting take place when the next CBS board meeting was scheduled in Toronto. LAG felt that our concerns had been submitted clearly in writing and hoped that CBS would have considered the need for an improved screening questionnaire before we met with them.

On December 4, 2009, representatives from CBS and LAG met in the boardroom of that 19th century building on Bloor Street, where the original Hospital for Sick Children was once housed, and where today some of the blood services for Ontario are located.

This meeting was conducted with utmost friendliness on all sides, but it was as informative as it was alarming. Both authors of this chapter were present, and every effort is made to summarize the discussion as fairly as possible. The LAG delegation presented the CBS group with copies of Pamela Weintraub's *Cure Unknown* (updated 2009 edition) and the documentary film *Under Our Skin*. These two items caused dramatic changes in State and federal law and polices within the US, following their release. Weintraub's book is a magisterial portrait of the evolution of Lyme disease in the US and the medico-political developments involved in testing and treatment.

LAG representatives explained that these two items played a significant role in the decision by a number of jurisdictions in the US to enact legislation designed specifically to further research and awareness campaigns into the existence and dangers of Chronic Lyme disease and to protect physicians' ability to treat Lyme disease, when using long-term antibiotic treatment. At the time of going to press, 16 States in the US enacted various types of legislative, policy, or financial support measures in aid of Lyme disease, as did the US Senate and Congress (see items appended to chapter 1); several more are pending. Weintraub's exhaustively referenced book, and the interviews with the leading Lyme researchers shown in the documentary, contradict with verifiable evidence the IDSA's dismissal of Lyme disease as "difficult to catch and easy to treat," as stated in their now discredited 2006 guidelines; in fact, this information proves that Lyme disease is ***easy to catch and hard to treat*** and usually leads to very serious disability and can cause death.

Given that the regulatory systems in Canada and the US work closely together, and must do so under NAFTA and other agreements, such as the mandatory reciprocal recognition between the Canadian and American medical associations, CBS should see the recent legislative and policy developments in the US as a red flag, and these developments should also be alarming to the Canadian government, as they are extremely important public health measures relevant to the whole continent.

Even though Health Canada and the Canadian Public Health Laboratory Network complacently continue to adhere to the discredited 2006 IDSA guidelines, LAG feels that the CBS must be vigilant about blood safety and needs to take appropriate action to implement screening for Lyme and other tick-borne disease. In view of the clearly defined responsibilities of the CBS, it is the CBS that can and must tell Health Canada what is needed—not the other way around.

Present were from CBS: Jean-Paul Bedard, Vice President of Public Affairs, Dr. Dana Devine, Vice-President, Medical, Scientific and Research Affairs, research and development director whose work includes a focus on "pathogen inactivation/ reduction procedures" in donated blood. Dr. Margaret Fearon, Medical Director, CBS. Also present were Stephanie Kelly, Senior Manager, Public Affairs of CBS and Lorna Tessier of Public Affairs.

The Lyme Action Group had asked Dr. Jozef Krop to attend; he is an ILADS trained physician with a large Chronic Lyme practice in Mississauga, which according to the CMAJ studies, is one of the Lyme tick-endemic areas in Canada; he is the author of chapter 7. Also attending was Dr. Doug Wilson (Professor Emeritus of Medicine, MacMaster University, himself a Lyme patient and a member of LAG). The following members of LAG were present: Karin Klouman (recovered Lyme patient, author of chapter 8); Rob Manten (former regular blood donor, Lyme patient); John Morgan (formerly a regular blood donor, once a blood recipient, now a Lyme patient), Wally Barr (also a former blood donor and Lyme patient), Helke Ferrie (medical science writer, publisher, and editor of this book), and Eleanor Johnston (also with Citizens for Choice in Health Care).

Representing the national patient support group, CanLyme was Rossana Magnotta, who was trained as a medical laboratory technologist; she is a board member of CanLyme, and now is the widow of Gabe Magnotta, whose tragic story is mentioned in Chapter 1 and dedication. He died of complications from Chronic Lyme disease less than three weeks after this meeting with CBS, as reported on CBC radio and in various national and local newspapers.

The Lyme Action Group's members provided up-to-date maps from reports by the US Centers for Disease Control, showing how Lyme disease has become a continental American epidemic—a fact still ignored in Canada. Some group members related how they have been repeatedly asked to donate blood again, even though they had been diagnosed with active Lyme disease and had informed the blood service clinics involved of their changed health status. One of them may have become infected with Lyme disease through a blood transfusion several years ago; his symptoms emerged shortly after that transfusion.

Dr. Krop described three of his most seriously ill Chronic Lyme patients whose history was strongly suggestive of the possibility of Lyme infection through a blood transfusion; in each case the onset of the classic Lyme symptoms had followed almost immediately after the transfusion event, and all three patients had no exposure to the outside at the time, nor did they develop the classic rash. The CBS representatives suggested Dr. Krop provide the details on each patient to enable them to track that transfusion event and contact the donor for further possible investigation and notification. LAG members felt that since the testing mandated for Lyme in Canada has an extremely high rate of false-negatives, such a call-back investigation was unlikely to yield useful information.

Mrs. Magnotta told the heart-breaking story of her husband's infection, already suspicious of Lyme at that time, and the inability to find any doctor who knew even the most basic facts about Lyme disease; their subsequent pointless exercise with Canada's testing procedure which "proved" him to be free of Lyme; the inexorable breakdown of her husband's health, as the original infection became full-blown Chronic Lyme; the final confirmation of that Lyme infection—but too late—from a US-based laboratory, and the fact that, ironically, their dog was correctly and promptly diagnosed with Lyme by their vet, properly treated, and cured.

Karin Klouman made a presentation based on a written submission handed to the CBS representatives. The chief issue of for LAG, she said, was supported by Justice Krever's statement that '*action to reduce risk should not await scientific certainty.*' She went on to say: "*It is our position, that the CBS to date has failed to follow this recommendation, in regard to the very possible risk of tick-borne organisms contaminating our blood supply. From our correspondence with the CBS to date LAG understands the CBS' position to be that there is not enough scientific evidence linking the spread of Lyme disease to blood transfusions. … However, Justice Krever … stated that upon learning of even a* ***potential risk*** *to the safety of the blood supply 'the CBS should cause the recipients to be informed, even in circumstances where the risk is* ***theoretical****.' This is a recommendation that the CBS appears to not follow, in regard to the threat of Lyme disease. Justice Krever in his evaluation of the AIDS/HIV blood scandal in Canada concluded that even 'When there was* ***reasonable evidence*** *that serious infectious disease could be transmitted by blood, the principal actors in the blood supply system in*

Canada refrained from taking essential preventive measures until causation had been proved with ***scientific certainty.*** *The result was a national public health disaster.'"*

Karin Klouman presented also on an important new report, not previously mentioned during the correspondence with CBS. This report from Rhode Island dealt specifically with Babesia, known to be acquired through transfusion. Since the Lyme disease-causing bacterium generally is accompanied by other co-infecting bacteria, and frequently by Babesia, its presence and transfusability should be treated as a red flag suggesting the potential presence of the Lyme spirochete as well, or that efforts must be made to understand when the Lyme spirochete actually becomes detectable in blood.

Karin Klouman explained: "*... in most cases [Borrelia burgdorferi, i.e. Lyme causing spirochetes], occur as a co-infection with* ***other*** *tick-borne organisms, such as (but not limited to) Babesia microti and Anaplasma phagocytophilum,* ***both*** *of which have already been proven to transmit through blood transfusions, sometimes with fatal results... There is currently a wealth of evidence in the scientific Literature on Transfusion Transmitted Babesiosis (TTB) (including a case in* ***Ontario****), but we would particularly like to refer you to one recent study. In 2007 the numbers of diagnosed TTB cases accounted for a full 10% of the total clinical Babesiosis cases that were reported in Rhode Island. The conclusion of this Rhode Island study is that 'The current screening method of omitting donors with a history of Babesiosis may be effective in preventing some, but not all, cases of TTB and current processing of blood products does not eradicate this parasite. Thus, a better screening test is needed. The most logical position for the CBS would be to screen all potential donors for Lyme disease by* ***introducing a new clinical screening interview****, with some very specifically formulated questions, aimed at ruling out donors that potentially could be infected by tick-borne organisms. The CBS' current clinical interview only identifies the acute and febrile form of a tick-borne illness and is, therefore, not of much use in screening for Chronic Lyme disease or other TBDs. This approach clearly fails to take into consideration the relapsing nature of almost all the TBDs.*

"However, this situation could easily be rectified by implementing a new or expanded interview process, designed to specifically look for symptoms of tick-borne illnesses. Such an interview should target those donors that have had exposure to ticks and also screen for well-known Ld and other TBD symptoms: such as, but not limited to; recurring flu like symptoms, severe brain-fog, aching joints, unexplained and persistent headaches, skin rashes. Chronic health conditions

should also raise the suspicion of a possible infection by tick-borne organisms: such as, but again not limited to MS, ALS, Rheumatoid Arthritis, early onset Alzheimer's, Chronic Fatigue, Fibromyalgia. A diagnosis of any such condition, therefore, needs to be considered as a reason for deferral."

Mention was made also of the recent discovery connecting Chronic Fatigue Syndrome with a virus known at present as XMRV. It is clear, that the safety of the blood supply is becoming increasingly tied to the complexity of disease causation.

Dr. Dana Devine, the Vice-president of CBS's Medical, Scientific and Research Affairs, made a PowerPoint presentation (slides appended to this chapter with Dr. Devine's kind permission) focused on a technology under development called "pathogen inactivation or reduction." Dr. Devine explained, that donor blood contamination has a long history. Pointing to this Devil's Staircase of escalating pathogen threats to donated blood since the 1930s, she said, "We will never get to the end of this, but need something more than a never-ending *reactive* strategy." What is needed now, everybody agrees, she explained, is a comprehensive strategy of pathogen reduction or inactivation that "takes them all out, from all blood products." Indeed, this is the current frontier in this line of research.

The dangerous contaminants found in donor blood include bacteria, viruses, parasites and prions. Dr. Devine explained that the protective interventions undertaken twenty years ago, following the Krever Commission, were directed against HIV and Hepatitis C contamination in donor blood, and these efforts were very successful. However, such actions take time to implement, she said, ranging from four to twenty years (!), depending on the difficulties involved, the interests of private companies that invest in their development, and government negotiations with the private sector for which the profits involved are often considered too limited. Dr. Devine made it clear that there were numerous technical problems to be overcome and that presently used pathogen reduction strategies only work on some blood products and that a lot more research was needed.

After the meeting, a quick internet search revealed that this pathogen reduction/inactivation technology has been under development since 1996 with the major pharmaceutical player then being Baxter and Steritech. A report on this technology in the *International Journal of Hematology* in 2002 was very encouraging and announced the commencement of animal and human studies. By 2008 the reports were somewhat disappointing because some blood products, treated with these emerging technologies, were now known to result in the host's production of antibodies to such transfusions. That is a mostly fatal complication.

A 2009 report by McMaster University experts entitled "Protecting the blood supply from emerging pathogens: The role of pathogen inactivation" reported that currently "only 10–15% of all transfusions associated mortalities" are now due to transfusion-transmitted infections. The "new technologies have evolved over the past decade to treat cellular blood components as well as plasma [which] have begun to be used in Europe…" The review concludes, "in order for pathogen inactivation technologies to become widely accepted, they must be shown to be both cost effective and not associated with new risks to recipients." In other words, we still have a long way to go. Indeed, Dr. Devine informed everyone at the meeting, that the first pilot project, pending Health Canada's approval, might start by the fall of 2010.

From LAG's perspective, that 10–15% figure has to be way too low, because the whole problem of Lyme and associated co-infections being transmitted through blood products flies under the current radar. This is surely one of the "known unknowns," to which Donald Rumsfeld's amusing observation refers.

Following up on this meeting, LAG observed on this point in a letter of December 12, 2009: *"Even under the most favorable circumstances, however, it seems that such a 'pilot project' cannot be up and running, until a year from now—and that the timeline you are realistically looking at (for generally implementing an inactivation/reduction method) could be 4 years thereafter. We are, therefore, looking at another 4–5 years of our blood supply remaining unprotected against the organisms that cause TBDs. This is a grave concern for us and we urge you, in the meantime, to implement an improved screening interview, to protect Canadians against Transfusion Transmitted Tick-Borne Diseases."*

Returning to the events of that meeting on December 4, Dr. Devine's presentation was followed by another by Dr. Margaret Fearon, the Executive Medical Director of the CBS. She informed the group that CBS and Health Canada are in the planning stages of a field-study to establish the extent of Lyme disease in Canada. When asked how people would be tested, she replied that the standard tests would be used!

Well! The truth is, that we need that two-tiered ELISA + Western blot confirmation testing like the proverbial hole in the head, as explained in chapter 1. In view of the fact that, specially for surveillance purposes, the US CDC changed their Lyme disease case definition in 2008 and dropped that restrictive and misleading ELISA + Western blot two-tier approach, it is astounding that Health Canada would, two years later, still even consider the use of this obsolete surveillance method! This appears absurd, given that Health Canada insists it is following CDC standards—the inconsistencies are mounting. The changed surveillance case definition can be viewed at www.cdc.gov/ncphi/disss/nndss/casedef/lyme_disease_2008.htm

The Krever Report as a Biblical Commandment

LAG expressed considerable alarm because, if this study proceeds under the hopelessly flawed Canadian Public Health Laboratory Network's Lyme disease guidelines of 2007 (based on the legally compromised 2006 IDSA guidelines), the results are beyond doubt going to be an expensive perpetuation of the myth that there is "no Lyme in Canada": the population will continue to be at risk; the medical profession will continue to be misled; any advancement in policy will be even more unlikely. Those 2007 Canadian guidelines make no reference to the guidelines developed by the International Lyme and Associated Disease Society ILADS since 2001 and ignore the related research as well—just as the IDSA was found to have done during that anti-trust investigation. Indeed, such a field-study would be the cause of a false sense of security and result in even more harm to the public. Such a study, if it were to be published, would not only already be outdated at the time of its publication, being based on grossly incomplete scientific information, but it would also tragically delay development of necessary services for Canadians.

However, since CBS has a duty to cooperate with its regulator—Health Canada and with the Canadian Public Health Laboratory Network—CBS would be expected to follow the IDSA-informed Canadian 2007 guidelines. Nevertheless, it appears to us, that CBS has a far greater duty to the public and must protest adherence to such legally and clinically insupportable guidelines, because CBS must follow the commandment given by Justice Krever, namely "**the safety of the blood supply is paramount—the principle of safety must transcend other principles and policies.**" CBS has a right and a duty to object to those flawed testing guidelines for Lyme. Since CBS is a member of the board of the Canadian Public Health Laboratory Networks, it has an obligation to raise such objections and insist on revised guidelines on being enacted and published.

Given the already often volatile relationship between the provinces and the federal government, such a flawed study would make it even easier for the provinces to abdicate their responsibility for a safe blood supply and a science-based, clinically justified medical policy on Lyme. As we have seen from the non-responses by ex-Minister David Caplan and the current Minister of Health and Long-Term Care, Hon. D. Matthews, they are very quick to ignore their legally anchored right and responsibility to influence Health Canada and the CBS processes in the public interest of their province. Such a flawed research study would support further inaction, and it would take a very long time to get the impact of such a flawed study out of the system.

It is crystal clear that Health Canada and the Public Health Agency of Canada are wedded to the 2006 IDSA guidelines, with regard to testing for Lyme disease. It is the adoption of these now wholly discredited guidelines that promoted the myth in Canada that Lyme is rare and that its chronic form is not a valid diagnosis and supposedly not due to infection. These guidelines have been exceptionally successful in keeping thousands of doctors ignorant of the truth of this pervasive and devastating disease.

Most importantly, it was this wholly inappropriate testing algorithm, invented and then forcefully promoted by the IDSA since 1994, that led to the anti-trust investigation of the guideline process by the Attorney General of Connecticut (starting originally in 1999 and commencing formally in 2006). The press release from the Attorney General's office of May 1, 2008, was part of the material LAG provided to the CBS delegation (see appended documents to chapter 1).

To make matters worse, since then, as of February 1, 2010, the Attorney General of Connecticut found evidence that the IDSA review panel he appointed to re-do those flawed guidelines, have attempted to bypass the mutually agreed-upon mandatory voting process. The vote was rigged (but discovered) to avoid the necessary re-write of those biased guidelines, and in order to bypass the admission that those guidelines are manifestly not in conformity with the evidence-based current science on diagnosis and treatment of Lyme disease.

In the follow-up letter to his meeting with the CBS, Karin Klouman wrote for LAG: *"We find the prospect of any CBS research using the currently mandated two-tier protocol (ELISA/Western Blot)* ***alarming****, as that choice would not be in keeping with the Krever recommendation that 'the safety of the blood- supply is paramount- the principle of safety must transcend other principles and policies'. This brings us back to our essential position, which we feel cannot be ignored and is of tremendous significance to public health: the CBS* ***must immediately implement an enhanced questionnaire and donor interview to screen for Lyme disease and other TBDs****, just as many other jurisdictions are already doing. This will rule out some donors and will be slightly more time consuming, but to quote your own website: 'A few minutes of caution is far better than a lifetime of regret'. It is, therefore, incumbent upon the CBS to ask* ***some very specific questions*** *intended to rule out those donors that might be infected by tick-borne organisms. This approach is* ***a simple and inexpensive measure*** *and although it would obviously not rule out all TBD infected donors, it would certainly be a vast improvement over the current system, which does not specifically screen for Lyme disease at all."*

Lest the reader think the Lyme Action Group too alarmist and unreasonable in their demand, it might be useful to see what the US Centers for Disease Control and the American Red Cross experts had to say back in 2002 at the Twenty-Sixth International Symposium on Blood Transfusion:

"New etiology agents of disease transmitted by ticks have emerged, while the geographic distribution of existing agents has expanded," researchers observed, then lamented the lack of decent tests for especially tick-borne diseases, and agreed during the discussion period involving those scientists from all over the world, that "probably the interview with the donor—much like in medical practice—just talking to the donor and getting a medical history, is the cheapest and the most fundamental way of getting to the nature of the medical problem—or in this case, maintaining the safety of the blood supply." This remark, interestingly, came from a research corporation, Cerus, located in Concord, California.

During the December 4, 2009, meeting with the CBS, Dr. Douglas Wilson asked: "How long does it take to change a screening questionnaire?"

"About a year. Health Canada has the final say," Dr. Devine replied.

"If something is a 'theoretical' risk, can't this be done more quickly?" Dr. Douglas Wilson inquired on behalf of LAG. Nobody had an answer.

However, the Krever Report does have one: "*When enhanced donor-screening measures are needed to identify new pathogens, the cost to the blood supply system may be a reduction in the numbers of donors… [But] If harm* ***can*** *occur, then it should be assumed that it* ***will*** *occur. If there are no measures that will entirely prevent the harm, measures that may only partially prevent transmission should be taken…*"

Prior to this meeting, Karin Klouman contacted Dr. Peter Ganz at Health Canada, Center for Biologic Evaluation, responsible for blood safety in Canada (www.usp.org). She asked Dr. Ganz whether the Krever Commission's report was in any way binding, or just a bunch of recommendations that may or may not be followed.

Dr. Ganz replied: "This is the Bible [for the CBS] and these [recommendations] are commandments."

Well, given the way the Bible's Old Testament Commandments have been so readily disregarded over the past millennia, the expectation that the CBS will obey *their* Bible is hopefully not too naive. Of course, ignoring commandments tends to carry consequences—for the victims as well as the perpetrators, and generally the consequences are far greater for the victims. While the CBS sorts all this out on the Lyme disease front, some practical advice might be in order for readers. Given what the authors of this book know about those national myths, that there is almost no Lyme disease in Canada, and that our blood supply is perfectly safe, the following might be worth considering:

1. Avoid using blood transfusions if at all possible. Unless you are in an emergency situation where a transfusion is unavoidable, make arrangements with your family doctor or surgeon to collect your own blood well ahead of time and store it until the day of your surgery.
2. If you develop recurring flu-like symptoms following a blood transfusion, get tested for Lyme disease—in the US, for the time being, until Canada makes up-to-date testing available. See Chapter 10 for reliable information on testing and consult the Resources section.
3. If you have family members or friends who have a chronic disease (many of which may be caused by Lyme spirochetes and their co-infections) or have been frequently ill with relapsing and unexplained fevers, suggest they read this book before considering donating blood and, in the case of chronic disease patients, get properly tested.

Justice Krever did his very best to place the public interest above all other considerations. The CBS undoubtedly wish to do their very best also in running the daily business of the nation's blood supply. However, inherent in this system is a conflict between what Justice Krever defined as the standard of safety on the one hand, and on the other hand the increasing need for enough blood which, unfortunately, may contain also more and more emerging blood-borne disease agents. That inherent conflict is strongly—and inappropriately—supported by a Lyme disease testing process mandated for Canada's laboratories that hides the dangers presented by this infectious disease.

The legitimate—and non-negotiable—demand the Lyme Action Group presented, namely to update the donor questionnaire, so as to rule out many of those donors who are likely to have been infected by a tick-borne disease agent, does not harmonize well with the CBS' desire for enough donors to meet the demand for blood. However serious this conflict may be, in the long run the most intelligent, the safest and least expensive in human and financial costs is undoubtedly to follow Justice Krever's commandments. Another blood scandal is unthinkable.

■

Postscript

As this book was going to press, Karin Klouman received a call on February 9, 2010, from Stephanie Kelly, Senior Manager, Public Affairs CBS, stating that the Canadian Blood Services "is committed" to bringing LAG's position on the need to amend the current blood-donor interview (to screen for Lyme and other Tick-Borne diseases) to a "working committee meeting" in the spring of 2010. Dr. Margaret Fearon, Executive Medical Director, CBS, Kelly said, will present all of the evidence LAG had provided on the likely contamination of Canada's blood supply with tick-borne organisms to that working committee. A specific date is not set, Kelly said, but offered the assurance that the CBS is taking all of LAG's concerns "very seriously."

Sources

(These include the sources provided in the correspondence with the CBS by LAG.)

Badon SJ *et al.* American Red Cross Blood Services, Farmington, Connecticut. Survival of *Borrelia burgdorferi* in blood products. *Transfusion*, 1989, Vol. 29 (7): 581-583

Banerjee SN, Banerjee M., Fernando K, Scott JD, Mann R & Morshed G, Presence of spirochete causing Lyme disease, *Borrelia burgdorferi*, in the blacklegged tick, *Ixodes scapularis*, in southern Ontario; CMAJ, May 30, 2000; 162 (11) 2000

Blajchman MA, Protecting the blood supply from emerging pathogens: The role of pathogen inactivation," *Transfusion Clinique et Biologique*, online prepublication edition May 7, 2009

Canadian Institute of Public Health Inspectors, *Fact Sheet on Lyme Disease* (available in public health offices)

Corbin F 3rd, Pathogen inactivation of blood components: current status and introduction of an approach using riboflavin as a photosensitizer, *International Journal of Hematology*, Aug 2002, 76 Suppl. 2:253-7

Gabitzsch ES, Piesman J, Dolan MC, Sykes CM, & Zeidner MS, Transfer of ***Borrelia Burgdorferi*** s.s. Infection via Blood Transfusion in a Murine Model, Centers for Disease Control and Prevention, Division of Vector-Borne Infectious Diseases, Bacterial Zoonoses Branch, Foothills Campus, Fort Collins, Colorado, *Journal of Parasitology,* 92/4, August 2006.

Johnson SE, Swaminathan B, Moore P, Broome CV, Parvin M., Borrelia burgdorferi: survival in experimentally infected human blood processed for transfusion. Meningitis and Special Pathogens Branch, Centers for Disease Control, Atlanta, Georgia 30333. 1990.

Kain KC, Jassoum SB, Fong IW & Hannach B, Transfusion-transmitted babesiosis in Ontario: first reported case in Canada, CMAJ • June 12, 2001; 164 (12) 2001

Leiby, D.A. *et al.* Relationship between tick bites and the seroprevalence of Babesia microti and Anaplasma phagocytophila (previously Ehrlichia sp.) in blood donors, *Transfusion* vol. 42 (12):1585 ff, December 14, 2002

Leiby, D.A. & Holland, J. H., Babesiosis and blood transfusion: flying under the radar, *Vox Sang* Vol. 90 (3):157 ff, April 1990

Lux JZ, Weiss J, Linden JV, Kessler D, Herwaldt BL, Wong SJ, Keithly J, Della-Latta P &. Scully BE, Transfusion-Associated Babesiosis after Heart Transplant,

Morbidity and Mortality Weekly Report, October 3, 2008, vol. 57, no SS-10; US Centre for Disease Control.

Nadelman RB, Sherer C, Mack L, Pavia CS, Wormser GP, Survival of Borrelia burgdorferi in human blood stored under blood banking conditions. *Transfusion*, 1990, May 30(4):298-301.

Nadelman RB *et al.* Survival of Borrelia burgdorferi in human blood stored under blood banking conditions. *Transfusion*, 1990, Vol. 30 (4): 298-301

Picard A. *The Gift of Death—Confronting Canada's Taunted Blood Tragedy*, Harper, 1998

Scott JD, Fernando K, Durden LA & Morshed MG. Lyme Disease Spirochete, *Borrelia burgdorferi*, Endemic in Epicenter at Turkey Point, Ontario, *J. of Medical Entomology*, Volume 41 (2):226-230 , 2004

Scott JD, Lee M-K, Fernando K, Jorgensen DR, Durden LA & Morshed MG. Rapid introduction of Lyme Disease Spirochete, *Borrelia burgdorferi*, sensu stricto, in *Ixodes scapuloris* (*Acari: Ixodidae*) established at Turkey Point Provincial Park, Ontario, Canada. *Journal of Vector Ecology*, Vol. 33(1):64–69. 2008.

Sibinga Th.S. & Dodd RY, eds. *Transmissible Diseases and Blood Transfusion: Proceedings of the Twenty-Sixth International Symposium on Blood Transfusion, Groningen, NL*, Kluwer Academic Publishers, 2002

Smith, H.V. *et al.* A Lyme borreliosis human serosurvey of asymptomatic adults in Ireland, *Zentralblatt for Bakteriologie*, Vol. 275 (3):382 ff, Aug. 1991

Solheim BG, Pathogen reduction of blood components, *Transfus. Apher. Sci.* August: 39 (1): 75-82; E-publication July 3, 2008

Spencer P. *The Krever Commission Recommendations* (and excerpt) on Longwoods Publishing website, accessed Nov. 11, 2009.

"Under Our Skin—There's No Medicine For Someone Like You," documentary film 2008—www.underourksin.com

Weintraub, P. *Cure Unknown—Inside the Lyme Disease Epidemic*, St. Martin's Press, 2009

Wilson K, MD. The Krever Commission—10 Years Later. CMAJ, Nov. 20, 2007, vol. 177 (11) Commentary. A Lyme borreliosis human serosurvey of asymptomatic adults in Ireland.

Zentralbl Bakteriol. 1991 Aug;275(3):382-9, http://www.ncbi.nlm.nih.gov/pubmed/1741921

American Red Cross: "Lyme disease—If this is a chronic condition you cannot donate. If you were treated with antibiotics and completely recovered, you can donate 12 months after the last dose of antibiotics was taken."

UCSF Blood Center: "Permanent Deferrals—The following conditions would permanently disqualify an individual as an allogenic or designated blood donor… Babesiosis… Lyme disease"

NY Blood Center: "Lyme Disease—**1.** If no signs of symptoms: Defer until treatment is completed. **2.** If signs or symptoms: Defer for six months whether or not treatment was received."

Guidelines for the Blood Transfusion Services in the UK for Lyme disease: "Must not donate if infected."

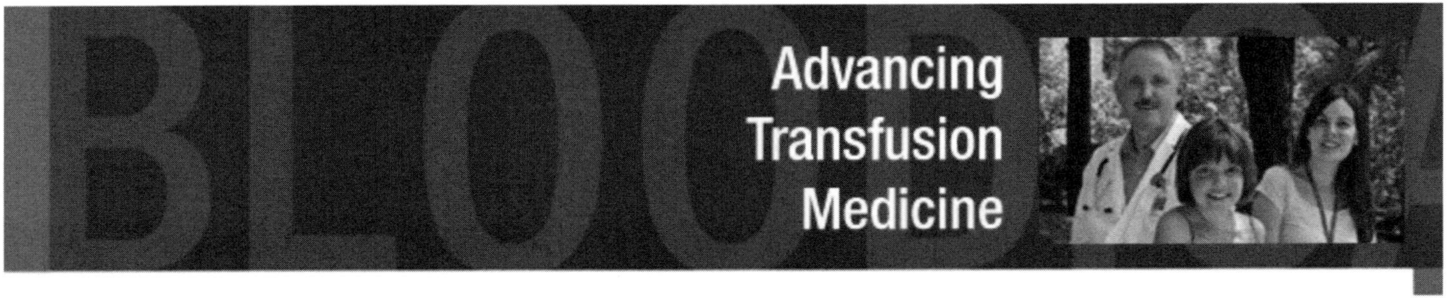

Blood Borne Pathogens: Strategies to Improve Blood Safety

Dana Devine, Ph.D.

Vice President, Medical, Scientific & Research Affairs

Lyme Action Group Meeting

December 4, 2009

1

Canadian Blood Services

it's in you to give

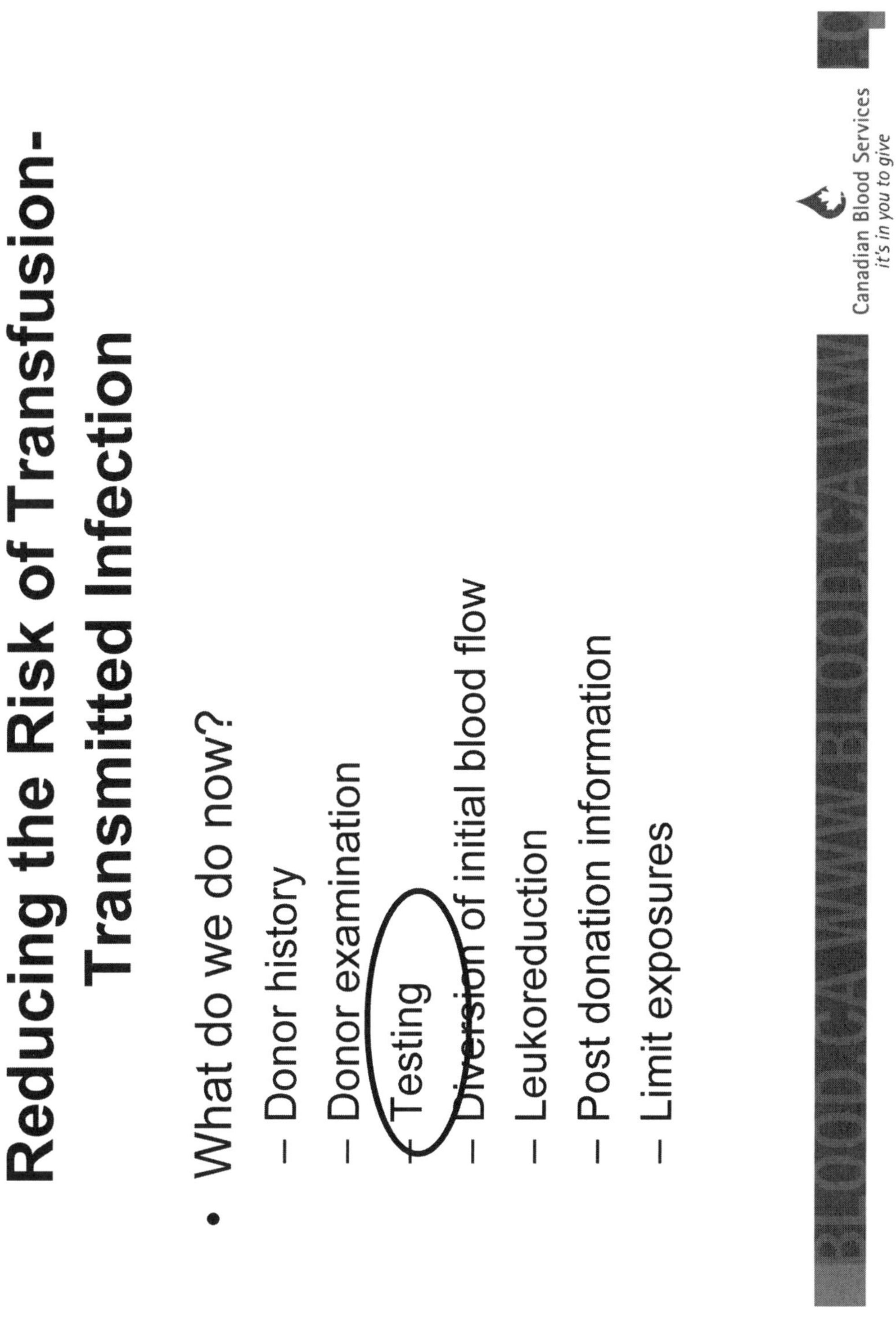
Reducing the Risk of Transfusion-Transmitted Infection
• What do we do now?
– Donor history
– Donor examination
– Testing
– Diversion of initial blood flow
– Leukoreduction
– Post donation information
– Limit exposures
Canadian Blood Services
it's in you to give
BLOOD.CA WWW.BLOOD.CA WWW

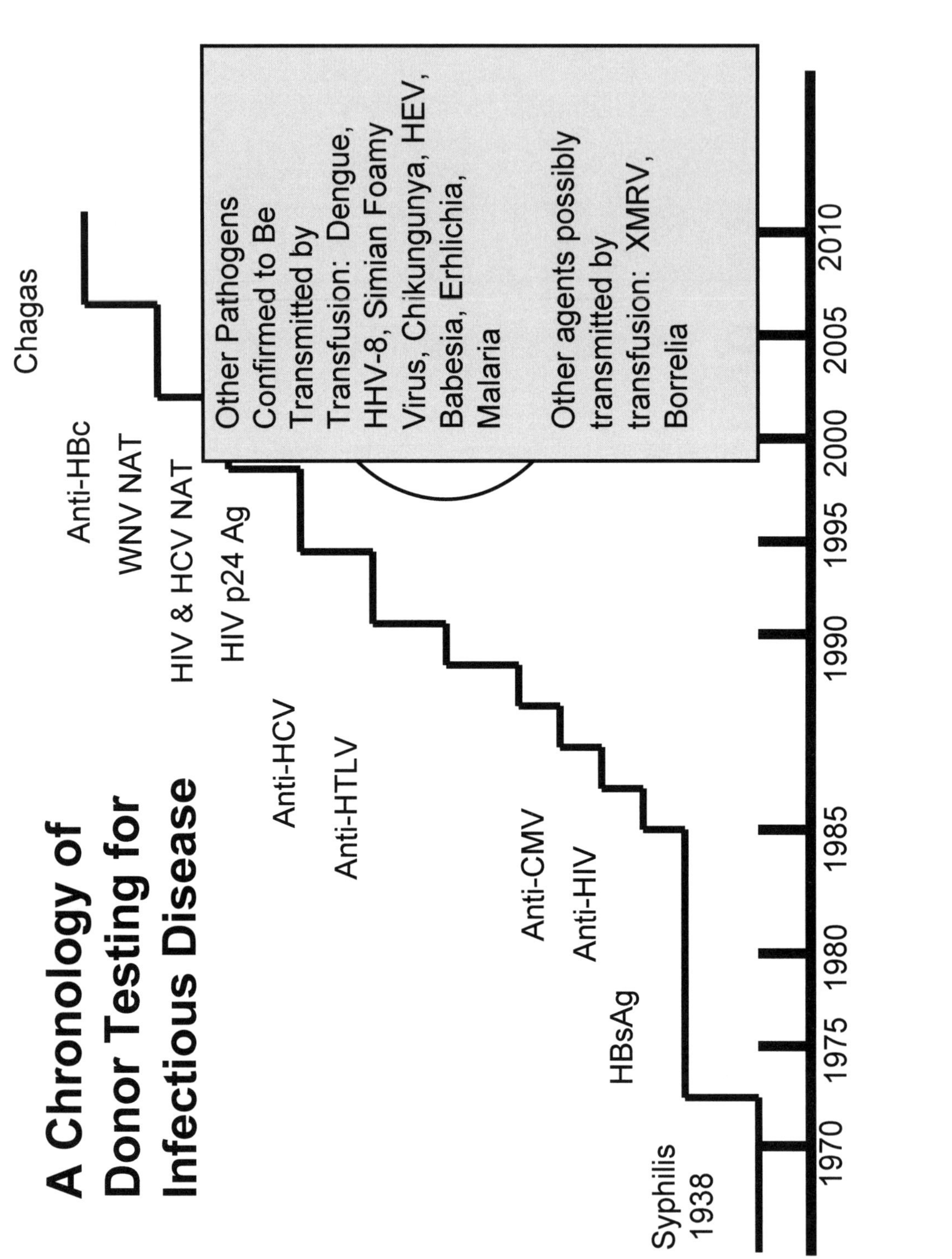
A Chronology of Donor Testing for Infectious Disease
Syphilis 1938
HBsAg
Anti-HIV
Anti-CMV
Anti-HTLV
Anti-HCV
HIV p24 Ag
HIV & HCV NAT
WNV NAT
Anti-HBc
Chagas
Other Pathogens Confirmed to Be Transmitted by Transfusion: Dengue, HHV-8, Simian Foamy Virus, Chikungunya, HEV, Babesia, Erhlichia, Malaria
Other agents possibly transmitted by transfusion: XMRV, Borrelia
1970
1975
1980
1985
1990
1995
2000
2005
2010

Pathogen Inactivation of Blood

An alternative strategy to additional testing.

Canadian Blood Services
it's in you to give

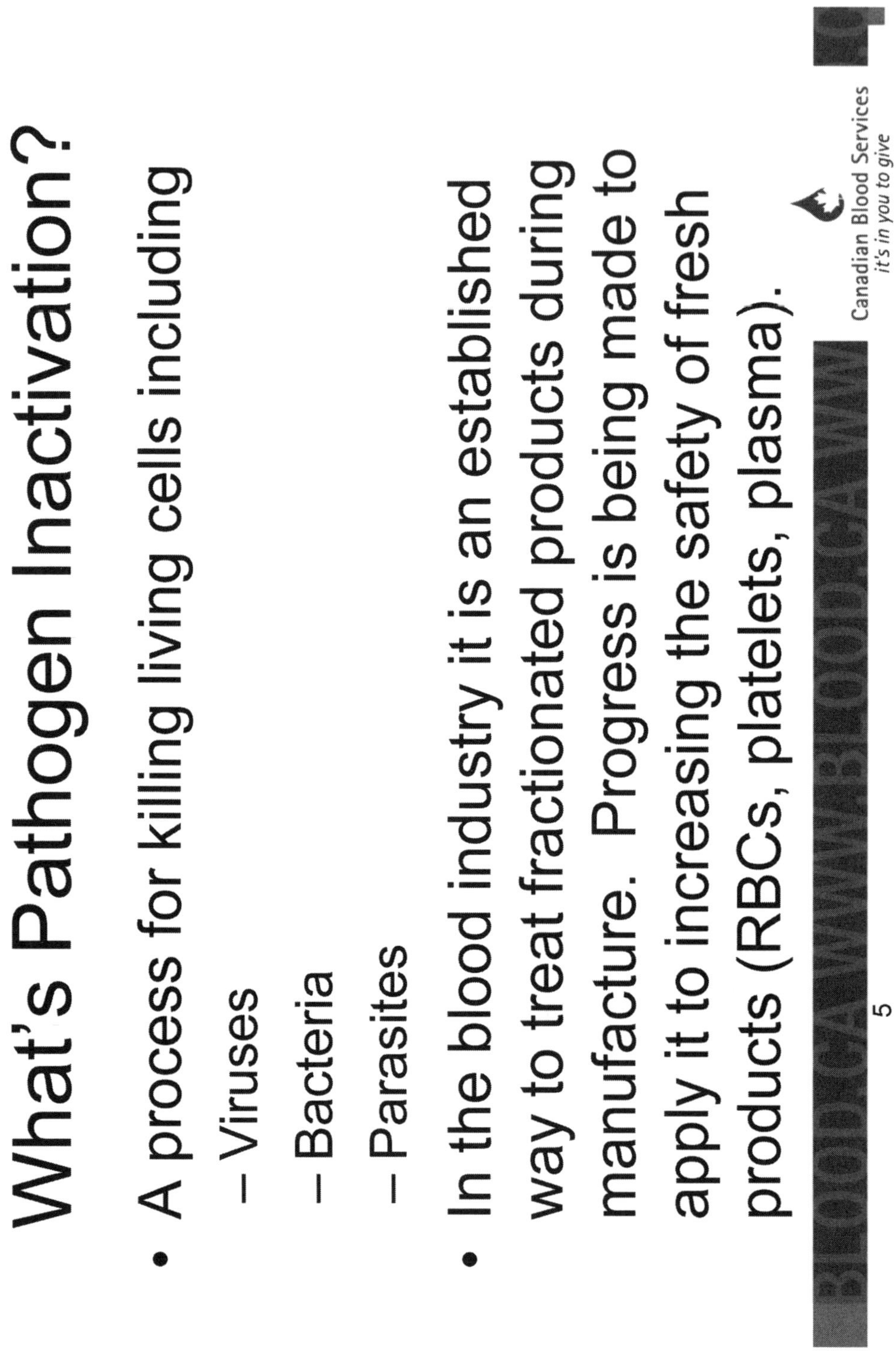
What's Pathogen Inactivation?
• A process for killing living cells including
– Viruses
– Bacteria
– Parasites
• In the blood industry it is an established way to treat fractionated products during manufacture. Progress is being made to apply it to increasing the safety of fresh products (RBCs, platelets, plasma).
Canadian Blood Services
it's in you to give
5

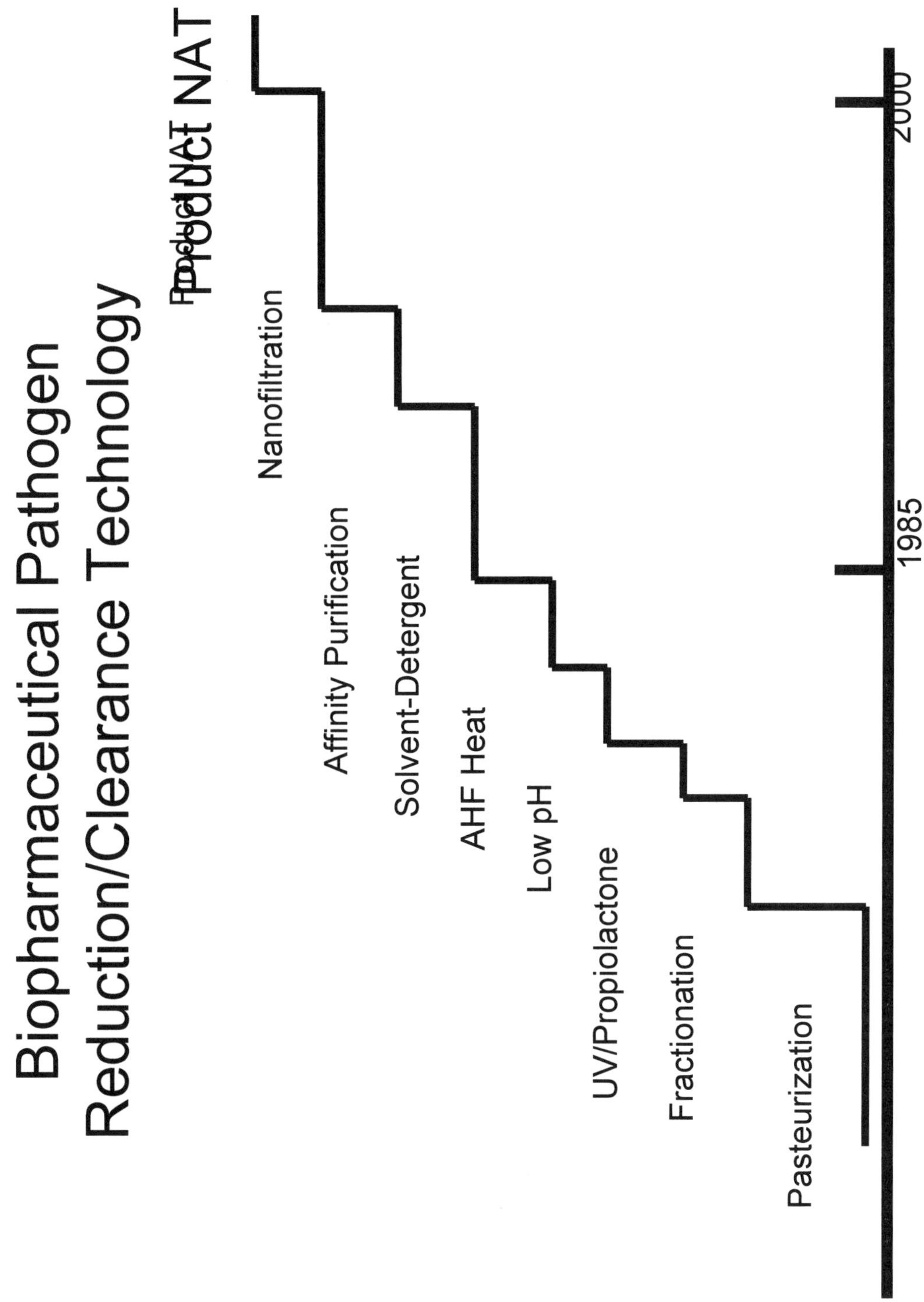
Biopharmaceutical Pathogen
Reduction/Clearance Technology
Pasteurization
Fractionation
UV/Propiolactone
Low pH
AHF Heat
Solvent-Detergent
Affinity Purification
Nanofiltration
Product NAT
1985
2000

Fractionated Plasma Products

These methods are very effective:

No transmission of HIV, HBV, or HCV by a virally inactivated plasma derivative has been documented for two decades.

BLOOD.CA WWW.BLOOD.CA WWW

Canadian Blood Services
it's in you to give

So, How Does It Work?
A Small Biology Review

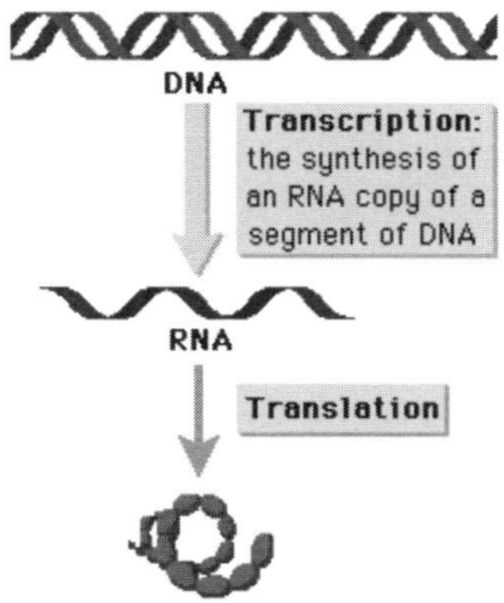

- 'The Central Dogma of Biology'
  - DNA (genes)
  - Transcribed to RNA
  - Translated to protein

BLOOD.CA WWW.BLOOD.CA WWW

8

Canadian Blood Services
it's in you to give

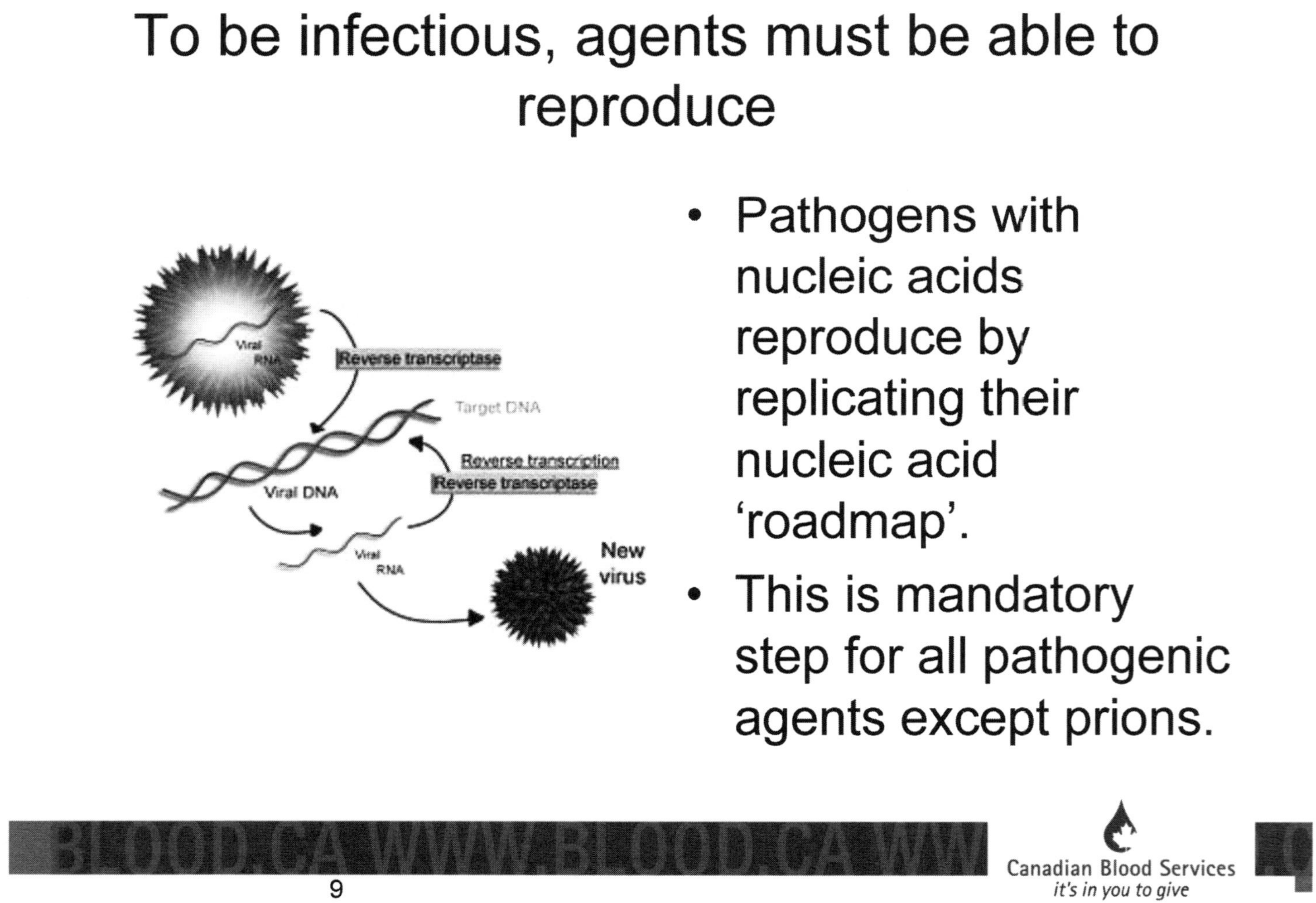
To be infectious, agents must be able to reproduce
Viral RNA
Reverse transcriptase
Target DNA
Reverse transcription
Reverse transcriptase
Viral DNA
Viral RNA
New virus
• Pathogens with nucleic acids reproduce by replicating their nucleic acid 'roadmap'.
• This is mandatory step for all pathogenic agents except prions.
BLOOD.CA WWW.BLOOD.CA WW
9
Canadian Blood Services
it's in you to give

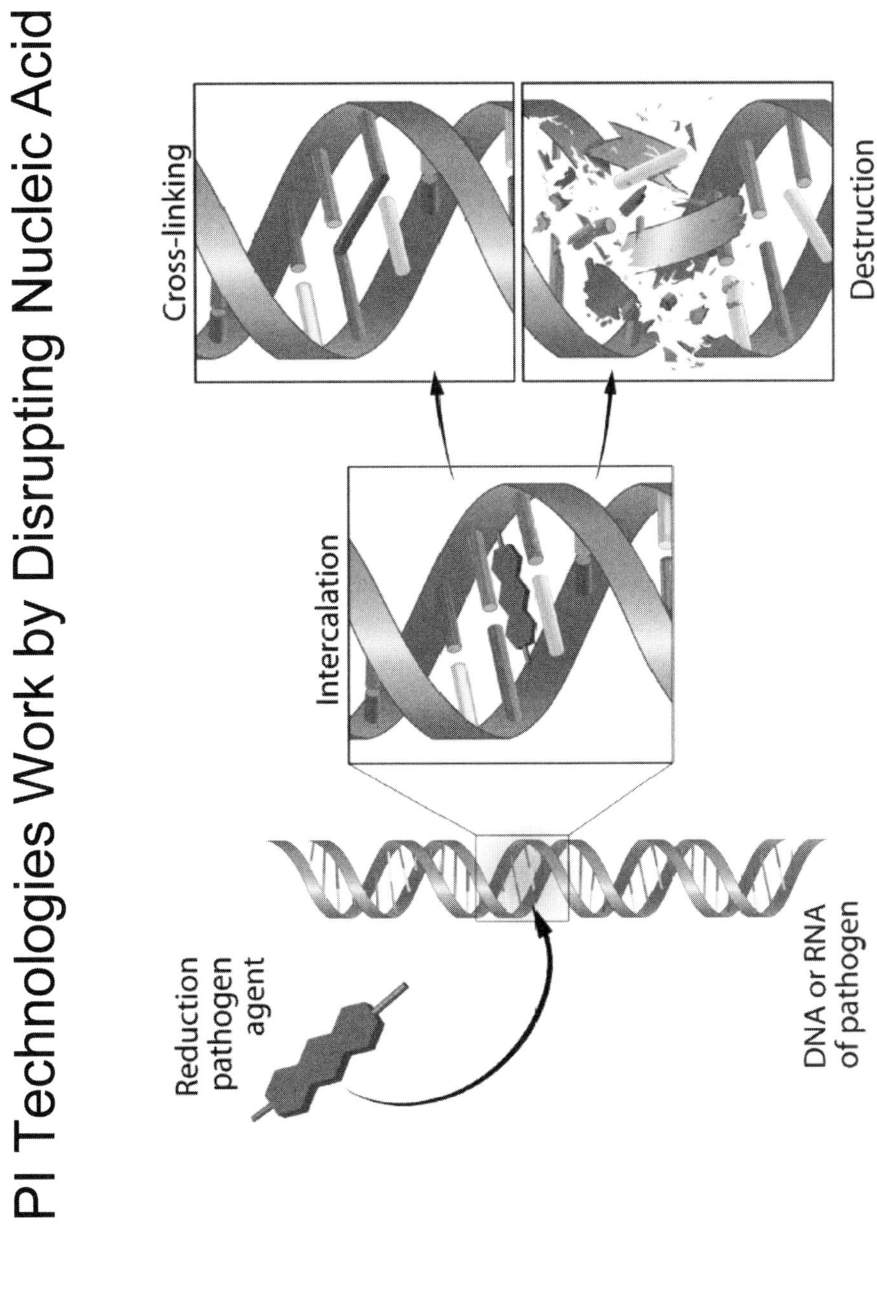
PI Technologies Work by Disrupting Nucleic Acid
Reduction pathogen agent
DNA or RNA of pathogen
Intercalation
Cross-linking
Destruction

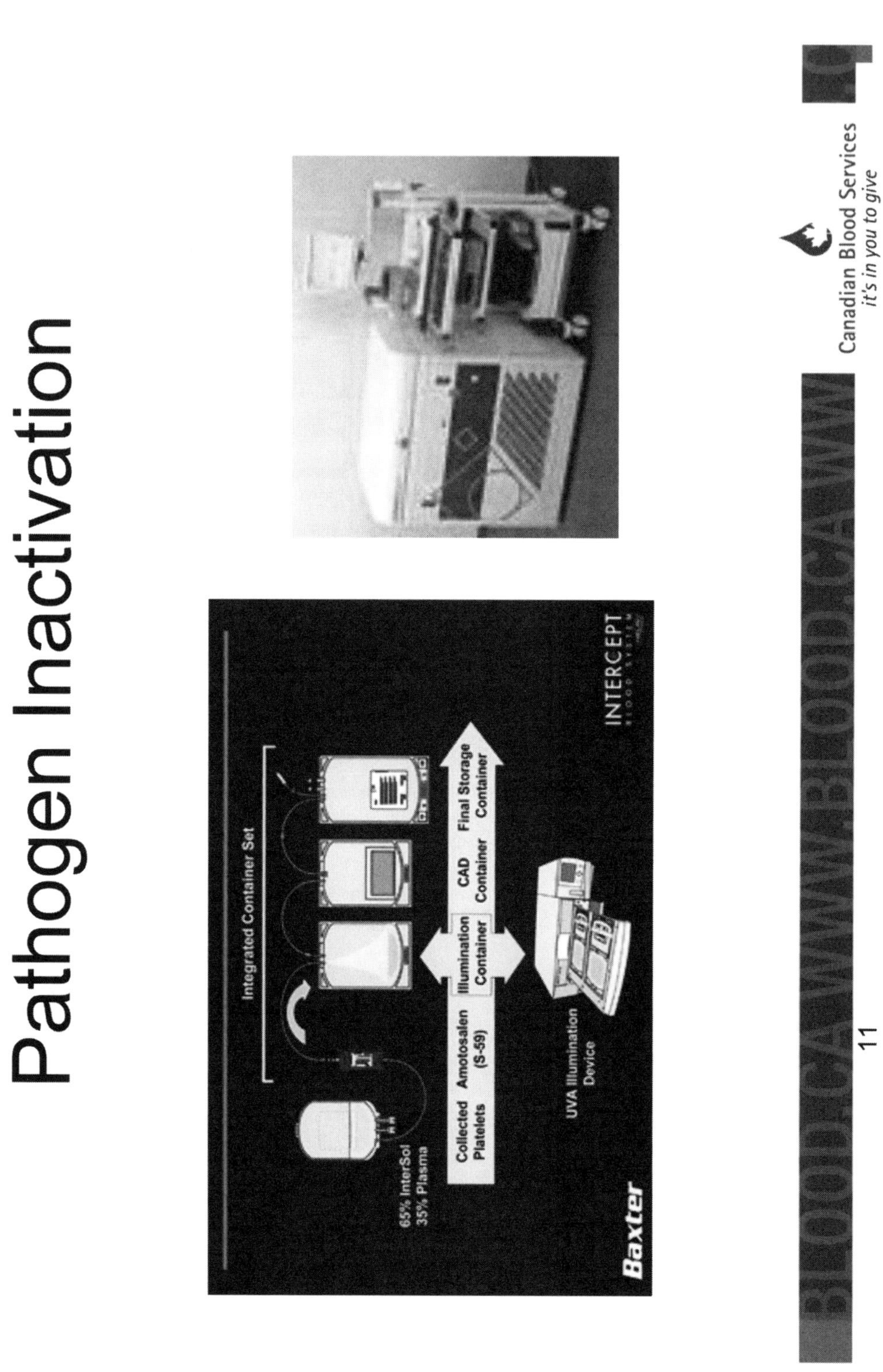
Pathogen Inactivation
Integrated Container Set
65% InterSol
35% Plasma
Collected Platelets
Amotosalen (S-59)
Illumination Container
CAD Container
Final Storage Container
UVA Illumination Device
INTERCEPT
Baxter
Canadian Blood Services
it's in you to give
11

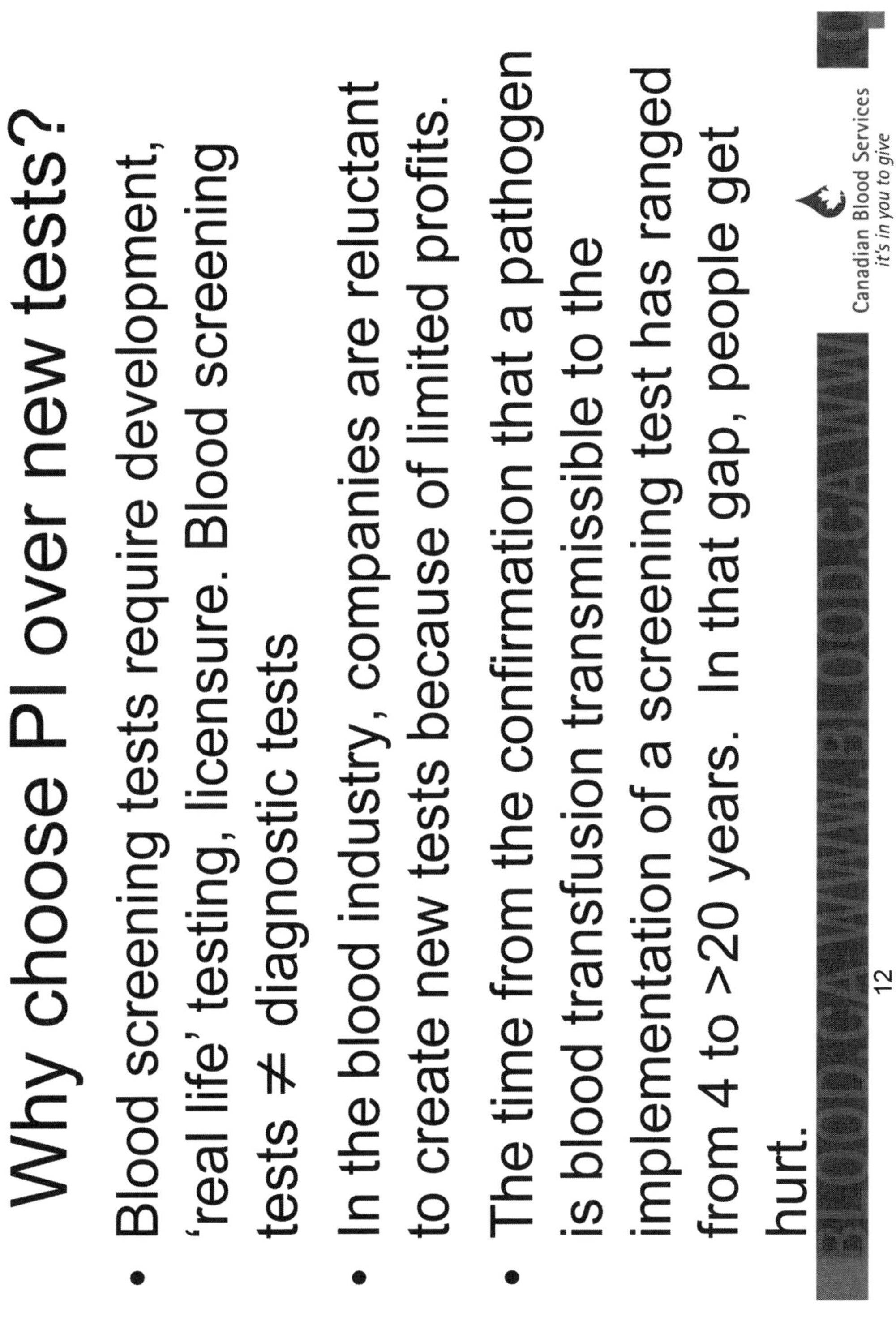
Why choose PI over new tests?
• Blood screening tests require development, 'real life' testing, licensure. Blood screening tests ≠ diagnostic tests
• In the blood industry, companies are reluctant to create new tests because of limited profits.
• The time from the confirmation that a pathogen is blood transfusion transmissible to the implementation of a screening test has ranged from 4 to >20 years. In that gap, people get hurt.
Canadian Blood Services
it's in you to give
12

CBS Actions & Plans for Pathogen Inactivation

- Consensus conference in March 2007 recommended movement to PI when appropriate technologies were available.
- Beginning this past spring the evaluation of PI technologies presently licensed in Europe began in the CBS development lab in Vancouver.
- Discussions with Health Canada on the path to licensure in Canada are scheduled for mid-December.
- To date technologies exist for plasma and platelet inactivation. Our initial target for PI implementation will be apheresis platelets.

WWW.BLOOD.CA WWW.BLOOD.CA WWW

Canadian Blood Services
it's in you to give

OH, CANADA

5

The "Politicks" of Lyme Disease[1]

By Paul Haefling, M.A., LL.B

Chronic ("late stage") Lyme Disease in Canada: "Conflicts" in Diagnosis, Treatment and Research

The Canadian protocols in the form of "guidelines" for diagnosing and treating Lyme disease, particularly late-stage or Chronic Lyme disease, are woefully inadequate and incomplete, and need to be changed immediately to protect people diagnosed with Lyme disease. The official protocol document in Canada is entitled, "The Laboratory diagnosis of Lyme borreliosis: Guidelines from the Canadian Public Health Laboratory Network." It first appeared in December 2006 and was later printed and published in March–April 2007.[2] That document opens with these observations:

> Lyme borreliosis is uncommonly seen in Canada. Most cases have occurred in close proximity to small geographical areas where infected ticks have become established. Although few cases are seen, thousands of patients are tested yearly. Unless patients are carefully selected and an appropriately sensitive and specific testing algorithm is applied, large numbers of patients without Lyme borreliosis will be diagnosed. The Canadian Public Health Laboratory Network has developed the present guidelines to assist physicians in assessing patients for Lyme borreliosis, and to help guide the choice and interpretation of laboratory testing.

Right from the start, that document's aim is to tell doctors: Lyme disease is not widespread, and you should be sceptical when confronted by persons with complaints or symptoms that could indicate or suggest a Lyme bacterial infection. The *Guidelines* go on to describe a few areas in Canada that are considered to have established tick populations (those being considered as "endemic" areas because they are known habitats for the *Ixodes scapularis* tick carrying the Lyme bacterium, *Borrelia burgdorferi*). But, the authors of the *Guidelines* then go on to say:

---

1 The comments and opinions expressed in this document are those of the author, and such views may not be shared by others. Nothing in this Brief is to be read or taken as medical advice. For that, please see and consult your family doctor.

2 *Can J Infect Dis Med Microbiol* Vol 18, No 2, March–April 2007.

> Although it is possible to be bitten by an infected tick anywhere in Canada, the chances of being bitten and subsequently infected are considered low in areas where populations are not established.[3]

Again, the message to doctors is to minimize the potential that they could encounter patients infected with the Lyme disease bacterium by asserting that Lyme disease is not widespread in Canada and that the chances of a patient being bitten are very limited. All that the authors seem to be saying is that, in some populous parts of Canada, the disease-carrying ticks are endemic, and, thus, there is a higher probability of being bitten and possibly becoming infected. In fact, research shows that persons can be infected almost anywhere because migratory birds disperse vector ticks from the U.S. and Central America across Canada, many of which are infected tick species carrying *Borrelia burgdorferi* bacteria, as well as other zoonotic pathogens that can result in co-infections for human hosts who may be bitten.[4] As early as 1991, researchers published the *Borrelia burgdorferi* infection rate for the Long Point area, which is another endemic area in Ontario along the north shore of Lake Erie,[5] but other federally funded studies dealing with established populations of *Ixodes scapularis* ticks (the known most commonly infected species) have not been published. One must ask: Why are infection rates for all other endemic tick areas not being published?

It is primarily through withholding or lack of information that the present state of knowledge about Lyme disease is so inadequate and incomplete. Most importantly, lack of knowledge about Lyme disease, and about chronic or persistent Lyme disease in particular has left hundreds of persons in Canada infected with *Borrelia burgdorferi* to suffer needlessly from a disease that is known to be treatable.

While conceding the reality that people have been and can be bitten and become infected anywhere in Canada, the emphasis in the Canadian *Guidelines* document still rests with the proposition that there is a greater probability or likelihood of being bitten and being infected in human populous areas that are endemic for vector ticks. Unfortunately, one consequence of that restricted viewpoint in the

3 Endemic areas, so-called, for the ticks in Canada are described as being concentrated in British Columbia "on the lower mainland, on Vancouver Island and the Fraser Valley," and in "a small number of localities along the shore of Lake Erie and Lake Ontario," and "near Lunenburg and Bedford in Nova Scotia."

4 See, for example, findings and references in: Morshed *et al.*, "Lyme Disease Spirochete, *Borrelia burgdorferi*, endemic at Epicenter in Rondeau Provincial Park, Ontario," *J. Med. Entomol.* 40 (I) 91–94, January 2003.

5 Lindsay, L.R., *et al.*, "Apparent incompetence of *Dermacentor variabilis* (Acari: Ixodiae) and flea (Insecta: Siphonaptera) as vectors of *Borrelia burgdorferi* in an *Ixodes dammini* [=*I. scapularis*] endemic area of Ontario, Canada," *J. Med. Entomol.* 1991; 28: 750–753.

Guidelines' approach is that numbers of Lyme disease patients report having been told by a doctor that they could not have a Lyme disease infection if they are not living in or have not visited one of the endemic areas listed by the *Guidelines'* authors. The *Guidelines'* point of view about the limited prevalence of ticks and the underlying suggestion that the tick vector for Lyme disease in Canada has some kind of boundaries or geographic limits must, however, be viewed with skepticism when one considers that at least 13 different established populations of *I. Scapularis* have been identified in Canada.[6] The U.S. Centers for Disease Control (CDC) has, since 1997, been reporting recorded and recognized cases of Lyme disease as far north as the State of Alaska, which lies between the 55° and 70° (north) latitudes, the same latitudes shared by Canada's northern territories. The CDC statistics refer to "Alaska Native" cases, and it is not clear how many of those are indigenous cases of individual infections, as opposed to infections acquired through travel.

When the Canadian *Guidelines* state that "Lyme borreliosis is uncommonly seen," or "few cases are seen" or refer to a "low pretest likelihood of Lyme disease," the authors are again suggesting that clinicians have reason to be sceptical about encountering Lyme disease, but such claims are misleading and must not be accepted unquestioningly by clinicians because real-life infectious and other geographic data belie those conclusions.[7] As a statistical matter, the U.S. Centers for Disease Control (CDC) recorded in 2007 and recently reported that there were more than 27,000 Lyme disease cases in the U.S. That organization also estimates that the number of probable occurrences of Lyme bacterial infections in the U.S.A. could be more than ten times the number of reported cases because of the belief that Lyme disease cases there are being missed, by being under-reported and sometimes misdiagnosed.[8] There is no reason to believe that the percentage probabilities or proportional case numbers differ greatly in Canada. As a result, while there were 62 Lyme disease cases reported for Ontario in 2007, the number of actual cases in all of Canada that are missed, through being under-reported or not diagnosed, and, thus, presently not counted, would probably number in many hundreds or into thousands. The municipal region adjacent to where the author lives, in 2008, had

6 See Ogden, N.H. *et al.*: "Role of Migratory Birds in Introduction and Range Expansion of *Ixodes scapularis* ticks and of *Borrelia burgdorferi* and *Anaplasma phagocytophilium* in Canada." Appl. Environ. Microbiol., Vol. 74, 2008.

7 A group of Lyme patients in Ontario who keep in touch via the internet had contact from a person living in or near the James Bay lowlands who had been recently diagnosed as being positive for Lyme disease.

8 See: "Surveillance for Lyme Disease—United States, 1992-2006," in *Morbidity and Mortality Weekly Reports (MMWR)*, October 3, 2008 / 57 (SS10); 1-9.

10 reported and confirmed cases of Lyme disease.[9] Although the data on the number of Lyme disease cases across Canada is collected and required to be reported, federal public health officials have suggested that the available data can be acquired only through individual provinces and territories. Why is information not collected and available nationally? What is there to be kept secret when an issue of public health has arisen?

The Canadian *Guidelines* document also makes reference to distinctions to be made among stages of Lyme disease infections, such as early ("acute"), "disseminated" and finally "late" or "chronic" (although the last word appears once only) stages of Lyme disease. But the typologies and descriptions of symptoms is confusing (or "confused") because various common symptoms and patient complaints can arise at any stage of the disease. The *Guidelines'* distinctions thus are not likely to be immediately of benefit or help to physicians or patients because the latter apparently can and do often present without having any recollection of having been bitten by an infected tick or any sign of the classic symptom: most often described as "a rash." There are in the *Guidelines* some listed possible aggregated symptoms suggested for "late" Lyme disease but the authors do not extensively cover any other late symptoms, which is one of the most serious major flaws in the *Guidelines* and the subject of many complaints made by the Canadian Lyme Disease Foundation ("CanLyme"), an organization (among whose members are Lyme disease patients) which advocates for patients and disseminates information about the disease. There are other studies, too, that suggest low reliability for the Canadian *Guidelines* document, especially concerning the lack of sensitivity. The *Guidelines* document refers (with little emphasis and almost in passing) to the necessity for a clinical assessment in diagnosing Lyme disease, but the *Guidelines* authors also insist adamantly on the use of a confirmatory two-stage serological testing procedure. There, the lack of sensitivity indeed is brought into question.

On February 10, 2009, the Canadian Lyme Disease Foundation ("CanLyme") announced that it had received a private donation of $500,000 from an Ontario family to go towards funding an independent research facility to investigate the prevalence and nature of Lyme disease infection in Canada. In a news release announcing that grant, CanLyme President, Mr. Jim Wilson, on behalf of the Foundation made these observations:

> "This family struggled within the Canadian health care system, as are thousands of Canadians, and were let down by poor testing and a false confidence within the

9 *Waterloo Region Record*, pg B2, Saturday, April 25, 2009, reported: "Last year, 10 Waterloo Region residents had confirmed cases of Lyme disease."

> medical community that Lyme disease is rare in Canada. The medical leadership in Canada, including the federal and provincial governments, are letting us down. Doctors and patients are not told of the serious limitations of the tests used—limitations acknowledged by the global science community."
>
> Lyme disease is a bacterial infection carried by ticks. Ticks are brought into Canada in the hundreds of millions each season on migratory birds and are spread randomly across Canada following migratory bird flyways. You do not need to live in or have visited a known endemic area to become infected as some government agencies and medical organizations suggest.
>
> Inadequate testing, inconsistent reporting criteria, limited surveillance and poor clinical diagnostic knowledge have resulted in less than 50 cases of Lyme disease being reported yearly in Canada. On the other hand, the United States reports over 25,000 cases of Lyme disease annually—mainly in states adjacent to the Canadian border. Due to under-reporting the U.S. Centers for Disease Control estimates that annual cases in the U.S. could actually be 200,000. The European Union confirms in excess of 85,000 cases annually.
>
> Lyme disease, the fastest growing infectious disease in the northern hemisphere, is known as the "Great Imitator." It is a multi-system, multi-organ infection and can cause numerous symptoms including extreme fatigue, arthritis, heart abnormalities, bowel and digestive problems, abnormal skin sensations, muscle weakness or jerking, eyesight or hearing abnormalities, cognitive and memory difficulties, dementia, and in some cases paralysis.
>
> Lyme disease is commonly misdiagnosed as rheumatoid arthritis, Multiple Sclerosis, Lupus, Parkinson's disease, irritable bowel, fibromyalgia, and chronic fatigue. CanLyme says research, including postmortem study, is required utilizing all of today's technology to determine how frequently these other diagnoses are in fact caused by Lyme disease. We know a percentage are in fact Lyme disease, what we don't know is what that percentage is.

The symptoms and conditions described in the CanLyme news release are typical of the experiences reported by many Lyme patients. As was mentioned, when they initially visit the doctor, many are told they could not have Lyme disease if they are not living in an endemic area. Those patients sometimes describe having a general feeling of malaise, lacking specificity, or they also describe experiencing "brain fog," as well as short-term memory loss, including difficulty in remembering and concentrating, as well as flu-like symptoms, dizziness or imbalance, blurred vision, aching or weak muscles and joints, stomach pains or intestinal discomfort, and, often, they say those symptoms occur together or in succession. Some of those are also the kinds of symptoms that are also looked upon clinically as presenting symptoms for chronic fatigue syndrome and fibromyalgia.

The Canadian Public Health Laboratory Network's *Guidelines* document omits such references and does not make any such connections or links for physicians to consider. The *Guidelines* document instead describes categories of symptoms of illness relating to "acute," "disseminated" and "late stage" Lyme disease depending on the timing and severity of infection but such symptoms may occur at any point when a person is infected. In contrast to the research results accessible through the CanLyme organization, the *Guidelines* document suggests that "Lyme borreliosis is uncommonly seen in Canada" and only "in close proximity to small geographical areas where infected ticks have become established." It makes no reference to the possibility that Lyme disease could be missed or misdiagnosed clinically because of shared symptomatologies. Instead, the *Guidelines'* authors suggest that "unless patients are carefully selected and an appropriately sensitive and specific testing algorithm is applied, large numbers of patients without Lyme borreliosis will be incorrectly diagnosed." They, therefore, ignore the U.S. CDC's position that Lyme disease must be clinically diagnosed, and, again, they adamantly insist that any Lyme disease diagnosis must be subject to a two-stage confirmatory serological test. The *Guidelines'* authors purport to offer guidance "to assist physicians in assessing patients for Lyme borreliosis, and to help guide the choice and interpretation of laboratory testing." But, as the CanLyme organization suggests, the Canadian experience using the *Guidelines* as a resource for diagnosing and treating Lyme disease patients, most notably those with Chronic Lyme disease, has been ineffectual and unworthy.

In this Brief, for reasons that follow, the conclusion is reached that the Canadian *Guidelines* must be given a "failed" grade as an aid to diagnosing and treating for both physicians and patients alike. The failure to offer information that is clear and unequivocal or to give adequate and accurate advice to physicians can be seen from the fact that the *Guidelines* fail to note, for example, that co-morbidity can occur, meaning that some patients, who may never have manifested the classic or typical sign of infection, described sometimes also as a "bull's eye rash," and later are diagnosed as positive for *Borrelia burgdorferi,* may also have other, serious co-infections. That is to say, they may test positive with some other secondary bacterial or viral infection.[10] Contrary to existing information and evidence available through

10 See: "other Lyme-like illness" and "coinfections complicate the diagnosis and treatment of Lyme Disease": www.canlyme.com/coinf.html.

CanLyme research links, the *Guidelines'* authors offer this assertion: "A patient with typical findings of multiple sclerosis [MS] or chronic fatigue syndrome [CFS] without objective findings is highly unlikely to have Lyme disease, and both the physician and patient should be dissuaded from serological testing." In fact, CanLyme research sources suggest that such presenting symptoms can give rise to the very situation in which a clinical diagnosis is necessary to determine if Lyme disease may be present, while serological testing could potentially be supportive or used as an adjunct to rule in or rule out the presence of Lyme disease bacteria.

It is also known that some Canadian patients, who originally tested negative, have later been diagnosed as having *Borrelia burgdorferi,* after further and more accurate (usually U.S.) testing was done that showed them to be positive for Lyme disease. At least one Ontario Lyme disease patient[11] is known to have tested "positive" in Canada a number of years ago, based on an initial (ELISA) laboratory test report issued by the Ontario Public Health Laboratory. That report asserted on the same page indicating a "positive" ELISA test: "no evidence of infection." As a result, with no recommended follow-up Western blot test, patient "H" began to receive treatment several years later and only after further, more accurate and effective (U.S.) testing. The one obvious conclusion is that Canadian testing is indeed flawed and inadequate. It is also a fact that the *Guidelines* document offers inaccurate and misleading information in suggesting that persons who present with MS or CFS symptoms, but may not be living in an endemic location, for example, are "unlikely to have Lyme disease" and do not need to be tested serologically. In point of fact, the *Guidelines'* advice and comment on that is exactly the opposite from advice contained in the new clinical definition and guidelines on chronic fatigue syndrome and fibromyalgia (CFS/FM), recently published. The latter guidelines suggest that clinicians who diagnose and treat such cases must first eliminate the possibility that a patient may have Lyme disease.[12] How can that ever be accomplished with any degree of accuracy if our laboratory testing regime in Canada so often generates unreliable results?

Test results from two-tiered serological testing often can be unreliable because *B. burgdorferi* spirochetes and cystic forms (a seemingly dormant form of the bacteria) often can be hidden in body tissues without a patient's showing human immune response from a serological test. The fact that patients can and do test positive, after having been more accurately tested and diagnosed (out-of-country), for

11 Now known as patient "H" (with permission).

12 See references in Alison C. Bested *et al. Hope and Help for Chronic Fatigue Syndrome and Fibromyalgia,* 2d ed.(2008), Cumberland House, Nashville, TN, pp. 12–15.

late-stage or Chronic Lyme disease is itself evidence that methods and procedures used for diagnosing and testing in Canada are inadequate, often wrong and, plainly, in many cases, simply wasteful and ineffectual. But, the real resulting harm is to patients. Such failings mean that patients who later have been found to be suffering from late-stage or Chronic Lyme disease, could have been (but were not) successfully treated earlier. As a result, the inadequate testing regime in Canada likely has caused such persons to suffer longer, with deeper and much more complex and serious and difficult to treat symptoms of late-stage, Chronic Lyme disease.

The Canadian *Guidelines* document, while purporting to offer assistance and help for physicians and patients, contains no mention of the fact that post-mortem studies of some patients who had dementia as a result of Alzheimer's disease were found to be positive in tests (post-mortem tissue studies) showing the presence of Lyme *borreliae*.[13] At least two of those studies had been completed and reported prior to publication of the Canadian Public Health Laboratory Network's *Guidelines* document on Lyme disease. That kind of omission (the silence of the *Guidelines* on the potential link between Alzheimer's disease and Chronic Lyme neuroborreliosis) is damning evidence, to say the least. Such an omission prompts one to ask these questions: On what research and science were the Canadian *Guidelines* based? and How is it that such significant clinical research findings could have been ignored or overlooked? More recently, the Canadian Alzheimer's Society (January, 2009) issued a news release that referenced results of a preliminary study indicating that approximately 500,000 Canadians now are living with Alzheimer's or a related disease, but, even more astonishingly, that report noted that more than 71,000 of those persons are under age 65 and 50,000 of those, under age 60.[14] It does not require a great stretch of imagination to suggest that, statistically, some proportion of those patients may be suffering from symptoms that can be linked to late-stage, Chronic Lyme disease, and that they may be in a febrile state only as a result of never having been properly treated, that is, diagnosed and tested, in Canada to rule in or rule out the presence of Chronic Lyme neuroborreliosis. The *Guidelines'* failure to acknowledge Lyme disease and Alzheimer's links and the dismissive comments denying possible links between Lyme disease and other serious health conditions, such as

13 See: Judith Miklossy et al: "*Borrelia burgdorferi* persists in the brain in Chronic Lyme neuroborreliosis and may be associated with Alzheimer disease": Journal of Alzheimer Disease 6 (2004); 639-649; also see: Alan B. MacDonald, "Dementia caused by *Borrelia* infection of the central nervous system": Columbia University LDA National Scientific Meeting, October 20, 2006; and now see: MacDonald, A.B. "Alzheimer's neuroborreliosis with trans-synaptic spread of infection and neurofibrillary tangles derived from intraneuronal spirochetes": Medical Hypothesis, 2007, 68, 822-825.

14 *Rising Tide: The Impact of Dementia on Canadian Society:* www.alzheimer.ca.

chronic fatigue syndrome (CFS) and MS, for example, in the face of contrary evidence allows one to ask the question: What clinical and diagnostic experience or skills do the *Guidelines'* authors have?

The real problem in this situation lies with the inadequacies of present-day serological testing for chronic or persistent Lyme disease. The *Guidelines'* requirement for a two-stage testing approach (an initial ELISA test, but only if and when there is some "clinical" evidence such as a rash and with a possible time or location for tick exposure, to be followed by a Western blot test but only if the ELISA test shows positive) is apparently copied from an almost identical set of procedures established in the U.S. by the Infectious Diseases Society of America (IDSA) that had also been accepted and recognized as the official diagnostic standard used by the U.S. Centers for Disease Control (CDC). The Canadian *Guidelines'* "Recommendations" concerning the approach to testing show that, in both the U.S. and Canada, the same fallacies concerning diagnosing and treating of Chronic Lyme disease are prevalent: in fact, both appear to deny that Chronic Lyme disease even exists. One group of researchers in the U.S. has gone so far as to suggest that patients who complain of or present with symptoms of "chronic" (also referred to as "late-stage" or "persistent") Lyme disease, after they had been treated for Lyme disease previously with antibiotics, are unlikely to continue to have any *Borrelia burgdorferi* infection. But, that group seems to ignore the fact that the Lyme bacteria can change form and hide its presence. Those researchers suggest, instead, that such patients may suffer from a psychiatric disorder or from what they call "post-Lyme syndrome," which is said to be an "autoimmune disorder." However, post-Lyme syndrome has never been defined. In other words, they seem to suggest that there is no such thing as "chronic" or "persistent" or "late-stage" Lyme disease after initial short-course antibiotic treatment, and that those who complain that they continue to have Chronic Lyme disease and symptoms of Lyme disease instead have post-Lyme Syndrome (which, it seems, they see as some kind of an autogenous disease, or some other autoinfectious novel condition, in which the patient has somehow caused the Lyme disease symptoms to recrudesce, or by some means has reintroduced or replicated the symptoms, but not the Lyme bacterial disease, within themselves). To date, there appears to be no acceptable or credible research evidence to support such a bizarre and far-fetched hypothesis. But, there is laboratory and scientific evidence that Chronic Lyme disease exists and that *Borrelia burgdorferi* bacteria cause that disease.

The Canadian *Guidelines* document, however, does acknowledge that there are deficiencies in the two-stage serological testing procedure, which is one of the recurring complaints made by organizations like the Canadian Lyme Disease Foundation (CanLyme), as well as the International Lyme and Associated Diseases Society (ILADS).[15] The latter is a professional medical society whose members are physicians, researchers and other health care providers, all of whom work in the area of managing and treating Lyme disease. The latter organization also offers medical training and accreditation in the U.S.A., as well as diagnostic and treating guidelines information for physicians and researchers, which includes, for example, reference to possible polymicrobial infections that may be encountered in individuals with Lyme disease. The ILADS organization's guideline also recognizes and offers practice suggestions and treatment recommendations for "persistent" or "chronic" Lyme disease.

The most startling omission in the *Guidelines* (Canada) and in guidelines published in the U.S. by IDSA (the Infectious Diseases Society of America) is the silence about, and absence of any reference to, the use of an IgG or IgM Western blot test for a human immune response to "Osp A" (or "Osp B" or "Osp C") protein ("Osp" means "outer surface protein"). Apparently, it has been known since the 1990s that there are species-specific proteins of the Lyme bacterium and that the outer surface protein from the *Borrelia burgdorferi* spirochete form of the bacteria can, as testing on certain bands shows, yield a specific human antibody immune response, to the degree that the finding of that kind of human immune response in the presence of the bacterial protein can be considered as "a marker" (a confirmatory test) that indicates the presence of the Spirochaetales bacterial infection.[16] The reason for the omission (as it appears) is that the science and knowledge was somehow kept "hidden" from diagnostic consideration... while private bodies involved in two separate commercial projects were attempting to use the knowledge to aid in their development of a vaccine against Lyme disease.[17] That apparently failed because of resulting complications to some patients who received vaccinations and participated in testing. In March of 2002, a domestic vaccine was withdrawn in Canada.

Yet another recent chapter in the history of Lyme disease "conflicts" came to light in May of 2008 following an investigation by the Office of the Attorney General

15 http://www.canlyme.ca/ and http://www.ilads.org.

16 http://www.lymediseaseassociation.org/ "POLITICS"/"Conflicts of Interest": footnote references 21, 22, 23, 53, 54, 73 in *Conflicts of Interest in Lyme Disease: Laboratory Testing, Vaccination, and Treatment Guidelines*, 2001: Lyme Disease Association Inc.

17 See footnote references 66, 67, 74 in *Conflicts of Interest in Lyme Disease, supra.*

for the State of Connecticut, which found that a number of persons who had participated in developing the IDSA (Infectious Diseases Society of America) treating protocols for Lyme disease that are used in the U.S.A. also had connections with interested third parties through ties to the pharmaceutical and insurance industries there.[18] As a result (through a compulsory process), the IDSA has undertaken steps for reviewing and re-writing the U.S. Lyme disease diagnostic and treating protocols, which process is now under way in the U.S.A. and is to be overseen by a neutral referee. Canada, however, continues to hue to the old path in which our public health agencies hold a belief in and reliance upon the earlier impugned guidelines and practice standards that now are, presumably, disgraced in the U.S.A. In view of what transpired in the U.S.A., why is Canada still using a treating and diagnostic approach that was tainted by scandal?

One serious consequence resulting from adherence to the practice standards in the Canadian *Guidelines* document is that medical governing bodies responsible for practice oversight of doctors in at least two provinces[19] also continue to hold allegiance to the same sets of limited and questionable practice standards. The B.C. and Ontario colleges have investigated physician members who dared to treat Chronic Lyme disease patients in accordance with ILADS practice standards or known best practices that have been used and adopted in the U.S.A. and some E-U countries. In Ontario, a number of patient files were seized in October of 2008 after investigators from the Ontario College made entry to a physician's office. One of the files taken was the confidential file of patient "H." A number of patients were in the doctor's office at the time of the raid by the Ontario College, and, since then, many of those patients have banded together to form a support group, calling themselves the "Lyme Action Group."[20] They identify their purpose as being to raise funds to support a defence for the physician and also to lobby governments and spread information publicly about Lyme disease in Canada. One other result of that raid on the doctor's office is that the Ontario College of Physicians and Surgeons has had possession of patient "H's" file, including results of the initial Canadian ELISA test for Lyme disease: reported "positive," but with a comment of "no evidence of infection." Thus, the Ontario College now has before it clear evidence showing the kind

18 **http://www.ct.gov/AG/cwp/view.asp**: "Attorney General's Investigation Reveals Flawed Lyme Disease Guideline Process, IDSA Agrees to Reassess Guidelines, Install Independent Arbiter." (May 1, 2008).

19 The British Columbia College of Physicians and Surgeons and the College of Physicians and Surgeons of Ontario, in particular.

20 **Lymeactiongroup.blogspot.com**

of slipshod laboratory testing that can occur in Canada, as certainly was apparent in that case. All indicators now are pointing to the fact that public health and medical governing bodies in Canada have begun taking sides in what is obviously an area of professional disagreement ("conflict") over Lyme disease treatment and diagnostic approaches. But, in so doing, those public bodies may be creating risk and jeopardizing the health and well-being of patients living with chronic or late-stage Lyme disease, rather than (as the governing statutes require) assisting physicians in attempting to return those patients to a state of better health. Such actions by government bodies, including the publication of the inapt Canadian *Guidelines*, obviously have the effect of inhibiting and interfering with the ability of physicians and clinicians to undertake and fulfill their professional responsibilities to their Lyme disease patients. This situation is untenable and unacceptable. It is most emphatically not a situation where an exercise of statutory powers can or should be permitted to run wild, with no apparent accountability, and, ultimately, with detriment to patients.

Added to the finding that "undisclosed financial interests" warranted "a reassessment of IDSA guidelines," the report of the investigation completed in May of 2008 by the State of Connecticut Attorney General's Office also made the following additional findings:[21]

- The IDSA's 2000 and 2006 Lyme disease panels refused to accept or meaningfully consider information regarding the existence of Chronic Lyme disease, once removing a panelist from the 2000 panel who dissented from the group's position on Chronic Lyme disease to achieve "consensus";
- The IDSA blocked appointment of scientists and physicians with divergent views on Chronic Lyme who sought to serve on the 2006 guidelines panel by informing them that the panel was fully staffed, even though it was later expanded.

In Canada, there have been repeated complaints through the Canadian Lyme Disease Foundation, as well as through the Ontario Lyme Disease Association of a similar nature, to the effect that dissenting voices and alternative research findings about Lyme disease are being stifled and ignored by public health officials. Such complaints followed from a conference held by the Public Health Agency of Canada (PHAC) in March of 2006 at which Canada's public health officials, laboratory personnel and a smaller number of "CanLyme" representatives attended, including

21 See footnote 18 *supra*.

experts from the U.S. brought in by the latter. Not surprisingly, while that meeting was intended initially to lead to agreement among those groups on a whole range of laboratory, clinical and surveillance guidelines pertaining to Lyme disease in Canada, no consensus emerged. Although a resolution was passed and an understanding reached that committees were to be struck to follow up and create a set of "made in Canada guidelines," nothing like that happened. Instead, what happened shortly after was that the Canadian *Guidelines* as they now exist were produced and published unilaterally by the Canadian Public Health Laboratory Network. Forgetting the cynicism that provoked, their action undermines the credibility of public health officials in the eyes of the wider community concerned about Lyme disease. That is, the *Guidelines* now used in Canada came to be published without any formal or direct input from CanLyme, which offers alternate views and which represents patients, researchers and medical practitioners and others whose interest is to work for the betterment of Canadians suffering with Lyme disease. That situation must now be corrected.

As an example of what went seriously wrong at that point, CanLyme had been pressing for recognition of Chronic Lyme disease as an emergent serious public health problem, and Canlyme also urged abandoning the necessity for the initial (most often inaccurate) ELISA screening test in favour of a more comprehensive and sensitive form of Western blot test (referenced earlier) to be used to measure human immune response to *Borrelia burgdorferi.* Such testing would require and mandate inclusion of the specific test bands used to detect a human immune response to Osp A and the other proteins specific to Lyme disease. CanLyme's President, Mr. Jim Wilson, continues to question why there has been so little research on Lyme disease when nearly one billion dollars has been paid by Canadians through taxes, money that has been used up and invested elsewhere, which was the amount paid out in 2005–2006 by our federal government through the Canadian Institutes of Health Research. In the absence of effective and timely federal actions, CanLyme recently created its own research organization to focus on independent, evidence-based research into Lyme disease.

One serious concern that arises, given the "conflicts" experience in the U.S., is whether or not Canada should continue its present approach to health research funding since that often channels government spending into private, for-profit activities and ultimately into corporate hands (that being the locus of all of the problems uncovered by the A-G for the State of Connecticut.). Given the nature of Canada's system of public health care through non-profit insurance, surely it is more logical and reasonable to argue that the public health system in Canada and, thus, the

Canadian government, should itself directly undertake and support and oversee research into Lyme disease as a major public health issue. New research should lead to licensing arrangements to permit re-capture of some public research spending, rather than simply having our federal government giving up or handing over proprietary rights that may come from such research and the public expenditures on health research. New and better avenues of Lyme disease research must be undertaken in the interests both of Canadians now diagnosed with Lyme disease and of countless others who may, unsuspectingly, have acquired the disease but (given our failed testing protocols) have no confirmation of that. We are at this moment truly at a crossroads in Canada in regard to research on Lyme disease.

The 2007 Canadian *Guidelines* are being surpassed and overtaken by other developments that could simplify or lead to better results in serological testing for Lyme disease. In 2006, as an example, the U.S. Food and Drug Administration approved a new test[22] that enables veterinarians to screen dogs for several tick-borne diseases, including Lyme disease, through a simple blood test that also simultaneously screens for heartworm and, in addition to Lyme disease, can uncover canine forms of anaplasmosis and ehrlichiosis. Surely, one must ask: Why is not the same type of testing and measurement technology capable of being adapted and put to use for human testing? On February 23, 2009, as another example, the *Journal of Clinical Pathology* first published an on-line report concerning a Scottish research project that resulted in increasing the sensitivity of testing for Lyme disease through the use of a "single mixed antigen" for IgG Western blot testing, which improved the predictive value of that test.[23] Such information holds out hope and promise for the initial diagnosing of Lyme disease and for tracking long-term sufferers from Chronic Lyme disease because it apparently improves accuracy in testing for both sero-positivity and sero-negativity.

What has been written thus far in this Brief makes it appear that the status quo (the doctor "do-little" and "do nothing") current approach to Lyme disease diagnosis, treatment and research is ineffectual. Those activities that have been undertaken through research agencies that report to the Public Health Agency of Canada to date achieved very little. Through the development, publication and dissemination of the Canadian *Guidelines,* physicians have not been assisted but rather (because their professional governing bodies have relied on that document) they are being inhibited in regard to vigorously and actively treating Lyme disease patients without fear of being investigated and prosecuted for doing so. One other major

22 See report: http://www.dogflu.ca/03012007/15/new_tick_test_available_for_dogs.

23 See: http://dx.doi.org/10.1136/jcp.2008.063461.

problem in Canada is that no single, comprehensive, accurate and up-to-date source of information exists, such as a clearing house for physicians, to which they and others can turn for accurate, current and complete practice information or reports of research. If, as the *Guidelines* purported, the intention was to provide information and content to be used by physicians and relied upon for clinical diagnostic and treatment purposes, such content and information must surely be in the form of a document that is accurate, comprehensive, evidence-based and reliable. But, as the foregoing critique suggests, the Canadian *Guidelines* document deserves a failing grade because it is little more than a political and polemical piece designed to support a particular point of view that is apparently intended to downplay the prevalence and risks of Lyme disease in Canada, and, as well, its effect has been to sow seeds of doubt and confusion. If our Canadian public health officials are intent upon and serious about offering support and guidance, they must be compelled to act and be allowed to fulfill their duties and responsibilities to produce and deliver what is now needed in Canada if only because the issue of potential risk of harm to patients with Lyme disease (those diagnosed and persons yet undiagnosed) is grave and serious. Rather than allowing for any open-ended debate or professional dialogue, the normative, or prescriptive and mandatory, approach the *Guidelines* process to date has taken, instead of assisting physicians, really acts as an unnecessary impediment, and, indeed, it threatens physician-patient relationships by withholding access to and even ignoring results from recent reliable research and evidence that could assist doctors. In Canada, the genie is now out of the bottle, and there is a growing awareness and concern about the spread and prevalence of Lyme disease among members of the Canadian public.[24] If our public health institutions honestly and genuinely mean to fulfill the statutory duties and responsibilities with which they are charged, and if there is to be any reasonable hope of either arresting or coping with the spread of Chronic Lyme disease in Canada, those agencies must reform their practices and undertake a true leadership role and provide guidance for Canadian professionals and the public, as well as undertaking research and the delivery of the full array of health services that are needed by Lyme disease patients.

Canadian Health Care Structures and Organizations Need Reform

Canada's health care system involves both the federal and provincial levels of government, but the Lyme disease *Guidelines* process described earlier, that is, the

24 In part, that can be attributed to numerous screenings across Canada of the award-winning film documentary entitled, *Under our Skin.*

process of preparing and disseminating information about Lyme disease, in this instance, originated with the Federal Government at Ottawa. Such an activity eventually reaches the hands of provincial health authorities, as well as doctors, nurses, and other hospital-care personnel who work in each province. There is a complex legislative framework and, at the federal government level, everything begins with and follows from what our federal Parliament has determined in different statutes to be the fundamental principles and governing framework for the Canadian system of public health care. The system in Canada, as most people know and understand, is entirely different and distinct from the manner in which health services are organized and structured in the U.S.A. where the system is essentially based on the provision of private and, most often, "for profit" health care services. To understand the differing principles that operate here in Canada and to understand how distinctive our publicly funded health care system is from that in the U.S.A., it is worthwhile to begin by looking at the *Canada Health Act* ("the Act").[25]

The governing principles stated as the legislated aims and objectives of the Canadian health care system are outlined in a long preamble to the *Canada Health Act,* and it refers specifically to some of the guiding principles and objectives that Parliament has recognized, among which are the following:

- that Canadians can achieve further improvements in their well-being through combining individual lifestyles that emphasize fitness, prevention of disease and health promotion with collective action against the social, environmental and occupational causes of disease, and that they desire a system of health services that will promote physical and mental health and protection against disease;
- that future improvements in health will require the cooperative partnership of governments, health professionals, voluntary organizations and individual Canadians;
- that continued access to quality health care without financial or other barriers will be critical to maintaining and improving the health and well-being of Canadians… .

The fundamental underpinning for achieving those public health initiatives and objectives is our fiscal system involving federal-provincial transfer arrangements for funding our public health care facilities and services as those are laid out in that statute. The *Canada Health Act's* "program criteria" are stated as principles to be

25 R.S. C.1985, c. C-6, as amended.

adhered to as part of the fiscal transfer arrangements, and those, too, are intended to guide the administration and the operation of our provincial insured health care systems on the basis of not-for-profit and public administration. Those criteria declare that the Canadian health care system that operates in each province must follow the principles of "comprehensiveness," "universality," "portability" and "accessibility," as those characteristics are defined in the *Act*.[26] The *Canada Health Act* also clearly identifies and specifies as the principal goals of the Canadian health care system these objects:

> 3. It is hereby declared that the primary objective of Canadian health care is *to protect, promote and restore the physical and mental well-being of residents of Canada and to facilitate reasonable access to health services without financial or other barriers.* (Emphasis added.)

Those goals describe what are the objective, program or task-oriented actions and outcomes that are to be undertaken and achieved. That is, the *Act's* objective is not just philosophical or idealistic but is directed to creating services and structures capable of achieving practical, program- or action-oriented results through systemic measures that foster and support those objectives. Those are, in summary, the bedrock principles that underlie measures to be taken to implement the objects and intentions of our Canadian Parliament.

One can say that any activities or undertakings that foster those goals are desirable and consistent with the principles of the *Canada Health Act,* which would be a good thing, but that any activities that run counter to, or serve to undermine, hinder or thwart the achievement of those objectives would lead to bad outcomes which, at all times, should and must be discouraged and avoided as leading to unacceptable and unworthy results. The words Parliament chose to use in s.3 to describe the objects of our Canadian health care system are mandatory and also serve as directives that must be read as being the underpinnings for other agencies or institutions and the programs and activities that are undertaken by those bodies to serve the purposes and objects of the *Canada Health Act.* The *Canada Health Act* also defines in s.2 what are "insured health services," meaning "hospital services," which are defined to include both in-patient and out-patient "services that are medically necessary for the purpose of maintaining health, preventing disease or diagnosing or treating an injury, illness or disability." Among such services are listed

26 R.S. C.1985, c. C-6: S 8, 9, 10, 11, 12.

"laboratory, radiological and other diagnostic procedures, together with the necessary interpretations." The *Act* also defines "physician services" to mean "any medically required services rendered by medical practitioners." The *Canada Health Act* also names "the Minister of Health" as the person ultimately in charge of and responsible for the operation and administration of the Canadian health care system and, thus, the *Act* charges the Minister of Health with the oversight of all of the *Canada Health Act's* provisions and other related legislation passed by Parliament.

A separate statute, the *Department of Health Act, 1996* also specifically and more particularly defines various "Powers, Duties and Functions of the Health Minister," among which are the following:[27]

> 4(1) The powers, duties and functions of the Minister extend to and include all matters over which Parliament has jurisdiction relating to the promotion and preservation of the health of the people of Canada not by law assigned to any other department, board or agency of the Government of Canada.
>
> (2) Without restricting the generality of subsection (1), the Minister's powers, duties and functions relating to health include the following matters:
>
> ....
>
> (a. 1) the promotion and preservation of the physical, mental and social well being of the people of Canada;
>
> (b) the protection of the people of Canada against risks to health and the spreading of diseases;
>
> (c) investigation and research into public health, including the monitoring of diseases;
>
> ....
>
> (h) subject to the *Statistics Act,* the collection, analysis, interpretation, publication and distribution of information relating to public health; and
> (i) cooperation with provincial authorities with a view to the coordination of efforts made or proposed for preserving and improving public health.

The responsibility last-listed clearly is to be seen as intended to encourage and permit federal-provincial collaboration in programs aimed at addressing emergent public health issues, which would include issues such as the spread of Lyme disease

27 C.8, s.4.

in Canada. In that regard, the *Department of Health Act* also specifically states, in s. 4.1., that "the Minister shall coordinate the activities of, and establish strategic priorities for, any board or agency for which the Minister is responsible," and it states, as well, that "those powers, duties and functions" may (subject to the Minister's terms and conditions) be delegated to the Deputy Minister of Health. In other words, that *Act* indicates that the duties of the Minister and Deputy Minister encompass and include oversight of all activities of the Health Department, which, presumably, must include the federal government's obligation to acknowledge and respond to emergent issues, such as to address the expanding scope of and managing of acute and chronic disease in Canada and the need for developing adequate and effective diagnostic and treatment protocols to undertake measures necessary to address any situation that creates a health risk for Canadians.

Similar duties and responsibilities are acknowledged and identified in the *Public Health Agency of Canada Act, 2006.*[28] The responsibility for and the administration of that *Act* (in s.4) is also invested with the Minister of Health:

> 4. The Minister presides over the Agency and has the management and direction of it.

Save for "the power to make regulations," the Minister may delegate other functions, "subject to any terms and conditions that the Minister specifies" (s.5). The "Chief Public Health Officer" is designated in the *Act* as the deputy head of the Agency, and the person so appointed must be "a health professional" who has qualifications in the field of public health.

In the preamble of the *Public Health Agency of Canada Act, 2006,* Parliament specifies clearly that the Canadian Public Health Agency is intended to function as a "hands on," actively participating body in the fulfilment of all measures and programs to be undertaken by the federal government in the public health field. For example, the program purposes and objectives specified in the preamble to the *Public Health Agency Act* are stated in the following terms:

> … the Government of Canada wishes to take public health measures, including measures relating to health protection and promotion, population health assessment, health surveillance, disease and injury prevention, and public health emergency preparedness and response;

28 S.C., c.5

> … the Government of Canada wishes to foster collaboration within the field of public health and to coordinate federal policies and programs in the area of public health;
>
> … the Government of Canada wishes to promote cooperation and consultation in the field of public health with provincial and territorial governments;
>
> … the Government of Canada also wishes to foster cooperation in that field with foreign governments and international organizations, as well as other interested persons or organizations;
>
> … the Government of Canada considers that the creation of a public health agency for Canada and the appointment of a Chief Public Health Officer will contribute to federal efforts to identify and reduce public health risk factors and to support national readiness for public health threats.

Sadly, as this Brief concludes, not all of those objects have been or are being served in respect of the growing prevalence of Lyme disease, and, particularly, its spread among growing numbers of patients living with Chronic Lyme disease in Canada. The further sad fact is that Chronic Lyme disease was, at one time, never even recognized, but, now, is probably being under-recognized. The *Guidelines* for Lyme disease in Canada were expediently borrowed and copied from the U.S. But, the U.S. standards have been found to be corrupt, that is, flawed and tainted by third-party influences. Also, by covertly appropriating a known, identifiable bacterial protein assay capable of eliciting a human immune response, the same flawed U.S. guidelines process, which Canada adopted, hid a reliable diagnostic model and bacterial identification test. All of the same deficiencies cast doubt on the credibility and reliability of Canada's *Guidelines.* The effect is that, in both Canada and the U.S., there is currently no universally accepted, credible and reliable protocol on which patients or their physicians can rely as a basis for properly diagnosing and treating Lyme disease. In the three-year period since the establishment of the Canadian Public Health Agency, it seems that very little else has been done or achieved that can count as a success in regard to diagnosing and treating Lyme disease, and in particular, Chronic Lyme disease, or in meeting Parliament's stated objectives in the field of public health care in relation to that disease.

The final piece of relevant legislation is the *Canadian Institutes of Health Research Act, 2000,*[29] which statute establishes the model and approach for medical

---

29 S.C. 2000, c.6

research undertakings for Canada (previously under the auspices of the Medical Research Council). The present *Act* allows for the creation of new research institutes to be set up through a corporation whose president is appointed by the Governor-in-Council. The research functions are farmed out and funded through a 20-member "governing council." The *Act* also allows for inter- and intra-corporate research undertakings, each with separate advisory boards, whose members and their staffs may be paid through the public purse. That *Act* specifies that research activities should be undertaken with "a transparent approach" so as to "facilitate accountability to Canadians" and must take "ethical issues" into consideration. The statute's aims, as stated in the preamble, are for "the creation of new scientific knowledge based on research that meets the highest international standards of excellence" and "the development and implementation of innovative policy and practice." The "objectives" stated in s.4 of the *Act* suggest that the research to be undertaken will pertain to all aspects of health and "include bio-medical research, clinical research ... environmental influences on health, and other research as required." All of that effort is to be directed to "addressing emerging health opportunities, threats and challenges and accelerating the discovery of cures and treatments and improvements to health care, prevention and wellness strategies."

Aside from the very thorough recent vector surveillance field studies and research analyses undertaken with cooperation by the Public Health Agency, the Canadian Wildlife Centre, participating zoonotic diseases agencies and university biology and entomology research departments,[30] no other kind of public research activity has to date offered hope or measures that would hold out possible relief and treatment success for Canadians suffering with Lyme disease. In spite of what may appear as necessary major reforms in health research services and activities in Canada, and what was promised at the time, the spread of Lyme disease, with each passing year, is emerging as a major threat to public health in this country, as well as in the U.S., Europe and Asia. But, Lyme disease, it seems, is not yet seriously "on the radar" for our institutional research bodies in Canada. Where is there any posting of Lyme disease research being undertaken, or of any articles or research abstracts to give up-to-date information and reporting about diagnosing and treating Lyme disease that would indicate that diagnosing and treating and halting the spread of that disease

30 See, for instance: Ogden, N.H. et al. "*Ixodes scapularis* Ticks Collected by Passive Surveillance in Canada: Analysis of Geographic Distribution and Infection with Lyme Borreliosis Agent *Borrelia burgdorferi* in *J. Med. Entomol.* 43(3) 600-609 (2006); and see: Ogden, N.H. *et al.* "Role of Migratory Birds in Introduction and Range Expansion of *Ixodes scapularis* Ticks and of *Borrelia burgdorferi* and *Anaplasma phagocytophiliu m* in Canada" in Applied and Environmental Microbiology, Mar. 2008. p. 1780-1790.

is going to receive the attention it needs in Canada? The Public Health Agency's activities in the case of Lyme disease treatment seem to extend no further than having issued and published the Canadian Lyme disease *Guidelines*. But, those, like the U.S. diagnostic and treating protocols, are disgraced and have had little or no positive impact for Lyme patients. Also, it is clear that the *Guidelines* document downplays and discounts the seriousness of the spreading in Canada of the Lyme bacterium, contrary to the approach that is needed today. Those *Guidelines,* if only because they aped the disgraced U.S. standards, need to be discarded and be replaced immediately.

Now is the right time for action and attention by the Minister of Health. The need for measures to arrest the threat to public health from the spread of Lyme disease is growing. We know the Public Health Agency convened a meeting in March of 2006, at which CanLyme experts and representatives were also present, for the purpose of establishing criteria to be used for a made-in-Canada diagnostic and treatment protocol for Lyme disease. That, it appears, was the specific mandate given to public health officials prior to that meeting. The March, 2006, conference did not result in agreement on either diagnostic criteria or treatment modes. From a set of notes subsequently made public by PHAC attendees, it seems there was to have been a continuing dialogue, through committees, on the establishment of criteria for diagnosing and treating Lyme disease. But, the Public Health Agency's post-conference notes appear to indicate that there was agreement at the March, 2006, meeting only about the need for continuing surveillance of Lyme disease. It seems that was then taken up by the authors of the *Guidelines* document to mean that surveillance information and studies on tick habitats and their prevalence in Canada was to be given emphasis. Sadly, in the absence of agreement on the real areas of need, including developing practice information that physicians could rely on for diagnostic and treatment purposes, the authors simply adopted the flawed IDSA/CDC guidelines criteria developed and now disgraced in the U.S.A. The Canadian version was issued without any hesitation or any further consultation with organizations such as CanLyme. The consequences have been that patients and physicians still do not have any appropriate needed guidance relating to diagnosing and treating Lyme disease. For reasons difficult to understand, responsible public health officials have remained silent on those matters ever since. It is plain and obvious from all of the preceding that the Minister of Health and representatives of the Public Health Agency of Canada owe an explanation to Canadians as to what went wrong, and, especially, to those persons who may be suffering silently and needlessly with Lyme disease symptoms but without receiving treatment, including persons suffering today who may be undiagnosed largely as a result of the fact that the *Guidelines* document has downplayed the scope and significance of Lyme disease in Canada. Those Canadians, too, are owed an explanation, and they need to see action taken. In this Brief, the writer is seeking and asking for an undertaking from the Minister of Health that this situation of neglect through inaction can and will be remedied immediately and will never be repeated. What can be done? How can that be assured?

The Minister of Health should assume responsibility, first, to intervene and investigate to discover why it has taken so long in Canada to advance the cause of properly diagnosing and treating Lyme disease in all of its manifestations. Senior Health Department officials should then be directed to re-open and re-establish communications with professional research bodies and representatives of the Canadian Lyme Disease Foundation (CanLyme) with the intention and objective of empanelling a new committee, to include representatives from patient-related groups like CanLyme, and other interested and knowledgeable professionals and individuals for the purpose of establishing a new set of "made in Canada" practice standards and criteria for diagnosing and treating Lyme disease, through investigation into all the known and possible manifestations of Lyme disease. The Minister must, as well, begin by adopting and directing attention to treatment and diagnostic methods known to be effective and worthy of promotion through scientific, evidence-based research that is reported as being underway in Canada, the U.S. and E-U countries. As one example, the Minister of Health, through the public health laboratory and other reporting agencies, should immediately order adoption of Western blot testing that uses and relies on the IgG/IgM bands specific to "Osp A." Without sounding unduly alarmist, physicians, the provincial colleges and other medical and nursing associations should be alerted to the potential that Lyme disease in Canada is likely far more prevalent than earlier indications have suggested, and, simultaneously, those groups should be informed about newer, better and more accurate diagnostic and treatment procedures to be introduced as soon as possible. As well, high-level representatives designated by the Minister of Health should immediately undertake to consult and collaborate with representatives of provincial health ministries to undertake appropriate professional information programs and options to introduce programs to train, as quickly as possible, every physician who wishes to learn about known best-practice approaches and techniques for diagnosing and treating Lyme disease, including exposure to teaching methods offered through ILADS and by affording them opportunities for accreditation. The current small number of "Lyme literate doctors" (LLDs) practising in Canada are the persons most likely to have access to, and to have with them to bring, the most up-to-date knowledge and experience. Those LLDs should be asked or recruited to undertake to write curricula for such programs of training for Canada. Rather than seeking to harass and prosecute our Lyme-literate doctors, the provincial colleges should look to those physicians as the key resource personnel for the interim. But, that is not all, since those steps alone may not be enough to bring about all needed and immediate changes. The Minister of Health must, finally, undertake also to retain personal oversight or create a specialist national oversight body for managing research on all of the public health issues surrounding the emergence of Lyme disease in Canada.

The Role of Canada's Attorney General

The federal response also needs to address and recognize numerous medico-legal issues that arise as a result of the sorry history of managing Chronic Lyme disease in Canada up to this point.

The Minister of Justice is also Canada's Attorney General, pursuant to the *Department of Justice Act, R.S.,* c. J-2 ("the *Act*"). The Minister is also "the legal member of the Queen's Privy Council for Canada" and, as such, is empowered to "see that the administration of public affairs is in accordance with the law," and the Minister also is vested with authority to exercise "the superintendence of all matters connected with the administration of justice in Canada, not within the jurisdiction of the governments of the provinces."[31] In cases where there are or may be legal issues pertaining to any other government departments, the *Act* says the Attorney General of Canada "shall advise the heads of the several departments of the Government on all matters of law connected with such departments." In addition, the Attorney General is empowered in subsection 5(d) to undertake "the regulation and conduct of all litigation for or against the Crown or any department, in respect of any subject within the authority or jurisdiction of Canada." The conflicts that have already been mentioned concerning the Canadian experience with the *Guidelines* and its problems in relation to diagnosing and treating Lyme disease outlined earlier undoubtedly disclose a variety of legal issues, some of which are subtle and some others that are obvious and potentially litigious in nature. The apparent arrogance of officials linked to the adoption and unilateral publication of the Lyme disease *Guidelines* document, for example, appears to have shown little regard for the fate of patients in this country suffering with Lyme disease from the

31 *Department of Justice Act*, ss.4(a) and (b).

fact of having hastily adopted and borrowed information from U.S. treating guidelines. Those are now disgraced and defunct because of conflicts of interest. In Canada, too, many related questions arise and corrective measures are needed.

The weight of all the evidence arising from and underlying the preceding critique of the *Guidelines* helps to shed light on "who's wrong" and "who's responsible" for the continuing conflicts in viewpoints, rather than adopting and embracing the better approach involving collaboration among all groups concerned about Lyme disease in Canada. But, some questions of a legal nature need answers. Were there any links or interests on the part of Canadian officials who unilaterally took over the responsibility for publishing the Canadian *Guidelines* akin to the kinds of personal and professional conflicts of interest discovered in the U.S. situation? And, in turn, that kind of question invites others: Are there any legislated conflict of interest rules in place to require full disclosure of personal interest or professional ties on the part of persons who may not be public office holders in Canada but are influential participants in federal public health policy initiatives and activities? Where persons or agencies who report to the Minister of Health or the Department of Health may be examined or questioned, it is surely within the purview of the Attorney General of Canada to investigate and give advice to that other ministry on such matters.

The situation here is one in which there is a conflict and controversy concerning appropriate treating and diagnostic services in respect of persons with Lyme disease. But, the situation here is also one which sees the Department of Health and the Public Health Agency failing or being unwilling or unable to provide accurate, up-to-date and unbiased guidance, support and direction for physicians and health practitioners in diagnosing and treating patients with Lyme disease. That situation raises many kinds of medico-legal issues. Because the Canadian *Guidelines* are so deficient and incomplete, persons diagnosed with Lyme disease, particularly Chronic Lyme disease, have in fact been denied adequate health services because physicians and clinicians are lacking the kinds of specific, accurate and complete information they need in order to offer competent and timely treatment. In one sample case referred to (that of patient "H"), the testing system in this country failed and that person continues in a chronic state, no doubt owing to a botched Canadian ELISA test result, without any recommendation for an initial screening with a Western blot test. There may be other persons who were initially tested and diagnosed as negative for Lyme disease but who, in fact, are positive but were missed because the present-day testing protocol is deficient and inadequate. There is voluminous information and evidence that is ignored or not provided to physicians in the *Guidelines,* such as the fact that Lyme disease sometimes can be refractory, and that

Borrelia burgdorferi is a polymorphous micro-organism that is able to hide itself in human tissue in a cystic form, rather than a spirochetal form, all of which simply means that Lyme disease, in its differing manifestations, can be persistent and chronic and very difficult to detect and treat.[32] Surely, for most Canadians, it is preferable, and their choice would be, that all persons suffering with Lyme disease should be returned to health, to be able to lead productive lives and to be self-supporting and able to care for themselves, rather than to remain chronically ill. It is also likely to be far less costly for our public health system to provide effective diagnosis and treatment than it is to pay for the costs of long-term, chronic care.

The Canadian *Guidelines* document merely duplicates the CDC/IDSA protocol. But that fact alone raises other difficult legal questions: Was the U.S. guideline model chosen for reasons of expediency? Was that done unwittingly or was that a result of wilful action or blind neglect of duty and was that choice taken without regard to potential harm to individual Canadians? There is in this instance an obvious duty of care because, through publication of the *Guidelines,* the Public Health Agency of Canada made the choice to implement a protocol for the purpose of addressing the case requirements for diagnosing and treatment of persons infected with the Lyme disease bacterium. But, as this Brief points out, the chosen *Guidelines* obviously failed to do that in any adequate or effective way. That same choice (the decision to adopt the U.S. standards and the situation that created) also brings to the forefront the fact that there is a public (institutional) as well as an individual duty of care in this set of circumstances. The Canadian *Guidelines* document was intended and written and adopted as a definitive, prescriptive and detailed directive for physicians, to which at least two of the provincial colleges have chosen to adhere in the course of investigating doctors who have undertaken to treat chronic states of Lyme disease. The Canadian *Guidelines* were intended and written as if they contained, and were to be relied upon as containing, complete and determinative statements about diagnosing and treating Lyme disease. The *Guidelines* document's many ascertainable shortcomings and failings as a diagnostic and treating protocol have already been commented on and noted earlier in this brief. To what effect?

---

32 For a scientific description of the morphology and investigational complexities of the cystic form of *Borrelia burgdorferi,* see: Brorson, S.H., "*Invitro* Conversion of *Borrelia burgdorferi* to Cystic Forms in Spinal Fluid and Transformation to Mobile Spirochetes by Incubation" in Infection 26 (1998) No. 3. Also, Balfour, A. in the British Medical Journal reported "dark-field" microscopic views of spirochaetes discharging spherical granules and "morphing" in liver tissue: http://www.drerniemurakami.com/attachments/DCysts.pdf.)

In his report made following the investigation into the U.S. treating protocols, the Attorney General for the State of Connecticut suggested that the U.S. guidelines had "sweeping and significant impacts on Lyme disease medical care," and it observed that the U.S. guidelines panel had "undercut its credibility" when it stacked the panel membership with individuals who had financial interests linked to pharmaceutical companies and insurance companies in what we now know are the key areas of Lyme disease conflicts. The A-G for Connecticut went so far as to say, "Medical societies that publish such guidelines have a legal and moral duty to use exacting safeguards and scientific standards."[33] As in the U.S., the situation here in Canada begs similar kinds of questions: Who's interests were served? Was any third-party interest served, and was there any improper conduct on the part of anyone in Canada? How (assuming there may be a finding that there were no improprieties) is anyone able otherwise to account for the Canadian *Guidelines'* fiasco outlined in this Brief?

Other questions concern the matter of the nexus, or relationship, between persons with Lyme disease who may be or were or are at risk of harm and the agencies who created the *Guidelines* and who owed a duty of care in the circumstances. The persons actually or potentially at risk of harm are those with Lyme disease, whether diagnosed or not, including persons who may yet be found to be in need of treatment for Lyme disease. In the circumstances here, the diagnosis and treatment of Lyme disease is the very subject-matter chosen and intended to be addressed by the Public Health Laboratory Network through its authorship and by the Public Health Agency through its adoption of the *Guidelines*.

In recognizing and acknowledging in Canada the need for adequate and proper diagnostic and treatment services to combat Chronic Lyme disease, one is confronted with the case circumstances of all individuals whom the *Guidelines'* fiasco has potentially negatively affected. Every Canadian has equality rights that are guaranteed under the Canadian Constitution. In particular, the *Charter of Rights and Freedoms,* in the two following *Charter* sections, declares unequivocally:

> 7. Everyone has the right to life, liberty and security of the person and the right not to be deprived thereof except in accordance with the principles of fundamental justice.

33 *Supra*, footnote 17.

and

15. Every individual is equal before and under the law and has the right to the equal protection and equal benefit of the law without discrimination, and, in particular, without discrimination based on race, national or ethnic origin, colour, religion, sex, age or mental or physical disability.

The Supreme Court of Canada in one recent case provided the following interpretation to indicate what it is that would amount to an infringement upon those equality rights:

> If a benefit program excludes a particular group in a way that undercuts the overall purpose of the program, then it is likely to be discriminatory: it amounts to an arbitrary exclusion of a particular group.[34]

The *Public Health Agency Act* allows for the introduction of a variety of programs and measures that could apply for all Canadians, but, in the situation here, the denial of such rights occurred because the *Guidelines* were intended to introduce detailed information and measures specific to the diagnosing and treatment of one group of Canadians: persons with Lyme disease. But, as this Brief indicates, the Canadian *Guidelines* are too minimalist, inaccurate and insufficient, as well as ineffectual and prospectively harmful to achieve that purpose. If there is any doubt or question as to whether or not the stated *Charter* protections could apply in the case of Lyme disease patients, and, in particular, those with Chronic Lyme disease, one need only contemplate and imagine the degree of outrage and the levels of public outcry that would arise in Canada if patients suffering with cancer, diabetes, heart disease, or other debilitating and potentially terminal illnesses were to be denied access to accurate and appropriate diagnostic and treatment services. This has been a disgraceful chapter in our history. The Canada *Health Act's* promises and the duties it and related statutes create in the case of Canadians with Lyme disease have not yet been met or fulfilled.

This brief ends with a direct appeal to the Attorney General and Minister of Justice of Canada to intervene officially and formally. That intervention must include a full investigation into the circumstances that led to implementing the inapt and ineffective Canadian Lyme disease *Guidelines.* Canadians then need the Minister's

34 *Auton (Guardian ad litem of) v. British Columbia (Attorney General),* [2004] 3 S.C.R. 657; (2004), 245 D.L.R. (4th) 1; [2005] W.W.R. 189; (2004), 124 C.R.R. (2d) 135; (2004), 34 C.B.L.R. (4th) 24.

intervention to promote and recommend measures to ensure that all of the applicable and referenced governing legislation will be fully understood, followed and applied properly for the future benefit of all Canadians. The objectives must also be to restore all persons suffering with Lyme disease to their proper status as persons for whom medical-health services are at least equivalent to the levels and kinds of services received or offered and available to other Canadians with a serious disease. This would mean ensuring that all Canadians, as well as persons with Lyme disease, will be able to benefit from the availability of enhanced diagnostic and treatment services and methods. A further aspect of such legislative objectives should be to restore physicians and others providing health services to their proper role of primary clinical case managers with freedom to choose, from within available, tested and reliable guidelines, the best diagnostic and treatment methods that can be offered, and, ultimately, to give recognition of the right for them to assert and fulfill their professional practice responsibilities by allowing them to offer services that best benefit and will promote the health and well being of all Lyme disease patients whom they may be called upon to treat without any fear of reprisals.

Note to the Reader

This chapter was originally composed in May 2009, "Lyme Disease Awareness Month," as a personal brief to the Minister of Health and the Attorney General of Canada and has been distributed widely among Lyme patients throughout Canada.

OPENING THE CLOSED MIND

6

By David Cubberley

What follows these remarks is a series of letters I wrote, in my capacity as the MLA (NDP) for Saanich South in British Columbia, to the medical licensing authority in British Columbia. On behalf of people living in British Columbia and many of my constituents who suffer from Lyme disease, I challenged the College's acceptance of Lyme disease 'guidelines' developed by the Infectious Diseases Society of America (IDSA). Those guidelines define Lyme disease for doctors, tell them when and where to expect it, how to detect it, what treatment to use, and for exactly how long. They are tightly prescriptive, as the many Canadians suffering from untreated Lyme sadly come to understand. These guidelines effectively tie doctors' hands, do their thinking for them, and create a basis for policing their actions—should they decline to go along. These guidelines are in many ways unprecedented in their effect to remove the use of individual powers of empirical observation, which are integral to the art of doctoring. These guidelines replace clinical judgment with formulae for a multi-systemic disease that is only just beginning to be understood.

The IDSA guidelines also provide infectious disease specialists in Canada with a rationale for denying or ignoring the fact that Lyme disease can be a persistent (chronic) infection. This enables doctors to refuse patients access to longer courses of antibiotic therapy. Antibiotics are the only known effective therapy for borrelia, and longer courses are the only way to get rid of or reduce the debilitating effects of Chronic Lyme. These guidelines, and the claims on which they rest are said to be based supposedly on "evidence" generated by "science." However, what qualified as "evidence" is so selective as to be skewed, so narrow as to be inadequate for generalization. In some places the "evidence" has holes large enough to spit through: for example, the IDSA-required bullseye rash is so infrequent, it cannot be justified as a "diagnostic marker" for all patients—and yet, there it is as a basic requirement for diagnosis! Some elements of the advocated testing regimen are so bizarre, that no justification can be found for it. For example, why the need for a two-step test protocol, with step one less sensitive to Lyme than step two, and why are just about all the most Lyme-specific bands missing from the Western blot test? The guideline writers took an evidence-holiday!

Science works by being open to continual criticism from observations that better interpret and explain the "evidence" observed. Society learns over time by having many minds test the matter at hand, and yesterday's idea of what we're doing and why is refined by today's discoveries. Usually, when there is significant controversy and doubt, science doesn't rush to definitive conclusions. But the science in Lyme disease diagnosis and treatment, as codified by the IDSA, attempts to freeze discussion for all time regardless of our actual state of knowledge about this disease. There have been over 18,000 scientific articles written on borrelia, most of which don't support the conclusions drawn by the guideline writers. But for them any contradictory observation and the documented treatment experience of physicians are irrelevant.

What is remarkable is just how effective this manipulation of science through guideline creation is when launched and supported through the bureaucracies of modern medicine. Because Lyme is an emerging epidemic involving a tricky, relatively new-to-Canada microbe, our physicians know little or nothing about it from medical school or their clinical practice. They are thus positioned by lack of knowledge to be Lyme-blind and to take as gospel what they are told by their overseers in the public health and medical licensing agencies—and these agencies speak as one voice on Lyme in consistent sound bites, such as "infrequent" or "rare." Lyme patients are even frequently told to their faces: "There's no Lyme in B.C." Or more aggressively: "If you think you have Lyme, you're part of a cult." None of this is evidence-based, but is very effective in suppressing consideration of Lyme as an explanation of symptoms. Quite simply, doctors do not look for Lyme, and these guidelines steer doctors away from even thinking about looking for it. The message is clear that the authorities expect doctors not to diagnose Lyme disease.

It's easy enough to cultivate the belief that Lyme is infrequent and should rarely be considered as an explanation of symptoms, except along the very narrow path beginning with a bullseye rash followed by inappropriate testing. Very few patients get diagnosed using those markers: three to five a year at most in the whole of tick-infested British Columbia. Realistically, few doctors have seen enough Lyme to accord it much status as a health threat, relative to what they are used to seeing, namely heart disease, diabetes and cancer. And if you tell doctors they need evidence of a tick bite, and must see a classic erythema migrans rash, before considering Lyme, then most Lyme cases are, of course, missed. Nor would most doctors risk their medical license by going to bat for people whose suspected illness doesn't meet criteria endorsed by the licensing authority—especially if it is already known that they go after doctors who take Lyme seriously and disregard the guidelines. Doctors who think for themselves and practice medicine as it should be practiced tend to become targets for disciplinary action, as we found out in British Columbia. Nor would most consider prescribing a longer course of antibiotic therapy, because the power to do that is thought to belong only to infectious disease specialists—who, of course, would generally be members of the IDSA cabal, who reject such treatment categorically. The net result for infected patients is indifference or outright hostility, manifested as a refusal to diagnose from symptoms and consider treatment. For the patient, all this amounts to a life-sentence in the living hell of Chronic Lyme disease.

What follows here are my letters to the College of Physicians and Surgeons which were written in the latter part of my term as a member of the B.C. Legislature. The most recent letters were written after I left provincial politics and joined the Canadian Lyme Disease Foundation as a director. Let me declare my bias, if it be a bias: I am an advocate for prompt diagnosis and sustained treatment of Lyme disease, both as new infection and in the chronic form that inevitably develops because the approved "guidelines" miss nearly all newly infected Lyme cases. I'm placing myself squarely on the side of patients and those few brave doctors willing to treat them beyond those clinically and scientifically indefensible guidelines. In the course of my four years as MLA, I came to realize that we aren't dealing with a simple mistake, but rather a deep-seated bias that has fully institutionalized itself. This won't change until forced to do so. The challenge of advocacy is to figure out how to marshal the necessary force needed to achieve fundamental change. My letters are an attempt to put those Emperors on notice that we know they will be naked soon!

The simple fact is that we have imported a problem created in the hothouse of free enterprise medicine to the south of us, which combines a policy favorable to private insurers with the settling of scores in disputes between schools of thought in medicine. In the Lyme disease arena this dispute was "won" by the IDSA which has been found by legal investigation to have stacked the guideline committee and cooked the evidence. Academic doctors can profit from the drugs and vaccines that flow from such a doctored disease definition, and such conflicts of interest were also to be found among the IDSA guideline committee members. In addition, private insurance companies have an interest in standardizing treatment such as to minimize their financial obligations to patients. These forced the creation of these inappropriately restrictive guidelines for a complex infectious disease, ignored most of the science on Lyme disease, and marginalized the experience of treating physicians and the symptoms of the patients suffering from Lyme disease.

Is it not astonishing, that the knowledge acquired by doctors practicing medicine as an art, learning through observation and experiment, was disallowed as "evidence" by those who developed the guidelines? Should our medical licensing and public health authorities not be outraged to learn that a professional society writing care-guidelines has flaunted public interest and produced cooked material not worthy of the name of science?

Canada has not only internalized the toxic byproduct of an American dispute over a disease which in the rest of the world is generally appropriately treated, and has, thereby inflicted even greater harm on Canadian patients than that suffered by patients in the USA. Our single-payer public health system has no equivalent to the American private health insurance market and those HMOs that rule patients' lives in the US. But when the door to treatment is closed for Canadians, the way the IDSA Lyme guidelines succeeded in doing, then there is no way for sick people in Canada to gain access to medically necessary and effective care. Here, patients run into a Berlin wall of indifference, and encounter a closed medical mind. In Canada, patients with Chronic Lyme either live with severe pain and disability, or they sell their homes, go the United States and buy access to antibiotics through the private market in health care. What an ugly paradox: denied diagnosis and treatment under U.S. guidelines in Canada's public healthcare system, you have to go to the home of private medicine for therapy!

This is a travesty for our public health plan. We must keep faith with its mission to make effective care available without regard for ability to pay. Canada is committed to this policy by law, and now is clearly in breach of the law by accepting those tainted guidelines. In effect, the IDSA Lyme guidelines de-insure Canadians who are infected with Lyme bacteria. Ready available, affordable, effective antibiotic therapies are being denied to sick people on grounds that are not consistent with published science or even with medical common sense!

Legislators in 17 states in the US have either passed legislation or protective regulation to enable Lyme patients to bypass the IDSA guidelines and thus enable them to obtain long-term antibiotics; Lyme-literate treating doctors are protected in those jurisdictions from IDSA-justified harassment, and insurance companies are prohibited from denying benefits on the grounds that Chronic Lyme disease doesn't exist.

Medical licensing authorities in Canada and the US, as self-governing professional bodies, certainly may advise doctors on "best practices" in medicine and to police malpractice. But they have a corresponding responsibility to serve the public interest, which in our health care system means ensuring that citizens have access to medically effective care and to guard against any arbitrary restriction of access to care. My letters discuss this issue in more detail.

In Canada, so far as I can tell, our authorities have simply accepted those IDSA guidelines uncritically as truth. I received just one single reply, and it was to my first letter to the B.C. College. It was not a response to the substance of my letter, but merely forwarded a copy of that junk-science IDSA guideline of 2006 which simply denies the existence of Chronic Lyme disease. In my view, that means our medical licensing authorities have failed the public interest with regards to Lyme disease. They never bothered to inform doctors in B.C. that there is a controversy concerning the IDSA, and that the Attorney General of Connecticut conducted an anti-trust investigation which found the IDSA guideline panel guilty of financial conflicts of interest and scientific misconduct. These facts were published in the relevant medical journals, but the BC College took no position on them.

We are dealing with an unacceptable systemic bias when the responsible agencies don't care to inform doctors, legislators, patients, or the general public that treatment guidelines have been placed in question by a legal investigation. The suppression of this knowledge in Canada should be grounds for the provincial Minister of Health to take action so that a publicly accessible critical analysis of imported guidelines takes place and, if necessary, develop made-in-Canada diagnostic and treatment guidelines. The Minister must by law ensure that the public interest is served by self-regulating societies, such as the College of Physicians and Surgeons in B.C. Today, the public interest is not served with respect to Lyme disease, and we are facing an emerging infectious disease of potentially epidemic proportions.

David Cubberley, MLA
(Saanich South)
Parliament Buildings
Victoria, B.C. V8V 1X4

Community Office:
301 - 3939 Quadra Street
Victoria, B.C. V8X 1J5
Phone: 250 952-4418
Fax: 250 952-4566

Province of
British Columbia
Legislative Assembly

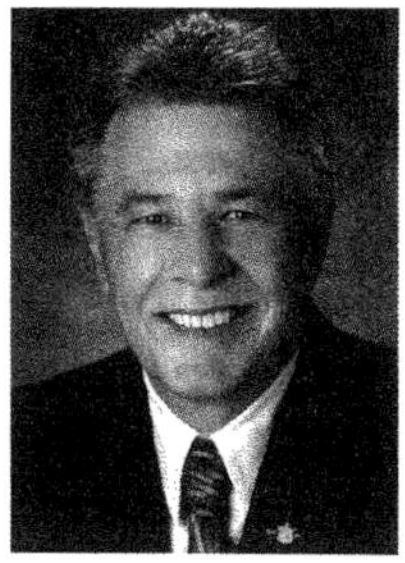
David Cubberley, MLA
(Saanich South)

December 18, 2008

Dr. A Dodek, President and Members of the Council
College of Physicians and Surgeons of British Columbia
400 858 Beatty Street
Vancouver, BC V6B 1C1

Dear Dr. Dodek and Council Members:

I write to express my deep concern about the advice on diagnosing Lyme disease in the October 2008 Bulletin, which reinforces the prevailing lack of awareness among B.C. doctors. The approach recommended actually contradicts the policy of the B.C. Ministry of Health and the B.C. Centre for Disease Control, which state that Lyme disease is to be diagnosed from patient symptoms and that diagnosis is not dependent 'in most cases' upon a positive blood test.
"Your doctor will probably be able to tell if you have Lyme disease based on your symptoms and whether you may have been exposed to deer ticks. In most cases, blood tests to diagnose Lyme disease are not necessary." B.C. HealthGuide, MoH, p. 110. "Lyme disease should be diagnosed through a clinical evaluation of the patient's symptoms and risk of exposure to infected ticks. A blood test may also be administered…but this should not be interpreted in the absence of a clinical diagnosis." BC Centre for Disease Control, February 29, 2008, news release.
The Bulletin implies that diagnosis of Lyme disease depends upon a positive blood test, which in B. C. is known to be unreliable due to its high level of false negatives (unreliable serology is presumably why the CDC makes 'symptoms' the basis of diagnosis). This error would be bad enough, but the College Bulletin compounds it by making testing for Lyme depend in turn upon the patient presenting with evidence of a tick bite and a bull's-eye rash. Only some of those bitten by an infected tick ever develop a discernible bull's-eye rash, while many who ultimately test positive for Lyme don't recall a tick bite or a rash.

There is robust evidence from long-term patients that B.C. doctors lack the knowledge of symptoms to diagnose Lyme disease clinically, which means most people are not promptly cured and go on to develop debilitating late-stage Lyme disease. There is a pressing need for all those responsible for medical practice in B.C. to develop a focus on raising doctor awareness of

/2…..

-2-

Lyme's symptoms. The College's advice makes a bad situation worse – it reinforces doctor ignorance of the incidence, symptoms, diagnosis and effective treatment of an infectious disease that is clearly on the rise across North America. It also repeats the claim that Lyme is infrequent in B.C., which further encourages doctors not to learn how to recognize it. Of course we have only a few 'proven' cases a year – most instances of Lyme infection will be missed with an approach that depends on unreliable indicators (i.e. bull's-eye rash, blood test).What most patients who present with Lyme symptoms hear from their doctors is that 'it's very rare' or that 'we don't have it here'. This attitude is so widespread as to constitute a barrier to accessing timely medical care – an obligation of our public healthcare system. Until doctors are given the basic tools to recognize the symptoms of Lyme and its multiple coinfections, healthcare resources will be wasted as patients are serially misdiagnosed with diseases they don't have and are condemned to live with the debilitating physiological and neurological effects of chronic Lyme disease.

The College Bulletin doesn't even mention the primary symptoms doctors should be aware of (persistent flu-like symptoms, aches and pains in the joints, disorientation and fatigue). Nor does it mention Lyme's mimicking of other diseases, or the growing likelihood of complex coinfections like Babbesia. All these omissions work to ensure that Lyme continues to be under-diagnosed in a province where its incidence is on the rise.

Finally, the College compounds the harm to Lyme sufferers by perpetuating the claim that chronic Lyme disease "remains controversial", meaning that it may in fact not exist. This equates to a life-sentence for anyone undiagnosed in the early stages (which is virtually everyone contracting Lyme in B.C. today) when a relatively short course of antibiotics may have nipped the infection in the bud. The only thing missing here is a reiteration of the standing caution that long-term antibiotics are unnecessary and dangerous, which closes the door to the only treatment that has proven effective for those debilitated by chronic Lyme disease. But implying that chronic or late-stage Lyme doesn't exist has pretty much the same effect anyway, doesn't it!

What I see from collecting case histories of people with chronic or late-stage Lyme disease are clear patterns of under-diagnosis, lack of awareness of symptoms, failure to promptly treat, failure to recognize flaws in serological testing, failure to monitor and tailor antibiotic treatment to the severity of the Lyme infection, and refusal to allow long-term or intravenous antibiotic treatments for chronic Lyme sufferers even when there is serological evidence of disease. These patterns in my view add up to a systemic failure to provide timely access to medically necessary

/3.....

-3-

care. The net result is untold human suffering coupled with the financial hardship for many of having to seek appropriate care out of country. I would be pleased to have the opportunity to present a number of case histories directly to the College Board, so that it might become more informed about the devastating impacts in human lives.

I am sure the College is sincerely committed to 'excellence in medical practice', so I request formally that it correct the impressions left in the October issue, that it acknowledge the deficiencies in current practice as regards Lyme disease, and that it work with all agencies overseeing infectious diseases to equip B.C. doctors with the knowledge required for timely clinical diagnosis.

Sincerely yours,

David Cubberley

David Cubberley, MLA
Saanich South

DC/ljn
pc/files
pc/Minister George Abbott
Dr. Perry Kendall
Jim Wilson, et al
BCGEU -701

COLLEGE OF PHYSICIANS & SURGEONS OF BRITISH COLUMBIA

January 6, 2009

JAN 2 1 2009

Mr. David Cubberley, MLA
(Saanich South)
Parliament Buildings
Victoria, BC V8V 1X4

Dear Mr. Cubberley:

We are writing in response to your letter of December 18, 2008 addressed to the President, Dr. A. Dodek, and the members of the Council of the College of Physicians & Surgeons of British Columbia. Your letter was reviewed by the Executive Committee of the College at its meeting on December 19, 2008.

Your letter appears to have been prompted by a brief article in the October 2008 issue of the College *Quarterly* entitled "Uncommon conditions do occur – Lyme Disease". Unfortunately, you appear to have missed the primary point of the article, namely that uncommon, even rare, conditions do occur and hence physicians should always be considering uncommon and rare diseases as a part of their differential diagnosis as they assess patients. The general symptoms of Lyme Disease are very non-specific, including fever, headache, muscle and joint pains, fatigue, skin rashes, and occasionally weakness of the muscles of the face. Such symptoms can herald numerous disorders of varying etiology. Hence, considering a full differential diagnosis is an imperative, as is appropriate assessment of the patient, including appropriate laboratory investigations, including an ELISA test and a Western Blot Test, if appropriate in the clinical circumstances.

Currently, the College is co-involved with the B.C. Centre for Disease Control in a research survey of British Columbia physicians' understanding of the diagnosis and treatment of Lyme Disease. The results of this research will assist in tailoring further continuing professional development for physicians in the province.

In your letter, you take issue with the College's comment that "chronic Lyme Disease remains controversial." We are enclosing a copy of the referenced review article published in the New England Journal of Medicine, 14 October 2007.

COLLEGE OF PHYSICIANS & SURGEONS OF BRITISH COLUMBIA

MR. DAVID CUBBERLEY, MLA - 2 - JANUARY 6, 2009

The Executive Committee has considered your offer to present a number of case histories directly to the College Board (Council). The Committee has respectfully declined your offer.

Yours truly,

D. H. Blackman, MD, CCFP
Deputy Registrar

DHB/ak
Encl

Copy: **The Honourable George Abbott**
Minister of Health Services

Copy: **Dr. Perry R.W. Kendall**
Provincial Health Officer

David Cubberley, MLA
(Saanich South)
Parliament Buildings
Victoria, B.C. V8V 1X4

Community Office:
301 - 3939 Quadra Street
Victoria, B.C. V8X 1J5
Phone: 250 952-4418
Fax: 250 952-4566

Province of
British Columbia
Legislative Assembly

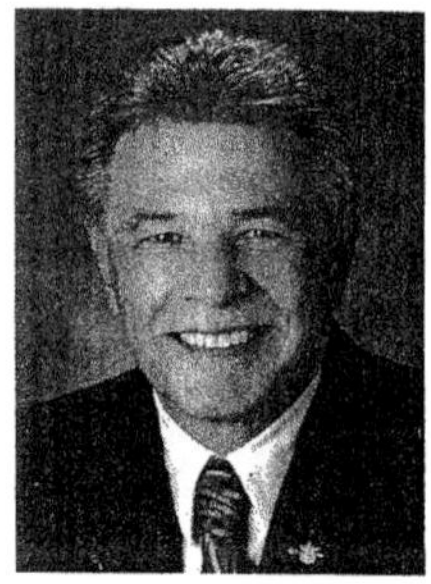

David Cubberley, MLA
(Saanich South)

March 2, 2009

Dr. A Dodek, President and Members of the Council
College of Physicians and Surgeons of British Columbia
400 858 Beatty Street
Vancouver, BC V6B 1C1

Dear Dr. Dodek and Council Members:

Thanks for your response to my December 18th letter regarding comments on Lyme disease diagnosis and treatment in the October 2008 College bulletin. I expressed concern that your advice to doctors was at odds with advice to patients from the B.C. Centre for Disease Control and the Ministry of Health's Healthguide. Both state that Lyme disease is to be diagnosed from symptoms and is not dependent upon either a detectable rash or a positive blood test; they also tell patients that B.C. doctors are equipped to provide this diagnosis. Your response states that I missed the point of your article, i.e. that "uncommon, even rare, conditions do occur and hence physicians should always be considering uncommon and rare diseases as part of their differential diagnosis". I suggested that calling Lyme 'rare' tells doctors they're unlikely to see it, while advising them that diagnosis and treatment require both a bull's-eye rash and a confirmatory ELISA test means that a majority of infected patients go undetected and untreated.

Your letter did not respond to the substance of mine, and you did not comment on the disparity between your position on Lyme diagnosis and that of the BC CDC and the Ministry of Health. This is a significant problem for patients in B.C., because the College's guidelines determine whether and when patients with Lyme are diagnosed and effectively treated. If these guidelines are flawed (as your advice about rash and test indicate they are) many patients will not receive diagnosis and the medically necessary care they're entitled to. If doctors are uninformed about Lyme symptoms, causes, and the unreliability of tests like the ELISA, they are more likely to diagnose Fibromyalgia, MS, CFS or any of a number of other illnesses sharing some symptoms with Lyme. These diagnoses would all miss the opportunity to treat Lyme infection effectively in its early stage when it's most curable. There is ample evidence that infected B.C. patients are not being diagnosed and treated when they present with Lyme symptoms, meaning they are doomed to untold horror and suffering from living with chronic Lyme disease.

Is characterizing Lyme disease as "uncommon, even rare" appropriate in light of the 20,000 new cases a year reported in the U.S.A., which the U.S. CDC says understates actual incidence by a factor of ten? Even the paper you sent me arguing against 'chronic' Lyme disease begins by

2/.....

-2-

recognizing Lyme as 'the most common tick-borne infection in the North American hemisphere' and 'a serious public health problem.' Lyme is the fastest rising infectious disease in North America and – unless ticks, deer and birds are somehow held in check by guards at the Canada/US border – it cannot be 'uncommon, even rare' here in B.C. Given that many British Columbians have acquired it walking the West Coast Trail, vacationing at Shawnigan Lake, or gardening in the suburban savannahs of Saanich, it's hardly rare or uncommon. The number of cases reported annually in B.C. is absurdly low given the incidence in Washington and Oregon – epidemiologically this fact alone should pique our concern and trigger a review of clinical practice guidelines and test regimes in B.C.

My central point was that Lyme will be under-diagnosed if physicians are told to rely on seeing a bull's-eye rash (not present in many cases of infection) and a positive ELISA test, which is inaccurate at the outset of infection and gets worse over time as bacteria leave the bloodstream for better hiding places. What happens to all those people who lack the rash and therefore don't even get to the inaccurate test, or those who have the rash but test negative when they're in fact positive? This inevitability appears to be of no concern to the College, but it is a serious public health issue with an untold number of victims. My offer to acquaint you with a few of the cases I've come across would include examples of BC doctors refusing to consider Lyme diagnosis even when a tick bite and EM rash are present, at times defiantly telling patients "there's no Lyme in British Columbia!" Sadly, this is not an "uncommon, even rare" event, but rather reflects what many see as a systemic bias against clinical diagnosis and effective treatment of Lyme disease.

The article you sent me – A Critical Appraisal of 'Chronic Lyme Disease' – argues there's no such thing as a 'chronic' phase of Lyme disease and claims there's no evidence that long-term antibiotic treatment can be justified as therapy. This is consistent with beliefs embedded in the 2006 Infectious Disease Society of America (IDSA) guidelines, which under your aegis govern patient access to care in B.C. These beliefs are actively enforced by our Infectious Disease Specialists, who refuse to permit long-term or IV antibiotic treatment of patients even when there is serological and/or symptomatic evidence of persistent Lyme disease. This denies Lyme-sufferers access to the only clinically effective response to a debilitating infectious illness, forcing them outside public healthcare in Canada and into for-profit care in the USA – where they must pay out-of-pocket for treatments that often prove effective in restoring their health over the long term.

I was surprised to note that the article you sent was coauthored by (among others) Doctors Gary P. Wormser, Eugene D. Shapiro, and Allen C. Steere, former Chair and members respectively of the IDSA panel that drafted the 2006 IDSA guidelines. I wonder if you're aware that these guidelines are now subject to complete review by an entirely new panel whose work is to be 'refereed' by medical ethicist Dr. Howard A. Brody? This unusual step follows a lengthy antitrust investigation by Connecticut Attorney General Richard Blumenthal, which unearthed conflicts of interest and serious breaches of procedure and guidelines. Blumenthal concluded that **"the IDSA's 2006 Lyme disease guideline panel undercut its credibility by allowing individuals with financial interests – in drug companies, Lyme disease diagnostic tests, patents and consulting arrangements with insurance companies – to exclude divergent**

/3.....

-3-

medical evidence and opinion" (emphasis added). The new panel is mandated to include members representing the entire spectrum of opinion on Lyme disease diagnosis and treatment, because the previous panel's composition reflected only the beliefs of chronic-Lyme deniers. Time will tell whether the IDSA will see fit to meet ethical and scientific standards in generating future guidelines. However, in the current circumstances, is it appropriate for the College to circulate conjectural articles co-authored by persons who failed to meet their own professional society's procedural standards for generating clinical practice guidelines?

Given the tainted process and bias against considering the supporting science and clinical practice experience of physicians who treat chronic Lyme with longer term antibiotic therapies, I wonder if the College has informed B.C. doctors of the guideline review and alerted them to their opportunity to participate? Given that British Columbia doctors are bound by guidelines created in another country, it would seem important to participate openly in any process affecting them. I would hope that a self-governing professional body like the College would ensure its members knew about the investigation and the mandated review of the guidelines.

I also think it's important that the College consider the substance of Blumenthal's findings, as they speak directly to the issue of whether confidence in the 2006 guidelines is warranted, and to the diligence and duty of care owed citizens of B.C. and Canada. Blumenthal summarized the public interest by noting that the guidelines have "sweeping and significant impacts on Lyme disease medical care" and "are commonly applied by insurance companies in restricting coverage for long-term antibiotic treatment or other medical care and also strongly influence physician treatment decisions." He also notes that "**medical societies that publish such guidelines have a legal and moral duty to use exacting safeguards and scientific standards**" (emphasis added). The investigation found the IDSA and its panel deficient, even derelict in meeting this legal and moral duty.

The 2006 IDSA guidelines tightly restrict a for-profit insurer's obligation to pay for patient treatment. Blumenthal notes that "insurance companies have denied coverage for long-term antibiotic treatment relying on these guidelines as justification" and that "the guidelines are also widely cited for conclusions that chronic Lyme disease is non-existent". These guidelines serve the same function in Canada's public healthcare system – although the insurers here (i.e. the governments and people of Canada) have never promoted chronic-Lyme denial and remain financially responsible for the serial misdiagnoses that ensue when doctors are taught not to see Lyme.

Science cannot be said to support the contention that chronic Lyme doesn't exist, because as Blumenthal's investigation showed, the IDSA panel simply refused to consider any science or clinical experience that didn't confirm a conclusion it had already drawn. The guidelines are, in fact, tendentious claims not substantiated by the panel's deliberations, nor are they confirmed 'scientifically' by the material presented in the article by Drs Wormser et al (which is, to be kind, 'selective'). Of the over 19,000 articles on Lyme disease, the panel cited just 405, nearly half of which were written by the guidelines authors! Given the divergence of medical and scientific opinion on these matters, a society creating clinical practice guidelines has an ethical obligation to ensure a very 'clean' and transparent process in working them up. Blumenthal's investigation

/4.....

-4-

determined there was anything but a defensible process behind the writing of these guidelines.

Rather, he found that "the IDSA's guideline panel improperly ignored or minimized consideration of alternative medical opinion and evidence regarding chronic Lyme disease." The IDSA's Lyme guideline process also "**lacked important procedural safeguards**". Among the most troubling of the flaws and manipulations tolerated or endorsed by the IDSA are the following:

"The IDSA **failed to conduct a conflicts of interest review** for any of the panelists prior to their appointment". Several members had undisclosed financial interests.

"The IDSA **failed to follow its own procedures** for appointing the 2006 panel chairman and members, **enabling the Chairman, who held a bias regarding the existence of chronic Lyme, to handpick a likeminded panel without scrutiny by or formal approval of the IDSA's oversight committee**".

"The IDSA's 2000 and 2006 Lyme disease panels **refused to accept or meaningfully consider information regarding the existence of chronic Lyme disease**".

"The IDSA **blocked appointment of scientists and physicians with divergent views on chronic Lyme** who sought to serve on the 2006 guidelines panel".

"The IDSA **portrayed another medical association's** [American Academy of Neurology (AAN)] **Lyme disease guidelines as corroborating its own** when it knew that the two panels shared several authors, including the chairmen of both groups, and were working on guidelines at the same time. In allowing its panelists to serve on both groups at the same time, **IDSA violated its own conflicts of interest policy.**"

The impropriety of doing these things will surely be evident to members of the College of Physicians and Surgeons in British Columbia. The IDSA compounded its failure to complete 'due diligence' by further attempting to promote the idea of an independent confirming opinion.

"When IDSA learned of the improper links between its panel and the AAN's panel, instead of enforcing its conflict of interest policy, it aggressively sought the AAN's endorsement to 'strengthen' its guidelines impact. The AAN panel – particularly members who had also served on the IDSA panel – worked equally hard to win AAN's backing of IDSA's conclusions."

"The two entities sought to portray each other's guidelines as separate and independent when the facts call into question that contention."

(All of the above quotes are drawn from Attorney General Richard Blumenthal's May 1, 2008 news release, copy appended, emphases added).

An abject lack of process-integrity on the part of the IDSA panel and the numerous failures by the IDSA to exercise ethical oversight of a committee operating in its name cast serious doubt on the 2006 IDSA guidelines. They raise questions about trusting this organization to develop any guidelines with the necessary respect for science and an appropriate degree of objectivity. As these guidelines affect the practice of doctors and lives of patients in B.C., should the B.C.

/5.....

-5-

College not be treating them with a greater degree of caution and skepticism? In the College's view, should any individual consulting with private insurers regarding Lyme treatment, or holding patents on particular tests or treatments for Lyme infection, be allowed to participate in developing guidelines? Perhaps a crisis of organizational ethics of this kind should lead a self-governing professional body in a separate country to undertake its own review of clinical practice guidelines for Lyme diagnosis and treatment? Perhaps the least-substantiated parts of the guidelines should be subject to a College initiated review, given the likelihood of systemic error: i.e., making an erythema migrans rash (only present sometimes) a precondition for allowing an ELISA test (flawed) as a further precondition for doing a Western blot test (also flawed) as a further precondition for even considering Lyme diagnosis, leading at best to approval of a one-size-fits-all course of antibiotic therapy (contradicted by science and evidence).

I would urge that, in the public interest, the College distance itself from the many scientifically unsupported components of the 2006 IDSA guidelines, and that it mandate made-in-Canada guidelines formulated from fair consideration of all scientific evidence – including the clinical practice experience of physicians who treat Lyme beyond the existing guidelines. As the 2006 guidelines remain in force, some steps could be undertaken in the interim in order to ensure more prompt diagnosis and effective treatment of infected patients:

- Make diagnosis from symptoms the recommended approach and treat tests as confirmatory only. Comprehensively review whether the ELISA test should be retained as an initial screen for Lyme infection given its inaccuracy. Implement an appropriate test regime and ensure that doctors understand the limitations of all tests for detecting Lyme infection. Ensure doctors understand that ELISA reliability decreases the longer after initial infection it is used. Refocus physician attention on symptom awareness and draw on the extensive experience of doctors with enough experience in Lyme diagnosis to develop skill among those who lack it.

- Revise the guideline mandating a fixed course of antibiotic therapy in every diagnosed case to mandate a variable course (based on monitoring) with a set minimum length. This would take account of patient variability in response due to personal health and differing levels of infection, and it would recognize the rising incidence of co-infections, such as babesia, bartonella, Rocky Mountain spotted fever, and others that often complicate treatment.

- Initiate training for GP's to increase their knowledge of Lyme and co-infection signs and symptoms and to assist with their differential diagnosis, so that diseases without known cause or cure like Fibromyalgia, MS, or Parkinson's aren't the default option. Ensure that doctors understand that a bull's-eye rash doesn't occur in all cases of Lyme, and that proof of being bitten by a tick isn't a necessary condition for diagnosis. Ensure doctors understand their reporting obligations under public health legislation. And invite B.C. doctors with experience and skill in diagnosing Lyme and co-infections from symptoms to assist in developing and delivering the training.

/6.....

-6-

- Initiate a colloquium on the issue of chronic Lyme disease and the effectiveness of long-term antibiotic therapy. Allow the clinical practice experience of doctors treating patients with longer courses to be part of the discussion. Publish the results and invite comment from those who have received such treatments.

- Work with public health agencies to develop and implement a public education program focused on school-aged children, to raise awareness of the spread of tick-borne infection and the safeguards useful in protecting children when they play in areas inhabited by ticks. Develop a protocol for what parents should do when a child has a tick attached to the body and what doctors should do when encountering ticks on the body. Ensure that under no circumstances is the tick just thrown away or Lyme diagnosis summarily rejected.

Action in these areas might begin to reverse the damage being done under the flawed IDSA guidelines, which miss so much Lyme infection by design, and risk so much Lyme relapse due to a non-patient-specific prescription for antibiotic treatment. I would once again offer to work collaboratively with you in raising the College Board's awareness of the under-diagnosis and ineffective treatment of early-stage Lyme disease in B.C., and of the horrendous consequences of categorically refusing antibiotic therapies for patients with persistent Lyme disease. Many people, young and old, are having to exhaust their family's life savings to buy therapies in the United States that should be supplied here under Medicare. Interestingly, most if not all of these patients find improvement when they have access to antibiotic and other therapies not allowed under the current guidelines. As agencies and decision makers responsible for the public interest, should we not be learning from the experience of doctors in supplying care to patients?

Sincerely,

David Cubberley
MLA, Saanich South

DC/ljn
pc/files
Hon. George Abbott
Dr. Perry Kendall
Hon. Leona Aglukkaq
Dr. R Brunhan, BC CDC
Denise Savoie, MP
Dr. Keith Martin, MP
Judy Wasylycia-Leis, MP
Adrian Dix, MLA

7 A DOCTOR'S PERSPECTIVE

By Dr. Jozef Krop, MD, FAAEM

In Canada a public health crisis is unfolding with increasing rapidity. Not only is it affecting the lives of tens of thousands of people, but it also seriously endangers the blood supply in Canada and North America. This public health crisis is caused by Lyme disease, an infectious disease which, in especially its chronic form, is all but ignored by those government departments that have the duty to protect the public from the spread of such a disease. Government-mandated testing is totally inappropriate due to the high false negatives; therefore, a key tool for accurate surveillance and treatment options is missing. Most doctors in Canada do not even know about this crisis, nor are they encouraged to educate themselves about correct diagnosis and treatment of Lyme disease, but often those doctors who chose to treat especially Chronic Lyme patients, are intimidated by their licensing and public health authorities. This situation is especially alarming because this lack of a patient-centered policy stands in marked contrast to the available facts in the medical scientific literature. Modern medicine knows how to prevent Lyme disease and how to treat it in its acute and chronic forms.

I have practised medicine for over 40 years and over 30 of those in Canada. I began practising Environmental Medicine 29 years ago when I took the appropriate training from the American Academy of Environmental Medicine (AAEM) of which I am a Fellow.

My understanding of medicine underwent a considerable evolution over the years. I outlined what I learned, especially from my patients, in the preface to my book *Healing the Planet One Patient at a Time: A Primer in Environmental Medicine* (KOS Publishing, third edition 2008). My understanding of medicine continues to evolve.

About 7 years ago, I also began treating patients with Lyme disease, mostly chronic cases. This infectious disease became very important in my practice because the symptoms of *Chronic Lyme* so often resemble and overlap with the symptoms I was familiar with from patients suffering from Multiple Chemical Sensitivity (MCS), or Environmental Illness (EI); often these chronically ill patients proved to be suffering from both conditions.

My work for patients with MCS, as well as my work for patients suffering from Chronic Lyme disease, has resulted in my twice being threatened with the loss of my medical license by the regulatory authority of the province in which I practice, namely the College of Physicians and Surgeons of Ontario (CPSO). Currently, an investigation of my practice is in the deliberation stage and yet another disciplinary hearing may be ordered, even though my lawyer has clearly demonstrated that my practice meets the standard of my peers treating Chronic Lyme disease. The outcome of this CPSO action is likely to set a precedent for anyone else practising in this field.

The first disciplinary investigation by the CPSO began in 1989, without patient complaint, and was focused on my diagnosis and treatment of MCS, which according to the CPSO, did not exist. The existence of the AAEM, whose physician members come from all over the world and focus on treating MCS, did not give the CPSO pause for thought, nor did positive patient outcome. The excellent results I obtained with very sick people through the use of the protocols developed by environmental medicine researchers in North America and Europe was of no interest to them either. The defence testimony from my peers, many of whom are members of the AAEM and other university-affiliated experts, nearly all of who treated MCS patients themselves, was also dismissed as irrelevant because of the supposed lack of scientific validity of the MCS "hypothesis."

In 2008, the CPSO once again commenced with a Section 75 (a) investigation (which refers to the relevant part in Ontario's Regulated Health Professions Act) and did so, once again, without patient complaint, and again only because the CPSO apparently questions the very existence of *Chronic Lyme* disease and, therefore, questions the fact that I treat what supposedly does not exist. Again, the fact that I am trained by the International Lyme and Associated Diseases Society (ILADS) and have excellent results using their protocols, seems to be of no interest. The CPSO has apparently accepted the IDSA-based views on Lyme disease.

The existence of *acute* Lyme disease cannot rationally be doubted, so the CPSO has chosen to frame this investigation as a question of my competence to treat infectious disease. This is similar to the approach taken when they attempted to show that I was not competent to treat allergy and, therefore, could be charged with essentially misinterpreting the signs and symptoms of MCS as some kind of "environmental allergy" which they asserted was of questionable scientific validity. MCS is, of course, not a classic allergy but an immune dysregulation that affects always more than one bodily system; the causes include exposures in various ways, acute or prolonged, to substances known to be toxic, such as pesticides, mercury amalgam dental fillings, the many poisons included in everything from laundry detergent to hair shampoo, cosmetics, paints, solvents, glues in building materials, and water contaminated with chlorine and fluoride, etc. Furthermore, the after-effects of infectious pathogens may also trigger MCS symptoms, such as food and mould sensitivities etc.

By asserting that a disease or condition does not exist, the CPSO, and any other regulatory body elsewhere in Canada, can effectively insist that the doctor who treats what *they* say does not exist, may be found guilty of "failing to maintain the standard of practice" because that standard, as unilaterally interpreted by the CPSO-chosen experts, does not include that condition. This can set precedents that warn other physicians not to practice in the area. This exercise in the *arbitrary* setting of standards moves a regulatory authority out of the domain of medicine as a science and places it, and its captive member practitioners, under the control of a virtually totalitarian system of medical politics. In both instances, MCS and Lyme disease, the legitimate disciplinary powers of this regulatory authority were used, and are being used, to attempt to establish standards of practice and to quash innovation and the application of new medical insights and therapies. Thus, positive patient outcome ceases to be important in medical regulation.

When medicine becomes political, it always abandons the patient—and tries to force the doctor to do the same. I learned this through personal experience. Not only does this situation obstruct medical advances in diagnosis and clinical application of new discoveries and threaten the livelihood of the doctor, but it also has a chilling effect on the entire medical profession and intimidates other doctors from learning about these new areas. The most tragic of all is the way patients' rights and lives are simply disregarded.

My first disciplinary investigations caused great suffering to MCS patients back then, and the same is true for Chronic Lyme patients now who are quite rightly fearful of not receiving the treatment they know they need. In most cases they have already been to many other doctors who could not help them. These disciplinary investigations also had a negative impact on those doctors who in the 1980s were beginning to work on the cutting edge of medical research in the field of the environment's impact on health; at that time, they were doing so, encouraged by both federal and provincial health authorities as well as university departments, which also were beginning to investigate these phenomena. Not surprisingly, the use of disciplinary powers, to attempt to enforce the status quo and prevent innovation based on well-supported patient-centered approaches, impeded the developments in environmental health in this country.

This current investigation into the treatment of Chronic Lyme disease is understandably having a chilling effect again, this time on those few doctors in Canada who are Lyme disease-literate and face these seriously ill patients daily, like I do.

The denial of MCS began in 1989 when the CPSO started its first inquiry and subsequently conducted an investigation into my diagnosis and treatment of patients with environmental and chemical sensitivity. When the disciplinary hearings began in 1994, the allegations made against me included my having recommended to my MCS patients the use of water and air filtration, eating organically grown foods to avoid pesticides, avoiding the usual toxic products used in homes and offices, not to use or be exposed to perfumes, and the use of oral and intravenous vitamin and mineral supplements for immune support, the use of acupuncture, as well as various detoxification protocols and non-invasive testing methods.

However, the CPSO's prosecution dismissed the very notion of food and environmental allergies/sensitivities as a trigger for MCS symptoms to be without scientific basis—and they were not willing to engage with the scientific publications offered by the defence. For me, the important issue was not the scientific debate, but the results my therapeutic methods achieved with very sick patients. Interestingly, during these disciplinary hearings, nearly every member of the panel was drinking bottled water.

My defence lawyers formally introduced more than 120 items of research from the standard medical literature, including more than 100 controlled studies, all in support of my diagnostic and treatment protocols, and most were part of the formal record when the trial ended. The CPSO's prosecution lawyers introduced various items from the medical literature—opinion pieces and only one single outdated and then already discredited study. Yet, the prosecution did not formally include any of even those supposedly supportive materials in the record. Consequently, the disciplinary panel did not have *any* scientific material presented by prosecution to justify their final decision on me. The supreme irony was that their unsupported decision was that my diagnostic and therapeutic methods had "no scientific merit," but were only based on *my* "beliefs."

What the CPSO's prosecution lawyers did do, however, in an apparent attempt to change that inquiry into MCS into a discussion of allergy treatment generally, was to call "expert" witnesses, who according to an affidavit filed by my lawyer on December 3, 1995, had received large grants from several international drug companies for standard allergy treatment research. Those grants had resulted in the availability of drugs which environmental medicine protocols render unnecessary when a patient's so-called allergic symptoms are shown to be induced by exposure to environmental toxins. None of those CPSO-selected experts treated MCS patients.

Today, the provinces of Quebec and Ontario have passed legislation against the cosmetic use of pesticides. Countless institutions, from banks to schools and hospitals, have no-fragrance policies. Recently, federal MPs from all three parties have had their blood tested which showed the presence of carcinogens and neurotoxins known to be present in their daily environments. Public awareness of sensitivity to food additives and toxic chemicals is now general, and the availability of green products and organic foods has become commonplace. The general understanding of what constitutes a healthy diet has dramatically improved in just one decade, and the need for some nutritional supplements is part of the general knowledge and common practice in doctors' offices and even recommended by the various Cancer Societies. Furthermore, the practice of acupuncture is now being regulated under the Regulated Health Professions Act.

In December 2000, Ontario's government passed into law the so-called "Health Freedom Bill," championed by MPP Monte Kwinter, to amend the provincial Medicine Act; this amendment was intended to protect responsible innovation in medical practice, and the bill was supported by the entire legislative assembly. (MPP Kwinter once said, "We all take our vitamins.") The passage of that bill did not stop the CPSO from reprimanding me for the diagnosis and treatment of MCS in 2002. This legislative amendment was in keeping with the 1991 legal decision known as *Brett* which protects responsible minority opinions (see detailed discussion in chapter 1).

That environmental toxins are largely causative of cancer and promote especially most chronic diseases, is information that can now be found almost daily in our media and medical textbooks. The intravenous use of vitamin C in the treatment of cancer has even become the subject of research in Canadian universities and the results have been published in our flagship publication, the *Canadian Medical Association Journal*. Indeed, it was amusing to learn that even before I was finally reprimanded in 2002 for having "failed to maintain the standard of practice," the washrooms in the CPSO building at 80 College Street in Toronto had notices advising visitors of a low no-fragrance policy for the building.

Ironically, the last day of my disciplinary hearing was also the day on which the international consensus statement on the diagnostic criteria of MCS was published. That was on June 19, 1999. I was one of the doctors who signed that statement while I was still in the discipline process intended to discredit MCS.

My family and I, as well as my patients, and many of my colleagues, had to endure an abusive process lasting 14 years, exacting a horrendous personal and financial toll; the days I spent working on my defence should have been spent treating sick people and advancing the field of environmental and nutritional medicine. The income I lost as a result of this unavoidable preoccupation with the legal process caused great hardship to my family. My children grew up basically only knowing their father involved in a huge fight to preserve his practice and defend the integrity of environmental medical practice. The legal cost of my defence exceeded $1 million and was covered almost entirely by donations from patients and like-minded friends. And all this was without any evidence of a single patient having been harmed—on the contrary: all this took place in the context of excellent patient outcome due to the protocols developed by environmental medicine practitioners and researchers internationally.

Had I not fought strenuously to defend good medicine, complementary therapies, and positive patient outcome, it would not have been safe for my colleagues to continue to offer such innovative therapies.

The CPSO's case against me ended in 2002 with a reprimand. The penalty finding stated that *"While [Dr. Krop] may hold strong beliefs in the appropriateness of his diagnostic methods [on MCS], his diagnostic conclusions, and his methods of treatment, he must make it clear to his patients that they are simply that—beliefs. He must be candid in stating that they are unsupported by scientifically-acceptable evidence."* This finding was based on the panel's opinion, regardless of the fact that no published scientific evidence to support this opinion was provided by the prosecution.

Less than five years later, the Canadian Human Rights court ruled in 2007 that MCS is not only real, but also that Canadians are entitled to be appropriately treated for it and be accommodated in the workplace as may be necessary.

Today, the issue of contention is *Chronic Lyme* disease for the diagnosis and treatment of which the CPSO has been investigating me. This time, my competence in the treatment of Lyme and tick-borne diseases is being questioned because I recognize, diagnose, and treat *Chronic* Lyme disease. Again, the fact that I am trained by ILADS and maintain my professional education with them appears to be irrelevant to the CPSO.

The regulatory authorities are, however, only part of the problem. There is currently in Canada no unified policy on this threat to public health. Nearly every province has a Lyme patients' support group working to raise awareness about the urgency of this problem with their ministries of health and with the public. A patient-centered national policy is urgently needed so that prompt attention is paid by all medical authorities to this rising epidemic and services become available rapidly.

As will be explained later, the government's required testing is so flawed as to conceal the true scale of this epidemic. This deficient testing has therefore also delayed the availability of appropriate treatment and study. Corrective action with regard to testing or X-rays used in other conditions has been taken in other provinces when the need arose; corrective action must be taken for Lyme disease.

My decision to make this matter public is based on my conviction that only with wide-spread public awareness can medical practice be freed from the sometimes misguided influence of our medical regulatory system, which is neither patient-centered, nor apparently aware of the public health implications of their policies and practices. The CPSO's current actions suppress progress with regard to the availability of accurate testing and effective treatments for Lyme disease. Patients are suffering unnecessarily. I am also deeply concerned about Canada's blood supply; this country has been through such a trauma once before and we know how to avoid it this time—or we ought to know.

Lyme disease is the fastest growing vector-borne disease in North America and Europe. Strangely, concerted efforts exist, especially in North America, to avoid facing the fact of this epidemic. However, as awareness has increased over the past few years, several jurisdictions have passed legislation or regulation to protect doctors treating Chronic Lyme disease using long-term antibiotic therapy and promoting education and research. (See material appended to chapter 1.) In Canada, our national medical journal, the CMAJ published important facts on Lyme disease and its prevalence in Canada as long ago as May of 2000 which has been largely ignored. In contrast, veterinarians will acknowledge freely that Lyme disease is endemic throughout Canada and consequently, as cats, dogs, and horses become victims of Lyme disease in both its acute and chronic forms, veterinarians are better informed about it and treat it far more effectively in their animal patients than most medical doctors do—or can—in human beings. I was not too surprised when the medical inspector, chosen by the CPSO to evaluate my treatment of Chronic Lyme patients, turned out to be an IDSA-affiliated infectious disease expert who is on record publicly, doubting that *Chronic* Lyme disease exists and denying the wide-spread presence of Lyme-infected ticks in Canada; he stated that people who think they have Chronic Lyme disease, "probably have something else."

In 2002, I first became aware that Lyme disease had long-term chronic consequences for the human population when not diagnosed and treated adequately in its acute form. Doctors tend to remember more vividly those patients whom they could not help as fully as they had hoped to. In over three decades of medical practice I have seen thousands of chronic conditions related to toxic environmental exposures. Most of them I helped, but I could not forget those severe, chronic, and outright bizarre symptoms in those patients I was unable to help. I realized that in some of my MCS patients there appeared to be something else at work, besides the clearly identifiable and measurable sensitivities to environmental toxins. Their immune systems were fighting something else *as well*. Eventually, my search for a solution for the problems these patients continued to face, led me to a conference on Lyme disease, and so I joined the International Lyme and Associated Diseases Society (ILADS) and obtained training and certification in diagnosing and treating Chronic Lyme disease. I re-checked some of those previous patients who had not responded fully to the treatment I had offered as long ago as 20 years, and to my surprise their tests were positive for Lyme. I now began to understand some of those previous treatment failures.

I learned through ILADS that many chronic, degenerative diseases can be caused by the tick-borne pathogen *Borrelia burgdorferi* but are misdiagnosed and incorrectly treated due to a lack of knowledge about this specific pathogen, its co-infections, the failure to use Lyme-specific appropriate testing, and not knowing how to interpret the results. Treating my first patient successfully for Chronic Lyme—which took four years—was so very difficult in part because she had been very ill for many years and also because of the near-total lack of knowledgeable collegial support; there were at that time no doctors in Ontario that I know of who knew how to treat Chronic Lyme disease. As a result, I consulted extensively with an experienced Lyme-literate medical doctor in the U.S.A. and continued attending conferences.

I am always extremely happy to see my patients regain their health and resume functioning lives. That is what it is to be a doctor. It is absolutely thrilling to observe especially very sick people get back to health. That is why I am so fiercely angry, because I know there are so many desperate patients who through their own careful research suspect they have Chronic Lyme, but they cannot get the treatment they need in Canada. In fact, they cannot even get the appropriate testing! Worst of all, their concerns are dismissed out of hand by their doctors, and even the specialists to whom they are referred, who tell them time and again: "There is no Lyme disease in Canada." For patients suspecting they are sick with Lyme disease it is nearly impossible to find a Lyme-literate doctor in this country. Should one of such patients manage to get confirmatory test results for Lyme from a US-based or European laboratory, they will find to their amazement that their Canadian doctors will generally reject these results and tell them, for example: "You don't have Lyme, you have Multiple sclerosis." Not being trained to deal with Lyme disease, doctors don't generally know that its chronic form can mimic multiple sclerosis to perfection.

Indeed, Lyme disease has been dubbed in the medical literature "the Great Imitator." Many patients who have been diagnosed with chronic fatigue syndrome, Fibromyalgia, one of the many forms of arthritis, Multiple Sclerosis, scleroderma, Crohn's disease, Lou Gehrig's, depression, some forms of schizophrenia and autism, and many other illnesses of so-called "idiopathic" (unknown) origin, can have their symptoms reversed through early and accurate investigation and treatment for the identifiable, persistent infections that may be the actual cause of their illness. I have personally treated patients who have consulted me with established diagnoses of Multiple sclerosis and who, upon further investigation and testing, turned out to be positive for Lyme. With appropriate antibiotic treatment they threw away their canes and returned to a normal life. In fact, scientific literature reports that about 50% of people with MS are positive for Lyme Borreliosis.

Why should the ignorance and arrogance of some members of the medical establishment deny these patients treatment that could return them to health? There are several reasons for this situation.

The first problem is that there is a controversy among doctors in North America over the existence of *Chronic* Lyme disease. How many patients have been consigned to life-long, disabling illness, as a result of this deplorable spat among doctors, can only be imagined. Patients treated for Lyme with a 2–4 week therapy protocol, prescribed by a doctor who is willing to ignore persisting symptoms, are denied further antibiotic treatment as a result of the doctrine that long-term infection with the Lyme spirochete, *Borrelia burgdorferi,* and associated tick-borne pathogens, is rare or nonexistent, and that the range of persistent symptoms is probably from an autoimmune reaction and not from chronic infection—never mind the observable facts, which can in most cases be verified by laboratory tests (not necessarily those available in Canada, though).

Orthodoxy has decreed that "true" Lyme patients must have evidence of a tick bite and the classic rash—which actually fewer than 50% of patients, later proven to have Chronic Lyme disease, are able to recall. Furthermore, they are expected to have been in an area known to be endemic for Lyme-carrying ticks, even though ticks are not the only mode of transmission. Unless these conditions are met, Lyme disease is rarely considered by doctors adhering to this orthodoxy as part of a differential diagnosis when the patient presents with symptoms consistent with Lyme disease.

The second problem is that most doctors are not aware of the connection between many chronic degenerative diseases and a possible underlying Lyme spirochete infection. This lack of education is a strange characteristic of the world of Lyme, which is actually a rather classic infectious disease and should be easily understood, given the long history supporting infectious disease research. The other infamous spirochetal bacterium causes syphilis, a disease medicine has learned how to handle very well, and its victims often also need long-term antibiotic treatment which is known to be successful. There, are in fact, a total of seven human spirochetal diseases and all share a characteristic set of similarities, including the necessity of long-term antibiotic treatment in certain cases.

The third problem is that the ELISA or EIA tests available in Ontario, which are covered by OHIP, are diagnostically unreliable and misleading due to the preponderance of false negative results. The provision of the ELISA test is based on the recommendations of the Canadian Public Health Laboratory Network Guidelines of 2007, which apply in all Canadian provinces; these are themselves based on the now discredited 2006 IDSA guidelines. Public laboratories here do not inform doctors that a negative test does not exclude Lyme disease, as those labs in other countries do whose results are reliable. However, regardless of tests, Lyme is first and foremost a clinical diagnosis. Nor can an Ontario-based doctor order further confirmatory tests in Canada if the patient's ELISA test was negative, so our system effectively rules out Lyme patients and, therefore, can maintain the fiction that Lyme is rare in Canada. Appropriate testing is simply not available, unless the patient is willing to have them done outside Canada at considerable personal expense. Then, of course, the next problem arises: how to find a Lyme-literate doctor in Canada. There are very few of us.

Lyme Disease became politicized in the U.S.A. when it reached epidemic proportions. I refer the reader to the detailed discussion and appended documents in chapter 1. Within this background of controversy, the CPSO commenced its present investigation into my practice. Meanwhile, I get phone calls every day from patients across the country who are desperate for treatment. This delay is unacceptable because the illness becomes much more difficult and expensive to treat. Most patients have to travel to those parts of the U.S.A. where Lyme disease doctors are not as persecuted as in other areas. Some travel to Europe, where, especially in Germany, Lyme disease is treated generally more appropriately.

Medical doctors across Canada are refusing to become involved with Chronic Lyme patients at all, for fear of investigation by their provincial College of Physicians and Surgeons. Some try to offer whatever help they can, but do so quietly and under the radar as long as possible. Patients struggling with serious health conditions do not want to be "protected" from access to well-documented therapies practiced with good verifiable results in other jurisdictions. They find that unacceptable, as do I. We have now reached a situation in Canada, where Lyme patients are protective of their Lyme-literate doctors and tend to be reluctant to use their names publicly in order to shield them from coming to the attention of their regulatory bodies.

In my native Poland, I lived for many years under the power of a police state where people lived in fear and they were encouraged to report on each other. I immigrated in 1972 to Canada, never dreaming I would be subjected twice to similar tactics here, and by my own medical authorities. Today, a system of fear is contaminating medicine, and doctors cannot necessarily treat patients according to the very best available knowledge.

The solution to this Lyme disease epidemic is simple: make proper testing available to doctors and only they—not laboratory technicians—must be able to decide which tests to order, because the testing methods are still evolving, doctors and the public must be educated about this disease and its many manifestations, especially about the many illnesses it mimics; testing for Lyme infection must become part of every routine differential diagnosis when suspecting a standard chronic disease; it is imperative to start a public awareness campaign so appropriate preventive action can be taken against this epidemic. In general, doctors everywhere are understandably preoccupied with the diagnosis and treatment of acute infectious disease; they are not provided with sufficient information to enable them to appreciate the chronic forms of infection of which there are many more besides Chronic Lyme, such as cell-deficient organisms also called stealth infections.

Medical science developed the tools for dealing with infectious disease epidemics over the past 150 years. We know how to do this right. Above all, we cannot permit that scientific advance is simply ignored. Our professional oath demands that, first we consider the well-being of the patient.

The advent of environmental medicine and Chronic Lyme disease were new challenges offered to medicine, but theoretically they were predictable. New medical conditions must be assumed to emerge from time to time. Bacteria, viruses and other pathogens are known to respond and adapt with great rapidity, to their own advantage, in changing host circumstances. The novel observations of doctors will always be the starting point for any advance in medicine, and this requires respect and encouragement, not denial. A helpful and effective regulatory system ought to promote innovation and protect creativity. As Justice O'Leary observed in the Brett decision in 1991: "If it be misconduct to use methods and techniques that are foreign to or disapproved of by the vast majority in the profession, the profession might never progress."

■

Postscript

In October 2009, I attended the annual ILADS conference in Washington DC. I witnessed a miracle when I met the young woman who is at the centre of the heart-wrenching documentary film "Under Our Skin—There is No Medicine for Someone Like You" referenced below. She was attending the conference and was totally cured. As the event progressed, I witnessed the second miracle as one of the speakers walked to the podium unaided by crutches or a wheelchair. It was Dr. Dave Martz, also featured in that same documentary and in more detail in Pamela Weintraub's book on Lyme in the USA (see below). He was originally an oncologist and now is a leading expert in Lyme disease and a member of ILADS. Diagnosed with ALS (Lou Gehrig's disease), he suffered from this progressive and debilitating illness for many years. He has now completely regained his health and the use of his body after successful, if lengthy, treatment for Chronic Lyme disease.

Examples of Testing for Lyme Disease in Ontario and the USA—on the same Patients

No 1: Patient B—The **Ontario Public Health Laboratory Report** of July 2005 shows, on the basis of the ELISA test, which was negative that there was supposedly "no evidence of infection."

In August (one month later) the **IGeneX and the USA's Centre For Disease Control** report that the patient ***does*** have Lyme and further states, at the bottom of each sheet of that report, that the "*diagnosis should not be based on laboratory tests alone. Results should be interpreted inconjunction with clinical symptoms and patient history*." The Ontario test neglected to state this, thereby causing a serious interpretive problem for Ontario physicians untrained in diagnosing Lyme Disease. Had this patient not been re-tested in the US, no treatment would likely have been the result, especially since most doctors in Ontario do not know that the diagnosis and treatment choice must first and foremost be dictated by the patient's symptoms and the entire clinical picture. This patient would then have most likely proceeded to be ill with Chronic Lyme Disease.

No 2: Patient H—The **Ontario Public Health Laboratory Test** Report of September 2003 indicates the presence of infection based on the ELISA test. Western blot confirmation was automatically performed. It was negative. Without physican consultation, the case was dismissed as negative. No further tests are permitted.

In June of 2007, ***4 years later***, when this patient finally was able to get a doctor to re-test because of debilitating symptoms, the **IGeneX and CDC** test reports confirm the clinical picture by showing the presence of Lyme. This case had by now progressed to the chronic state, which could have been avoided through proper education and a wider choice of tests and more timely re-testing years earlier.

Note: There is no other test available in Ontario to assist in treatment choice if the clinical symptoms and patient history compel the physician to treat the patient for Lyme Disease. Numerous tests exist which are more sensitive than the ELISA and Western blot—but they are not available in Ontario. The medical training in Lyme Disease is also available for doctors in the US and Europe, but not in Canada. Recently, the CDC in the US changed its testing requirements to make the ELISA optional, but Canada has not taken note.

Sources and Recommended Reading

Ashford, N., MD & Miller, C., MD. *Chemical Exposures: Low Levels and High Stakes*, second edition, Van Nostrand Reinhold, 1998.

This is the classic book on the evolution of environmental medicine in North America. The Ontario and federal governments' involvement in the initial population-based research on environmentally induced illness is also discussed. My practice served as one of the index practices for these investigations

Banerjee, S.N. et al. Presence of spirochete causing Lyme disease, *Borrelia burgdorferi*, in the blacklegged tick, *Ixodes scapularis*, in southern Ontario. CMAJ, May 30, 2000, vol. 162 (11) p. 1567-1569. Also see editorial in this issue on Lyme disease and its potential as an epidemic.

Canadian Human Rights Commission Report on Environmental Sensitivities, May 2007

Part I: M.E. Sears, *The Medical Perspective on Environmental Sensitivities*

Part II: C. Wilkie & D. Baker, *Accommodation for Environmental Sensitivities: Legal Perspective* (Download from the website of the Canadian Human Rights Commission)

Canadian Medical Association Journal (the CMAJ is free on-line) series on environmental medicine, vol. 166, nos. 8-13, 2002

Ferrie, H., *Multiple Chemical Sensitivity—A Report Prepared for the Ministry of Human Resources, Government of Canada*, October 2003. Download from www.mcs-global.org/technicalpapers

Ferrie, H. *Dispatches from the War Zone of Environmental Health—Information from the Files of A Medical Science Reporter*, KOS, 2004

Ferrie, H. *What Part of No! Don't They Understand? rescuing Food and Medicine from Government Abuse: A Manifesto*, KOS 2008

Both these books can be downloaded for free from www.kospublishing.com; they contain several articles about my case and other doctors who had similar experiences

Glasnost—A Report to the Government and the People of Ontario Prepared by Doctors and Patients, 2001

Several medical associations and patient support groups compiled the then available information on doctors who were being prosecuted by the College of Physicians and Surgeons of Ontario in order to enforce standards of practice that were not in accord with the available scientific literature. The submission had stakeholder status in the government's 2001-2004 mandatory review of the Regulated Health Professions Act. My case is featured in this report. Download the report from www.freedomofchoiceinhealthcare.ca/Articles/GlasnostReport

Glover, W.A. et al., Insights into the Molecular Basis of L-Form Formation and Survival in *Escherichia coli*, *PLoS ONE* vol. 4(10), December 2009

Kilburn, K. H., *Chemical Brain Injury*, Van Nostrand, 1998.

The editor-in-chief the of *Archives of Environmental Health* summarizes the effects of environmental toxins on brain development and central nervous system function.

Krop, J. MD. *Healing the Planet One Patient At A Time—A Primer in Environmental Medicine,* KOS (2002) third edition 2008

Krop, J. MD. (French translation of the above) *Peril Chemique: Gare A Vous! Une premiere en medicine environmentale,* Les Editions Le Mieux-Etre, 2006

Krop, J. MD. (Polish) *Ratujmy sie—elementarz medycyny ekologicznej,* Oficyna Wydawniczo-Poligraficzna, 2007

Krop, J. MD. Submission to the World Commission on Environment and Development, *Our Common Future*, Oxford, 1987

Moriarty, T. J. et al, Real-Time High Resolution 3D Imagining of the Lyme Disease Spirochete Adhering to and Escaping from the Vasculature of a Living Host, *PLoS Pathogens*, vol. 4 (6) June 2008

Moynihan, R. & Cassels, A.. *Selling Sickness*, Nation Books, 2004.

Useful information on the interference of corporate and regulatory authorities in the practice of medicine and the research on which it is based.

"Multiple Chemical Sensitivity: a 1999 consensus," *Archives of Environmental Medicine*, Vol. 54(3)-147-149 (US National Institutes of Health publication)

Nicolson, G. L. , MD, et al. Chronic Fatigue Syndrome patients subsequently diagnosed with Lyme Disease Borrelia burgdorferi: evidence for Mycoplasma species co-infections, *Journal for Chronic Fatigue Syndrome*, vol. 14 (4):5-17, 2008

Nicolson, G.L., MD, Chronic infections in neurodegenerative and neurobehavioral disease, *Laboratory Medicine,* vol. 38 (5):291-299, 2008

Padayatty, S.J. et al. Intravenously administered vitamin C as cancer therapy: three cases. CMAJ, March 28, 2006, vol. 174 (7)—937-942

Radetsky, P., *Allergic to the Twentieth Century—The Explosion in Environmental Allergies: From Sick Buildings to Multiple Chemical Sensitivity*, Little, Brown & Co., 1997. One of the first books to provide an overview of the emerging problem of MCS in which the pioneering work of many of my colleagues from the American Academy of Environmental Medicine is described.

Randolph, T., *Environmental Medicine—Beginnings & Bibliographies of Clinical Ecology*, Clinical Ecology Publications1987. This is the essential, classic book describing the evolution of clinical practice, diagnosis and treatment for environmental illness by its pioneer, Dr. Randolph from the University of Chicago.

Schmid, G.P., Epidemiology and clinical similarities of human spirochetal diseases, *Review of Infectious Disease*, Vol. 11, Suppl. 6:S1460f, Sept.–Oct. 1989

Smith, R. & Lourie, B., *Slow Death by Rubber Duck—How the Toxic Chemistry of Everyday Life Affects Our Health*, Knopf, 2009. An up-to-date summary of environmentally linked illness in Canada.

"Under Our Skin—There is No Medicine for Someone Like You," a documentary film by Andy Abrahams Wilson, Open Eye Pictures, 2008, The DVD version is available from www.underourskin.com The film was nominated for an Oscar.

Weintraub. P., *Cure Unknown—Inside the Lyme Epidemic*, St. Martin's Press, 2009.

The currently definitive analysis of the medical politics of Lyme disease in America. This is a goldmine of medical references.

The so-called "Health Freedom Bill" or "Kwinter Bill" of the year 2000 states in Section 5.1 of the *Medicine Act* of Ontario: "A member [of the medical profession] shall not be found guilty of professional misconduct or of incompetence under sections 51 and 52 of the Health Professions Procedural Code solely on the basis that the member practices a therapy that is non-traditional or that departs from the prevailing medical practice, unless there is evidence that proves that the therapy poses a greater risk to a patient's health than the traditional or prevailing practice."

See *Hansard*, Ontario Government, October 5, 2009, submissions by myself and others on the proposed bill 179.

■

Krop Clinic Folks—Thanx!

By Louise Robillard, 2006

I dial the phone, you fit me in,
You're at the door when I walk in (Charlene)
You smile and say, enjoy your stay,
Before I leave, you make me pay! (Maria)

And when the girls aren't in their chair,
You fill the empty space left there (Mrs.Krop)
I'm eating so much better too,
My diet changed, it's thanx to you (Maya).

A zing, a beep, with all of that
You tell me where my Lyme is at (Wanda)
It may be dogs or may be trees
You tell me 'bout my allergies (Usha).

You squeeze, your prod, sometimes you poke
And what you're blowing ain't no smoke! (Elizabeth)
You hit your mark with expertise,
Blood flows, you say, ""I aim to please!" (Victor)

When all is done, I come to you (Dr. Krop)
You tally up the old, the new,
You set a protocol or two,
You tell me what I next should do.

Yes, Dr. Krop, without you there,
Like many more, I would despair,
Because for very long, you see,
I knew not what was wrong with me.

Through you, I now know it is Lyme,
I also know it will take time,
I know the challenge that I face,
I know the path that I must trace.

And stronger every day I grow,
And yes, each of those days I know,
That every morning when I wake,
It's a step forward that I take.

Your guidance is what pulls me through,
I'll make it now, because of you,
And all the rest of your team too,
Thank you, thank you, thank you ... THANK YOU!

A CHRONIC LYME DISEASE PATIENT'S PERSPECTIVE

8

By Karin Klouman

I am healthy and it seems like a miracle. My mind is working, I do not tremble and shake, nor do I stumble and fall and I no longer have episodes of those excruciating pain-attacks that used to keep me bed-ridden for weeks. I do not look like a skeleton anymore. In fact, many people in our little community will frequently cross the street in town to say they are amazed to see me looking so well. I tell my neighbours and my friends that I have finally beaten Lyme disease. However, I also explain that although I eventually received the medical treatment I needed, many people in Canada still do not get help, and in future even fewer might, given the currently prevalent health policy in Canada with regards to Chronic Lyme Disease.

My story is not unique, but follows the same path as most Chronic Lyme sufferers'. My health declined steadily, over 9 long years. During this time many well-meaning physicians offered various diagnoses and ordered subsequent treatments, but none of those measures helped. I myself had never heard of Lyme disease and none of the doctors I saw asked me if I had been in tick country.

By 2002 my health had deteriorated so severely that I was basically non-functional. Then finally, one doctor arrived at the diagnosis of Chronic Lyme disease through careful evaluation of all my multi-symptom complaints and by ordering numerous laboratory tests, some of which had to be sent out of the country.

Living In Hell With Undiagnosed Chronic Lyme Disease

In September of 1993 I attended a National Golden Retriever dog-show near Albany, New York. I had driven there with my husband, children, and dogs from Shelburne, Ontario. We took our dogs hiking through the surrounding bush during this visit. Shortly after returning home, I developed a high fever, a generalized hot-burning rash and a very sore throat. The result of a throat swab came back as negative for streptococcus and so I thought I had just contracted "the flu." One of my dogs that had competed in Albany at this time also started having health issues and after we arrived back at home I spent several days picking ticks off him.

In the following months, my flu-like symptoms mysteriously kept recurring. However, apart from those days, I managed to carry on with my busy life. Since I was otherwise healthy, I did not suspect that anything could be seriously wrong. As time went on, however, it became increasingly more difficult to ignore that my health was deteriorating. I had now also begun to have profuse menstrual bleeding and thus became anaemic. My joints were aching and I was experiencing increasingly frequent migraine attacks. I also had developed recurring, oozing skin lesions and a troublesome essential tremor.

Then, in early 1995, I came down with another feverish, flu-like episode. This one was especially frightening, since it was accompanied by vivid hallucinations. I initially thought this incident had been caused by the high fever, however, in the following weeks more such episodes occurred. When I was not "seeing" things, I was "hearing" music playing in my head. I also began experiencing severe insomnia.

I consulted my family doctor who diagnosed me as being severely depressed and prescribed antidepressants. However, the various medications that I tried over the next months did not help. Whenever I tried to discuss my increasingly serious health issues with my family doctor, she dismissed these concerns. I was told that if I just stayed on the antidepressants, I would "soon" also begin to feel physically better. However, my extremely heavy, long menstrual periods could no longer be ignored. So, in June of 1996, I had a hysterectomy. Following the surgery I suffered a significant pulmonary embolism and I spent several weeks in the hospital.

At this time I started seeing a psychotherapist, who is also a medical doctor and had an interest in the mind-body connection. It helped to have somebody to talk to who validated that I had serious health issues. By this time I suspected that the cocktail of anti-depressants, sedatives, and sleeping medications might be harmful, so I stopped taking all these drugs in late 1996, having also been encouraged to do so by my therapist.

My neurological problems, however, intensified at an alarming rate. My tremor had become very noticeable and I could not control my intense shaking. I also suffered from bizarre episodes of numbness in my face and limbs. I next began to stumble and occasionally I also fell. My migraine attacks were becoming stroke-like in intensity, as I frequently lost the ability to speak and even see. These headaches were always accompanied by severe neck-pain. My painful joints were also becoming a serious issue and I was beginning to suffer from intense attacks of Fibromyalgia. Furthermore, there were recurring oozing skin lesions which became especially troublesome. Sometimes, I also suffered from a generalized burning rash that would suddenly appear and then equally suddenly disappear, within minutes.

In 1998 I started having severe back pain, and one day I put my back right out. Again I consulted the family doctor, who was more interested in finding out how I was coping with my depression. She dismissed my concerns about my back as well as my serious kidney stone attacks and only acknowledged both problems as real when they had been definitively diagnosed at the hospital emergency department. I consulted an orthopaedic surgeon and was immediately operated on for a severely herniated disc.

Meanwhile, despite years of therapy, I was still frequently hallucinating and although I knew that these were not reality-based events, I was still becoming very anxious. I was also experiencing scary moments of complete cognitive dysfunction. Having always been an articulate person, words were now escaping me, in mid-conversation. I started having difficulties writing coherently and I forgot how to spell even simple words. Sometimes, I inexplicably could not recall my children's names. At other times, I suddenly could not understand how to use a phone. Next, driving became difficult, since I had problems interpreting basic traffic signs. I decided to stop driving, after I once came to a traffic-light and had no idea what the *green* light meant.

By the year 2000, I had almost stopped consulting my family-doctor for the myriad of health issues that were plaguing me. Instead, I asked my psychotherapist if he could refer me to an environmental doctor that I had heard about. I was in desperate shape when I met Dr. Jozef Krop for the first time.

On my initial appointment, in the summer of 2000, Dr Krop took a most exhaustively detailed history, followed by what seemed to be a myriad of tests which showed that I suffered from a severe mould-allergy, *Candida albicans* overgrowth, mercury toxicity, and multiple food intolerances. He also discovered that I was suffering from several chemical sensitivities. All these findings made sense because they were confirmed by daily experience and I took steps to limit exposure to the various toxic environmental triggers. However, I still did not get much better.

The next crisis occurred when I was hospitalized for stomach pains, caused by a partial obstruction. I was then diagnosed with Crohn's disease, but the medication prescribed caused many severe side-effects, including haemorrhaging. I was becoming very weak with chronic anaemia and I therefore stopped those medications. Instead, I tried to control this condition by diet, but only with limited success: I was now losing weight at an alarming rate. Yet another health problem now began to appear: I started having episodes of very rapid heart-beat, combined each time with a drastic fall in blood pressure.

My multi-system health-issues were bewildering, both to myself as well as to the many physicians I had seen over several years. Dr. Krop was the only doctor that did not give up; he continued to take careful note of all my complaints, asking lots of questions and always running more tests, saying he was certain there must be *something* we were missing.

A Controversial Diagnosis

In the spring of 2002 Dr. Krop finally asked me a pivotal question:" *Have you ever been bitten by a tick?*" I answered that, to my knowledge, this had happened once: in my teenage years, I had found a tick attached to me when I lived in East Africa. Dr. Krop next wanted to know exactly when my health had started to deteriorate so drastically and I remembered my recurring flu-like episodes, which had started shortly after that trip to Albany, in 1993. He then asked: "*Could you have been exposed to ticks there*?" I then clearly recalled the hikes through the bush, wearing summer clothes and open-toed sandals. I also remembered how one of my dogs had fallen ill and that I had removed numerous ticks from him.

Now I was finally tested for Lyme disease. The Canadian ELISA result came back positive for the tick-borne organisms *Erlichia* (now *Anaplasma*) and *Babesia*; this was then followed up with a positive Bowman antigen test for *Borellia.* Later on, I also had repeated positive *Borrelia* Western Blot results. To my astonishment I learned, however, that OHIP would not cover any of the further laboratory work, beyond the first ELISA screening. To diagnose this well-known infectious disease I had to pay well over one thousand dollars out of my own pocket. I found this quite disturbing, especially since the *Canadian Medical Association Journal* had, starting in the late 1990s, already identified Lyme disease to be of urgent concern in this country.

I was, however, still very lucky, in that my very first blood test indicated the presence of *two* tick-borne organisms. The findings of both *Erlichia* and *Babesia* indicated that l might, therefore, also be infected by *Borrelia burgdorferi*, the causative agent for Lyme disease. It is a well-documented fact that the same ticks often carry all three organisms. Today, however, the only screening test for Lyme in Canada is a simple ELISA test that *only* looks for evidence of *Borrelia burgdoferi* and does not consider any of the other tick-borne organisms to be of importance. Therefore, the vast majority of Lyme patients in Canada remain undiagnosed, since the ELISA test is known to be notoriously unreliable as a screening test for *Borrelia* alone.

Dr. Krop was now able to make sense of everything he had learned and told me that I had the clinical signs of Chronic Lyme disease. However, I still needed more information and began investigating the various opinions on the diagnosis of Lyme disease, as well as the different schools of thought regarding the best treatment for this condition. I must add, that Dr. Krop very clearly informed me of the potential dangers of long-term antibiotic treatment that he recommended.

I knew nothing about Lyme and being a rather cautious person I did not immediately accept the recommended course of treatment. Given my many years of experience with doctors and severe illness, the next weeks were, therefore, spent reading all the medical papers I could locate on Lyme disease. It was both an enormous relief and a complete shock to repeatedly recognize my own symptoms in the Lyme literature.

In August of 2002 I again collapsed, with excruciating neck and head pain. I could not open my eyes, nor move my neck and I had developed the usual oozing lesions, all over my face. I was rushed to the local hospital where the seriousness of my condition was recognized and I was pumped full of morphine.

Despite my repeated requests, the hospital refused to confirm Dr. Krop's Lyme diagnosis by ordering the appropriate tests, justifying this by insisting that *"We do **not** have Lyme in Canada."* The basic (and in this case inappropriate) blood-work showed normal values and the hospital doctors concluded that I must have "a virus." Heavily drugged, I spent many days in hospital and thereafter was sent home with orders to take strong pain killers as needed.

By this time I had no doubt that Dr. Krop had arrived at the correct diagnosis, especially as I was now able to compare his thorough investigation, his painstakingly long interviews and multiple blood-tests with the hospital's astonishing opinion that *there is no Lyme in Canada,*—and so I drew my own conclusion.

At this time, I had also been referred to an infectious disease-specialist. After one interview this doctor wrote a letter, agreeing that I fit the clinical picture of Lyme disease. Later, however, the one and only blood-test he had ordered came back negative. Strangely, based exclusively on this, the specialist concluded that I did *not* have Lyme disease. He chose to dismiss all the other positive results, which had been obtained from standard Canadian *and* US laboratories. I simply could not accept his opinion. This specialist had only seen me for a few minutes, and the clinical interview as well as the physical examination had been performed by a medical student. Furthermore, after only one blood-test, he appeared to disregard my complex, multi-system clinical picture which was so thoroughly documented. He also provided me with absolutely no alternative answers for why I was so ill.

All I had learned about Lyme, which included the official information from Health Canada as well as many published reports from the US Centers for Disease Control, had taught me that this is a difficult diagnosis to make. Multiple factors, the most important one being the *clinical history* of the patient, must be taken into account. The consensus is that *any* laboratory tests (ELISA, EIA, Antigen capture, Western Blots), although *helpful*, must never be the sole criteria for a Lyme disease diagnosis.

Treatment and Recovery—Not For the Faint-hearted

Before treatment commenced, I was fully aware that there are two very different, well-recognized protocols for treating Lyme disease within the scientific medical community:

There is one medical opinion, put forward by the Infectious Disease Society of America (IDSA), which recommends only a few short weeks of antibiotics. This school of thought believes that any long-term symptoms which might linger, after a relatively short-term antibiotic treatment, are due to something called "post-Lyme syndrome" and *not* a result of a lingering and persistent infection. As I researched this approach, I also found out that it was the opinion most strongly supported by the medical insurance industry.

The other school of thought, represented by the International Lyme and Associated Diseases Society (ILADS), was the one Dr. Krop recommended. This treatment-plan prefers a more aggressive approach by employing the use of long-term antibiotics, until all symptoms of Lyme disease have disappeared. That protocol is based on the findings of numerous Lyme experts who are all physicians working in Lyme-endemic areas. These doctors have seen most of their clients dramatically improve as a result of their long-term treatment approach, and many of their Lyme patients have also achieved "sustained remissions." I discovered that the insurance industry vigorously opposes this school of thought.

Having read numerous scientific articles about the two widely differing medical opinions regarding the treatment for Lyme, I chose to follow Dr. Krop's advice. He also started closely consulting a well-known Lyme expert in the States who remained available to advise on my treatment. I felt I was in very good hands.

Due to the various allergies and sensitivities to pharmaceutical drugs ,which I had developed over the years, effective treatment for me involved having a 'peripherally inserted central catheter' (a PICC-line) inserted at St. Joseph's Hospital, in Toronto, to enable the required long-term intravenous treatment with antibiotics. In September of 2002, I was started on a daily regimen of intravenous Doxycycline. I luckily was accepted as a patient by our local community nursing organization.

These home-care nurses provided wonderful support and were available at a moment's notice, always ready to offer advice and to help out.

After just a few short days of antibiotics I started having seizures, which I now learned was my first so-called "Herxheimer" reaction. I was rushed to the hospital, where an EEG exam showed some minor abnormalities. I also had some abnormal spikes in my liver enzyme values. The interpretation was that this was a massive "die-off" of the *Borrelia* spirochetes, which was resulting in large amounts of the associated neuro-toxins being released into the blood stream. My head and neck pain was excruciating, my sore throat returned. I was extremely ill. But then, after a few days, all the symptoms stopped as suddenly as they had started. I remained on Doxycyline and was rapidly beginning to feel much better. My blood-work showed that the liver enzyme counts had returned to normal. As treatment progressed, my Crohn's symptoms were the first to disappear. Then the brain-fog was lifting. I was not losing my words anymore in mid-sentence, and traffic signs again made perfect sense to me. My skin lesions and the mysterious rash disappeared next.

Exactly one month later I, however, experienced another ferocious Herxheimer reaction. This lasted a few days and thereafter I once more felt well. Now I also noticed that, in addition to my generally improved mental health, my joint pains were also almost gone. Another significant set-back, however, happened at this time: I suffered a pulmonary embolism, during a PICC-line change. Luckily, no major damage resulted, but I remained in hospital for some days, while my condition was monitored.

And so I very slowly crept towards recovery. The Herxheimer reactions occurred like clockwork: Every month, without fail, I became extremely sick for a few days, but after seven long months these hellish episodes also disappeared. I had now entered my first remission and the PICC-line was removed in May of 2003. I felt remarkably strong and healthy, once more.

Unfortunately this remission did not last very long: after only 6 months of feeling well *all* my symptoms recurred, and soon the intravenous antibiotic regime had to be started all over. Again, I suffered through Herxheimer reactions, but these eventually grew less intense, with each passing month.

I was prescribed a complex combination of antibiotics this time. Metronidazole, Zithromax, and Doxycyline became the mainstays of my treatment targeting the various stages of the *Borrelia* organism, as well as the *Erlichia* and *Babesia* infections. I was repeatedly treated with the antifungal drug Diflucan. All these drugs are potentially toxic to the liver, the activities of which were constantly monitored and I was prescribed for long-term use many vitamin and herbal supplements to further protect liver function. I was also on injectable Fragmin to stop any further blood clotting incidents.

Throughout this period, I always felt well looked after and was always closely followed up with routine blood tests. All indications were that, despite having severe Herxheimers, I tolerated the IV antibiotic treatment well.

During my worst Herxheimer episodes it was my doctor, Dr. Krop, who occasionally wondered if we should abort the treatment, but I absolutely refused to give up. Since I was clearly experiencing a steady improvement and could track my own progress more reliably than any outsider ever could, I was not about to throw in the towel, before the battle was fully won. I was lucky that I had a compassionate doctor who was willing to listen to the patient. Despite the seemingly endless treatment and several set-backs, I never lost hope. As time went by, I kept up with the reading and kept abreast of all the new scientific articles and medical information I could find regarding the treatment of Chronic Lyme disease. My case was undoubtedly similar to many others.

I fully understand the complexity and difficulty involved in treating this disease: the major organism that is being targeted can and *will* morph into many different forms, from the dormant cysts to the very active spirochetes.

I was on antibiotic intravenous treatments for over four years, with some remissions and short-term breaks. My last significant Herxheimer event occurred in December of 2006. Following it, we maintained intravenous antibiotic treatment for three full months, before finally ending the treatment. Since March 2007, I have not received any more antibiotic treatment.

I am still monitored closely by Dr Krop, with regular check-ups every 3 months and I have remained healthy. My debilitating neurological symptoms have all disappeared. I believe I am as "cured" as any Chronic Lyme patient can *ever* hope to be and the reward of being strong and fully functional again has been well worth the long battle it took to get my health back.

Many people in Canada, however, may never get the opportunity that I was offered due to the fundamentally irrational attitude currently prevailing in the medical community on the subject of Chronic Lyme disease. Although *my* battle has finally been won, the war against Lyme Disease in Canada is only beginning.

Canada's Lyme Disease Policy And What's Wrong With It

I am one of the very few lucky Chronic Lyme patients in Canada: I was finally correctly diagnosed and then received the appropriate treatment. Most people in the same situation as mine remain chronically ill and are never treated; they are simply not heard by the Canadian medical establishment.

I had a lot working to my advantage: I was an assertive patient who was quite certain that there was something seriously wrong with me, and I stubbornly refused to admit defeat. But most Lyme patients are so beaten down into hopelessness that they no longer have the strength to keep up this seemingly endless fight. Worst of all, most do not have the resources that became available to me:

First and foremost, I had a doctor who was willing to listen and who persistently sought the underlying cause for my escalating health problems. Dr. Krop also did not hesitate in prescribing aggressive treatment for Lyme disease, since it was based on the well-documented medical research and clinical experience gathered by many renowned Lyme experts.

Secondly, I had a fully supportive husband and children. Without the constant care and encouragement of my family, I doubt I would have had the will to pursue the long battle to get better.

Finally, I had a whole team of professionals pulling for me; in addition to my doctor and the hard-working staff at his clinic, I also had a compassionate psychotherapist supporting me with whom I could discuss my neuro-psychiatric Lyme issues, without being given a knee-jerk prescription for anti-depressants. I also had the invaluable expertise of truly dedicated home-care nurses.

However, the sad fact is that very few people in Canada have access to such an extensive support-network. This is an infectious disease—something our medical system ought to know how to handle effectively. However, most Lyme patients will likely remain permanently disabled with little or no hope of recovery. Many of the chronically ill Lyme patients in Canada will not get the opportunity of being tested correctly for Lyme disease. Our Canadian physicians, for the most part, unfortunately remain uninformed about the relatively common occurrence of Lyme disease in Canada. While our population is warned incessantly about the dangers of the "flu," and we are bombarded with information about West Nile Virus and H1N1, very little attention is paid to Lyme.

This near-total ignorance is alarming because of the clear evidence that Lyme is now becoming an emerging epidemic in North America, as identified by US government agencies, such as the Centers for Disease Control. There currently are over 28,000 new cases diagnosed annually in the US and the distribution is widespread across the continent. However, the largest incidence of Lyme is still reported from the Northeastern and North-central states, many of which border on Canada.

Indeed, the facts on Lyme in Canada are reported in the *Canadian Medical Association Journal* since the year 2000. As discussed in this book, wildlife and migratory birds carrying Lyme-causing bacteria know no borders and human cross-border travel is also common, all of which increase the opportunities for Canadians to contract Lyme disease. Yet, our doctors remain largely uninformed about Lyme disease, while there is only a most inadequate government policy in place to deal with the well-documented increasing risk of Lyme disease spreading among Canadians. Finally, Health Canada continues to downplay the impact of this disease on the population. Even though this is an infectious disease and therefore by its nature of great danger to the entire population, nothing seems to awaken our governments from their slumber of inaction. As a result, the number of undiagnosed and Chronic Lyme sufferers in Canada is growing annually.

The cost to our healthcare system and our social service networks will be huge in the years to come. It is, in my opinion, high time that the Canadian medical establishment wakes up and realizes the enormous cumulative human and monetary cost inflicted on our society by ignoring the growing incidence of Lyme disease cases.

Treating a chronically ill person with pharmaceuticals, only targeting various symptoms without getting to the underlying cause, while also having to support such a patient on long-term disability, will in the end be far more expensive to society than accurately diagnosing and treating Lyme disease.

The reported number of Lyme disease cases in Canada is likely seriously underestimated. Those few patients who finally do get some sort of clinical recognition of Lyme are often screened by only one single ELISA-antibody test, which produces mostly false negatives. Many will, therefore, be told that they do *not* have Lyme disease, when they in fact may very well be infected, but cannot have this checked correctly. The ELISA screen is used in Canada as a first-line investigative tool, even though it was originally developed for Lyme tick surveillance purposes, not for diagnosis. According to international medical opinion, this test is almost never useful by itself, due to its known tendency to produce false negatives. The ELISA is not sensitive enough to serve as an adequate screen, and there are many patients with full-blown Lyme who will test negative on ELISA, but who will still have fully diagnostically positive results on Western Blot.

The Western blot test is considered a far superior screening tool. However, this test is not available to Canadians and this, therefore, causes many patients to send their blood-work, at their own considerable expense, to US laboratories or even to Europe. Health Canada and their provincial health departments have thus abandoned our Lyme patients.

An especially alarming recent development is the current trend towards discrediting those few doctors in Canada who are willing and trained to treat Lyme patients. This is happening despite the fact that these doctors have taken the trouble to obtain this specialized training in the treatment of this disease and continuously share new information as research institutions produce it. What is now under attack is a doctor's fundamental right to use an internationally recognized and scientifically documented protocol for the diagnosis and treatment of *any* illness. What is, therefore, *also* under attack is the patient's equally fundamental right to choose a scientifically-recognized treatment for what should by now be well-understood disease. Astonishingly, more and more Lyme doctors are now threatened by disciplinary actions from their licensing authorities for following a carefully developed medical treatment that is internationally recognized.

One has to wonder if this might have anything to do with the medical insurance industry's vigorous opposition to the long-term antibiotic treatment for Chronic Lyme. We must consider such potential conflicts of interest and as patients we must be vigilant against any such trend, which contaminates the practice of good medicine.

If the practice of medicine is more and more influenced by economically powerful non-medical lobby groups (such as the insurance industry), instead of being based on the experience of those doctors who work with the ill patients, then the very fundamentals of our health-care system are threatened.

Although I am now healthy, I am deeply troubled by what the future will hold for all those other people struggling with Lyme disease in Canada. My hope is that eventually all Lyme patients in this country will be treated with the same compassionate and effective care as I was.

Recommended Sources

Joseph Burrascano. MD. *Advanced topics in Lyme disease, diagnostic hints and treatment guidelines for Lyme and other tick-borne illnesses, 16th edition,* 2008. www.ILADS.org

"Lyme disease controversy spreading across Canada," August 6, 2008. www.cbc.ca/health

Fact sheet on Lyme Disease (in public health offices) by the Canadian Institute of Public Health Inspectors. www.ciphi.ca

Columbia University Lyme Disease Research Information. www.columbia-lyme.org/index.html

Morbidity and Mortality Weekly Report, October 3, 2008, vol. 57, no SS-10, US Centre for Disease Control.

Diagnosis and appropriate treatment of Lyme and its associated diseases, International Lyme and Associated Diseases Society (ILADS) www.ILADS.org

B. A. Fallon MD, et al. A randomized, placebo-controlled trial of repeated IV antibiotic therapy for Lyme encephalopathy, *Neurology*, 70:992-1003, 2008.

The Lyme Disease Controversy; Lyme and Tick-Borne Diseases Research Center, http://www.columbialyme.org/patients/controversies.html

Brian A. Fallon, M.D., et al. Regional Cerebral; Blood Flow and Cognitive Deficits in Chronic Lyme Disease, *The Journal of Neuropsychiatry and Clinical Neurosciences*, August 2003.

Anna J. Henningson et al. Neuroborreliosis—an epidemiological, clinical, and health economical study from an endemic area in the south-east of Sweden, *Clinical Microbiology and Infection*, online pre-publication version, September 29, 2009.

BUTTERFLY

By Louise D. Marshall, 2007

The curtain fell down
I lost the light
the darkness brought
a terrible fright
for once in my life
I had to fight
for the essence
of my very life
when wellness came
I saw the light
so, so bright.
Like a butterfly
all anew
I flew away
from a big dark cocoon.

Medical Hypotheses 72 (2009) 153–156

Contents lists available at ScienceDirect

Medical Hypotheses

journal homepage: www.elsevier.com/locate/mehy

Clinical trials validate the severity of persistent Lyme disease symptoms

Daniel J. Cameron *

First Medical Associates, 175 Main Street, Mt. Kisco, New York 10549, United States

ARTICLE INFO

Article history:
Received 25 August 2008
Accepted 4 September 2008

SUMMARY

Background: Persistent Lyme Disease Symptoms (PLDS) have included fatigue, headaches, poor concentration and memory, lightheadedness, joint pain, and mood disturbances. Evidence-based guidelines committees disagree over the severity of PLDS. The 2004 International Lyme and Associated Diseases Society (ILADS) concluded that PLDS are severe. The 2006 Infectious Disease Society of America (IDSA) guidelines committee concluded that PLDS are nothing more than the "aches and pains of daily living" and an ad hoc International Lyme group concluded that PLDS are "symptoms common in persons who have never had Lyme disease."

Hypothesis: Clinical trials validate the severity of persistent Lyme disease symptoms.

Evaluation of the Hypothesis: There are 22 standardized instruments used to measure the severity of PLDS among the four published National Institutes of Health (NIH) sponsored double-blind randomized placebo-controlled trials (RCTs).

Validating the hypothesis: All four NIH sponsored RCTs validate the severity of PLDS. PLDS are as severe as symptoms seen in other serious chronic illnesses, and result in a quality of life lower than for the general population as determined by 22 standardized measures of QOL, including fatigue, pain, role function, psychopathology, and cognition. None of the four RCTs support the IDSA hypothesis that PLDS are nothing more than "the aches and pains of daily living" nor the ad hoc International Lyme group conclusion that PLDS are "symptoms common in persons who have never had Lyme disease."

Implications of the hypothesis: If the QOL of life for these patients is as poor as for patients with other serious chronic diseases, their symptoms need to be addressed by their doctors. Studies differ as to the precise cause of PLDS, the most effective treatments, and whether a cure is possible. But the fact that there is disagreement is not a license for physicians to ignore or turn away patients complaining of PLDS, or to dismiss their symptoms as purely psychosomatic. For physicians, the goal or purpose of treating PLDS should be the same as their purpose in treating other chronic illnesses that result in a poor QOL: vigorous pursuit of a cure, and where a cure proves impossible, amelioration of patients' symptoms and suffering. Even if this hypothesis fails to be apply to more than a fraction of the total Lyme disease population, this still represents a significant number of patients, and these findings could address a neglected aspect of caring for patients with Lyme disease.

Background

Persistent Lyme Disease symptoms (PLDS) have included fatigue, headaches, poor concentration and memory, lightheadedness, sleep disturbance, joint pain, and mood disturbances. Two retrospective cohorts support the need to assess PLDS. Thirty-four percent of LD patients in a massachusetts population-based retrospective cohort were symptomatic an average of 6.2 years after treatment [7]. Sixty-two percent of LD patients in a retrospective Westchester cohort were symptomatic an average of 3.2 years after treatment [8]. The cost for individuals with PLDS beyond human suffering can be estimated to be $16,199 per year for clinically defined late-stage Lyme disease in Maryland's Eastern Shore [9]. Ninety-five percent of the cost was indirect medical costs, non-medical costs, and productivity losses.

Evidence-based guidelines committees disagree on the severity of PLDS. The 2004 International Lyme and Associated Diseases Society (ILADS) guidelines committee concluded that PLDS are severe [5]. By contrast, the 2006 Infectious Disease Society of America (IDSA) guidelines committee concluded that PLDS are nothing more than "the aches and pains of daily living" [6] and an hoc international Lyme disease group concluded that PLDS are "symptoms common in persons who have never had Lyme disease "[4].

* Tel.: +914 666 4665; fax: +914 666 6271.
E-mail address: Cameron@Lymeproject.com

0306-9877/$ - see front matter © 2008 Elsevier Ltd. All rights reserved.
doi:10.1016/j.mehy.2008.09.030

Hypothesis

Clinical trials validate the severity of persistent Lyme disease symptoms.

Evaluation of the hypothesis

To be plausible, the "severity of PLDS" hypothesis should be measureable with standardized instruments. There were 22 standardized instruments used to measure the severity of PLDS among the four published NIH sponsored double-blind randomized placebo-controlled trial (RCTs) (1–3). Eleven instruments assessed QOL (1, 3), fatigue (2, 3), pain (1, 3), role function (1), and psychopathology (1, 3) of PLDS. Eleven other instruments assessed cognitive function of PLDS (1–3).

Quality of life

The Fallon and two Klempner RCTs assessed QOL using the medical outcomes study (MOS) 36-item short-form general health survey (SF-36) (1, 3). Thirty-six questions assessed the physical component summary (PCS) and mental component summary (MCS) of QOL. The PCS assessed the ability to perform daily physical activities, e. g., self care, walking, climbing stairs, and vigorous activities; degree to which individual performs typical work/daily activities; intensity, duration, and frequency of bodily pain, and limitations in usual activities due to pain; and personal evaluation of general health, including current and prior health and health outlook. The MCS assessed the personal evaluation of energy and tiredness; the ability to develop, maintain, and nurture social relationships, including family, friends and marital functioning; degree to which emotional problems limit work/daily activities; and a person's emotional, cognitive, and intellectual status.

Fatigue

The Fallon and two Klempner RCTs assessed fatigue using a reliable, well studied, modified version of the self-administered fatigue severity scale, FSS-11 [10].

Fibromyalgia Impact questionnaire

The two Klempner RCTs measured the severity of PLDS using a modified version of the fibromyalgia impact questionnaire (FIQ). The FIQ "measures difficulties with activities of daily living and symptoms of pain, fatigue, morning tiredness, stiffness, job difficulty, depression, and anxiety along with amount of work missed and overall well-being during the past week" [11].

Ability to perform usual activities

The two Klempner RCTs measured the ability to participate in daily activities using the MOS for role functioning. The role functioning scale measured limitations in daily activities including having to take frequent rests and the need for special assistance [12].

Pain

The Fallon RCT measured the McGill pain questionnaire-short-form (SF-MPQ) [13]. The SF-MPQ uses word descriptors and an intensity scale to generate a score. The words include the sensory qualities of the pain (e.g., throbbing, sharp, stabbing), the affects of the pain (e.g., sickening, blinding, grueling), the overall experience of the pain (e.g., annoying, intense, unbearable), and miscellaneous characteristics of the pain (e.g., radiating, piercing, nagging). The SF-MPQ has been used for pain assessment in patients with arthritis [12]. The Fallon RCT also measured pain using a visual analogue scale (VAS) consisting of a line 10 cm in length, with end points labeled no pain to severe pain. The patient places a mark on the line corresponding to the intensity of the pain. The two Klempner RCTs assessed the severity of pain using the MOS. 'The effect of pain was measured based on its impact on mood, walking ability, sleep, normal work, recreational activity, and life enjoyment using a 5-point Likert-type scale anchored to the frequency of symptoms" [12].

Psychological measures

The Fallon RCT assessed three psychopathology measures. The Beck Depression Inventory (BDI) is an estimate of the severity of depression [14]. The zung anxiety scale [15] is a measure of anxiety. The SCL-90 GSI is a self-reported measure of psychological distress. The SCL-90 GSI is a eight dimension measure: anxiety, agoraphobia, depression, somatic symptoms, distrust and interpersonal sensitivity, anger hostility as well as sleeping disorders [16].

Cognitive function

The Krupp RCT measured the severity of impairment of cognition using the alpha-arithmetic (A–A) Test, a reaction time task. The A–A test was considered to be a sensitive measure of cognitive impairment. Patients with Lyme disease demonstrated slower performances (i.e., greater impairment) on the A–A Test compared to healthy controls in prior studies [17]. The two Klempner RCTs assessed the severity of cognition using an MOS scale which measures problems with reasoning, concentration, confusion, forgetfulness, maintaining attention, and slowed thinking. The Fallon RCT assessed cognition using individual scales and an index based on the following six domains: "motor function (finger tapping, simple reaction time, choice reaction time), psychomotor function (Trail Making A&B; Digit Symbol), attention (Continuous Performance Test, Stroop task), memory (Buschke Selective Reminding Test [verbal memory]; Benton Visual Retention Test [visual memory]), working memory (A, Not B Logical Reasoning Test; N-Back Test), and verbal fluency (Controlled Oral Word Association Test and Category Fluency Test)" [3].

Findings from standardized testing

Quality of life

The SF-36 measure of PCS was 37.1, 33, and 35.8 for the Fallon and two Klempner RCTs respectively. For comparison, the PCS for common chronic conditions are as follows: diabetes (42), heart disease (39), sciatica (46), cancer not skin-related (41), depression (45), osteoarthritis (39), and rheumatoid arthritis (42) [18]. The mean PCS score for the general population of the United States and for the Fallon RCT is 50 and 55.9, respectively.

The SF-36 measure of MCS was 39.2, 43.4, and 46.7 for the Fallon and two Klempner RCTs respectively. For comparison, the MCS for common chronic conditions are as follows: diabetes (48), heart disease (49), sciatica (48), cancer not skin-related (49), depression (37), osteoarthritis (49), and rheumatoid arthritis (48) [18]. The mean MSC score for the general population of the United States and for the Fallon RCT is 50 and 56.2, respectively.

Fatigue

The modified version of the self-administered Fatigue Severity Scale, FSS-11 was 5.5 and 5.2 for the Krupp and Fallon RCTs respectively. Severe fatigue has been defined as an elevated score (⩾4.0) on the FSS-11 [2]. The means score for the FSS-11 was 2.1 for controls in the Fallon RCT [3].

Fibromyalgia Impact questionnaire

The fibromyalgia impact questionnaire was 47.9 for the two Klempner RCTs. The average score for the general population is 14 (1), whereas the average fibromyalgia patient scores about 50 and severely afflicted patients are usually 70-plus [19].

Ability to perform usual activities

The role functioning scale using MOS was 53.5 and 56.0 for the two Klempner RCTs. The role functioning was 44.5 and 12 for chronic tension-type headaches and the general population respectively [20].

Pain

The SF-MPQ measure of pain (13) was 11.6 in the Fallon RCT compared to 1.1 for controls. The VAS measure of pain was 5.2 compared to 0.1 for controls. The MOS measure of pain was 49.4 and 63.0 for the two Klempner RCTs. The pain was 54.3 and 13.5 for chronic tension-type headaches and controls respectively [20].

Psychological measures

All three psychopathology measures for Lyme disease patients in the Fallon RCT were worse than controls. The BDI of 12.8 for patients with PLDS was worse than the average score of l.9 for controls. The zung anxiety scale for PLDS of 49.6 showed a higher level of anxiety among Lyme patients than the scores for controls of 32.9. The SCL-90 GSI measure of psychological distress for PLDS of 63.9 was worse than the scores for controls of 42.6.

Cognitive function

The nine measures of cognitive function in the Fallon RCT were significantly worse than controls. The cognitive measure of MOS of 54.2 and 53.3 for the two Klempner RCTs was also significantly less than controls. The alpha-arithmetic (A–A) Test measure of cognitive function in the Krupp RCT of 4.1 was only mildly worse than healthy controls and less than anticipated from other Lyme disease populations [17].

Table 1
Severity of persistent Lyme disease symptoms (PLDS) for four NIH sponsored RCTs.

Study	Year	Size	Patient population	Primary outcome variable	Severity of PLDS	
					Cases	Controls
Klempner (1)	2001	78	Seropositive LD with persistent symptoms in Northeast (NE) US	SF-36 quality of life (QOL), mean (SD)		
				PCS	33.1 (9.9)	
				MCS	43.4 (11.6)	
				Medical outcome study (MOS), mean (SD)		
				Pain	49.9 (24.3)	
				Cognition	54.2 (21.5)	
				Role functioning	53.5 (33.4)	
				Fibromyalalgia impact questionnaire – FIQ, mean (SD)	58.4 (19.7)	
				Psychopathology measure, mean (SD)	11.2 (7.1)	
				Depression (BDI)		
Klempner (1)	2001	51	Seronegative LD with persistent symptoms in NE US	SF-36 QOL, mean (SD)		
				PCS	35.8 (8.6)	
				MCS	46.7 (9.7)	
				MOS score, mean (SD)		
				Pain	63.0 (21.6)	
				Cognition	53.3 (20.0)	
				Role functioning	56.0 (32.9)	
				Fibromyalalgia impact questionnaire – FIQ, mean (SD)	47.9 (15.2) 12.9 (7.2)	
				Psychopathology measure, mean (SD)		
				Depression (BDI)		
Krupp (2)	2003	55	LD with disabling fatigue in NE US	Fatigue, mean (SD)	5.7 (1.4)	
				Cognitive function, mean (SD)	4.1 (1.7)	
Fallon (3)	2007	37	LD with cognitive dysfunction NE US	Fatigue,% (SD)	5.2 (1.5)	2.1 (0.5)
				Neurocognitive results mean, (SD)		
				Motor	−0.23 (1.34)	0.58 (0.63)
				Psychomotor	−0.21 (0.75)	0.98 (0.75)
				Attention	−0.12 (0.76)	0.35 (0.85)
				Memory total	−0.75 (1.07)	0.56 (0.43)
				Buschke	−1.13 (1.33)	0.38 (0.76)
				Benton	−0.36 (1.21)	0.73 (0.46)
				Workin memory	−0.92 (1.09)	0.34 (0.69)
				Fluency	−0.73 (0.94)	0.48 (0.66)
				Index	−0.49 (0.63)	0.55 (0.40)
				SF-36 QOL, mean (SD)		
				Physical component summary (PCS)	37.1 (8.6)	55.9 (3.6)
				Mental component summary (MCS)	39.2 (11.6)	56.2 (2.9)
				Pain, mean (SD)		
				McGill	11.6 (7.8)	1.1 (2.5)
				Visual analogue scale	5.2 (3.1)	0.1 (0.2)
				Psychopathology measures, mean (SD)		
				Depression	12.8 (8.6)	1.9 (2.4)
				Anxiety (zung index)	49.6 (11.6)	32.9 (6.7)
				Global (GSI of SCL-90)	63.5 (11.5)	42.6 (7.2)

Validating the hypothesis

All four NIH sponsored RCTs validate the severity of PLDS Table 1 [5]. PLDS are as severe as symptoms seen in other serious chronic illnesses and result in a QOL lower than that of the general population as determined by 22 standardized measures (1, 3), fatigue (2, 3), pain (1, 3), role function (1), psychopathology (1, 3), and cognition [1–3]. None of the four RCTs support the IDSA hypothesis that PLDS are nothing more than "the aches and pains of daily living"(6) nor the ad hoc International Lyme group conclusion that PLDS are "symptoms common in persons who have never had Lyme disease" [4].

Implications of the hypothesis

If the QOL of life for these patients is as poor as for patients with other serious chronic diseases, their symptoms need to be addressed by their doctors. Studies differ as to the precise cause of PLDS, the most effective treatments, and whether a cure is possible. But the fact that there is disagreement is not a license for physicians to ignore or turn away patients complaining of PLDS, or to dismiss their symptoms as purely psychosomatic. For physicians, the goal or purpose of treating PLDS should be the same as their purpose in treating other chronic illnesses that result in a poor QOL: vigorous pursuit of a cure, and where a cure proves impossible, amelioration of patients' symptoms and suffering. Even if this hypothesis fails to be apply to more than a fraction of the total Lyme disease population, this still represents a significant number of patients, and these findings could address a neglected aspect of caring for patients with Lyme disease.

References

[1] Klempner MS, Hu LT, Evans J, et al. Two controlled trials of antibiotic treatment in patients with persistent symptoms and a history of Lyme disease. N Engl J Med 2001;345(2):85–92.

[2] Krupp LB, Hyman LG, Grimson R, et al. Study and treatment of post Lyme disease (STOP-LD): a randomized double masked clinical trial. Neurology 2003;60(12):1923–30.

[3] Fallon BA, Keilp JG, Corbera KM, et al. A randomized, placebo-controlled trial of repeated IV antibiotic therapy for Lyme encephalopathy. Neurology 2008;70(13):992–1003.

[4] Feder Jr HM, Johnson BJ, O'Connell S, et al. A critical appraisal of "chronic Lyme disease". N Engl J Med 2007;357(14):1422–30.

[5] Cameron D, Gaito A, Harris N, et al. Evidence-based guidelines for the management of Lyme disease. Expert Rev Anti Infect Ther 2004;2(1 Suppl):S1–S13.

[6] Wormser GP, Dattwyler RJ, Shapiro ED, et al. The clinical assessment, treatment, and prevention of lyme disease, human granulocytic anaplasmosis, and babesiosis: clinical practice guidelines by the Infectious Diseases Society of America. Clin Infect Dis 2006;43(9):1089–134.

[7] Shadick NA, Phillips CB, Logigian EL, et al. The long-term clinical outcomes of Lyme disease. A population-based retrospective cohort study. Ann Intern Med 1994;121(8):560–7.

[8] Asch ES, Bujak DI, Weiss M, Peterson MG, Weinstein A. Lyme disease: an infectious and postinfectious syndrome. J Rheumatol 1994;21(3):454–61.

[9] Zhang X, Meltzer MI, Pena CA, Hopkins AB, Wroth L, Fix AD. Economic impact of Lyme disease. Emerg Infect Dis 2006;12(4):653–60.

[10] Krupp LB, LaRocca NG, Muir-Nash J, Steinberg AD. The fatigue severity scale. Application to patients with multiple sclerosis and systemic lupus erythematosus. Arch Neurol 1989;46(10):1121–3.

[11] Burckhardt CS, Jones KD. Effects of chronic widespread pain on the health status and quality of life of women after breast cancer surgery. Health Qual Life Outcomes 2005;3:30.

[12] Kaplan RF, Trevino RP, Johnson GM, et al. Cognitive function in post-treatment Lyme disease: do additional antibiotics help? Neurology 2003;60(12):1916–22.

[13] Melzack R. The short-form McGill pain questionnaire. Pain 1987;30(2):191–7.

[14] Beck AT, Beamesderfer A. Assessment of depression: the depression inventory. Mod Probl Pharmacopsychiatry 1974;7(0):151–69.

[15] Zung WW. A rating instrument for anxiety disorders. Psychosomatics 1971;12(6):371–9.

[16] Derogatis LR, Rickels K, Rock AF. The SCL-90 and the MMPI: a step in the validation of a new self-report scale. Br J Psychiatry 1976;128:280–9.

[17] Pollina DA, Sliwinski M, Squires NK, Krupp LB. Cognitive processing speed in Lyme disease. Neuropsychiatry Neuropsychol Behav Neurol 1999;12(1):72–8.

[18] Ware JE, Kosinski M. SF-36 Physical & Mental Health Summary Scores: A Manual for Users of Version 1. 2nd ed. 1994. p. 1-238.

[19] Bennett R. The fibromyalgia impact questionnaire (FIQ): a review of its development, current version, operating characteristics and uses. Clin Exp Rheumatol 2005;23(5 Suppl 39):S154–62.

[20] Holroyd KA, Stensland M, Lipchik GL, Hill KR, O'Donnell FS, Cordingley G. Psychosocial correlates and impact of chronic tension-type headaches. Headache 2000;40(1):3–16.

Medical Hypotheses 72 (2009) 688–691

Contents lists available at ScienceDirect

Medical Hypotheses

journal homepage: www.elsevier.com/locate/mehy

Insufficient evidence to deny antibiotic treatment to chronic Lyme disease patients

Daniel J. Cameron *

First Medical Associates, Medicine, 175 Main Street, Mount Kisco, NY 10549, USA

ARTICLE INFO

Article history:
Received 5 January 2009
Accepted 7 January 2009

SUMMARY

Background: The severity, length of illness, and cost of chronic Lyme disease (CLD) have been well described. A number of oral, intravenous, and intramuscular antibiotics have been prescribed for CLD. Surprisingly few antibiotic schedules prescribed for the treatment of CLD have been evaluated in randomized double-blind placebo-controlled clinical trials (RCTs). Physicians have increasingly turned to clinical treatment guideline (CPG) panels to judge the mixed results of the evidence. Two CPG panels have looked at the evidence only to reach opposite conclusions: (1) antibiotic therapy for CLD is not effective and (2) antibiotic therapy for CLD is effective. Physicians have been advised by guideline developers to use clinical discretion in diagnosing and treating CLD. Nevertheless, many health insurers – relying exclusively upon only one CPG – have a policy of automatically denying antibiotics to CLD patients regardless of the specifics of each case or the recommendations of the patient's physician.

Hypotheses: This paper examined the eight limitations of the evidence used to conclude that antibiotics therapy for CLD is not effective in forming the following hypothesis: insufficient evidence to deny antibiotic treatment to CLD patients.

Evidence for the Hypothesis: There are eight limitations that support the hypothesis: (1) the power of the evidence is inadequate to draw definite conclusions, (2) the evidence is too heterogeneous to make strong recommendations, (3) the risk to an individual of facing a long-term debilitating illness has not been considered, (4) the risk to society of a growing chronically ill population has not been considered, (5) treatment delay has not been considered as a confounder, (6) co-infections have not been considered as a confounder, (7) the design of RCTs did not address the range of treatment options in an actual practice, and (8) the findings cannot be generalized to actual practice.

Implications of the hypotheses: This hypothesis suggests that physicians should consider the limitations of the evidence before denying antibiotic treatment for CLD. Physicians who deny antibiotic treatment to CLD patients might inform their patients that there are some clinicians who disagree with that position, and then offer to refer them for a second opinion to a doctor who could potentially present a different point of view. The hypothesis also suggests that health care insurers should consider the limitations of the evidence before adopting policies that routinely deny antibiotic treatment for CLD patients and should expand coverage of CLD to include clinical discretion for specific clinical situations.

Introduction

The number of individuals with Lyme disease (LD) continues to grow worldwide [1–3]. The number of LD cases reported each year in the US alone to the Centers for Disease Control and Prevention (CDC) nearly tripled from 1992 to 2007 to more than 27,000 [3]. The actual number of LD cases in the US has been estimated to be more than 270,000 per year assuming a 10-fold underreporting to the CDC [4]. The estimated incidence of 34,000 LD cases in Connecticut alone in 2004 was 24× the number reported to the CDC [5].

The severity, length of illness, and cost of chronic Lyme disease (CLD) have been well described. For patients who contract Lyme disease, the risk of developing CLD has been reported to be as high as 34–62% years in two cohorts after antibiotic treatment [6,7]. Onsets of illness of CLD averaged 4.7–9 years in National Institutes of Health (NIH) sponsored double-blind randomized placebo-controlled clinical trials (RCTs) [8,9]. The symptoms of CLD enrolled in RCTs were severe on all 22 standardized measures of fatigue [8,10], pain [8,11], psychopathology [8,11], cognition [8,10,11], role function [11,12], and quality of life [8,11]. The annual, average per-patient cost for CLD patients in the US has been estimated to be $1872 for direct medical costs and $14,327 for indirect medical costs, non-medical costs, and productivity losses [13].

A number of antibiotic treatments have been prescribed based on the evidence from non-placebo and comparator trials and case series for CLD including the following: (1) oral doxycycline, amoxicillin, cefuroxime, azithromycin, clarithomycin, penicillin VK [14,15], (2) intravenous ceftriaxone, cefotaxime, penicillin G [14,15], and (3) intramuscular benzathine penicillin [16]. These antibiotics have

* Tel.: +1 914 3251471; fax: +1 914 666 6271.
E-mail address: Cameron@LymeProject.com.

0306-9877/$ - see front matter © 2009 Elsevier Ltd. All rights reserved.
doi:10.1016/j.mehy.2009.01.017

been used singly or in combinations [14] or with antibiotics for co-infections such as atovaquone with azithromycin for *Babesia microti* [17]. Antibiotics have been prescribed for more than 30 days – and months if necessary – until CLD has resolved [8,14,18,19].

Surprisingly few antibiotic schedules described for the treatment of CLD have been evaluated in RCTs. The Krupp RCT concluded that 4 week of intravenous (IV) ceftriaxone was significantly more effective than placebo for fatigue (69% vs. 23%, $p = 0.001$) but not more effective for cognitive function and for an Outer surface protein A (OspA) laboratory measure of infection [10]. The Klempner RCTs concluded that 4 weeks of IV ceftriaxone followed by 8 weeks of oral doxycycline was not more effective than placebo for improving quality of life (QOL) [9]. The Fallon RCT concluded that 10 weeks of intravenous ceftriaxone was more effective than placebo for fatigue (67 vs. 25, $p = 0.05$) [8]. The Fallon RCT also concluded that the significant benefits in cognitive function after 10 weeks of intravenous ceftriaxone were not sustained 3 months after the end of antibiotic therapy [8]. I authored a RCT that concluded that oral amoxicillin for 3 months was significantly more effective than placebo (46 vs. 18, $p = 0.007$) [20].

Clinical practice guidelines (CPG) panels have looked at the evidence from these RCTs only to reach different conclusions. The Infectious Diseases Society of America (IDSA) [15] CPG panel concluded: antibiotic therapy for CLD is not effective [15]. The American Academy of Neurology (AAN) CPG panel [15] and the Ad Hoc International Lyme Disease Group echoed that recommendation [21]. The International Lyme and Associated Diseases (ILADS) CPG concluded: antibiotic therapy for CLD is effective. The opposing recommendations have been characterized as two standards of care [22] and clinical equipoise [23]. Clinical equipoise has been defined as the absence of consensus within the clinical community.

Physicians have been advised by guideline developers to use clinical discretion for particular patient or special clinical circumstances. IDSA's *Guide to the development of practice guidelines* advised the following: "Clinical discretion is of the utmost importance in the application of a guideline to individual patients, because no guideline can ever be specific enough to be applied in all situations" [24]. In a disclaimer, the IDSA CPG for LD advised caution in applying their CPG to individual patients: "It is important to realize that guidelines cannot always account for individual variation among patients. They are not intended to supplant physician judgment with respect to particular patients or special clinical situations" [25].

Nevertheless, health care insurers have published policies that deny antibiotics to CLD patients without taking into account specific clinical discretion for specific clinical situations. UnitedHealthcare [26], Cigna [27], Aetna [28], and BlueCross BlueShield of Wisconsin [29] are examples of insurers who have cited the IDSA CPG to deny more than 4 weeks of intravenous antibiotics without taking into account clinical judgment for specific clinical situations and IDSA CPG's own disclaimer [30].

Hypotheses

This paper examines the eight limitations of the evidence used to conclude that antibiotics therapy for CLD is not effective. The limitations lead to the following hypothesis: insufficient evidence to deny antibiotic treatment to CLD patients.

Evidence for the hypothesis

The power of the evidence is inadequate to draw definite conclusions

Only the Krupp RCT enrolled enough subjects to have sufficient power to draw definite conclusions on the treatment of CLD. The Krupp RCT [10] found 4 weeks of ceftriaxone was more effective than placebo for the primary outcome, fatigue (64% vs. 18.5%, $p < 0.001$). The Krupp RCT [10] was not able to demonstrate a treatment effect for cognition in part due to a differing power concern: "although the patients with Lyme disease showed cognitive slowing compared to healthy controls, these deficits were relatively mild, which may have contributed to the lack of a treatment effect on cognition" ([10], p. 1928). The Krupp RCT [10] did not reach the sample size estimated for the OspA laboratory measure of infection as there were only nine of 55 LD subjects (16%) that had an abnormal OspA at baseline. The actual sample sizes of 51, 78, 37, and 86 for the two Klempner [11], Fallon [8], and Cameron [20] RCTs, respectively, were less than the 194, 194, 45, and 118 recommended by power analysis to draw definite conclusions. The actual number of subjects in the treatment arms for all five trials combined equaled only 167 subjects [8,10,11].

The evidence is too heterogeneous to make strong recommendations

The success rates for the RCTs [8,10,11] were too heterogeneous to make strong recommendations. The success rates varied from as low as 37% and 41% for the two Klempner RCTs [11] on a QOL scale to as high as 64% and 67% for the Krupp and Fallon RCTs on a fatigue severity scale [8,10]. The Fallon RCT also reported moderate improvements on a cognitive index for both treatment and placebo. Antibiotics were more effective than placebo in improving cognitive function in the Fallon RCT at 3 months but the difference was not significant at 6 months [8]. The Cameron RCT concluded that oral amoxicillin for 3 months was significantly more effective than placebo (46 vs. 18, $p = 0.007$) [20]. The 37–67% success rates for the RCTs were also heterogeneous compared with the 63–100% success rates for comparator [31] and case series [18,19,32–34].

The risk to an individual of facing a long-term debilitating illness has not been considered

The 4% risk of a serious adverse event to an individual because of antibiotic treatment of CLD has not been weighed against the risk to an individual of facing a long-term debilitating illness. There were six serious adverse events for the 167 subjects in the treatment arms of the RCTs [8,10,11]. Four individuals developed serious events know to be related to antibiotics consisting of anaphylaxis [10], allergic reaction [8], and two cases of thrombus. Two individuals developed serious events that are not established events related to antibiotics – one individual with life-threatening pulmonary embolism [11] and a second with fever, anemia, and gastrointestinal bleeding [11]. The Cameron RCT concluded that a significant gain in the QOL for subjects randomized to amoxicillin without serious adverse events is consistent with the goal of improving patient's QOL and consequently worthy of further study. The risk of facing a long-term debilitating illness without antibiotic treatment was demonstrated by the two Klempner RCTs where subjects were ill an average of 4.7 years with a QOL "equivalent to those observed in patients with congestive heart failure or osteoarthritis and were more than 0.5 SD greater than the impairment observed in patients with type 2 diabetes or a recent myocardial infarction" ([11], p. 89). The risk of facing a long-term debilitating illness was confirmed in the Fallon RCT where subjects were ill an average of 9 years with a QOL as poor as subjects entering the two Klempner RCTs, severe fatigue, and pain "similar to those of postsurgery patients" ([35], p. 1127). The severity of the symptoms of CLD was validated in a review of four of the RCTs as determined by 22 standardized measures of QOL, including fatigue, pain, role function, psychopathology, and cognition [12].

The risk to society of a growing chronically ill population has not been considered

The risk to society of emerging resistant organisms has not been weighed against the risk to society of an emerging population saddled with CLD. The risk to society of overuse of antibiotics and emergence of multi-resistant infectious disease organisms [36] has received considerable attention. The risk to society of the emerging population of CLD has received less attention. The risk of developing CLD has been downplayed following reports that 88–95% of LD cases exhibiting an erythema migrans and Bell's palsy were successfully treated. Cohort studies of consecutively treated LD patients have shown that long-term outcomes were not nearly so successful. Thirty-four percent of a population-based, retrospective cohort study in Massachusetts had long-term sequelae from Lyme disease (arthritis or recurrent arthralgias, neurocognitive impairments, and neuropathy or myelopathy) a mean of 6.2 years after treatment [7]. Sixty-two percent of a cohort of 215 consecutively treated LD patients in Westchester County remained ill a mean of 3.2 years after treatment [6]. Mean durations of illness of 4.7–9 years for the two Klempner [11] and Fallon RCT [8] validate the risk to society of a growing chronically ill population [6,7].

The cost of a growing CLD population was significant using a Centers for Disease Control and Prevention (CDC) economic cost study of 'clinically defined late-stage LD' in Maryland's Eastern Shore. The average annual economic impact of LD was estimated to be $16,199 per patient, per year [13]. Ninety-five percent of the cost was indirect medical costs, non-medical costs, and productivity losses. The authors estimated the annual economic impact of LD to be ≈$203 million (in 2002 dollars) in the US based on the 23,763 cases reported to the CDC. The actual annual economic cost of LD could be as much as ≈$2 billion (in 2002 dollars) in the US based on CDC estimates that the actual number of LD cases is 10× higher than reported.

Treatment delay has not been considered as a confounder

None of the RCTs was able to address whether or not treatment delay was a confounder to explain the heterogeneous outcomes. The Fallon RCT described delays of 1.8 years without discussing whether the delay affected the outcome [8]. A similar delay in treatment of 1.8 years was reported in a consecutive case series of LD patients confirmed by IgG Western blot testing [37]. Treatment delay was strongly associated with treatment failure [37]. The Klempner RCT did not discuss whether any of the average onset of illness of 4.7 years was due to delayed treatment [11]. The Krupp RCT [10] did not report whether delays in treatment occurred.

Coinfections have not been considered as a confounder

None of the RCTs were able to resolve whether co-infections could explain their mixed outcome. The ticks that carry LD also carry co-infections known to cause diseases such as babesosis, anaplamosis, and ehrlichosis [38]. Krause reported an increased severity and duration of illness in patients co-infected with Lyme disease and babesiosis [17]. The Fallon RCT reported low positive IgG results for 10.8% of samples for of *Anaplasma phagocytophila* and an astonishing *27%* for *B. microti*. The Klempner RCT actively excluded subjects with evidence of co-infections [8].

The design of RCTs did not address the range of treatment options in an actual practice

None of the RCTs assessed the range of treatment options available in actual practice. All four RCTs were limited to fixed predefined interventions rather than the option to modify the antibiotic regimen as has been described in actual practice [14]. None of the RCTs incorporated symptomatic treatment into the protocol. CLD patients who are ill an average of 4.7–9 years with severe pain, fatigue, and a poor QOL might have benefited from symptomatic treatment combined with antibiotic therapy.[11] Fallon RCT's decision to drop a subject that required pain management illustrates the difficulty of designing RCTs to reflect the treatment options available in actual practice [8].

The findings cannot be generalized to actual practice

None of the RCTs discussed the difficulties encountered when attempting to generalize their data to actual practice. Following the Klempner RCT's report that, at the time of enrollment, study subjects had already been ill an average of 4.7 years and had already received an average of three courses of treatment, an analytical review by this author raised concerns about the generalizability of Klempner's conclusions, as follows: "Applying the findings to target populations with characteristics that differ from those included in these trials is inappropriate and may limit options for chronic Lyme disease patients who might benefit from antibiotic treatment" ([30], p. 12). The same generalizability issue could have been raised following the Fallon RCT wherein LD subjects had been symptomatic for an average of 9 years [8]. Fallon RCT raised an additional generalizability concern by noting that 3331 (99%) of the 3368 initial clinic contacts were excluded due to restrictive entrance criteria [8].

Test of the hypothesis

The hypothesis could be tested through new innovative trials of CLD that address the eight limitations discussed: the trials are better powered, the heterogeneity of results are reconciled, the risk to an individual of facing a long-term debilitating illness has been considered, the risk to society of a growing chronically ill population has been considered, treatment delays and co-infections have been considered as a confounder, trials are completed that address the range of treatment options in an actual practice, and findings can be generalized to actual practice.

Implications

This hypothesis suggests that physicians should consider the limitations of the evidence before denying antibiotic treatment for CLD. Physicians who continue to deny antibiotic treatment for CLD patients could let their patients know that there are clinicians and a professional society that consider the evidence insufficient to deny antibiotic treatment for this condition [14]. Shrier in a bioethical discussion of clinical equipoise came to the same conclusion as follows: "Rather than prohibiting the clinician from informing the patient of his or her personal beliefs, clinical equipoise simply asks the clinician to be honest, letting the patient know that a different but equally competent clinician might decide on a different course" [39].

The hypothesis also suggests that health care insurers consider the limitations of the evidence before adopting policies that deny antibiotic treatment for CLD patients. The hypothesis suggests that insurers should expand coverage of CLD to include clinical discretion for specific clinical situations.

Conflict of interest statement

The author is the President of ILADS, first author of the ILADS CPG, the principle investigator for one of the five RCTs, a clinician who treats Lyme disease patients, and an advocate of better evidence. He has no interests that conflict with that goal.

Author contribution

Article written solely by author.

Funding source

None.

Acknowledgment

Thanks to Staton Rabin for critical reading of the manuscript.

References

[1] Lyme disease - United States. MMWR Morb Mortal Wkly Rep 2002;51(2):29–31.

[2] Smith R, O'Connell S, Palmer S. Lyme disease surveillance in England and Wales, 1986–1998. Emerg Infect Dis 2000;6(4):404–7.

[3] Bacon RM, Kugeler KJ, Mead PS. Surveillance for Lyme disease - United States, 1992–2006. MMWR Surveill Summ 2008;57(10):1–9.

[4] Lyme disease - United States, 2001–2002. MMWR Morb Mortal Wkly Rep 2004;53(17):365–9.

[5] <http://www.ct.gov/ag/lib/ag/health/0129lyme.pdf>; p. 290 [accessed 12.4.08].

[6] Asch ES, Bujak DI, Weiss M, Peterson MG, Weinstein A. Lyme disease: an infectious and postinfectious syndrome. J Rheumatol 1994;21(3):454–61.

[7] Shadick NA, Phillips CB, Logigian EL, Steere AC, Kaplan RF, Berardi VP, et al. The long-term clinical outcomes of Lyme disease. A population-based retrospective cohort study. Ann Int Med 1994;121(8):560–7.

[8] Fallon BA, Keilp JG, Corbera KM, Petkova E, Britton CB, Dwyer E, et al. A randomized, placebo-controlled trial of repeated IV antibiotic therapy for Lyme encephalopathy. Neurology 2008;70(13):992–1003.

[9] Klempner MS. Controlled trials of antibiotic treatment in patients with post-treatment chronic Lyme disease. Vector Borne Zoonotic Dis 2002;2(4):255–63.

[10] Krupp LB, Hyman LG, Grimson R, Coyle PK, Melville P, Ahnn S, et al. Study and treatment of post Lyme disease (STOP-LD): a randomized double masked clinical trial. Neurology 2003;60(12):1923–30.

[11] Klempner MS, Hu LT, Evans J, Schmid CH, Johnson GM, Trevino RP, et al. Two controlled trials of antibiotic treatment in patients with persistent symptoms and a history of Lyme disease. N Engl J Med 2001;345(2):85–92.

[12] Cameron DJ. Clinical trials validate the severity of persistent Lyme disease symptoms. Med Hypotheses 2008.

[13] Zhang X, Meltzer MI, Pena CA, Hopkins AB, Wroth L, Fix AD. Economic impact of Lyme disease. Emerg Infect Dis 2006;12(4):653–60.

[14] Cameron D, Gaito A, Harris N, Bach G, Bellovin S, Bock K, et al. Evidence-based guidelines for the management of Lyme disease. Expert Rev Anti Infect Ther 2004;2(Suppl. 1):S1–13.

[15] Halperin JJ, Shapiro ED, Logigian E, Belman AL, Dotevall L, Wormser GP, et al. Practice parameter: treatment of nervous system Lyme disease (an evidence-based review): report of the Quality Standards Subcommittee of the American Academy of Neurology. Neurology 2007;69(1):91–102.

[16] Steere AC, Green J, Schoen RT, Taylor E, Hutchinson GJ, Rahn DW, et al. Successful parenteral penicillin therapy of established Lyme arthritis. N Engl J Med 1985;312(14):869–74.

[17] Krause PJ, Telford 3rd SR, Spielman A, Sikand V, Ryan R, Christianson D, et al. Concurrent Lyme disease and babesiosis. Evidence for increased severity and duration of illness. JAMA 1996;275(21):1657–60.

[18] Donta ST. Macrolide therapy of chronic Lyme disease. Med Sci Monit 2003;9(11):PI136–42.

[19] Donta ST. Tetracycline therapy for chronic Lyme disease. Clin Infect Dis 1997;25(Suppl. 1):S52–6.

[20] Cameron D. Severity of Lyme disease with persistent symptoms. Insights from a double-blind placebo-controlled clinical trial. Minerva Med 2008;99(5):489–96.

[21] Feder Jr HM, Johnson BJ, O'Connell S, Shapiro ED, Steere AC, Wormser GP, et al. A critical appraisal of "chronic Lyme disease". N Engl J Med 2007;357(14):1422–30.

[22] Johnson L, Stricker RB. Treatment of Lyme disease: a medicolegal assessment. Expert Rev Anti Infect Ther 2004;2(4):533–57.

[23] Cameron DJ. An appraisal of "chronic Lyme disease". N Engl J Med 2008;358(4):429–30 [author reply 430–421].

[24] Kish MA. Guide to development of practice guidelines. Clin Infect Dis 2001;32(6):851–4.

[25] Wormser GP, Dattwyler RJ, Shapiro ED, Halperin JJ, Steere AC, Klempner MS, et al. The clinical assessment, treatment, and prevention of lyme disease, human granulocytic anaplasmosis, and babesiosis: clinical practice guidelines by the Infectious Diseases Society of America. Clin Infect Dis 2006;43(9):1089–134.

[26] UnitedHealthCare. Treatment of chronic and recurrent Lyme disease. <http://www.unitedhealthcareonline.com/b2c/cmaIndexResult.do?channelId= 01622 8193392b010VgnVCM100000c520720a____&htmlFilePath=/ccmcontent/ProviderII/UHC/en-US/Assets/ProviderStaticFiles/ProviderStaticFilesHtml/MedicalPolicies/Treatment_of_Chronic_and_Recurrent_Lyme_Disease.htm>; [accessed 12.23.08].

[27] Cigna. Medical coverage policy Lyme disease treatment. <http://www.cigna.com/customer_care/healthcare_professional/coverage_positions/medical/mm_0400_coveragepositioncriteria_lyme_disease_treatment.pdf>; [accessed 12.23.08].

[28] Aetna: Clinical Policy Bulletin. Lyme disease and other tick-borne diseases. <http://www.aetna.com/cpb/medical/data/200_299/0215.html>; [accessed 12.23.08].

[29] BlueCross BlueShield of Wisconsin parenteral antibiotics for the treatment of Lyme disease. <http://www2.bluecrosswisconsin.com/provider/medpolicy/policies/MED/lyme.html>; [accessed 12.23.08].

[30] Cameron DJ. Generalizability in two clinical trials of Lyme disease. Epidemiol Perspect Innov 2006;3:12.

[31] Dattwyler RJ, Wormser GP, Rush TJ, Finkel MF, Schoen RT, Grunwaldt E, et al. A comparison of two treatment regimens of ceftriaxone in late Lyme disease. Wien Klin Wochenschr 2005;117(11–12):393–7.

[32] Logigian EL, Kaplan RF, Steere AC. Chronic neurologic manifestations of Lyme disease. N Engl J Med 1990;323(21):1438–44.

[33] Wahlberg P, Granlund H, Nyman D, Panelius J, Seppala I. Treatment of late Lyme borreliosis. J Infect 1994;29(3):255–61.

[34] Logigian EL, Kaplan RF, Steere AC. Successful treatment of Lyme encephalopathy with intravenous ceftriaxone. J Infect Dis 1999;180(2):377–83.

[35] Krupp LB, LaRocca NG, Muir-Nash J, Steinberg AD. The fatigue severity scale. Application to patients with multiple sclerosis and systemic lupus erythematosus. Arch Neurol 1989;46(10):1121–3.

[36] Levy SB. The 2000 Garrod lecture. Factors impacting on the problem of antibiotic resistance. J Antimicrob Chemother 2002;49(1):25–30.

[37] Cameron DJ. Consequences of treatment delay in Lyme disease. J Eval Clin Pract 2007;13(3):470–2.

[38] Swanson SJ, Neitzel D, Reed KD, Belongia EA. Coinfections acquired from ixodes ticks. Clin Microbiol Rev 2006;19(4):708–27.

[39] Shrier I. Uncertainty about clinical equipoise. CMAJ 2001;164(13):1831 [author reply 1831–2].

Special Articles

Lyme Disease: A Neuropsychiatric Illness

Brian A. Fallon, M.D., M.P.H., and Jenifer A. Nields, M.D.

Objective: Lyme disease is a multisystemic illness that can affect the central nervous system (CNS), causing neurologic and psychiatric symptoms. The goal of this article is to familiarize psychiatrists with this spirochetal illness. Method: Relevant books, articles, and abstracts from academic conferences were perused, and additional articles were located through computerized searches and reference sections from published articles. Results: Up to 40% of patients with Lyme disease develop neurologic involvement of either the peripheral or central nervous system. Dissemination to the CNS can occur within the first few weeks after skin infection. Like syphilis, Lyme disease may have a latency period of months to years before symptoms of late infection emerge. Early signs include meningitis, encephalitis, cranial neuritis, and radiculoneuropathies. Later, encephalomyelitis and encephalopathy may occur. A broad range of psychiatric reactions have been associated with Lyme disease including paranoia, dementia, schizophrenia, bipolar disorder, panic attacks, major depression, anorexia nervosa, and obsessive-compulsive disorder. Depressive states among patients with late Lyme disease are fairly common, ranging across studies from 26% to 66%. The microbiology of Borrelia burgdorferi *sheds light on why Lyme disease can be relapsing and remitting and why it can be refractory to normal immune surveillance and standard antibiotic regimens. Conclusions: Psychiatrists who work in endemic areas need to include Lyme disease in the differential diagnosis of any atypical psychiatric disorder. Further research is needed to identify better laboratory tests and to determine the appropriate manner (intravenous or oral) and length (weeks or months) of treatment among patients with neuropsychiatric involvement.*

(Am J Psychiatry 1994; 151:1571–1583)

Lyme disease (Lyme borreliosis), caused by the tick-borne spirochete *Borrelia burgdorferi,* may progress from an initial skin infection to a disabling multisystemic illness. Now the most common vector-borne infection in the United States, Lyme disease is increasing in incidence and geographic spread (1). The disease has dermatologic, arthritic, ophthalmologic, cardiac, neurologic, and psychiatric manifestations (2). In its protean manifestations, in its spirochetal etiology, and in its course (early skin localization and rapid invasion of the central nervous system [CNS]), Lyme disease is similar to syphilis (3). Like syphilis, early recognition is important to prevent an acute, treatable illness from becoming a chronic or relapsing one. Because current diagnostic tests are not always reliable, physicians must rely on clinical presentation as the basis for diagnosis. Because many of the symptoms of Lyme disease involve the CNS, patients with Lyme disease may be referred to psychiatrists both before and after diagnosis.

In this article, we present an overview of Lyme disease with a particular emphasis on its neuropsychiatric features.

Received March 16, 1992; revisions received Oct. 22, 1993, and March 30, 1994; accepted April 1, 1994. From the Department of Psychiatry, College of Physicians and Surgeons of Columbia University, New York; the Division of Therapeutics, New York State Psychiatric Institute; and the Department of Psychiatry, Yale University School of Medicine, New Haven, Conn. Address reprint requests to Dr. Fallon, New York State Psychiatric Institute, 722 West 168th St., Unit 13, New York, NY 10032.

Supported in part by a grant to Dr. Fallon from the Lyme Research Foundation, Inc.

The authors thank Drs. W. Burgdorfer, P.K. Coyle, D.F. Klein, M.R. Liebowitz, and R.T. Schoen for comments on earlier versions of this article.

LYME DISEASE

TRANSMISSION

Lyme disease is transmitted by an infected nymphal or adult female *Ixodes* tick. Smaller than the dog tick, the *Ixodes* tick may easily be missed on casual inspection. The bite is usually not painful. Transmission of the spirochete appears to require the tick to feed at least 12–24 hours (4). The ticks are most commonly carried by deer and by the white-footed mouse, but other carriers have been described as well.

DISTRIBUTION

Lyme disease has been reported throughout the United States and in numerous countries around the world. The geographic spread and the incidence in the United States have been rapidly increasing. For example, during 1992, 45 states reported 9,677 cases, representing a 19-fold increase over the 497 cases reported by 11 states in 1982 (5). The State of Connecticut, which in 1992 had the highest rate of Lyme disease in the country, reported between 1991 and 1992 a threefold increase in the proportion of infected ticks in four communities and a one and a half-fold increase in reported cases throughout the state (6). The most heavily affected areas include the Northeast (New York, New Jersey, Connecticut, Massachusetts, Rhode Island, Pennsylvania), the upper Midwest (Minnesota, Wisconsin), and the Pacific coastal region (California, Oregon).

HISTORY

Although Lyme disease was first described in the United States as an arthritic illness preceded by a rash (7), early reports in Europe described a primarily neurologic illness without any arthritis (8, 9). Psychiatric symptoms were described in some of these early reports.

In 1909 a Swedish physician described the classic Lyme rash, known as erythema chronicum migrans, noting that it developed at the site of an *Ixodes* tick bite (10). In 1922 two French doctors, Garin and Bujadoux, wrote a case entitled "Paralysis by Ticks," now thought to be the first report of Lyme meningoradiculitis (8). The patient developed erythema migrans after a tick bite, followed by radiculopathy, paralysis of a portion of one arm, anxiety, and meningitis. In 1930 Hellerstrom, of the Karolinska Institute, described a man who, 3 months after an erythema migrans rash, developed an encephalitis with psychotic symptoms, disorientation, and marked CSF abnormalities (11). In 1941 Bannwarth, a German neurologist, described the syndrome of chronic lymphocytic meningitis, which was characterized by radicular pains, lymphocytic meningitis, and peripheral nervous system involvement, especially facial palsy (9). The cases in all of these early reports, previously described as Garin-Bujadoux syndrome, Bannwarth's syndrome, and neuroborreliosis, are now considered to have been cases of Lyme disease.

In the United States, the first report of a tick-induced erythema migrans rash was in 1970 (12). In 1977 "Lyme arthritis" was described by Steere et al. (7); the article was based on an epidemiological investigation of an outbreak of presumed juvenile rheumatoid arthritis in Connecticut. In 1978 the link between Lyme arthritis and the bite of an *Ixodes* tick (13) was recognized. In 1982 Burgdorfer et al. isolated the etiologic agent of Lyme disease from an *Ixodes* tick—a spirochete now known as *B. burgdorferi* (14). Early in the history of Lyme disease, aspirin and nonsteroidal anti-inflammatory agents were used for symptoms that emerged after the erythema migrans rash (15). Subsequently, penicillin was shown to shorten the duration of illness, thus supporting an infectious etiology. While short courses (10 days) of oral or intravenous antibiotics were recommended at first, it is now recognized that some patients benefit from longer courses (6 weeks or longer) or repeated treatments (16–18).

TYPICAL CLINICAL MANIFESTATIONS OF LYME DISEASE

Within days or weeks after the bite of a tick infected with *B. burgdorferi,* a localized skin reaction may occur, consisting most typically of an erythematous annular rash (erythema migrans), which may enlarge to a size of 5 cm or greater. This early localized sign of infection may soon be followed by mild to severe flu-like symptoms.

Hematogenous dissemination may lead to early (weeks to months) heart, ophthalmologic, or nervous system involvement. Although second- or third-degree atrioventricular block is most common, rare reports of myopericarditis, left ventricle dysfunction, and cardiomegaly exist (19). Conjunctivitis can be an early manifestation of ocular involvement.

Within the first few weeks after skin infection, *B. burgdorferi* may disseminate to the CNS (20–22) where it may remain quiescent for months to years before producing symptoms (23). Because approximately one-third of infected patients do not recall the tick bite or rash and because the flu-like symptoms are nonspecific and may be mild (24), patients may not realize that they are infected until long after the initial bite. Neurologic problems, which occur in 15%–40% of patients (25), may be the presenting symptom. Early on, patients may experience headaches without any signs of inflammation in the CSF (18). Shortly thereafter, patients may develop meningitis, cranial neuritis, and motor or sensory radiculitis (26). With meningitis, symptoms may include recurrent severe headaches, stiff neck, photophobia, and, less commonly, nausea and vomiting. At this stage, objective signs are commonly present in the CSF (see the section on CNS laboratory tests). In less than half of the patients with meningitis, a mild encephalitis develops that is characterized by fluctuating disturbances of mood, concentration, memory, and sleep. Cranial neuritis, such as Bell's palsy, occurs in 5%–10% of patients with neurologic Lyme disease (27). Other signs of peripheral nerve involvement include sensory or motor radiculoneuropathies; objective abnormalities may be evident on nerve conduction studies. Symptoms of peripheral neuropathy typically include sharp shooting pains, areas of numbness, paresthesias, weakness, or fasciculations.

Later-stage illness (months to years after infection) generally affects the joints, eyes, skin, or CNS. Arthritic involvement begins with migratory arthralgias and, in 60% of untreated patients, develops into an inflammatory arthritis, typically affecting the large joints, such as the knee (28). Ophthalmologic involvement may consist of localized inflammation such as uveitis, iritis, or optic neuritis (29, 30). A late dermatologic manifestation of Lyme disease, acrodermatitis chronica atrophicans, is seen almost exclusively in Europe (31).

Late neurologic involvement may be manifested by encephalomyelitis or encephalopathy (18, 23, 32). Encephalomyelitis, an uncommon late manifestation of Lyme disease, may have quite severe and diverse presentations, including spastic paraparesis, transverse myelitis, cerebellar syndromes, hemiparesis, and movement disorders (18, 32). More common in late Lyme disease is an encephalopathy characterized by subtle to severe cognitive changes and a polyradiculoneuropathy (23). In this stage of illness, the CSF may appear normal (18, 21) (see section on CNS laboratory tests). Other accompanying symptoms of later infection include profound fatigue, sleep disturbance, photophobia, auditory hyperacusis, extreme irritability or emotional lability, word-finding problems, dyslexic-like errors when speaking or writing, and spatial disorientation (23, 33). Disturbances in other sensory modalities, such as taste and smell, have been reported (33, 34). These symptoms may fluctuate in intensity so that symptoms are present on some days but not others. The profile of persistent, marked fatigue and cognitive deficits associated with late-stage Lyme disease is similar to the symptom profile of the chronic fatigue syndrome (35). Whether the late-stage symptoms of Lyme disease are due to persistent infection or to a postinfectious immune activation is an important question that requires further elucidation.

Because patients with encephalopathy or encephalitis may experience marked mood lability, irritability, and sleep disturbance, the distinction between an organic mood disorder and a concomitant primary major depression may be quite difficult to make.

ATYPICAL NEUROLOGIC MANIFESTATIONS OF LYME DISEASE

Because the clinical spectrum of Lyme disease continues to expand, physicians who work in endemic areas should keep Lyme disease in the differential diagnosis of any atypical neurologic illness with multisystemic features. Case reports, for example, have linked a variety of neurologic syndromes to late Lyme disease; these include blindness (30), progressive dementias (32, 36, 37), seizure disorders (34, 38, 39), the Tullio phenomenon (40), strokes (41), extrapyramidal disorders (42), amyotrophic lateral sclerosis (43), Guillain-Barré syndrome (44), and progressive demyelinating-like syndromes mimicking multiple sclerosis (23).

CENTERS FOR DISEASE CONTROL (CDC) CRITERIA FOR DIAGNOSIS

Lyme disease surveillance by the CDC began in 1982, and in 1991 Lyme disease became nationally reportable. For epidemiologic surveillance studies (1), the CDC requires history of exposure in an endemic area and either 1) a physician-diagnosed erythema migrans rash of at least 5 cm in diameter or 2) laboratory confirmation of exposure to *B. burgdorferi* and at least one systemic manifestation. Systemic manifestations must be either musculoskeletal (arthritis), neurologic (lymphocytic meningitis, cranial neuritis, radiculopathy, encephalomyelitis with intrathecal antibody production), or cardiac (second- or third-degree atrioventricular conduction delays). Laboratory confirmation requires the isolation of *B. burgdorferi,* the demonstration of diagnostic levels of *B. burgdorferi* immunoglobulin (Ig) M or IgG antibodies in serum or CSF, or a rising specific antibody titer on serum samples taken from acutely ill and convalescent patients.

These criteria have been useful for epidemiologic studies, but not all patients with Lyme disease will meet this case definition. About one-third of patients do not recall the erythema migrans rash; serologic testing may be unreliable (45); and the clinical spectrum of Lyme disease continues to expand beyond the manifestations currently included in the CDC case definition.

LABORATORY TESTING

Because *B. burgdorferi* is difficult to culture, indirect methods are used to detect the presence of the spirochete. Currently available serologic tests, such as the enzyme-linked immunosorbent assay (ELISA) and the indirect immunofluorescence assay, rely on the immune response following exposure to *B. burgdorferi*, but they can be unreliable, with both false positive and false negative results (45). In a recent study, over half of the 45 laboratories studied reported falsely negative values in a known positive serum sample from a patient with Lyme disease (46). The Western blot is also often used to examine the serum for antibodies against epitopes that are specific for *B. burgdorferi* (e.g., 31 kD, 34 kD, or 39 kD bands). Other laboratory tools are emerging—such as urine antigen tests (47), cell-mediated immunoassay (48), immune complex assays (49), polymerase chain reaction assays (50, 51), and borreliacidal

LYME DISEASE

TABLE 1. Neuropsychological Test Results Among Patients With Disseminated Lyme Disease

Study	N	Diagnosis	Comparison Subjects	Neuropsychological Tests[a]	Results
Logigian et al. (23)	27	Late neurologic Lyme disease	None	California Verbal Learning Test, Wechsler Memory Scale, Wisconsin Card Sorting Test, Trail Making Test, Rey-Osterrieth Complex Figure Test, Finger Tapping Test, Hooper Visual Organization Test, Benton Face Discrimination Test, Boston Naming Test, Token Test, Oral Word Association Test	56% had memory deficits
Kaplan et al. (56)	20[b]	Lyme encephalopathy	11 fibromyalgia and 11 nonpsychotic depressed patients	California Verbal Learning Test, Wechsler Memory Scale, Rey-Osterrieth Complex Figure Test, MMPI, Beck Depression Inventory	Lyme disease patients were significantly more impaired on memory tests
Halperin et al. (27)	17	Neurologic Lyme disease	None	California Verbal Learning Test, Wechsler Memory Scale, Symbol Digit Modalities, Booklet Category Test, Block Design, Purdue Pegboard	Impaired memory, attention, conceptual ability, and motor function; improvement with antibiotics
Krupp et al. (57)	15	Late Lyme disease and cognitive symptoms	10 Healthy age- and sex-matched subjects	WAIS-R[c], Trail Making Test, Booklet Category Test, Oral Word Association Test, Wechsler Memory Scale, Selective Reminding Test	Lyme disease patients had significantly impaired verbal fluency and memory

[a]Neuropsychological tests were not administered by individuals who were blind to medical diagnosis.
[b]A subgroup of patients from the study by Logigian et al. (23).
[c]Subtests of information, vocabulary, similarities, digit span, block design, object assembly, and digit symbol.

antibody tests (52)—but these are not yet well standardized across laboratories.

Several *B. burgdorferi* antigens are shared by other spirochetes. For example, both *B. burgdorferi* and the etiologic agent of syphilis, *Treponema pallidum,* may cause a positive finding on the fluorescent treponemal antibody absorption test; results of nontreponemal tests, such as the rapid plasma reagin and Venereal Disease Research Laboratory tests, are usually negative in Lyme disease (18). Patients with syphilis or periodontal disease (oral spirochetes) may have falsely positive Lyme ELISA serologies and a common 41 kD antibody to flagellar antigen evident on Western blot.

Falsely negative test results may occur for a variety of reasons. If tested too soon after initial infection, the patient may not yet have mounted an antibody response (53). In addition, antibiotic treatment early in the infection may abrogate the humoral immune response (54). In some cases, free antibodies may not be detected because the borrelia antibodies are bound within circulating immune complexes (55). Finally, interlaboratory variability in antigenic standardization of Lyme assays may result in false negative as well as false positive results (46).

CNS LABORATORY TESTS FOR LYME DISEASE

The results of laboratory testing among patients with neurologic Lyme disease vary depending on the stage of the illness. In very early CNS involvement (meningismus) or late-stage infection (encephalopathy), the CSF may appear normal (18). When clinical signs of meningitis or encephalitis are present, a spinal tap may reveal a mononuclear pleocytosis, mildly increased protein, and, in some cases, an elevated IgG index or oligoclonal immunoglobulins. Intrathecal anti-*B. burgdorferi* antibody production is present in 70%–90% of patients with Lyme meningitis (18). Magnetic resonance imaging (MRI) studies may demonstrate punctate white matter lesions on T_2 weighted images, similar to those seen in demyelinating disorders, such as multiple sclerosis. EEG studies may show diffuse slowing or epileptic discharges, but this is uncommon.

In patients with late Lyme encephalopathy, results of brain MRI and EEG studies are generally normal. Functional brain imaging using quantitative brain perfusion single photon emission computed tomography (SPECT), however, may reveal hypoperfusion, particularly in the cerebral white matter, even in patients with no CSF or MRI abnormalities (E.L. Logigian et al., unpublished data, 1994). Objective deficits may be seen on neuropsychological testing (23, 27, 56, 57) (table 1). In about half of these patients, typical markers of CSF infection (pleocytosis, elevated protein, intrathecal antibody production) cannot be found (18). Current experimental research using sensitive ELISA and Western blot techniques has demonstrated the continued presence of spirochetal antigens among many patients with encephalopathy whose CSF otherwise tests normal (21). In some of these patients, results of standard antibody testing of both the serum and the CSF have been negative, but the immune complex dissociation assay revealed bound *B. burgdorferi*-specific antibody (58).

Given the limitations of diagnostic tests, clinicians need to consider clinical factors that would aid in the diagnosis of Lyme disease. These include a history of an erythema migrans rash or *Ixodes* tick bite, exposure to a Lyme endemic area, and the combination of neuropsychiatric and extraneural symptoms. Because Lyme disease is a multisystemic illness, patients whose neuropsychiatric symptoms start after a flu-like illness should be asked about a history of other symptoms of Lyme disease, including rashes, joint pains, arthritis, cardiac problems, changes in vision, and radicular pains or cranial nerve palsies.

NEUROPSYCHOLOGICAL FINDINGS

Most studies have found that patients with Lyme encephalopathy have subtle impairments in memory, concentration, learning, and conceptual ability. Typically, the deficits suggest frontal lobe involvement, affecting short-term memory, verbal fluency, or executive cognitive functions (table 1). Logigian et al. (23), in a study of 27 patients with chronic neurologic Lyme disease, found that 15 of the 27 had quantifiable memory deficits. In order to determine whether psychological factors might account for the memory impairment among Lyme disease patients, Kaplan et al. (56) compared 20 patients with Lyme encephalopathy with 11 fibromyalgia patients and 11 nonpsychotic depressed patients on a neuropsychological test battery. They found that the Lyme disease patients showed greater impairment on standardized memory tests than either of the comparison groups and that the impairment was independent of the number of somatic complaints and the presence of depression.

Cognitive impairments among patients with late Lyme encephalopathy often improve with antibiotic treatment (23, 27), suggesting that active spirochetal infection causes the encephalopathy. In Halperin et al.'s study (27) of patients with late Lyme borreliosis, serial neuropsychological testing before and after a course of intravenous antibiotics revealed marked improvement on tests of memory, attention and concentration, conceptual ability, and psychomotor and perceptual motor function. Noteworthy is that many patients with cognitive deficits did not have clinical evidence of focal CNS disease. Results of EEGs, CSF studies, and other laboratory investigations were often normal. MRI scans were abnormal in some of the patients with severe memory impairment, revealing hyperintense T_2 white matter lesions suggestive of edema or inflammation. Some patients with late Lyme encephalopathy continue to have residual neuropsychological deficits after antibiotic treatment.

Krupp et al. (57) compared 15 patients with Lyme disease who had complaints of persistent cognitive difficulty 6 months after antibiotic treatment to 10 healthy comparison subjects matched in age and education. Compared to the healthy subjects, the Lyme disease patients exhibited marked impairment on memory tests. In that study, the memory impairment was not correlated with serum or CSF anti-*B. burgdorferi* antibody titers and was not explained by MRI findings or depression. Fatigue, however, a nonspecific marker of chronic Lyme disease, was correlated with memory impairment; this suggested to the authors that the persistent encephalopathy could be an indirect effect of systemic infection elsewhere in the body. The authors noted that persistent neuropsychological deficits were somewhat more common among patients who had received only oral rather than intravenous therapy. In addition, of the six Lyme patients with no objective neuropsychological test deficits but subjective complaints of memory impairment, five had the highest depression scores of the entire group of 15, suggesting that depression in some Lyme patients may account for the subjective experience of cognitive dysfunction.

PSYCHIATRIC MANIFESTATIONS OF LYME DISEASE

A limited but ever increasing literature is beginning to suggest that psychiatric disorders may be part of the clinical profile of Lyme disease. Before reviewing this literature, we present the following case.

Ms. A, a previously healthy 18-year-old college freshman, suddenly developed severe and sustained anxiety, depersonalization, and panic attacks associated with insomnia and appetite loss. She consulted the university health services. After evaluation by both a psychologist and an internist, rest was recommended, under the assumption that these symptoms represented an adjustment reaction to being away from home. As her symptoms worsened, Ms. A began to fear that she was going crazy.

Two weeks later, Ms. A returned home on a medical leave of absence. An extensive medical workup revealed no abnormalities except for a positive Lyme ELISA titer. A Western blot for *B. burgdorferi* also came back positive. Ms. A insisted on getting a spinal tap. Although the cell count and total protein were normal, the CSF revealed IgG antibodies to *B. burgdorferi*. The diagnosis of CNS Lyme disease was made. The patient was treated with a 6-week course of intravenously administered antibiotics, and over the course of the following 3 months she felt 80% better.

Noteworthy in this case is that a diagnosis of Lyme disease was never considered by the college's counselor and internist. The private community physician also did not suspect Lyme disease, but because the patient lived in an endemic area and because Lyme disease is well-known as the "new great imitator" (59), this doctor included a Lyme test in the battery of blood tests. After the ELISA results came back positive, the patient recalled a large annular rash several months earlier that had been followed by a brief period of moderate headaches and uncharacteristic fatigue. Ms. A did not have any joint pain, radiculopathy, cranial nerve palsies, or cardiac symptoms. Her primary manifestation of Lyme disease was psychiatric. Because Ms. A's CSF studies demonstrated borrelial antibodies and because her psychiatric symptoms resolved so rapidly after intravenous antibiotic treatment, active CNS infection was presumed to have been the cause of the severe anxiety and depersonalization. Had Ms. A's serologic Lyme test results come back falsely negative, the diagnosis of Lyme disease would have been missed. It should be emphasized, however, that careful history taking by a clinician well-versed in the clinical spectrum of Lyme disease would have suggested the diagnosis even in the absence of positive serologic test results.

The psychiatrist's evaluation becomes complicated when psychiatric symptoms emerge after the patient has already received a standard course of antibiotic treatment. Such a situation developed with Ms. A.

One year later, Ms. A developed a return of anxiety with panic attacks and agoraphobia. In addition, she developed rare déjà vu episodes, repetitive musical hallucinations, and intrusive obsessional thoughts and images. Results of a repeat spinal tap were normal on routine testing with a nonreactive CSF ELISA for *B. burgdorferi* antibodies. An EEG after sleep deprivation revealed intermittent slowing in the right and left temporal areas with rare sharp waves. Ms. A was treated for 6 months with imipramine, with complete resolution of her panic attacks and agoraphobia. With time, the obsessional thoughts, déjà vu experiences, and musical hallucinations also resolved.

Although the panic disorder and obsessive-compulsive disorder may have been mere epiphenomena with the Lyme disease, the lack of a family history of these disorders and the normal premorbid history suggest that Lyme disease may have triggered these symptoms. Severe anxiety and panic attacks have been previously described in Lyme disease (60). Obsessive-compulsive disorder has been associated with CNS infections, such as the encephalitis epidemic of 1916–1922 (61), and has also been associated with Lyme disease (62); antineuronal antibodies triggered by systemic infection may induce certain subtypes of obsessive-compulsive disorder (63). Persistent infection could not be completely ruled out in Ms. A's case, given the fact that patients with late CNS Lyme disease may have no demonstrable CSF abnormalities on currently available testing. However, because of the absence of other systemic Lyme symptoms and the improvement with psychiatric medications, this patient has continued to be treated symptomatically and observed for the possible reemergence of signs of CNS infection.

Reviews

In 1990 two review articles appeared in Germany which suggested that psychiatric symptoms may be part of the picture of Lyme disease (64, 65). After an extensive review of the neurologic literature, Omasits et al. (64) concluded: "psychiatric manifestations can at times be predominant, ranging from agitated depressive states to the clinical picture of dementia." Kohler (65) described a staging of psychiatric symptoms, with depression occurring in early CNS disease and organic mood and psychotic disorders occurring in late-stage disease. Although Kohler's report was suggestive, there was no mention of prospectively collected data to support the staging description.

The sparse world literature on the psychiatric manifestations of Lyme borreliosis is methodologically limited. Most of the literature consists of case reports and uncontrolled small series. When standardized measures were used, they were generally self-report depression items that examined one point in time without a comparison group. Despite these marked methodological problems, the case reports and small series are provocative.

Psychiatric Case Reports

Case reports have linked Lyme disease to a vast array of neuropsychiatric symptoms, including paranoia (37, 62, 66–68), thought disorder (66), delusions (62, 66), auditory hallucinations (62, 67), olfactory hallucinations (34), visual hallucinations (69), stereotypies (67), anorexia nervosa (70), obsessions or compulsions (62, 70), major depression (37, 58, 64), disorientation (37, 69, 70), confusion (34, 37, 70), violent outbursts (62, 70), mood lability (60, 62, 67, 70), panic attacks (60, 62), mania (60, 62), personality changes (34, 37), catatonia (67), and dementia (36, 37). In three of these cases (66, 67, 69), it was not until the onset of a psychotic disorder that the patient was brought to medical attention. In two of these cases, no other symptoms of systemic Lyme disease were evident at initial presentation, although a careful history revealed neck and radicular pains 4–6 months earlier. Four patients were hospitalized for a psychiatric illness (62, 66, 67, 70) before it was recognized that the psychiatric symptoms might be caused by CNS Lyme disease. One patient's mania and movement disorder led to hospitalization for a neuropsychiatric evaluation, but Lyme disease was not considered and therefore not diagnosed until several months after discharge (60). Two patients had such extensive multisystemic symptoms that somatization disorder would have been hard to rule out had these two patients not had positive results on serologic tests and a normal premorbid history (60). Many of the patients had abnormalities noted on EEG, CSF, or structural brain imaging (34, 60, 62, 66–68, 70). In one patient (68), *B. burgdorferi* was successfully cultured from the CSF. In two other patients (37, 70), pathological studies of brain tissue revealed *B. burgdorferi*-like spirochetes.

Among the 11 well-described cases, nine patients were treated with intravenous antibiotics for presumed CNS infection (34, 60, 62, 66–68, 70). Duration of intravenous antibiotics ranged from 10 days (one course) to 29 weeks (three courses). Although all patients responded well to antibiotic treatment, relapses occurred in several patients (37, 60, 62, 68). One 47-year-old man with seropositive Lyme disease manifested primarily by depression and memory deficits had an initial excellent response to intravenously administered antibiotics; he relapsed 5 months later, was not re-treated, was institutionalized in a state psychiatric hospital with an organic mood syndrome and progressive frontal-type dementia, and died at age 52. The neuropathological examination revealed degeneration of the substantia nigra and thalamus, with spi-

BRIAN A. FALLON AND JENIFER A. NIELDS

TABLE 2. Psychiatric Disorders in Larger Series of Patients With Lyme Disease

Study	N	Diagnosis	Measures	Comparison Group	Results	Comments
Logigian et al. (23)	27	Late neurologic Lyme disease	MMPI (score >70 signified depression)	None	26% had extreme irritability; 33% were depressed	89% had encephalopathy
Barr et al. (71)	88	Lyme disease	Beck Depression Inventory, Spielberger anxiety scale	Seronegative patients	Significantly more depression among seropositive patients	
Belman et al. (72)	96 children	Neurologic Lyme disease	Neurologic examination	None	38% had behavioral changes (irritability, lability, poor attention)	Most common symptom was headaches
Krupp et al. (57)	15	Late Lyme disease and cognitive symptoms	Center for Epidemiologic Studies Depression Scale neuropsychological battery	10 healthy age- and sex-matched subjects	Lyme disease patients were significantly more depressed	The most depressed patients did not have abnormal neuropsychological findings
Fallon et al. (73)	51	Chronic, seropositive Lyme disease	Survey using DSM-III-R criteria	30 non-Lyme disease patients with arthritis	Lyme disease patients were significantly more likely to have DSM-III-R depression (66% versus 23%)	32% of Lyme disease patients reported panic attacks (versus 19% of comparison patients; n.s.)
Halperin et al. (27)	17	Neurologic Lyme disease	Beck Depression Inventory	None	Mean Beck scores did not show depression	Depressed patients may have been excluded from study
Kaplan et al. (56)	20[a]	Lyme encephalopathy	Beck Depression Inventory, MMPI	11 fibromyalgia and 11 nonpsychotic depressed patients	Mean Beck scores were not significantly different between groups	Only 13 of the 20 patients completed the Beck inventory
Reik et al. (74)	18	Neurologic Lyme disease	Clinical interview	None	39% had mood lability and irritability; 22% had marked depression	Lyme disease diagnosed by history of erythema migrans or Lyme disease arthritis
Ackermann et al. (32)	44	*Borrelia* encephalomyelitis	Clinical interview	None	12 patients had mild memory and mood problems; 2 patients had dementia-like deficits	Diagnosis based on intrathecal production of Bb antibodies and clinical features

[a]A subgroup of patients from the study by Logigian et al. (23).

rochetes evident in the substantia nigra (37). A flare-up of symptoms shortly after the initiation of antibiotics was reported in four of these patients (60, 62); in one case (62), the antibiotic treatment may have precipitated a manic episode. This treatment-initiated flare-up may reflect an inflammatory response to spirochetal lysis and antigen release, similar to the Jarisch Herxheimer reaction that occurs in the treatment of syphilis. In addition to worsening systemic symptoms (e.g., arthralgias, weakness, shooting pains), this reaction may include worsening neuropsychiatric symptoms, such as depression, anxiety, or photophobia (33).

Psychiatric Series

Nine reports (23, 27, 32, 56, 57, 71–74) of larger series of Lyme patients are summarized in table 2. Irritability, mood lability, or depression were reported in seven of the nine studies, with a frequency ranging from 26% to 66% of the sample. Of the four controlled studies, three (57, 71, 73) reported that depression was greater or more frequently reported by the Lyme disease group. Noteworthy is that all of these studies were composed of patients with disseminated Lyme disease, primarily with late neurologic symptoms consistent with encephalopathy. The patients with Lyme encephalomyelitis (32) showed the most extreme illness, with two patients suffering from dementia-like syndromes. The one study of children with neurologic Lyme disease (72) indicated that behavioral or mood disturbances were the second most common symptom, resulting in mood lability, decreased interest in play, or poor school performance. Six of the 96 children in this series were thought to have psychiatric disturbances unrelated to Lyme disease.

Three of the studies relied on a clinical interview for psychiatric assessment (32, 72, 74). One used a survey based on DSM-III-R (73). Five used standardized self-report instruments (23, 27, 56, 57, 71). In one survey of 51 seropositive patients (73), the cumulative frequency of DSM-III-R major depression since the onset of illness was three times higher among the Lyme patients than among a medically ill comparison group, even though the comparison group was both older and ill far longer. In addition, among the Lyme patients who reported major depression, most (90%) denied a prior history of depression. It should be noted that none of the nine published series used structured psychiatric diagnostic interviews, and six of the nine studies relied solely on self-report measures. Although all of the studies in table 2 have methodological flaws (small sample size, unclear inclusion/exclusion criteria, biased samples, use of nonstandardized instruments, retrospective or cross-sectional data rather than a prospective design, reliance on patient self-report rather than a structured clinical interview conducted by an individual who was blind to the patient's diagnosis), the preponderance of evidence supports the notion that Lyme disease may be associated with marked mood changes.

In order to investigate the extent to which CNS infection with *B. burgdorferi* may contribute to the association between depression and Lyme disease, biological studies of depressed patients with Lyme disease, examining the CSF for evidence of direct infection or immune modulators, should be conducted. As in the investigation of depression in other medical illnesses, the multifactorial etiology of depression in Lyme disease needs to be addressed through examination of such factors as severity of illness, extent of pain, degree of disability, concomitant central neurologic symptoms or signs, psychodynamic factors, socioeconomic stressors, and family and personal history of psychiatric illness. Brain imaging studies (regional cerebral blood flow, SPECT, positron emission tomography) looking for evidence of metabolic dysfunction would also be of considerable interest.

MICROBIOLOGY OF *B. BURGDORFERI*

The microbiology of *B. burgdorferi* sheds light on why Lyme disease is an illness that at times can be relapsing and remitting and that can be refractory to normal immune surveillance and standard antibiotic regimens. The causative agent of Lyme disease—the spirochete *B. burgdorferi*—has a long replication time, comparable in this respect to *Mycobacterium tuberculosis*. Rapidly transmitted throughout the body, *B. burgdorferi* is known to invade the CNS within the first few weeks after initial infection (20–22). *B. burgdorferi* is known to be neurotropic, leaving the CSF to adhere to glial cells or other brain tissue (75). Once in the CNS, *B. burgdorferi*, like *T. pallidum*, may remain latent, only to cause illness months to years later (23).

Much of the genetic material in *B. burgdorferi* is contained in plasmids (76), resulting in the possibility of significant antigenic variability. This includes marked variability in the expression of surface antigens, with consequent alterations in immunogenicity. Such changes could lead to resistance to normal immunologic functions—for example, through a failure of the *B. burgdorferi*-specific antibody to induce phagocytosis—as well as to evasion of routine laboratory detection. Recent animal research (77) has found that the spirochete may undergo genetic alteration once it is sequestered in the CNS, thus resulting in a new strain of spirochete that is different from the infecting peripheral spirochete. The remarkable strain variation of *B. burgdorferi* may account for the differences between the presentation of Lyme disease in Europe and in the United States (78–80). For example, in Continental Europe, arthritic involvement is less common, and most cases of neurologic Lyme disease have prominent CSF abnormalities. Late-stage neurologic Lyme disease in the United States, on the other hand, is less likely to show CSF abnormalities on routine testing (81).

During growth, *B. burgdorferi* appears to shed membranous material (blebs) from its surface. These blebs coat the spirochete and have been found free in the CSF, serum, and urine (21, 82, 83). The blebs appear to interact specifically with IgM molecules. It is hypothesized that in some cases, the blebs may bind all of the free circulating *B. burgdorferi*-specific IgM antibodies, thereby enabling the organism itself to escape immune surveillance. In addition, the blebs possess potent, nonspecific mitogenic activity that may cause an inappropriate and ineffective stimulation of the immune system. This could initiate autoimmune disease processes (84).

B. burgdorferi has been shown to be capable of persisting in human hosts despite extensive antibiotic treatment (17, 85–88). Because in vitro studies demonstrate that *B. burgdorferi* can be recovered from antibiotic-treated fibroblast monolayers (89) and because *B. burgdorferi* has been shown to lodge inside human fibroblasts (89), mouse macrophages (90), and human endothelial cells (91), researchers conclude that the intracellular location may enable the spirochete to remain inaccessible to antibiotics and normal immune surveillance. Sequestration in other antibiotic- and immunologically privileged sites (e.g., CNS, joints, anterior chamber of the eye) may also account for persistent illness despite antibiotic treatment (20).

Several features are known to contribute to an organism's resistance to standard lengths of antibiotic treatment. These features include an intracellular location (92), long replication time, genetic variability, and the ability to become sequestered in difficult-to-penetrate sites. *B. burgdorferi* appears to possess all of these characteristics.

PATHOGENESIS OF CNS LYME DISEASE

A consistent finding in pathological studies is that the spirochete *B. burgdorferi* is rarely recovered from the affected organ, such as the CNS. Features consistent with a focal vasculitis, however, have been found in both the central and the peripheral nervous systems of patients with neurologic Lyme disease (93, 94). Scientists now believe that a small number of organisms can cause significant neurologic dysfunction either through a *B. burgdorferi*-initiated immune response directed specifically against neural tissue or through the triggering of a nonspecific inflammatory response (93). The immune response may remain active when spirochetal antigens are still present, as in an ongoing infection, or when a postinfectious autoimmune process has been triggered against host tissue.

Evidence exists to support the role of both specific and nonspecific immune processes in the production of CNS Lyme disease. Evidence of specific processes includes the production of *B. burgdorferi*-specific immune complexes and T cell responses within the CSF (95, 96), autoantibodies to neural tissue (97), and cross-reactivity of *B. burgdorferi* antibodies with neural tissue (98). Evidence of nonspecific processes includes an elevation of neurotoxins, such as quinolinic acid, in the CSF of Lyme patients but not normal comparison subjects (99). Of particular interest is that nonspecific products of immune activation, such as kynurenines or quinolinic acid, can be excitotoxic to neurons and have been linked to memory loss (100), anxiety and depression (101), seizures (101), and the chronic fatigue syndrome (102). In HIV-infected patients, elevations of quinolinic acid in the CSF tend to be correlated with the degree of neuropsychological deficits (100). Further investigation in this area is needed.

LYME DISEASE AND SYPHILIS

Several authors have noted similarities between Lyme disease and syphilis (3, 59, 103). Both are caused by a spirochete: syphilis by *T. pallidum* and Lyme disease by *B. burgdorferi.* Both start with skin inoculation and a localized skin reaction, followed by a disseminated multisystemic infection. Both may progress in stages. Both can cause meningitis, encephalitis, cognitive deficits, cranial neuropathy, and vasculitis. Both diseases can, in rare cases, lead to the Tullio phenomenon (40), characterized by nausea and nystagmus in response to sound stimulation. (This syndrome was previously considered pathognomonic for syphilis.) Antibiotic treatment of both diseases may lead to an initial worsening of symptoms, including neuropsychiatric ones (33, 104). The mechanism of injury in both infections is thought to be primarily indirect: one of immunopathogenesis, not a direct effect of the spirochete itself.

Both *T. pallidum* and *B. burgdorferi* can rapidly invade the CNS, within the first few weeks after infection. Both spirochetes can remain latent for long periods of time before the onset of disease. Both spirochetes can pass through or between endothelial cells (105, 106), thereby enabling dissemination and extensive tissue involvement. Both may persist in the host to cause a chronic infection.

Unlike *T. pallidum*, which is generally transmitted from host to host, the Lyme spirochete is carried by a vector. Furthermore, radiculopathy and peripheral neuropathy are features of Lyme disease that syphilis does not share.

Neurosyphilis is known to be associated with memory problems, depression, mania, psychosis, and personality changes, such as irritability, emotional lability, and apathy (107). Recent evidence suggests that Lyme borreliosis, the "new great imitator" (59), may be associated with a similarly wide spectrum of psychiatric disorders. What Hollos and Ferenczi (108) wrote about syphilis in 1925 bears analogy to the present state of knowledge about Lyme disease:

> The psychical symptomatology of paresis is by no means only an intellectual deterioration. On the contrary, it contains almost all the mental symptoms that occur in other psychoses, very frequently the most characteristic symptoms of mania, of melancholia, of paranoia, and of dementia praecox. In many cases the diagnosis for a long time oscillates between a "functional psychosis" and paresis, and only the beginning of pupillary stiffness, a facial palsy, or the finding of a "positive Wasserman," is the determining factor.

FUTURE DIRECTIONS IN RESEARCH

There are two areas of major clinical significance in which current knowledge about Lyme disease remains incomplete: diagnosis and the optimal treatment for patients with persistent symptoms.

Because currently available serologic tests are not always reliable, Lyme disease remains a clinical diagnosis that is based on a constellation of typical patterns. Diagnostic difficulty arises when patients present with symptoms that are nonspecific or atypical for Lyme disease. If these patients test positive for *B. burgdorferi,* they may be told that they have falsely positive test results. If they test negative, they may be told that they clearly do not have Lyme disease. Although the latter conclusions may be accurate in many cases, the absence of reliable laboratory tests makes such conclusions impossible to draw definitively. Although the prevalence of patients with seronegative Lyme disease is not known, such patients clearly do exist (48, 55, 109). Faced with diagnostic uncertainty, some clinicians may choose not to treat in order to avoid the risks of antibiotic therapy (110). Other clinicians who work in endemic areas may recommend an empirical trial of antibiotics because of what they judge to be a greater risk that a potentially multisystemic chronic infection may progress if untreated (17).

Definitive treatment guidelines for Lyme disease have not been established because knowledge about this illness continues to evolve. However, because of the rapid CNS invasion, aggressive treatment is recommended as early as possible (18). General guidelines consist of 3–4 weeks of oral antibiotics for patients without evidence of central neurologic involvement or 4–6 weeks of intravenous antibiotics for patients with central neurologic involvement. In many cases, following these guidelines results in a remission of symptoms. However, in some cases, relapse occurs after antibiotics are stopped (23).

Because intravenous antibiotic treatment is expensive

and the need for long-term treatment is not yet proven, some insurance companies are now denying reimbursement for repeated courses of intravenously administered treatment; denial of reimbursement is based on the argument that the efficacy of long-term or repeated antibiotic treatment has not been established (111). Yet clinical experience suggests that some patients with central neurologic involvement may require repeated intravenously administered treatment. Several lines of evidence support this clinical observation. First, some patients with Lyme encephalopathy respond well to additional courses of antibiotics (23, 27). Second, several case reports document the persistence of the spirochete or symptoms in patients who have already had the recommended 4–6-week course of antibiotics (17, 85–88). Third, newer diagnostic techniques are able to detect the presence of *B. burgdorferi* antigens in some previously treated, persistently symptomatic patients (21). Fourth, as noted earlier, the microbiology of *B. burgdorferi* makes it clear why standard courses of antibiotics might be ineffective in some cases.

Some patients do not get better with repeated treatment. Persistent symptoms in these patients may result from permanent damage or from a postinfectious autoimmune process (112). Prospective microbiological and clinical studies are needed to identify risk factors that may predispose certain patients to develop chronic Lyme disease and to distinguish those patients who will respond to prolonged or repeated antibiotic treatment from those who will not.

CONCLUSIONS

The neuropsychiatric effects of many infectious illnesses, bacterial (neurosyphilis, tuberculosis), parasitic (neurocysticercosis, toxoplasmosis), fungal (coccidiomycoses, cryptococcosis), and viral (herpes simplex, HIV), are well known. Also well known are the prominent neuropsychiatric manifestations of illnesses, such as systemic lupus erythematosus and multiple sclerosis, that cause CNS inflammation. Early in the history of many of these illnesses, the psychiatric symptoms were thought to be functional in nature. Women suffering from multiple sclerosis were thought to be hysterical. Early depression and cognitive decline in patients with AIDS were thought to represent purely an emotional reaction to a serious illness. Later research provided objective evidence that CNS pathology caused by infection or inflammation was associated with each of these psychiatric syndromes.

The spectrum of neuropsychiatric syndromes associated with Lyme disease is only beginning to be elucidated by clinical studies and case reports. At the same time, biological studies and brain imaging techniques suggest a physiological basis for such syndromes through one or more of the following mechanisms: direct infection in the CNS; specific, localized autoimmune reactions; or secondary but centrally active immunologic responses to systemic infection.

This article emphasizes the biological substrate of the neuropsychiatric symptoms associated with Lyme disease. The complicated secondary emotional reactions to this illness that relate to particular aspects of its symptoms, including fluctuating course, bizarreness of symptoms, cognitive disability, chronic pain, and the uncertainties surrounding its diagnosis and management, have been discussed in greater detail elsewhere (33).

In addition to the dermatologic and arthritic manifestations, the breadth of neuropsychiatric symptoms in Lyme disease should be recognized. The lessons painfully learned in syphilis apply here: delays in diagnosis and treatment can result in a treatable, acute illness becoming a chronic one with, in some cases, devastating consequences.

REFERENCES

1. White DJ, Chang HG, Benach JL, Bosler EM, Meldrum SC, Means RG, Debbie JG, Birkhead GS, Morse DL: The geographic spread and temporal increase of the Lyme disease epidemic. JAMA 1991; 266:1230–1236
2. Burgdorfer W: Lyme Borreliosis: ten years after the discovery of the etiologic agent, Borrelia burgdorferi. Infection 1991; 4: 257–262
3. Lukehart SA, Marra C: A comparison of syphilis and Lyme disease: central nervous system involvement, in Lyme Disease: Molecular and Immunologic Approaches. Edited by Schutzer SE. Cold Spring Harbor, NY, Cold Spring Harbor Laboratory Press, 1992
4. Piesman J, Mather T, Sinskt R, Spielman A: Duration of tick attachment and Borrelia burgdorferi transmission. J Clin Microbiol 1987; 25:557–558
5. CDC: Lyme Disease—United States 1991–1992. MMWR 1993; 42:345–348
6. State of Connecticut Department of Public Health: Lyme Disease Update. Connecticut Epidemiologist 1993; 13:9–12
7. Steere AC, Malawista SE, Snydman DR, Shope RE, Andiman WA, Ross MR, Steele FM: Lyme arthritis: an epidemic of oligoarticular arthritis in children and adults in three Connecticut communities. Arthritis Rheum 1977; 20:7–17
8. Garin Ch, Bujadoux A: Paralysie par les tiques. J Med Lyon 1922; 3:765–767
9. Bannwarth A: Chronische lymphocytare meningitis, entzundliche polyneuritis and "rheumtisums." Arch Psychiatr Nervenkr 1941; 113:284–376
10. Afzelius A: Erythema chronicum migrans. Acta Derm Venereol (Stockh) 1921; 2:120–125
11. Hellerstrom M: Erythema chronicum migrans Afzelii. Acta Derm Venereol (Stockh) 1930; 11:315–321
12. Scrimenti RJ: Erythema chronicum migrans. Arch Dermatol 1970; 102:104–105
13. Steere AC, Broderick TF, Malawista SE: Erythema chronicum migrans and Lyme arthritis: epidemiologic evidence for a tick vector. Am J Epidemiol 1978; 108:312–321
14. Burgdorfer W, Barbour AG, Hayes SF, Benach JL, Brunwaldt E, Davis JP: Lyme disease—a tick-borne spirochetosis? Science 1982; 216:1317–1319
15. Gilliland BC, Petersdorf RG: Infectious arthritis, in Principles of Internal Medicine. Edited by Petersdorf RG, Adams RD, Braunwald E, Isselbacher KJ, Martin JB, Wilson JD. New York, McGraw-Hill, 1983
16. Lavoie PE, Lyme disease (Lyme Borreliosis), in Conn's Current Therapy 1991. Edited by Rakel RE. Philadelphia, WB Saunders, 1991
17. Liegner KB: Lyme disease: the sensible pursuit of answers. J Clin Microbiol 1993; 31:1961–1963

18. Coyle PK: Neurologic Lyme disease. Semin Neurol 1992; 12: 200–208
19. Reznick JW, Braunstein DB, Walsh RI, Smith C, Wolfson PM, Gierke IW, Gorelkin I, Chandler RW: Lyme carditis: electrophysiologic and histopathologic study. Am J Med 1986; 5:923–927
20. Luft BJ, Steinman CR, Neimark HC, Muralidhar B, Rush T, Finkel MF, Kunkel M, Dattwyler RJ: Invasion of the CNS by Bb in acute disseminated infection. JAMA 1992; 267:1364–1367
21. Coyle PK, Deng Z, Schutzer SE, Belman AL, Benach J, Krupp LB, Luft B: Detection of Borrelia burgdorferi antigens in cerebrospinal fluid. Neurology 1993; 43:1093–1097
22. Garcia-Monco JC, Villar BF, Alen JC, Benach JL: Borrelia burgdorferin in the central nervous system: experimental and clinical evidence for early invasion. J Infect Dis 1990; 161: 1187–1193
23. Logigian EL, Kaplan RF, Steere AC: Chronic neurologic manifestations of Lyme disease. N Engl J Med 1990; 323:1438–1444
24. Steere AC, Bartenhagen NH, Craft JE, Hutchinson GJ, Newman JH, Rahn DW, Sigal LH, Spieler PN, Stenn KS, Malawista SE: The early clinical manifestations of Lyme disease. Ann Intern Med 1983; 99:76–82
25. Reik L: Lyme Disease and the Nervous System. New York, Thieme, 1992
26. Pachner AR, Steere AC: The triad of neurologic manifestations of Lyme disease: meningitis, cranial neuritis, and radiculoneuritis. Neurology 1985; 35:47–53
27. Halperin JJ, Pass HL, Anand AK, Luft BJ, Volkman DJ, Dattwyler RJ: Nervous system abnormalities in Lyme disease. Ann NY Acad Sci 1988; 539:24–34
28. Steere AC, Malawista SE, Hardin JA, Ruddy S, Askenase PW, Andiman WA: Erythema chronicum migrans and Lyme arthritis: the enlarging clinical spectrum. Ann Intern Med 1977; 86: 685–698
29. Flach AJ, Lavoie PE: Episcleritis, conjunctivitis, and keratitis as ocular manifestations of Lyme disease. Ophthalmology 1990; 97:973–975
30. Steere AC, Duray PH, Danny JH, Kaufman MD, Wormser GP: Unilateral blindness caused by infection with Lyme disease spirochete, Borrelia burgdorferi. Ann Intern Med 1985; 103:382–384
31. Asbrink E, Hovmark A, Hederstedt B: The spirochetal etiology of acrodermatitis chronica atrophicans Herxheimer. Acta Derm Venereol (Stockh) 1984; 64:506–512
32. Ackermann R, Rehse-Kupper B, Gollmer E, Schmidt R: Chronic neurologic manifestations of Erythema migrans borreliosis. Ann NY Acad Sci 1988; 539:16–23
33. Fallon BA, Nields JA, Burrascano JJ, Liegner K, DelBene D, Liebowitz MR: The neuropsychiatric manifestations of Lyme borreliosis. Psychiatr Q 1992; 63:95–115
34. Reik L, Smith L, Khan A, Nelson W: Demyelinating encephalopathy in Lyme disease. Neurology 1985; 35:267–269
35. Krupp LB, Mendelson BW, Friedman R: An overview of chronic fatigue syndrome. J Clin Psychiatry 1991; 52:403–410
36. MacDonald AB, Miranda JM: Concurrent neocortical borreliosis and Alzheimer's disease. Hum Pathol 1987; 18:750–761
37. Waniek C, Prohovnik I, Kaufman MA: Rapid progressive frontal type dementia associated with Lyme disease and subcortical degeneration, in Abstracts of the VII Annual International Scientific Conference on Lyme Borreliosis. Hartford, Conn, Lyme Disease Foundation, 1994
38. Reik L, Burgdorfer W, Donaldson JO: Neurologic abnormalities in Lyme disease without erythema chronicum migrans. Am J Med 1986; 81:73–77
39. Brogan GX, Homan CS, Viccellio P: The enlarging clinical spectrum of Lyme disease: Lyme cerebral vasculitis, a new disease entity. Ann Emerg Med 1990; 19:572–576
40. Nields JA, Kveton JF: Tullio phenomenon and seronegative Lyme borreliosis (letter). Lancet 1991; 338:128–129
41. Kohler J, Kern U, Kaper J, Rhese-Kupper B, Thoden U: Chronic central nervous system involvement in Lyme borreliosis. Neurology 1988; 38:863–867
42. Kohlhepp W, Kuhn W, Kruger H: Extrapyramidal features in central Lyme borreliosis. Eur Neurol 1989; 29:150–155
43. Halperin JJ, Kaplan GP, Brazinsky S, Tsai TF, Cheng T, Ironside A, Wu P, Delfiner J, Golightly M, Brown RH: Immunologic reactivity against Borrelia burgdorferi in patients with motor neuron disease. Arch Neurol 1990; 47:586–594
44. Clavelou P, Beytout J, Vernay D, Aumaitre O, Dordain G, Tournilhac M: Neurologic manifestations of Lyme disease in the northern parts of the Auvergne (abstract). Neurology 1989; 39(suppl 1):350
45. Magnarelli LA: Laboratory diagnosis of Lyme disease. Rheum Dis Clin North Am 1989; 15:735–745
46. Bakken LL, Case KL, Callister SM, Bourdeau NJ, Schell RF: Performance of 45 laboratories participating in a proficiency testing program for Lyme disease serology. JAMA 1992; 268: 891–895
47. Hyde FW, Johnson RC, White TJ, Shelburne CE: Detection of antigens in urine of mice and humans infected with Borrelia burgdorferi, etiologic agent of Lyme disease. J Clin Microbiol 1989; 27:58–61
48. Dattwyler RJ, Volkman DJ, Luft BJ, Halperin JJ, Thomas J, Golightly MG: Seronegative Lyme disease. New Engl J Med 1988; 319:1441–1446
49. Schutzer SE, Coyle PK, Brunner M: Identification of specific borrelia burgdorferi components in circulating antigen-antibody complexes, in Lyme Disease: Molecular and Immunologic Approaches. Edited by Schutzer SE. Cold Spring Harbor, NY, Cold Spring Harbor Laboratory Press, 1992
50. Rosa PA, Schwan TG: A specific and sensitive assay for the Lyme disease spirochete, borrelia burgdorferi, using the polymerase chain reaction. J Infect Dis 1989; 160:1018–1029
51. Nocton JJ, Dressler F, Rutledge BJ, Rys PN, Persing DH, Steere AC: Detection of Borrelia burgdorferi DNA by polymerase chain reaction in synovial fluid from patients with Lyme arthritis. New Engl J Med 1994; 330:229–234
52. Callister SM, Schell RF, Lim LCL, Jobe DA, Case KL, Bryant GL, Molling PE: Detection of borreliacidal antibodies by flow cytometry. Arch Intern Med 1994; 154:1625–1632
53. Grodzicki RL, Steere AC: Comparison of immunoblotting and indirect enzyme-linked immunosorbent assay using different antigen preparations for diagnosing early Lyme disease. J Infect Dis 1988; 157:790–797
54. Shrestha M, Grodzicki RL, Steere AC: Diagnosing early Lyme disease. Am J Med 1985; 78:235–240
55. Schutzer SE, Coyle PK, Belman AL, Golightly MG, Drulle J: Sequestration of antibody to Borrelia burgdorferi in immune complexes in seronegative Lyme disease. Lancet 1990; 335: 312–315
56. Kaplan RF, Meadows ME, Vincent LC, Logigian EL, Steere AC: Memory impairment and depression in patients with Lyme encephalopathy: comparison with fibromyalgia and nonpsychotically depressed patients. Neurology 1992; 42:1263–1267
57. Krupp LB, Masur D, Schwartz J, Coyle PK, Langenbach LJ, Fernquist SK, Jandorf L, Halperin JJ: Cognitive functioning in late Lyme borreliosis. Arch Neurol 1991; 48:1125–1129
58. Coyle PK, Schutzer SE, Belman AL, Krupp LB, Dheng Z: Cerebrospinal fluid immunologic parameters in neurologic Lyme disease, in Lyme Disease: Molecular and Immunologic Approaches. Edited by Schutzer SE. Cold Spring Harbor, NY, Cold Spring Harbor Laboratory Press, 1992
59. Pachner AR: Neurologic manifestations of Lyme disease, the new "Great Imitator." Rev Infect Dis 1989; 11(suppl 6):S1482–S1486
60. Fallon BA, Nields JA, Parsons B, Liebowitz MR, Klein DF: Psychiatric manifestations of Lyme borreliosis. J Clin Psychiatry 1993; 54:263–268
61. von Economo C: Encephalitis Lethargica: Its Sequelae and Treatment. London, Oxford University Press, 1931, pp 118–131
62. Fallon BA, Schwartzberg M, Bransfield R, Zimmerman B, Scotti A, Weber CA, Liebowitz MR: Late stage neuropsychiatric Lyme disease: differential diagnosis and treatment. Psychosomatics (in press)

LYME DISEASE

63. Swedo SE, Leonard HL: Speculations on antineuronal antibody-mediated neuropsychiatric disorders of childhood. Pediatrics 1994; 93:323–326
64. Omasits M, Seiser A, Brainin M: Recurrent and relapsing borreliosis of the nervous system. Wien Klin Wochenschr 1990; 102:4–12
65. Kohler VJ: Lyme disease in neurology and psychiatry. Fortschr Med 1990; 108:191–194
66. Roelcke U, Barnett W, Wilder-Smith E, Sigmund D, Hacke W: Untreated neuroborreliosis: Bannwarth's syndrome evolving into acute schizophrenia-like psychosis. J Neurol 1992; 239: 129–131
67. Pfister HW, Preac-Mursic V, Wilske B, Rieder G, Forderreuther S, Schmidt S, Kapfhammer HP: Catatonic syndrome in acute severe encephalitis due to Borrelia burgdorferi infection. Neurology 1993; 43:433–435
68. Diringer MN, Halperin JJ, Dattwyler RJ: Lyme meningoencephalitis: report of a severe, penicillin-resistant case. Arthritis Rheum 1987; 30:705–707
69. Burrascand JJ: Lyme disease presenting as organic psychosis (abstract). Sixth Annual Lyme Disease Scientific Conference, 1993. Hartford, Conn, Lyme Disease Foundation
70. Pachner AR, Duray P, Steere AC: Central nervous system manifestations of Lyme disease. Arch Neurol 1989; 46:790–795
71. Barr WB, Hilton E, Warum F, Flash V, Solomon S: Assessment of depression in late Lyme disease (abstract). Neurology 1991; 41S:120
72. Belman AL, Iyer M, Coyle PK, Dattwyler R: Neurologic manifestations in children with North American Lyme disease. Neurology 1993; 43:2609–2614
73. Fallon BA, Nields JA, DelBene D, Liebowitz MR, Klein DF: Depression and Lyme disease: a controlled survey, in New Research Program and Abstracts, 144th Annual Meeting of the American Psychiatric Association. Washington, DC, APA, 1991
74. Reik L, Steere AC, Bartenhagen NH, Shope RE, Malawista SE: Neurologic abnormalities of Lyme disease. Medicine 1979; 58: 281–294
75. Garcia-Monco JC, Fernandez-Villar B, Benach JL: Adherence of the Lyme disease spirochete to glial cells and cells of glial origin. J Infect Dis 1989; 160:497–506
76. Barbour AG, Garon CF: Linear plasmids of the bacterium Borrelia burgdorferi have covalently closed ends. Science 1987; 237: 409–411
77. Pachner AR, Itano A: Borrelia burgdorferi infection of the brain: characterization of the organism and response to antibiotics and immune sera in the mouse model. Neurology 1990; 40:1535–1540
78. Hanrahan JP, Benach JL, Coleman JL, Bosler EM, Morse DL, Cameron DJ, Edelman R, Kaslow RA: J Infect Dis 1984; 150:489–596
79. Steere AC, Taylor E, Wilson ML, Levine JL, Spielman A: Longitudinal assessment of the clinical and epidemiological features of Lyme disease in a defined population. J Infect Dis 1986; 154:295–300
80. Schwan TG, Burgdorfer W, Garon CF: Changes in infectivity and plasmid profile of the Lyme disease spirochete, Borrelia burgdorferi, as a result of in vitro cultivation. Infect Immun 1988; 56:1831–1836
81. Coyle PK: Antigen detection and cerebrospinal fluid studies, in Lyme Disease. Edited by Coyle PK. Philadelphia, Mosby Year Book, 1992
82. Garon CF, Dorward DW, Corwin MD: Structural features of Borrelia burgdorferi—the Lyme disease spirochete: silver staining for nucleic acids. Scanning Microsc Suppl 1989; 3:109–115
83. Dorward DW, Schwan TG, Garon CF: Immune capture and detection of Borrelia burgdorferi antigens in urine, blood, or tissues from infected ticks, mice, dogs, and humans. J Clin Microbiol 1991; 29:1162–1170
84. Whitmire WM, Garon CF: Specific and nonspecific responses of murine B cells to membrane blebs of Borrelia burgdorferi. Infect Immun 1993; 61:1460–1467
85. Preac-Mursic V, Weber K, Pfister HW, Wilske B, Gross B, Baumann A, Prokop J: Survival of Borrelia burgdorferi in antibiotically treated patients with Lyme borreliosis. Infection 1989; 17: 355–359
86. Haupl T, Hahn G, Rittig M, Krause A, Schoerner C, Schonherr U, Kalden JR, Burmester GR: Persistence of Borrelia burgdorferi in ligamentous tissue from a patient with chronic Lyme borreliosis. Arthritis Rheum 1993; 36:1621–1626
87. Hassler D, Riedel K, Zorn J, Preac-Mursic V: Pulsed high-dose cefotaxime therapy in refractory Lyme borreliosis (letter). Lancet 1991; 338:193
88. Liegner KB, Shapiro JR, Ramsay D, Halperin AJ, Hogrefe W, Kong L: Recurrent erythema migrans despite extended antibiotic treatment with minocycline in a patient with persisting Borrelia burgdorferi infection. J Am Acad Dermatol 1993; 28:312–314
89. Georgilis K, Peacocke M, Klempner MS: Fibroblasts protect the Lyme disease spirochete, Borrelia burgdorferi, from ceftriaxone in vitro. J Infect Dis 1992; 166:440–444
90. Montgomery RR, Nathanson MH, Malawista SE: The fate of Borrelia burgdorferi in mouse macrophages: destruction, survival, recovery. J Immunol 1993; 150:909–915
91. Ma Y, Sturrock A, Weis JJ: Intracellular localization of Borrelia burgdorferi within human endothelial cells. Infect Immun 1991; 59:671–678
92. Mahmoud AF: The challenge of intracellular pathogens (editorial). N Engl J Med 1992; 326:761–762
93. Benach JL, Garcia Monco JC: Aspects of the pathogenesis of neuroborreliosis, in Lyme Disease: Molecular and Immunologic Approaches. Cold Spring Harbor, NY, Cold Spring Harbor Laboratory Press, 1992
94. Duray PH: Target organs of Borrelia burgdorferi infections: functional responses and histology, in Lyme disease: molecular and immunologic approaches. Edited by Schutzer SE. Cold Spring Harbor, NY, Cold Spring Harbor Laboratory Press, 1992
95. Coyle PK, Schutzer SE, Belman AL, Krupp LB, Golightly MG: Cerebrospinal fluid immune complexes in patients exposed to Borrelia burgdorferi: detection of Borrelia specific and non-specific complexes. Ann Neurol 1990; 28:739–744
96. Pachner AR, Steere AC, Sigal LH, Johnson CJ: Antigen-specific proliferation of CSF lymphocytes in Lyme disease. Neurology 1985; 35:1642–1644
97. Garcia-Monco JC, Coleman JL, Benach JL: Antibodies to myelin basic protein in Lyme disease patients. J Infect Dis 1988; 158:667–668
98. Sigal LH, Tatum AH: Lyme disease patients' serum contains IgM antibodies to Borrelia burgdorferi that cross react with neuronal antigens. Neurology 1988; 38:1439–1442
99. Halperin JJ, Heyes MP: Neuroactive kynurenines in Lyme borreliosis. Neurology 1992; 42:43–50
100. Heyes MP, Brew JB, Martin A, Price RW, Salazar AM, Sidtis JJ, Yergey JA, Mouradian MM, Sadler AE, Keilp J, Rubinow D, Markey SP: Quinolinic acid in cerebrospinal fluid and serum in HIV-I infection: relationship to clinical and neurological status. Ann Neurol 1991; 29:202–209
101. Lapin IP: Behavioral and convulsant effects of kynurenines, in Quinolinic Acid and the Kynurenines. Edited by Stone TW. Boca Raton, Fla, CRC Press, 1988
102. Heyes MP, Saito K, Crowley JS, Davis LE, Demitrack MA, Der M, Dilling LA Elia J, Kruesi MJP, Lackner A, Larsen SA, Lee K, Leonard HL, Markey SP, Martin A, Milstein S, Mouradian MM, Pranzatelli MR, Quearry BJ, Salazar A, Smith M, Strauss SE, Sunderland T, Swedo SW, Tourtellotte WW: Quinolinic acid and kynurenine pathway metabolism in inflammatory and non-inflammatory neurologic disease. Brain 1992; 115:1249–1273
103. Miklossy J, Kuntzer T, Bogousslavsky J, Regli F, Janzer RC: Meningovascular form of neuroborreliosis: similarities between neuropathological findings in a case of Lyme disease and those occurring in tertiary neurosyphilis. Acta Neuropathol 1990; 80: 568–572
104. Thomas EW: Syphilis: Its Course and Management. New York, Macmillan, 1949, pp 112–113
105. Comstock LE, Thomas DD: Penetration of endothelial cell

monolayers by Borrelia burgdorferi. Infect Immun 1989; 57: 1626–1628

106. Thomas DD, Navab M, Haake DA, Fogelman AM, Miller JN, Lovett MA: Treponema pallidum invades intercellular junctions of endothelial cell monolayers. Proc Natl Acad Sci USA 1988; 85:3608–3612
107. Rundell JR, Wise MG: Neurosyphilis: a psychiatric perspective. Psychosomatics 1985; 26:287–295
108. Hollos S, Ferenczi S: Psychoanalysis and the Psychic Disorder of General Paresis. New York, Nervous and Mental Disease Publishing Co, 1925, p 2
109. Keller TL, Halperin JJ, Whitman M: PCR detection of Borrelia burgdorferi DNA in cerebrospinal fluid of Lyme neuroborreliosis patients. Neurology 1992; 42:32–42
110. Appropriateness of parenteral antibiotic treatment for patients with presumed Lyme disease: a joint statement of the American College of Rheumatology and the Council of the Infectious Diseases Society of America. Ann Intern Med 1993; 119:518
111. Stevens S: Suits seen rising to force coverage of untested therapies. Physicians Financial News, Dec 15, 1993, pp 1, 36
112. Sigal LH: Possible autoimmune mechanisms in Lyme disease, in Lyme Disease: Molecular and Immunologic Approaches. Edited by Schutzer SE. Cold Spring Harbor, NY, Cold Spring Harbor Laboratory Press, 1992

MEDICAL MAYHEM AND MIRACLES

9

A Story of Pediatric Lyme Disease

By Linda Laidlaw, PhD

A Parent's Worst Nightmare

December 4, 2007—Video Diary

My daughter lies prone on a sofa, her face slack, eyes unfocused. She pokes at her eyes, prods her forehead, appearing to experience discomfort. She seems unaware of the video camera recording her, though a few months earlier she would have delighted in being recorded and would have wanted to see her image played back immediately. She sucks on and pulls at her shirt, puts her fingers in her mouth, the gestures of an infant rather than a girl who is nearly five. She no longer engages in conversations, though occasionally will echo others' words, or a phrase might slip through during a fleeting lucid moment. This formerly vibrant and curious four and a half year old girl appears as a profoundly disabled child. After a day spent in the children's Emergency ward earlier in the week, she awaits appointments with psychiatry and neurology. The pediatrician has warned me that her condition could be due to psychosis, or the result of constant absence seizures, and so the video diary is recorded to provide some evidence of what has been occurring. Soon the awaited "episode" begins and my daughter begins to laugh, although whatever is causing the laughter is not visible to an outside eye. The giggles are infectious at first, especially in contrast to the earlier lack of affect. But, after witnessing these laughing fits occur several times each day, they have come to seem more ominous ... yet another sign that my child is slowly losing her mind to an unknown disease. The laughter and accompanying restless movements continue for forty minutes until eventually the giggles die into something resembling shrieking, and then my daughter retreats back into silent, blank staring.

The preceding account, based on video recordings, attempts to provide a brief picture of my daughter Xian as she descended into illness. This chapter will present the story of her decline into what seemed an inexplicable and untreatable neurological illness, and the path that was necessary for her recovery. But this story is not hers alone, and so I will also share part of the larger story that is pediatric Lyme disease in North America. I am fully aware of the impact a book such as this can make, as it was only through another mother's willingness to share her son's Lyme story that I was finally provided with the necessary clues for my daughter to begin the slow road back to health and to the child she once was.

At the beginning of Xian's treatment, which came over a year after she had begun developing symptoms, I was offered a glimmer of hope, but we had been down too many wrong paths for me to truly believe my daughter could fully recover or that she even had an illness that could be treated. The best I was hoping for, quite truthfully, were the sort of improvements that would allow us to return to a semblance of a normal life: to be able to leave the house once again, for Xian to attend school, and for me to return to work. After her descent into what appeared to be a permanently altered state, with loss of memory, dementia, the loss of her ability to communicate normally, as well as the emergence of multiple physical problems, I assumed that there would be no escaping irreversible damage. No child could come back from such depths of disability. Or could they…?

Into the Twilight Zone

In retrospect, the very beginning of Xian's illness closely followed a trip to Vancouver Island, in May 2007. We'd had a busy start to the year, with travel to China in January to adopt Xian's then two year old little sister Rachel. Xian herself had been adopted from China as a 15 month old, and was very excited about the trip and about being a big sister. On the return from China, after the expected post-travel jet lag and settling in period, Xian was at the top of her form, happy to introduce her new little sister to friends, relatives, and her preschool program. Our family was managing so well with all the changes that in late spring we traveled to Vancouver Island to visit family members so that they could meet our new addition. Towards the end of the trip, I noticed that Xian had what appeared to be some odd red bites, but as she had spent some time cuddling with my sister's dogs, I assumed that she might have encountered a flea or two. I couldn't have told you what a tick looked like at that point, nor had I ever looked for one.

Xian's initial symptoms began several weeks later, though they were vague enough to be explained away as a new developmental stage, or perhaps some low level virus. She'd had what seemed to be a cold, with a heavy cough and mild fever. I considered taking her in to the pediatrician to have her cough checked out but it slowly eased. At the same time, Xian began to experience periods where she was sensitive to sound and suddenly became anxious and upset when she was in noisy locations. She began to act moody and irritable, unusual for her outside of illness or times when she was feeling stressed. At daycare, her caregivers mentioned that she seemed clingy and was easily upset, but we all assumed these changes could be attributed to her favorite caregivers being away on holiday.

A repeat trip to BC in August to visit Xian's grandparents marked further changes. She became even more sensitive to noise and no longer seemed to want to go on outings to places she'd formerly enjoyed. Even the prospect of a new toy purchase would not lure her into the car; she would rather stay indoors or outside in my parents' quiet and shaded backyard. At this point a new symptom emerged: inexplicable tantrums and screaming fits that would appear suddenly and end just as abruptly. Xian was unable to talk about them once they had passed and seemed as confused by her behaviour as everyone else was. During the trip there were times she seemed to be hearing and seeing things that made her laugh and which weren't connected to anything the rest of us were noticing, though my parents and I brushed off those first occurrences as being connected to an active imagination and even joked about her "imaginary friend." But by the time we returned to Edmonton, I had a sense that something odd was going on that went beyond a developmental phase, and because of Xian's extreme sound sensitivities and behaviour changes I decided to make the first of a long series of appointments with the pediatrician. She was referred to an audiologist to check whether the issues might be related to hearing difficulties (as by then she was also often not responding when spoken to), but her results were perfectly normal, and while she did have a large quantity of earwax removed by the nurse at the pediatrician's office, strangely enough, her sound sensitivities were immediately heightened after this procedure.

In September Xian moved into a new daycare room with the older preschool and kindergarten children. From the time Xian moved rooms she refused to put her belongings in their new spots, often wandered back into the old room, and spent a lot of time crying. The "new tantrums" also began to appear at daycare. The childcare workers and I initially assumed she was having difficulty with the transition, although her reactions seemed extreme compared to her responses to earlier changes. However, many of the difficulties were linked to another new symptom, one that she could compensate for at home and in more familiar environments but not in her new classroom—the loss of her short-term memory. What her caregivers and I had assumed was a refusal to adapt to change was in fact an inability to remember new routines or new locations for objects. By this point Xian also began to exhibit a decline in skills she had formerly mastered. She became increasingly sloppy when eating and now required assistance in dressing and toileting and seemed unable to focus on most tasks. Xian's tantrums became more frequent and even more intense, but because she was now suffering from extreme insomnia in addition to her other issues, her teachers, doctor and I assumed that sleep deprivation was the cause of the tantrums, mood swings, and decline in independence, even though the insomnia had in fact followed some of those changes. From early September Xian had become increasingly unable to fall asleep. She would lie in bed staring vacantly and was unable to tell me why she couldn't sleep or what was bothering her. No sleep remedies or even more substantial medications worked. Some nights she would simply sob inconsolably or repeatedly apologize. While at the time I interpreted the night time upsets as related to the daycare changes, I am certain now that she was becoming aware of her symptoms taking hold and was increasingly frightened by her experiences.

Because Xian's sensitivity to sound and light were increasing, her doctor suggested that perhaps Xian was experiencing an underlying sensory integration problem. At this point Xian's collection of symptoms was very perplexing and didn't really "fit" with my child as I knew her, but the explanations all seemed to make sense, although none of the solutions seemed to be making any difference. I had an increasing feeling in the pit of my stomach that there was something seriously wrong, especially since Xian also seem to be acting consistently with the very few times she'd been quite sick. My gut was telling me that I had an increasingly ill child, though no one seemed to be recognizing that, yet. I hoped it would simply be a matter of time until the cause of her problems was uncovered.

In late September Xian had several good weeks when her sleep and other symptoms improved a little and I began to hope that maybe whatever was afflicting her had simply run its course. Little did I know that we were experiencing what was to be the ongoing cycle of her illness—new symptoms followed by some improvements and then followed by another spiral downward into more severe illness and further loss of abilities.

By Halloween Xian was having longer periods of zoning out—periods of time when she appeared completely absent and would not respond to communication unless requests were repeated loudly. While previously she had been a "chatterbox," now she spoke very little, and would have days when, if pressed to respond, her answers would be one or two words. She was no longer able to answer any questions other than those involving a simple "yes" or "no." By this point, her three-year-old sister Rachel also knew that there was something wrong. She commented, "Xian's talking isn't working." Within weeks, Rachel observed, "Xian's playing isn't working." While Halloween had been one of Xian's favorite times of the year, our short excursion to children's events at a local mall seemed terrifying to her.

In mid fall Xian started having bladder problems. She had days when she couldn't seem to "go" at all and days where she had constant pain and urgency, although urine tests and an abdominal ultrasound revealed nothing. By late fall Xian had blood work done to check for thyroid function and other abnormalities that could be more common causes of developmental anomalies. Her pediatrician wondered if she might be experiencing absence seizures after seeing Xian completely unresponsive during a November appointment, and she was put on a waiting list for an EEG and a neurology appointment. By the end of November it was clear that the periods where she was unaware of what was going on around her were increasing. On some days her daycare teachers reported that she would suddenly "come to" hours after I had dropped her off and wonder where I was, and spent other days working on one activity like an automaton. Both at home and at daycare she was having more frequent episodes of disconnected laughing or screaming. At home, she began to spend hours laying on the couch in dim light, watching Dora—for some reason the only video program she would tolerate. By this point, Dora videos aside, she could no longer stand any noise at all in the house—TV, radio, appliances, and even conversation all seemed to cause her severe distress. My previously cuddly child could no longer bear physical touch, especially anywhere near her head or on her upper body. Her sense of taste, too, seemed changed and she would spit out or gag on previously favorite foods.

Mayhem

In December, with repeated fruitless doctor's appointments and Xian moving farther away from her normal behaviour and personality, and developing more troubling symptoms, I took her to Pediatric Emergency. There she received a CT scan, an EEG, a wider range of blood tests, and she was seen by a pediatric neurologist, who recognized that something appeared to be going on, though it also took some convincing on my part to prove to her that Xian was not "faking it." The neurologist did not believe Xian was having seizures, though she did ask me to videotape her at home to provide some evidence of the episodes of laughing, zoning out, and screaming. Xian was put on one waitlist for an MRI to check for brain tumors or other structural abnormalities, and another to receive a longer EEG, and was sent home. A week later, when Xian continued to decline even further, no longer recognizing me, we returned to the hospital again and I insisted she be admitted, hoping that someone would be able to figure out what was going on.

Xian spent nearly three weeks in the children's hospital, having the MRI, a lumbar puncture, a skin biopsy to check for mitochondrial diseases, dozens of additional tests, and was examined by many more specialists and medical residents. The cause of Xian's illness remained undetermined, although one of the specialists who examined her, a child psychiatrist, believed that whatever was going on seemed to have a component of delirium to it, as Xian's condition fluctuated from morning to evening and day by day. By then my daughter reminded me of a small Alzheimer's patient—during occasional lucid moments she would briefly recognize family members and engage in familiar activities, but at other times she was very confused and frantically repeated strange statements such as "I forgot to call you back!" and could only calm herself when I pretended to have her make a call at the ward pay phone. At other times she was entirely unresponsive, even when undergoing painful medical procedures such as an IV insertion for anesthesia. At the end of her hospital stay, when there seemed to be nothing further anyone was going to do, she was released home with a diagnosis of suspected "late onset autistic spectrum disorder" and an appointment to see a developmental pediatrician who specialized in autism. I was told by a medical resident that since they'd explored all of the "treatable common conditions," and most "treatable uncommon conditions," that Xian's medical investigations had moved into "untreatable uncommon conditions," which meant, effectively, that there was now little urgency to finding a cause. I was also told by several of Xian's doctors that I needed to stop expecting a diagnosis and told to stop researching conditions on the Internet. I asked if there was any chance of Xian recovering or being treated eventually, and was told there was little hope for cases like hers, and in fact it might be many years before a diagnosis would be found. Still, somehow I had a sense that Xian could recover if we could find the right answers—I knew my daughter was "still there" when she had her occasional lucid moment—and I sensed there was an urgency to her situation, even though her doctors no longer seemed to agree.

During her hospitalizations, it often seemed that the doctors and specialists didn't really listen when Xian's symptoms did not fit with what they already knew or the possible diagnoses they were considering. I repeatedly mentioned that she'd been completely well before summer, and though I worried she might have picked something up during our travel to China, Xian had certainly enjoyed the trip. I shared that we had traveled to Vancouver Island in the late spring and that things had not been quite right ever since. Some doctors wanted to attribute her condition to psychological trauma due to her return to China and visiting her sister's orphanage the preceding January. Others searched for genetic conditions such as Rett's disease and Fragile X Syndrome that would have likely shown signs earlier on and did not seem to accept the idea that she'd previously been a perfectly normal and healthy child. Still others were ready to blame me as somehow causing Xian's condition, something I discovered when I read her chart during long waits for appointments in the hospital. As a busy single parent who was by then unable to work at the job that provided our family income, and who had survived the rigors and scrutiny of two adoption homestudy processes and required post adoption follow up visits from social workers, the "Munchausen's By Proxy" listed in one of the initial differential diagnoses was too ridiculous for words. I later discovered that the parents of young Lyme patients are quite commonly accused of this "disease du jour" (see for example, Sherr, 2005).

When I insisted that I believed that Xian was "still in there," providing some examples of her lucid moments, and asked about her having some sort of bacterial, parasitic, or viral condition, I was told those would have been indicated in her lumbar puncture and I was assured by the pediatric infectious diseases team as well as the travel medicine specialist that she could not have any type of infection. By the time Xian was in hospital she was having drenching night sweats along with other visible symptoms. When I pointed out her wet sheets to a medical resident and one of her doctors, I was told that "she must have urinated" (she hadn't) or that maybe she was simply a sweaty child. (Xian later tested positive for *babesia duncani*, a Lyme co-infection known for causing heavy night sweats.)

After her release from hospital, Xian had appointments with additional specialists and was seen by the autism expert, who met with her during one of her slightly more lucid moments. While he thought Xian's condition was puzzling, he was quite certain that what was going on was not anything on the autistic spectrum. By this point Xian was also having increasing digestive issues, losing weight, and having swallowing difficulties. The autism doctor provided some ideas for elimination testing so I could see if particular foods were problematic. While it took months to sort out, Xian's illness had caused her to have gluten and fructose intolerances—severe enough that she would have seizure-like episodes about two hours after eating a meal that contained a high amount of either nutrient.

Beginning from her time in hospital when doctors had recommended trying out an anti-psychotic medication to see if it would alleviate any symptoms, Xian had begun having episodes of extreme rage in which she had terrifying hallucinations. These events were so severe that if she were not restrained she would slam her head or body into the floor and bite and scratch herself to the point of making blood flow. She would also lose bladder control during these episodes, become very flushed, and scream until she lost her voice. I believe that she experienced pain as well as disturbing images or sensations during these episodes because she would sometimes cry out, "Make it stop!" or "Help me!" or "Get Dr. ____" (her pediatrician) as the episode gained intensity and before she lost complete control. Her doctors seemed to believe that was going on was simply extreme temper tantrums, but they were like no tantrum I have ever witnessed.

While Xian had continued to have small ups and downs all along the course of her illness, in February she hit a new low, when her occasional lucid periods vanished completely. During her illness, she'd inexplicably retained the ability to draw (drawing had been an area where she had particular skill for her age before she became sick), but suddenly she could no longer grasp a pencil or a crayon, and her fingers clenched into hot fists. Her speech had also declined even further and now was slurred and difficult to understand on the rare occasions that she spoke, and Xian was no longer able to find the correct words. For example, if she wanted toast, she might say "butter," or simply, "I want it" and I would have to guess what it was she was requesting. She spoke only to get basic physical needs met and was often so confused that she would get lost in the house, unable to find the upstairs bathroom, or locate me if I moved to another room. While she'd experienced some difficulties with coordination on and off, now she would lean heavily on me as we walked, and she rarely had the energy to sit up or move around. Her severe insomnia had grown increasingly worse, and now on a good night she might sleep from midnight to 7 am, a far change from the 12 hours she had required before her illness began.

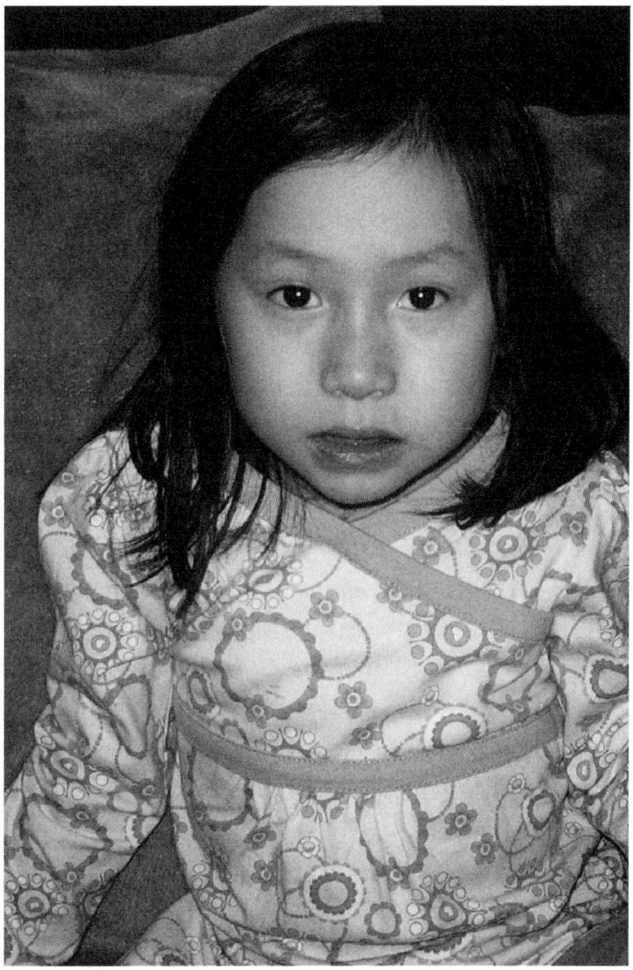

Xian Laidlaw in January 2008 as her illness increasingly impaired her language and cognitive abilities.

In April, Xian's raging episodes dramatically increased in frequency and duration so that her days alternated from extremes of lethargy to raging episodes and then back. At this point I knew that we were not going to be able to continue to manage without some sort of assistance, as it was rarely possible to leave the house or to find someone who was up to the challenge of providing respite so I could do necessary errands like buying groceries. I took Xian to Emergency yet again, where she was admitted overnight. A resident informed me that she was certain Xian had a psychiatric illness and that probably "play therapy" was in order, though I'd informed her that Xian was no longer communicating or playing. When Xian eventually had one of her episodes in the pediatric ward, the child psychiatrist who happened to be present commented that an EEG (electroencephalogram) might be a good idea. Instead, the team of specialists decided that she should spend three weeks in a child psychiatric ward for observation, at another hospital, although three psychoactive medications that had been used experimentally in earlier months had actually worsened her symptoms during the time Xian had used them. Her doctors told me that they were returning to a late onset autistic spectrum disorder diagnosis, despite the lack of agreement from the autism specialist who was suddenly no longer the right expert. When I questioned the ASD diagnosis and asked for further exploration of possibilities, I was told I needed to start to accept that my daughter had an unknown condition that was not treatable. Child psychiatry could help with accessing autism services, and help with the "severe behaviour issues," I was told, and I was informed that we had no other options within the medical system except to have her admitted to the child psychiatric ward.

With much reluctance (the child psychiatry ward was not set up for younger children, and they rarely had patients as young as Xian) I agreed, on the condition that Xian could at first attend as a day patient, and that I could stay with her when they wanted her there overnight, and there were also plans arranged to have some metabolic testing done, as requested by the metabolic specialist who had examined her. Xian's time in child psychiatry did not result in any new revelations and after Xian completed the metabolic testing I decided to take her home, as she had regressed even further while she was there and had injured herself when she had been placed on her own in a time out room during one of her screaming/hallucination episodes. At that point, seeing her become more detached and worrying about what might happen when I could not be present, I was also concerned that being on the ward might remind Xian of her early life in her orphanage, since the physical space was indeed similar. (And it likely did, as Xian has insisted very recently that during her illness I returned her to her orphanage in China and she remembers me going into an elevator with a suitcase, and her shoes being taken away—two events that did take place during her stay in the ward. Fortunately thus far, this is the only memory she has retained of the experience.)

Saved by a Reading and a Teenage Boy

It was alongside Xian's stay in child psychiatry that I happened to read a newspaper and encountered some letters to the editor that, after Xian returned home, eventually led me back to an article about a teenage boy, Ed Sperling, who'd experienced what his mother had called "a living death" (see http://www.canada.com/edmontonjournal/news/story.html?id=3ab6db90-51bf-4b58-af9c-4b3ee54af289&k=2658). Despite the age difference, something about his story was hauntingly familiar, and seemed to echo what had been happening to Xian. I decided that I had little to lose by trying to contact this family and within hours I was talking to Janet Sperling, who provided me with an IgeneX blood testing kit to send to the California lab specializing in tick-borne illness. In that first conversation with Janet, suddenly a number of the puzzling aspects of Xian's mystery illness seemed to have a possible explanation. At the very least, I might be pursuing yet another dead-end, but there was little to lose to explore one last possibility. What was interesting, as we eventually compared notes, was the discovery that Xian and Ed son had been seen by at least a half dozen of the same pediatric specialists and were tested for a number of the same rare conditions, such as Juvenile Huntington's Disease. Both had been patients in the same acute care and psychiatric hospital settings. Yet, no one had made a connection between Ed's condition and Xian's, although Janet and her husband had informed all of their son's specialists of his recovery after Lyme treatment and had publicized his story widely.

While awaiting Xian's test results I did more research and also contacted a Lyme specialist in Seattle who had trained with a well-known Connecticut pediatric Lyme specialist. Within minutes, after hearing a summary of the details of Xian's case, she told me she needed to see Xian as quickly as possible. While travel to Seattle with a very ill and disabled child was difficult, it was the beginning, finally, of Xian's path to recovery.

Miracles

As I write now, a little over a year from Xian's entry into Lyme treatment on multiple antibiotics, my daughter is close to a full recovery. Her memory has returned and her speech is back to what it was before she got sick, and she has returned to spending hours creating complex drawings, making elaborate crafts and playing actively with her sister and friends. Her remaining issues are those that are more connected with the effects of her illness, trying to interpret memories of her strange experiences when ill as they emerge, dealing with "lost time" (e.g. she was unaware that she had turned five while she was sick), and having more fears at night. While we have continued to struggle to get Canadian Lyme treatment and recognition of her illness, with the help of a US Lyme specialist, a retired Canadian Lyme specialist and several sympathetic Canadian doctors, Xian has slowly shed the layers of the disease that had her in its grasp. Her recovery was much like Lavoie's (cited in Weintraub, 2008) onion analogy—where slowly, treatment stripped away the symptoms caused by the infection. During her initial stages of treatment, Xian experienced what is common to many Lyme sufferers—severe Jarisch-Herxheimer-like reactions, where her symptoms got initially worse, and then better, in an often rocky roller coaster ride as the first months passed. Still, each as the weeks went by she slowly regained old skills and shed symptoms, first gaining energy and losing fatigue, and then gradually regaining her speech, which returned with her initially sounding much like a stroke-victim, slurred, stuttering, and difficult to understand. As she improved, I brought her to see some of her Canadian doctors and mentioned her Lyme treatment, and while we are still a long way away from having easy access to Canadian treatment and clear recognition

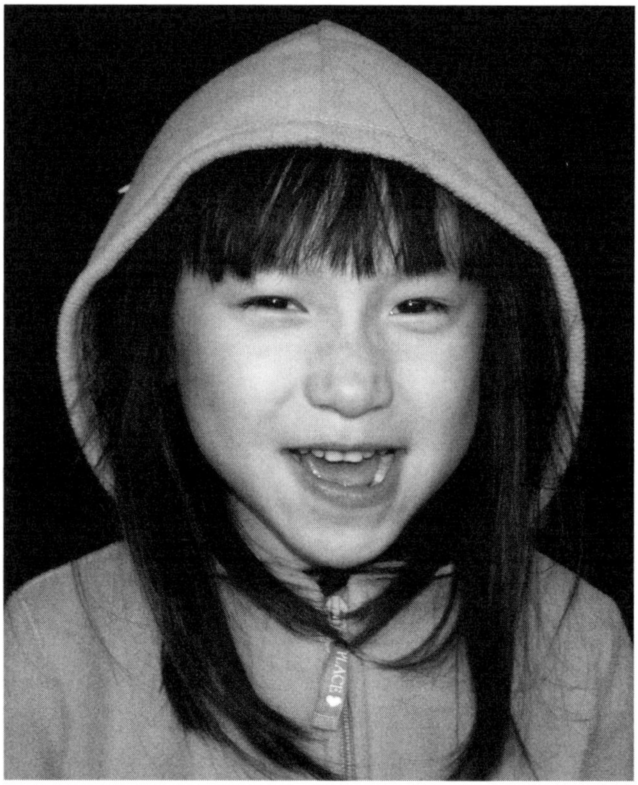

Xian in May, 2009, well on the road to recovery on antibiotics.

of Xian's illness, there are now many medical witnesses to the fact that she is recovering on treatment for Lyme and co-infections. A number of her tests and medical records now include the words "suspected Lyme disease," which seems to be progress, however small. While there are still some unknowns for her in terms of her future and whether or not she will be able to keep this illness at bay permanently, I now have my daughter back. What continues to play on my thoughts, however, is that if it hadn't been for me reading about Ed Sperling's case, Xian may never have recovered and would have been sentenced to a slow, painful demise. Not one doctor in Canada had explored the possibility of tick-borne illness, and essentially, the Canadian medical system had abandoned her by the time I decided to take her to the US, a sad irony for a child who had already survived abandonment and infancy in a poor orphanage in China, and whose country had allowed her to be adopted and come to Canada for what was supposed to be a better life.

Children and Lyme: The Larger Story

I was told that whatever it was my daughter was suffering from, it had to be something exceedingly rare. However, what seems to be rare is the recognition of pediatric Lyme cases in Canada. In a recent interview, US pediatric Lyme specialist Dr. Charles Ray Jones mentions that he has treated Canadian children from all provinces among the thousands of his young patients (see Interview with the Extraordinary Dr. Jones, 2009). While accurate Lyme statistics are hard to acquire given the lack of diagnoses in Canada, gauging from the cases that have been mentioned recently within the Canadian media, Xian is not alone in contracting this illness, nor alone in encountering difficulties getting Canadian treatment (see Knox, 2008, for a particularly compelling example in a story about fifteen year old Nicole Bottle). Unfortunately, if pediatricians and doctors rely on the Canadian Pediatric Guidelines (see Halperin & Lang, 2009), they will be unlikely to diagnose or successfully treat cases like my daughter's, as the guidelines present this illness as uncommon in Canada, focus on diagnosis through the *erythema migrans* (Bull's Eye) rash, emphasize the likelihood of false positive results in testing, and limit treatment to eight weeks, stating:

> There are physicians who believe that Lyme disease is commonly underdiagnosed, and that a significant number of patients with a wide variety of symptoms would benefit from prolonged courses of parenteral antibiotics. There are no scientifically valid data to support this and, therefore, it is not recommended.

While my observations are anecdotal, I can say with confidence that Xian had only reached the very early stages of recovery after eight weeks of oral antibiotics and never had intravenous antibiotics even suggested as an option, and I am quite certain she would have ended any improvements had her treatment been completed at that early point. The first of the "bigger" signs that she was getting better and making cognitive improvements appeared after she had been receiving antibiotics for over three months and it was close to a year of treatment until she showed the biggest gains. When she began to plateau on one antibiotic combination in her tenth month of treatment, a switch to a new combination created observable improvements within days. And since as her mother, I might be suspected of not being an objective observer, I have ensured that there are records provided by outside professionals, who have documented each stage of her recovery, through speech and language assessment and cognitive tests. As well, since Xian attended daycare and school, her child care workers and educators have also observed and recorded her changes, and in fact, often they are the ones to alert me to particular improvements they notice.

Canadian Pediatric Guidelines aside, an additional factor that can delay diagnosis are collections of symptoms that differ somewhat from the better known Lyme cases in the endemic areas of the Eastern U.S. Unlike the historically familiar pediatric cases, where a group of children who all had juvenile arthritis symptoms, in Lyme, Connecticut, were the first recognized cases in North America (see Weintraub, 2008), my daughter did not exhibit joint or muscle issues in the early stages of her illness; these appeared, and only to a milder extent, once she had been ill for close to a year. In most of the Lyme information available, neurological involvement is commonly noted as part of chronic, late Lyme disease (for one example see the information posted at the Columbia University Lyme and Tick-Borne Diseases Research Center at http://www.columbia-lyme.org/patients/ld_lyme_symptoms.html). For Xian, however, the earliest symptoms were neurological and these continued to predominate all through her illness. While to my knowledge there have not been any Canadian pediatric Lyme studies done (the disease would have to be diagnosed and recognized, for that to occur), my daughter's Lyme specialist mentioned that she has been seeing a large number of predominantly neurological Lyme cases in her Western Canadian patients. Her theory is that perhaps the variant of borrelia in this region is more similar to that found in European areas known for early onset neurological Lyme disease.

However, with Lyme now being acknowledged as an emerging disease in Canada (Ogden, Lindsay, Morshed, Sockett & Artsob, 2009) and with children recognized as a particularly vulnerable population (see Interview..., 2009; CDC, 2004), parents and doctors would be well advised to become more familiar with the wider array of symptoms frequently present in undiagnosed children. While children may exhibit similar physical symptoms to those of adults, neurological, cognitive and behavioral symptoms may be more evident through performance at school or in similar settings, in sudden decline or increasing difficulties. My daughter's earliest symptoms, had we known enough to recognize them, were clearly evident when she was at daycare and involved in preschool activities. Hamlen and Kliman (2007) list sixteen such symptoms, such as "deficits with memory," "emotional and uncharacteristic behavioral presentation," and "executive function impairment," in a report for school psychologists. Over the time she became ill and over the process of her recovery, Xian has exhibited all of the symptoms listed. While supposedly my daughter's undiagnosed illness had a unique presentation and I was told that it had to be something exceedingly rare and difficult to diagnose, even the strangest of her neurological symptoms (Lyme "rage" and hallucinations) can be found in many easily accessed Lyme documents through ILADs (International Lyme and Associated Diseases Society) based websites, and while pediatric information is more difficult to find, several helpful resources do exist (see, for example, Corson's 2008 pediatric Lyme presentation, available on-line).

A Call for Change

If, as stated by Ogden et al, "Lyme disease is emerging in Canada" (p. 1224), more families will inevitably encounter this complex and difficult illness in the future. For parents of children who are on the receiving end of this illness, obtaining an accurate diagnosis and adequate and appropriate treatment can present a huge challenge. In my daughter's case, even her dramatic recovery with Lyme and co-infection treatment has not been enough to convince her pediatrician to risk treating for longer than the pediatric infectious diseases doctors have advised, although I am certainly grateful for whatever support she has given. The personal risks for doctors treating children seem to be much greater than in dealing with adult Lyme cases, and in my daughter's situation any doctors who have been involved have also had to spend much time addressing the concerns of our Canadian pharmacists who are also unfamiliar with pediatric Lyme treatment. Much of my daughter's treatment and recovery is due to the involvement of a US Lyme specialist and was paid for out of pocket. While Xian's pediatrician has been open to referring her to a practicing Canadian Lyme specialist, thus far, we have not been able to find one that is willing to take on a pediatric case. In our experience, the doctors willing to go against the advice of the Canadian pediatric Lyme guidelines or look into the ILADS approach to treatment are few and far between, and those who may be willing to treat do not want to be publicly known because of the risks involved. While living through my daughter's illness has been a significant trauma, often it feels as though we are being doubly punished by a medical system that will not openly deal with her illness and that will not offer any safety net in terms of her future, should she need a longer course of treatment or experience a future relapse.

While, in the end, my daughter's story is one with a miraculous, happy ending rivaling those of the fairy tales she loves, I am left with this: her recovery was only possible because I would not back down as a parent, and because I was fortunate to learn about a disease that no one had thought to mention, before it was too late. If I had not had the knowledge, resources, and stamina to continue to question the answers we were given and I had not been able to find the financial resources to pay for U.S. testing and initial treatment, I probably would have lost my daughter forever, either through death or insurmountable disability. And so, I end this chapter with questions:

- What will it take for better Lyme diagnostic processes in Canada?
- What will it take to ensure adequate Lyme treatment in Canada for all children (and bigger people, too)?
- How many more childhoods have to be lost before there is hope for all children who contract this disease?
- Who will be willing to do what it takes to stand up for those who cannot advocate for themselves?

I wait, hopeful that there are doctors and politicians who might rise to the challenge, and I hope that in sharing her story, my daughter's lost years, lost celebrations and lost birthdays will not be in vain.

References

Centers for Disease Control and Prevention (CDC). (2004). Lyme disease—United States, 1992–1998. *MMWR Morb Mortal Wkly Report* 53: 365-9.

Columbia University Medical Center. Lyme and Tick-Borne Diseases Research Center. (2009). Available: http://www.columbia-lyme.org/patients/ld_lyme_symptoms.html

Corson, A.F. (2008). June 2006 Pediatric Lyme Talk, revised 5/28/08. Available: http://www.lymepa.org/html/dr_ann_f_corson_april_24_20_2.html

Halperin, S & Lang, B. (2009). Lyme disease in Canada: Q and A for pediatricians. Infectious Diseases and Immunization Committee, Canadian Pediatric Society. *Pediatric Child Health* 14(3):103-5.

Hamlen, R.A. & Kliman, D.S. (2007). Lyme disease: Etiology, neuropsychological sequelae and educational impact. *Pediatric School Psychology* 35(5):34-35.

Interview with the Extraordinary Dr. Jones. (2009). Posted July 28, 2009 on the Lyme Disease Research Database. Available: http://lyme-disease-research-database.com/lyme_disease_blog_files/charles-ray-jones.html

Knox, J. (2008). Desperate parents seek controversial treatment for their ailing daughter. *Times* Colomnist, Wednesday, October 1, 2008. Available: http://www.canada.com/victoriatimescolonist/news/story.html?id=f11089c1-c908-4b90-b9f8-3d748daa9200

Ogden, N.H., Lindsay, L.R., Morshed, M., Sockett, P. & Artsob, H. (2009). The emergence of Lyme disease in Canada. CMAJ 180(12): 1221-1224.

Sherr, V. (2005). Munchausen's Syndrome by Proxy and Lyme disease: Medical misogyny or diagnostic mystery? *Medical Hypotheses* 65 (5): 440-447.

Sinemma, J. (2008). Teen's 'living death' was Lyme disease, family says. *The Edmonton Journal,* April 4, 2008. Available: http://www.canada.com/edmonton-journal/news/story.html?id=3ab6db90-51bf-4b58-af9c-4b3ee54af289&k=2658

Weintraub, P. (2008). *Cure Unknown: Inside the Lyme epidemic*. New York: St. Martin's Press.

Acknowledgement

I would like to acknowledge the Children's Bridge International Adoption Consultants who published an early version of my daughter's story in their newsletter (Children's Bridge Newsletter—volume 49, December 2008. Available: http://wwww.childrens bridge.com).

Pediatric Overview: The Children of Lyme Disease

Charles Ray Jones, MD
Pediatrician, Private Practice, New Haven, CT

Current research indicates that the Lyme disease bacteria, Borrelia burgdorferi, can be transmitted within hours after an infected tick attachment. Failure of parents and teachers to recognize Lyme disease early in its course can result in a child developing a chronic difficult to treat infection in the brain, eyes, joints, heart and elsewhere in the body. In my experience treating 5,000+ children birth to 18 with Lyme disease, 50% have no tick attachment history, 10% or less have an erythema migrans (bullseye rash) history, but all have a history of living in or having visited a Lyme endemic area and have a decline in the way they play and perform in school. They are tired, wilt easily, have dark circles under their eyes and are sick.

Lyme disease has a profound negative impact on a child's life, cognitive function and ability to perform maximally in school. Severe fatigue unrelieved by rest results in decreased stamina and a decreased ability to play and to do school work. Insomnia, headaches, nausea, abdominal pain, impaired concentration, poor short-term memory, an inability to sustain attention, confusion, uncharacteristic behavior outbursts and mood swings, fevers/chills, joint pain, dizziness, noise and light sensitivity, and difficulty thinking, expressing thoughts, reading, writing, and making decisions as well as a feeling of being overwhelmed by schoolwork plague a child with Lyme disease. Pain and impaired cognitive function make it difficult to sustain attention and to learn and recall new material.

Although Lyme is usually transmitted by Ixodes scapularis (deer) and Lyme-like STARI (Southern tick-associated rash illness) by Amblyomma americanum (lone star) ticks, it can also be transmitted in utero and through breast milk. These children, frequently floppy with poor muscle tone, are irritable and ill early in their lives with frequent fevers, increased incidence of ear and throat infections, pneumonia, joint and body pain. They have gastroesophageal reflux, small windpipes (tracheomalacia), cataracts and other eye problems, developmental delay, learning disabilities, and psychiatric problems. All respond to months or years of continuous antibiotic therapy.

When Lyme disease is a possible diagnosis, the children should be evaluated by a Lyme knowledgeable physician who will continue antibiotic therapy until all Lyme symptoms resolve. In most circumstances, *Ixodes scapularis* tick attachment should be treated with one month of antibiotic therapy.

Lyme Disease in the Eye: A Pediatric and Adolescent Perspective

Eric L. Singman, MD, PhD, Neuro-Opthalmologist
Director, Family Eye Group, Lancaster, PA

Lyme disease is a significant infectious disease that has become much more common lately with the encroachment of human development on natural areas. Adolescents and children are probably at a higher risk for this illness because they spend more time in areas where they might suffer a bite from a tick carrying the infectious spirochete (Borrelia burgdorferi). As a neuro-ophthalmologist, I see Lyme disease patients presenting with a number of ocular findings, including optic neuritis, anterior uveitis, keratitis, dry eye, and episcleritis. Furthermore, these patients seem to have central nervous defects, including hyperintense white matter lesions of the brain and even an arachnoiditis leading to intracranial hypertension. Because of the neurasthenic effects of this illness, patients often present with reading difficulties such as fatigue, tearing, letters running together, or double vision.

Lyme disease can mimic so many diseases, including multiple sclerosis, chronic fatigue syndrome and fibromyalgia. Therefore, a young patient's health care team must ensure that the patient has been correctly diagnosed. Intracranial hypertension is a difficult diagnosis, particularly when it presents in an uncommon way.

If Lyme disease attacks the optic nerve, it can lead to blindness. For this reason, examining just the eyes might not elucidate the etiology of a child's or adolescent's vision problems. Neuro- ophthalmologists are particularly trained in examining the entire visual pathway.

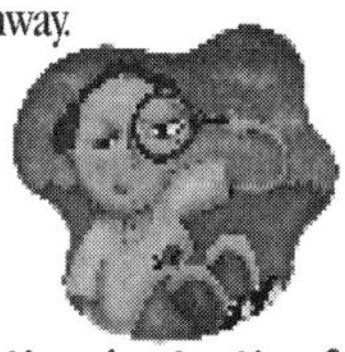

Special thanks to the following organizations for supporting the publication of this brochure:

IGeneX, Inc.

www.IGENEX.COM

A specialty immunology laboratory and research facility, providing personalized service to over 1,000 private practice physicians, hospitals, and other clinical reference laboratories throughout the U.S. and Canada. Telephone (800) 832-3200.

North Jersey Lyme Support Group

(201) 825-6978

Emotional Needs of Children and Their Families: Psychotherapy and Family Therapy Support

Sandy Berenbaum, LCSW, BCD
Brewster, New York

Lyme disease, particularly if it is chronic, affects the lives of children and adolescents in three major areas: Family, School, Peers.

The family might find the Lyme patient to be irritable and jumpy, depressed or anxious, and constantly complaining. Disturbances in eating and sleeping patterns are common. In adolescents, the role of hormones further complicates the picture. Mood swings often accompany physical complaints. School issues can be considerable, and vary from day to day. Fatigue, cognitive and mood problems, and symptoms that might be seen as ADD or AD/HD may get in the way of school attendance and academic performance.

Children with Lyme often complain about feeling isolated. Profound fatigue can limit, or prevent, socialization. Peers often fail to understand the variations in the levels of functioning from day to day, resulting in their not believing their friends when they complain of their Lyme symptoms. The Lyme patients' lives are further complicated by trips to the doctor, pills they have to take, blood work and other diagnostics. Their experience of life sets them apart from their peers, and the gap that is created can be very difficult to bridge.

Psychotherapy and family therapy with a Lyme-literate psychotherapist can help in the process of recovery from Lyme disease through developing in patients and parents:

- An understanding of the nature of the illness, and strategies to deal with it.
- The ability to cope with the flare of symptoms and side effects of medications, yet function at the highest possible level.
- The ability of parents to advocate on the child's behalf in school.
- Enhanced communications and problem-solving, within and outside of the family.

Lyme disease is a medical illness that calls for non-medical strategies, to assure the growth and success of your children.

For Further Reading on School Issues

Smith, P. The Effects of Lyme Disease on Students, Schools and School Policy. School Leader, New Jersey School Boards Association, Sept/Oct 2004.
see http://lymediseaseassocation.org/Schools.html

Neuropsychiatric Effects of Lyme Disease on Children and Adolescents

Brian Fallon, MD
Director, Lyme Disease Program, New York State Psychiatric Institute
Associate Professor, Clinical Psychiatry, Columbia University, NY

Children with Lyme disease may develop neuropsychiatric symptoms affecting mood, thinking, and behavior. The infection itself may have direct effects on the brain or indirect effects through the activation of the immune system which produces substances which affect the brain. For example, marked fatigue would result in trouble paying attention or staying awake in class as well as struggles with parents about getting to school on time.

Common psychiatric presentations in younger children include irritability and increased separation anxiety or other fears. In older children, mood swings and anxiety attacks are more common. Less frequently, children may develop new onset motor or vocal tics, obsessive compulsive disorder, or rarely a regression that looks very much like an autistic spectrum disorder.

Common cognitive problems include trouble with visual and auditory attention and slower mental processing speed. Children with unrecognized Lyme disease may be misdiagnosed as having primary attention deficit disorder – a mistake that not only results in unnecessary school problems for the child but also may allow a treatable acute infection to become a more entrenched chronic one. For example, these children may have trouble directing or maintaining focus on what the teacher says in class or storing into memory what he/she reads. The decline in school performance alarms parents and may result in a lowering of the child's self-esteem such that he/she feels stupid - until the cause is identified. Neuropsychological testing may reveal that the child's IQ has declined considerably, with the performance subtests more heavily affected than the verbal subtests. School systems must make special accommodations for these medically-disabled children.

As an adjunct to the medical work-up of these children, brain SPECT scans can be helpful in differentiating primary psychiatric disorders from the secondary neuropsychiatric effects of a diffuse brain illness such as Lyme disease.

For Further Reading:

Tager FA, Fallon BA, Keilp J, Rissenberg M, Jones CR, Liebowitz MR. A controlled study of cognitive deficits in children with chronic Lyme disease. J Neuropsychiatry Clin Neurosci 2001 Fall;13(4):500-507.

Fallon BA, Kochevar JM, Gaito A, Nields J. The Underdiagnosis of Neuropsychiatric Lyme Disease in Children and Adults. In Diagnostic Dilemmas. Edited by David Tomb. Psychiatric Clinics of North America, 1998; 21: 693-703.

Gastrointestinal Lyme

Martin D. Fried, MD
Director, Pediatric Gastroenterology and Nutrition
Assistant Program Director, Department of Pediatrics
Jersey Shore Medical Center, Neptune, NJ

Lyme disease has been reported in the gastrointestinal tract of children and adolescents. Pediatric gastrointestinal Lyme disease may present as abdominal pain, vomiting, diarrhea, heartburn, blood in the stool, and it may mimic Crohn's disease or colitis. Blood tests for diagnosing Lyme disease may be negative while gastrointestinal and other Lyme disease symptoms persist. The diagnosis is made clinically on the basis of symptoms and by excluding other possible etiologies.

Once treatment has begun with antibiotics, most patients reported a decrease in the frequency and severity of their abdominal pain. In addition to antibiotics, a low fat diet further alleviated some of the abdominal symptoms associated with Lyme disease. In patients who reported having a crampy, colicky, below the belly button pain, treatment also included antispasmodic and anticholinergic medications.

After treatment was completed, some residual abdominal pain may persist for a couple of months at a markedly reduced level of severity. This diminished pain usually represents the activation and persistence of the immune system to fighting the infection even long after the infection is gone.

In addition to Lyme disease, other co-infections such as Bartonella, mycoplasma, H. pylori and babesia have been confirmed to occur in the GI tract.

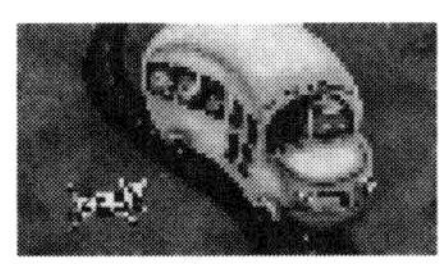

Endorsed by:

ILADS

International Lyme & Associated Diseases Society
A Professional Medical and Research Organization

This brochure is designed to provide practical and useful information on the subject matter covered. However, it is being distributed with the understanding that the LDA is not engaged in rendering medical or other professional services. If medical or other expert assistance is required, the services of a competent professional should be sought.

The Role of Co-Infections in Lyme Disease

Richard I. Horowitz, MD
Internist, Private Practice, Hyde Park, NY
Vice President, Board of Directors, International Lyme & Associated Diseases Society (ILADS)

There are several other organisms found in ticks which when transmitted alone, or in combination with Lyme disease, may account for increased severity of symptoms and or persistence of illness. These organisms cause diseases which include, but are not limited to, Ehrlichiosis, babesiosis, bartonellosis, Rocky Mountain spotted fever, Powassan encephalitis, Q fever, tick paralysis, anaplasmosis, and STARI.

Ehrlichiosis may cause high fevers, headaches, myalgias, and flu-like symptoms. Clinical laboratory findings may include positive antibody titers for Human Monocytic Ehrlichiosis (HME) and Human Granulocytic Ehrlichiosis (HGE now called anaplasmosis), with morulae in leukocytes (intracytoplasma colonies), and low white cell counts, low platelet counts with elevated liver functions in certain patients.

Babesia microti is an intracellular parasite found in red blood cells which causes a malarial like illness. Children may complain of intermittent fevers, chills, day and night sweats, as well as having an increased severity and duration of Lyme disease symptoms. Diagnosis is made by antibody titers (IFA), blood smear, DNA (PCR) and RNA analysis (FISH assay). Antibiotic treatments include atovaquone and azithromycin, and clindamycin and quinine.

Bartonella henselae are intracellular bacteria that can be transmitted either by a cat bite or scratch or a tick bite. When present in combination with Lyme disease, atypical presentations may result including visual problems, headaches, significant lymph node enlargement, resistant neurological deficits, and the new onset of a seizure disorder. Diagnosis is made by acute and convalescent antibody titers (IFA) and by PCR (DNA) analysis.

STARI, Southern-tick associated rash illness, also called Master's Disease, is a Lyme-like illness caused by Borrelia lonestari, bacteria carried by the lone star tick.

Continued severity and/or persistence of illness in a child or adolescent with Lyme disease necessitates searching for these other tick-borne diseases, both by titers and serial PCR's. Treatment regimens are still evolving, but significant clinical improvement may result once all overlapping co-infections are found and treated.

The Rheumatic Manifestations of Lyme Disease in Children

Andrea Gaito, MD, FACR
Past President, International Lyme & Associated Diseases Society
Rheumatolgist, Private Practice, Basking Ridge, NJ
Diplomate, American Board of Internal Medicine and Rheumatology

Lyme disease can cause a variety of arthritic manifestations in children that can mimic many other rheumatological disorders. It can present with monoarticular arthritis, but more commonly will develop into a migratory polyarthritis. Joint swelling frequently does not occur, but may occasionally be seen in late stages of the infection. Patients often complain of "traveling" arthritis. The most commonly involved joints are the knees, hips, neck, wrists, hands and temporomandibular joints.

It is not uncommon for a patient to have concomitant muscular pain. The muscle pain is most often found to be in a diffuse pattern, and not localized to the classic "trigger point" locations seen in fibromyalgia. Children with Lyme disease may also experience morning stiffness, rest pain and muscle weakness. Difficulties in the child's ability to participate in sports activities will be noticed. Inflammatory myopathies, such as dermatomyositis and polymyositis have also been documented in chronic Lyme disease.

The proper evaluation of these patients should include the appropriate serology for tick-borne disorders, accompanied by levels for antinuclear antibodies, rheumatoid factor, and creatinine kinase and sedimentation rate. Cross-reactive antibodies against the Lyme bacteria may yield low levels of false positive autoantibodies. Appropriate antibiotic treatment should be given until the joint and muscle symptoms dissipate. Partial treatment may result in the development of chronic arthritis.

Educating Children with Lyme Disease

Al Tagliabue, MEd
Director of Student Personnel
and Community Services, Jackson, NJ (Ret.)
Learning Consultant, Calais School

Pat Smith, BA
President, Lyme Disease Association, Inc.
Vice President of Political Affairs, International Lyme & Associated Diseases Society (ILADS)
Former President, Wall Township Board of Education, NJ
Former Chair, Governor's Lyme Disease Advisory Council, NJ

Children may display a multitude of medical symptoms that can make it impossible to keep up in class. Common educational problems for these students include memory loss, fatigue, depression and the inability to organize, focus and sustain attention. All of these factors have a negative impact on their ability to perform academically. Children whose illness affects school performance may qualify for special education accommodations or services.

Students with disabilities may receive services under either the Individuals with Disabilities Education Act, IDEA, where classification type depends on how severely the illness impacts learning ability or Section 504 of the 1973 Rehabilitation Act, civil rights legislation that prevents discrimination. Students qualify for 504 services if their medical condition "substantially limits" their ability to learn. Students with Lyme disease often fit into 504, due to their ever-shifting medical and educational condition. Schools preschool through college that receive federal funding must meet 504 requirements.*

School district special education policies adopted by the board of education should be examined. Policies that mandate a waiting period for home instruction do not apply to long term home instruction under an Individualized Education Program, IEP. IEP's should be written so that students with Lyme can attend school when medically able and be concurrently eligible for supplemental home tutors, or they can receive home instruction without a waiting period. An extended school year can be written into an IEP, and all subjects and subject levels that are offered in a school setting must be offered, with modifications as necessary, to a student on home instruction. The parent is an integral part of the child study team, and as such, must be informed and be an active participant in the process of making educational decisions for the student.

Resources
http:www.ideapractices.org
http://www.504idea.org
http://www.specialeducationadvocacy.com

Involvement of the Nervous System in Lyme Disease

Dorothy Pietrucha, MD, FAAP
Director, Division of Pediatric Neurology
Medical Director, Child Evaluation Center
Jersey Shore Medical Center, Neptune, NJ

The nervous system is frequently affected by Lyme disease. Both the central and peripheral nervous systems are at risk. Frequently, patients with Lyme disease develop an encephalopathy resulting in learning disabilities, difficulties with attention span, memory and word finding, and the patients complain of headache. Acutely, a person may also have a Lyme meningitis with inflammation of the covering over the brain and spinal cord. They may have an inflammation of the brain itself called encephalitis. Nerves can be involved, such as the 7th nerve causing a facial palsy, or peripheral nerves causing neuropathy with sensory changes and weakness. There have been rare cases of stroke, and patients may have seizures with Lyme disease. In children, we can also see increased pressure in the nervous system called pseudo tumor. This also results in headaches and may also affect vision. The muscles may be involved and this can cause weakness and pain.

Some diagnostic tests that may be helpful in evaluating the nervous system include an MRI of the brain, EEG, spinal tap, SPECT scan, EMG's and nerve conduction studies.

In addition to treating the Lyme disease with appropriate antibiotic therapy, medications may have to be given to help relieve some of the symptoms and the discomfort that patients have as a result of involvement of the nervous system. They may require anti-convulsants for seizures, diuretics to decrease the intracranial pressure, analgesics for pain, appropriate education intervention if there are learning problems, and physical therapy for weakness.

It is important for physicians and patients to recognize how frequently the central and peripheral nervous systems may be involved in Lyme disease.

Other recommended resources:

http://Columbia-Lyme.org
http://www.LymeNet.org
http://www.Lymeinfo.net
http://www.ILADS.org
http://www.IGeneX.com
http://www.LymeDiseaseAssociation.org

10

THE DIAGNOSIS AND TREATMENT OF CHRONIC LYME DISEASE

The International Lyme and Associated Diseases Society

Evidence-based guidelines for the management of Lyme disease

The ILADS Working Group
ILADS, P.O. Box 341461
Bethesda, MD 20827-1461, USA
www.ILADS.org

KEYWORDS:
antibiotics, *Babesia*, *Bartonella*, *Borrelia burgdorferi*, *Ehrlichia*, guidelines, Lyme disease, tickborne diseases

The International Lyme and Associated Diseases Society

The ILADS Working Group

Daniel Cameron, MD, MPH	Internal Medicine and Epidemiology, Mt. Kisco, New York
Andrea Gaito, MD	Rheumatology, Basking Ridge, New Jersey
Nick Harris, PhD	Immunology, Palo Alto, California
Gregory Bach, DO	Family and Integrative Medicine, Colmar, Pennsylvania
Sabra Bellovin, MD	Family Practice, Portsmouth, Virginia
Kenneth Bock, MD	Family Practice, Rhinebeck, New York
Steven Bock, MD	Family Practice Rhinebeck, New York
Joseph Burrascano, MD	Internal Medicine East Hampton, New York
Constance Dickey, RN	Registered Nurse Hampden, Maine
Richard Horowitz, MD	Internal Medicine Hyde Park, New York
Steven Phillips, MD	Internal Medicine Ridgefield, Connecticut
Laurence Meer-Scherrer, MD	Internal Medicine Flamatt, Switzerland
Bernard Raxlen, MD	Psychiatry Greenwich, Connecticut
Virginia Sherr, MD	Psychiatry Holland, Pennsylvania
Harold Smith, MD	Emergency Medicine Danville, Pennsylvania
Pat Smith	President, Lyme Disease Association, Inc. Jackson, New Jersey
Raphael Stricker, MD	Hematology and Immunotherapy San Francisco, California

Summary & disclaimer

These guidelines represent an evidence-based review of Lyme and associated tickborne diseases by the International Lyme and Associated Diseases Society (ILADS). Although the guidelines present evidence-based approaches to the diagnosis and treatment of Lyme and associated tickborne diseases, they were not intended to be a standard of medical care. Physicians must use their own judgment based on a thorough review of all available clinical information and the Lyme disease literature to decide on the best course of treatment for an individual patient.

Acknowledgements

ILADS would like to thank the Turn the Corner Foundation, New York, NY, for financial support of formulation of the guidelines; Medallion Media, Novato, CA, for editorial support of development of the guidelines; and the Lyme Disease Association, Inc., Jackson, NJ, for financial support of publication of the guidelines.

Table of contents

The International Lyme and Associated Diseases Society

Section I: Introduction to guidelines

This report, completed in November 2003, is intended to serve as a resource for physicians, public health officials and organizations involved in the evaluation and treatment of Lyme disease.

1. International Lyme and Associated Diseases Society (ILADS)

ILADS is an interdisciplinary organization of health science professionals established in 1999 to accomplish the following objectives:

- Analyze the medical literature, position statements and practice parameters related to Lyme and associated diseases
- Improve the management of these diseases through evaluation of established and innovative therapies
- Educate a broad range of healthcare providers and serve as an effective advocate for clinicians seeking cost-effective state-of-the-art treatment regimens

ILADS identified the need for new and expanded guidelines for the diagnosis and treatment of Lyme and associated diseases. In 2001, a working party was formed to evaluate current practices and to encourage new standards of care. This report, completed in November 2003, is intended to serve as a resource for physicians, public health officials and organizations involved in the evaluation and treatment of Lyme disease.

2. Chronic Lyme disease: a growing epidemic

The Centers for Disease Control and Prevention (CDC) consider Lyme disease the fastest growing vector-borne disease in the USA. By conservative estimate, the number of new Lyme disease infections per year may be ten times higher than the 17,730 cases reported to the CDC during 2000 [1,2].

The prevalence of chronic Lyme disease ranges from 34% in a population-based, retrospective cohort study [3] to 62% in a specialty clinic located in an area endemic for Lyme disease [4]. Clinic patients presented with arthralgia, arthritis, cardiac and neurologic symptoms [4].

A widening array of chronic presentations is associated with the Lyme spirochete, *Borrelia burgdorferi*. There are great challenges in determining optimal cost-effective means for appropriate diagnosis, clinical management and public health control of Lyme disease throughout the world. Additional problems include the identification and management of tickborne coinfections including *Ehrlichia*, *Babesia* and *Bartonella* species [5].

3. The need for new guidelines

Guidelines of the Infectious Disease Society of America (IDSA) fall short of meeting the needs for diagnosis and treatment of individuals with chronic Lyme disease [6]. The latest IDSA Guidelines (2000) fail to take into account the compelling, peer-reviewed, published evidence confirming persistent, recurrent and refractory Lyme disease and, in fact, deny its existence [6].

The IDSA's symptomatic approaches to Lyme disease are limited and exclude many individuals with persisting clinical and laboratory evidence of active *B. burgdorferi* infection. In addition, physicians treating individuals with Lyme and other tick-borne infections recognize the need for new guidelines to better serve the patient population [6].

Previous guidelines for management of Lyme disease have been published in the *New England Journal of Medicine* in 1990 by Rahn [7]; in *Conn's Current Therapy* in 1997 by Burrascano and in 1998 by Steere [8,9]; in Burrascano's Guidelines on the ILADS website (www.ilads.org); and in the *Journal of Infectious Diseases* by Wormser and colleagues in 2000 [6]. The ILADS Guidelines expand on these protocols using the evidence-based approach and Cochrane methodology employed by the IDSA [6,10].

Our goal is to present practitioners with practical and defensible guidelines for treating all individuals with Lyme disease including those with persistent, recurrent and relapsing symptoms of *B. burgdorferi* infection.

The ILADS Guidelines focus on which patients to evaluate, what tests to order, what antibiotics to use and what steps to take to ensure that concerns over antibiotic use are addressed.

The ILADS Working Group that formulated these guidelines included primary care clinicians, researchers, community healthcare providers and patient advocates. In developing these treatment guidelines, the group considered factors such as incidence of Lyme disease; severity of disease in terms of morbidity; comorbidities and determinants of when Lyme disease is most likely to become chronic; feasibility, efficacy and cost of antibiotic treatment; impact of antibiotic therapy on quality of life, including adverse drug events; and the potential for drug resistance to develop.

Because of the complexity and variability of Lyme disease symptoms, the guidelines are flexible. Treatment depends on the severity of each case, the patient's response to therapy and the physician's own clinical judgment.

4. A problem of definitions

Lyme disease was initially investigated by CDC epidemiologists focusing on erythema migrans, heart block, meningitis and arthritis. The ELISA test and later, the western blot, were introduced for seroepidemiologic studies. Chronic, persistent, recurrent and refractory Lyme disease were not included in these studies; consequently cases of chronic Lyme disease still go unrecognized.

For the purpose of the ILADS guidelines, 'chronic Lyme disease' is inclusive of persistent symptomatologies including fatigue, cognitive dysfunction, headaches, sleep disturbance and other neurologic features, such as demyelinating disease, peripheral neuropathy and sometimes motor neuron disease; neuropsychiatric presentations; cardiac presentations including electrical conduction delays and dilated cardiomyopathy; and musculoskeletal problems. Symptoms may continue despite 30 days of treatment (persistent Lyme disease). The patient may relapse in the absence of another tickbite or erythema migrans rash (recurrent Lyme disease), or be poorly responsive to antibiotic treatment (refractory Lyme disease).

By these definitions, almost two-thirds of 215 Lyme disease patients in a recent retrospective cohort from an endemic region had chronic Lyme disease [4]. Case definitions for Lyme disease have evolved and will continue to develop as a better understanding of chronic Lyme disease emerges to shape a common lexicon.

5. Competency and training

The appropriateness of treatment hinges on the clinician's experience in treating Lyme disease. Competence requires diagnostic and treatment skills heretofore not offered in medical school or postresidency training.

Clinicians more practiced in treating Lyme disease achieve better outcomes and encounter fewer complications because of an enhanced ability to interpret clinical data, the prompt prescription of antibiotics and the use of measures to reduce adverse events, e.g., employing acidophilus to replace normal intestinal flora that is depleted by antibiotics.

6. The increasing role of primary care

The primary care physician has an important role as the first and at times, the principal medical contact for the person with Lyme disease.

Primary care physicians focus on the resolution of symptoms, monitoring for side effects, maintenance or improvement of functional status and prevention of recurrent symptoms.

These guidelines incorporate the evidence used by primary care physicians for the care of patients with Lyme disease.

7. Highlights of guidelines

- Since there is currently no definitive test for Lyme disease, laboratory results should not be used to exclude an individual from treatment
- Lyme disease is a clinical diagnosis and tests should be used to support rather than supersede the physician's judgment
- The early use of antibiotics can prevent persistent, recurrent and refractory Lyme disease
- The duration of therapy should be guided by clinical response, rather than by an arbitrary (i.e., 30 day) treatment course
- The practice of stopping antibiotics to allow for delayed recovery is not recommended for persistent Lyme disease. In these cases, it is reasonable to continue treatment for several months after clinical and laboratory abnormalities have begun to resolve and symptoms have disappeared

Section II: New presentatons

Lyme disease was first described in 1977 as 'Lyme arthritis' among patients initially thought to have arthritis or juvenile rheumatoid arthritis [11]. It was later renamed 'Lyme disease' following recognition of a combination of cardiac, neurologic and rheumatologic presentations, including heart block, meningitis and Bell's palsy. For more than 10 years, variable symptomatic conditions have been recognized including encephalopathy and neuropsychiatric presentations.

8. Symptomatic presentation

Variable symptomatic presentations have been increasingly documented in Lyme disease, with the best example being encephalopathy [12]. Encephalopathic presentations were described in an initial cohort of 27 patients as a symptom complex including memory loss (81%), fatigue (74%), headache (48%), depression (37%), sleep disturbance (30%) and irritability (26%), often without objective markers [12]. Only two of the 27 patients presented with objective findings on lumbar puncture: one had pleocytosis (seven cells) and a second had an antibody index of greater than one [12].

Neuropsychiatric presentations in acute and chronic Lyme disease have been increasingly recognized and can include depression, anxiety and rage [13]. These are presumably related to persistent infection and are potentially reversible with antibiotics. Neuropsychiatric symptoms may reflect additional psychosocial processes including the stress of coping with a chronic illness.

Asch and colleagues found that more than half of 215 patients in a Lyme-endemic region had symptomatic presentations of chronic Lyme disease [4]. The patients presented with chronic fatigue, headaches and joint pain (but not headaches alone) in this retrospective cohort study.

9. Symptoms of Lyme disease

- Fatigue
- Low grade fevers, 'hot flashes' or chills
- Night sweats
- Sore throat
- Swollen glands
- Stiff neck
- Migrating arthralgias, stiffness and, less commonly, frank arthritis
- Myalgia
- Chest pain and palpitations
- Abdominal pain, nausea
- Diarrhea
- Sleep disturbance
- Poor concentration and memory loss
- Irritability and mood swings
- Depression
- Back pain
- Blurred vision and eye pain
- Jaw pain
- Testicular/pelvic pain
- Tinnitus
- Vertigo
- Cranial nerve disturbance (facial numbness, pain, tingling, palsy or optic neuritis)
- Headaches
- 'Lightheadedness'
- Dizziness

The International Lyme and Associated Diseases Society

10. Increasing evidence of persistent infection

Persistent, recurrent and refractory presentations from ongoing infection are the most feared of the long-term complications of Lyme disease.

Laboratory culture of *B. burgdorferi* has documented persistent infection in chronic Lyme disease patients, but the yields are quite low by current methods [14]. In fact, there is no reliable, commercially available culture assay that can confirm the eradication of the organism. Using experimental techniques, however, *B. burgdorferi* has been detected in virtually every organ in the body, and the spirochete has a strong predilection for the central nervous system. Oral antibiotic levels in the central nervous system are low, and this fact may necessitate the addition of drugs with good penetration across the blood–brain barrier [15], such as intravenous ceftriaxone or cefotaxime.

Most studies demonstrate a beneficial effect of antibiotics in the management of chronic Lyme disease, but the extent of optimal treatment is still uncertain [4,12,13,16–22]. Recent clinical trials questioning the benefits of antibiotics have been criticized for enrolling patients with refractory Lyme disease who were sick for a mean of 4.7 years despite an average of three courses of antibiotics, and for relying only on one treatment protocol (1 month of i.v. ceftriaxone followed by 2 months of low-dose oral doxycycline) [23]. In view of these methodological problems, persistent infection remains a continued concern for physicians.

11. Disappointing results of symptomatic treatment

A theoretical immune mechanism has been proposed to explain persistent symptoms in chronic Lyme disease, but no clinical or laboratory test can confirm this theory. The immune mechanism theory is based on physiological events (often in the form of cascades) that are not reversed by simply killing the infecting organism.

The presentation of chronic Lyme disease can be identical to that of other multisystem disorders, including systemic lupus erythematosus, rheumatoid arthritis and fibromyalgia. In the seminal article describing fibromyalgia in a Lyme disease population, antibiotic treatment failure and relapse of symptoms were considered to be proof of the absence of *B. burgdorferi* infection, and persistent symptoms were assumed to be due to postinfectious sequelae [24]. However, the failure of short-course (2–4 week) antibiotic treatment in 14 (94%) of 15 fibromyalgia patients is consistent with a persistent, inadequately treated infection with *B. burgdorferi* [24].

The increasing successes of repeated and prolonged antibiotic treatment in chronic Lyme disease are more consistent with a persistent infection mechanism.

12. Severity of chronic Lyme disease

For patients with chronic Lyme disease, the quality of life has been evaluated in a clinical trial sponsored by the National Institutes of Health (NIH) using a standardized questionnaire [23]. The quality of life of the 107 individuals with chronic Lyme disease was worse than that of patients with Type 2 diabetes or a recent heart attack, and equivalent to that of patients with congestive heart failure or osteoarthritis. Moreover, the average Lyme disease duration of 4.7 years in subjects enrolling in the study emphasized the chronic nature of the condition. Finally, the failure of 1 month of i.v. ceftriaxone followed by 2 months of oral doxycycline delineated the potential for a poor outcome in chronic Lyme disease [25].

Section III: Diagnostic concerns

The most important method for preventing chronic Lyme disease is recognition of the early manifestations of the disease.

13. Atypical early presentations

Early Lyme disease classically presents with a single erythema migrans (EM or 'bullseye') rash. The EM rash may be absent in over 50% of Lyme disease cases, however [25]. Patients should be made aware of the significance of a range of rashes beyond the classic EM, including multiple, flat, raised or blistering rashes. Central clearing was absent in over half of a series of EM rashes [26]. Rashes can also mimic other common presentations including a spider bite, ringworm, or cellulitis. One series of eleven EM rashes was misdiagnosed and treated as cellulitis, with all eleven patients showing clinical evidence of Lyme disease progression [27].

Physicians should be aware that fewer than 50% of all Lyme disease patients recall a tickbite [28]. Early Lyme disease should also be considered in an evaluation of 'off-season' onset when flu-like symptoms, fever and chills occur in the summer and fall. Early recognition of atypical early Lyme disease presentation is most likely to occur when the patient has been educated on this topic.

14. New chronic Lyme disease presentations

A detailed history may be helpful for suggesting a diagnosis of chronic Lyme disease. Headache, stiff neck, sleep disturbance and problems with memory and concentration are findings frequently associated with neurologic Lyme disease. Other clues to Lyme disease have been identified, although these have not been consistently present in each patient: numbness and tingling, muscle twitching, photosensitivity, hyperacusis, tinnitus, lightheadedness and depression.

Most patients diagnosed with chronic Lyme disease have an indolent onset and variable course. Neurologic and rheumatologic symptoms are characteristic, and increased severity of symptoms on wakening is common. Neuropsychiatric symptoms alone are more often seen in chronic than acute Lyme disease. Although many studies have found that such clinical features are often not unique to Lyme disease, the striking association of musculoskeletal and neuropsychiatric symptoms, the variability of these symptoms and their recurrent nature may support a diagnosis of the disease.

15. The limitations of physical findings

A comprehensive physical examination should be performed, with special attention to neurologic, rheumatologic and cardiac symptoms associated with Lyme disease.

Physical findings are nonspecific and often normal, but arthritis, meningitis and Bell's palsy may sometimes be noted. Available data suggest that objective evidence alone is inadequate to make treatment decisions, because a significant number of chronic Lyme disease cases may occur in symptomatic patients without objective features on examination or confirmatory laboratory testing.

Factors other than physical findings, such as a history of potential exposure, known tickbites, rashes or symptoms consistent with the typical multisystem presentation of Lyme disease, must also be considered in determining whether an individual patient is a candidate for antibiotic therapy.

16. Sensitivity limitations of testing

Treatment decisions should not be based routinely or exclusively on laboratory findings [2,25]. The two-tier diagnostic criteria, requiring both a positive ELISA and western blot, lacks sensitivity and leaves a significant number of individuals with Lyme disease undiagnosed and untreated [29,30]. These diagnostic criteria were intended to improve the specificity of tests to aid in identifying well-defined Lyme disease cases for research studies [31]. Though arbitrarily chosen, these criteria have been used as rigid diagnostic benchmarks that have prevented individuals with Lyme disease from obtaining treatment. Diagnosis of Lyme disease by two-tier confirmation fails to detect up to 90% of cases and does not distinguish between acute, chronic, or resolved infection [21].

The CDC considers a western blot positive if at least 5 of 10 IgG bands or 2 of 3 IgM bands are positive [31]. However, other definitions for western blot confirmation have been proposed to improve the test sensitivity [30,32–36]. In fact, several studies showed that sensitivity and specificity for both the IgM and IgG western blot range from 92 to 96% when only two specific bands are positive [34–36].

Lumbar puncture has also been disappointing as a diagnostic test to rule out concomitant central nervous system infection. In Lyme disease, evaluation of cerebrospinal fluid is unreliable for a diagnosis of encephalopathy and neuropathy because of poor sensitivity (see Section II.8). For example, pleocytosis was present in only one of 27 patients (sensitivity 3%) and with only seven cells [12]. The antibody index was positive (>1) in only one of 27 patients (sensitivity 3%) [12]. An index is the ratio between Lyme ELISA antibodies in the spinal fluid and Lyme ELISA antibodies in the serum. The proposed index of 1.3 would be expected to have even worse sensitivity.

Several additional tests for Lyme disease have been evaluated. These include antigen capture, urine antigen and polymerase chain reaction. Each has advantages and disadvantages in terms of convenience, cost, assay standardization, availability and reliability. These tests remain an option to identify people at high risk for persistent, recurrent and refractory Lyme disease but have not been standardized.

17. Seronegative Lyme disease

A patient who has tested seronegative may have a clinical presentation consistent with Lyme disease, especially if there is no evidence to indicate another illness.

Although many individuals do not have confirmatory serologic tests, surveillance studies show that these patients may have a similar risk of developing persistent, recurrent and refractory Lyme disease compared with the seropositive population. A prospective observational study of 1094 patients [21] and the Klempner clinical trials [23] found no difference in measured outcomes (e.g., success of retreatment) among seropositive or seronegative Lyme disease patients.

18. Continued importance of differential diagnosis

The differential diagnosis of Lyme disease requires consideration of both infectious and noninfectious etiologies. Among noninfectious causes are thyroid disease, degenerative arthritis, metabolic disorders (vitamin B12 deficiency, diabetes), heavy metal toxicity, vasculitis and primary psychiatric disorders.

Infectious causes can mimic certain aspects of the typical multisystem illness seen in chronic Lyme disease. These include viral syndromes such as parvovirus B19 or West Nile virus infection, and bacterial mimics such as relapsing fever, syphilis, leptospirosis and mycoplasma.

The clinical features of chronic Lyme disease can be indistinguishable from fibromyalgia and chronic fatigue syndrome. These illnesses must be closely scrutinized for the possibility of etiological *B. burgdorferi* infection.

19. Clinical judgment

Clinical judgment remains necessary in the diagnosis of late Lyme disease. A problem in some studies that relied on objective evidence was that treatment occurred too late, leaving the patient at risk for persistent and refractory Lyme disease.

As noted, time-honored beliefs in objective findings and two-tier serologic testing have not withstood close scrutiny [21,30,34,37]. Lyme disease should be suspected in patients with newly acquired or chronic symptoms (headaches, memory and concentration problems and joint pain). Management of patients diagnosed on the basis of clinical judgment needs to be tested further in prospective trials, and diagnostic reproducibility must be verified.

20. Testing for coinfection

Polymicrobial infection is a new concern for individuals with Lyme disease, and coinfection is increasingly reported in critically ill individuals [25,38]. Although *B. burgdorferi* remains the most common pathogen in tickborne illnesses, coinfections including *Ehrlichia* and *Babesia* strains are increasingly noted in patients with Lyme disease, particularly in those with chronic illness. *Bartonella* is another organism that is carried by the same ticks that are infected with *B. burgdorferi,* and evidence suggests that it is a potential coinfecting agent in Lyme disease [25].

Recent animal and human studies suggest that Lyme disease may be more severe and resistant to therapy in coinfected patients [25,38]. Thus, concurrent testing and treatment for coinfection is mandatory in Lyme disease patients.

The International Lyme and Associated Diseases Society

Section IV: Treatment considerations

Since Lyme disease can become persistent, recurrent and refractory even in the face of antibiotic therapy, evaluation and treatment must be prompt and aggressive.

21. Prompt use of antibiotics

Although no well designed studies have been carried out, the available data support the prompt use of antibiotics to prevent chronic Lyme disease. Antibiotic therapy may need to be initiated upon suspicion of the diagnosis, even without definitive proof. Neither the optimal antibiotic dose nor the duration of therapy has been standardized, but limited data suggest a benefit from increased dosages and longer treatment, comparable to the data on tuberculosis and leprosy which are caused by similarly slow-growing pathogens [25].

22. Choosing an antibiotic

In acute Lyme disease, the choice of antibiotics should be tailored to the individual and take into account the severity of the disease as well as the patient's age, ability to tolerate side effects, clinical features, allergy profile, comorbidities, prior exposure, epidemiologic setting and cost.

Conversely, persistent and refractory Lyme disease treatment is more likely to include intravenous and/or intramuscular antibiotics. The choices depend in part on the patient's response to antibiotic therapy and on the success of antibiotics in treating other Lyme disease patients (see below).

Therapy usually starts with oral antibiotics, and some experts recommend high dosages. The choice of antibiotic therapy is guided by weighing the greater activity of intravenous antibiotics in the central nervous system against the lower cost and easy administration of oral antibiotics for *B. burgdorferi*.

23. Oral antibiotic options

For many Lyme disease patients, there is no clear advantage of parenteral therapy. Along with cost considerations and pressure to treat patients with Lyme disease with the least intervention, there is growing interest in the use of oral therapy.

First-line drug therapies for Lyme disease may include (in alphabetical order): oral amoxicillin, azithromycin [39–41], cefuroxime [42], clarithromycin [43], doxycycline and tetracycline. These antibiotics have similar favorable results in comparative trials of early Lyme disease. In one study, azithromycin performed slightly less well when compared to amoxicillin and doxycycline. However, the efficacy of azithromycin was underestimated because the antibiotic was only given for 10 days [39].

One study has suggested that oral doxycycline (100 mg twice daily for 30 days) is as effective as intravenous ceftriaxone (2 g daily for 30 days) in early disseminated Lyme disease [40]. Two European studies have demonstrated similar efficacy of oral doxycycline and parenteral penicillin and ceftriaxone in early Lyme disease [44,45].

There are no studies comparing oral with intravenous antibiotics for persistent, recurrent and refractory Lyme disease.

24. Intravenous antibiotic options

It is common practice to consider intravenous antibiotics upon failure of oral medications in patients with persistent, recurrent or refractory Lyme disease, and as the first line of therapy for certain conditions, (i.e., encephalitis, meningitis, optic neuritis, joint effusions and heart block).

Ideally, the intravenous antibiotic should be selected on the basis of *in vitro* sensitivity testing or clinical experience [101]. Intravenous antibiotics are also justified by concern for penetration into the central nervous system [15].

Until recently, ceftriaxone, cefotaxime and penicillin were the only intravenous antibiotics routinely studied for use in Lyme disease. Intravenous imipenem, azithromycin and doxycycline have an adequate antispirochetal spectrum of activity and may represent suitable alternative therapies. However, the latter two drugs are often considered for intravenous use only if they are not tolerated orally.

There is a paucity of data on alternative intravenous antibiotics, and their success is less predictable in chronic Lyme disease.

25. Intramuscular antibiotic options

Intramuscular benzathine penicillin (1.2 to 2.4 million units per week) is sometimes effective in patients who do not respond to oral and intravenous antibiotics. If intramuscular benzathine penicillin is used, long-term therapy may be necessary due to the low serum concentration of this form of penicillin [46]. Luft and colleagues report, "It was demonstrated that while *B. burgdorferi* may be sensitive to relatively small concentrations of penicillin and ceftriaxone, the organism is killed slowly. This implies that, as in syphilis, prolonged blood levels of these drugs may be necessary in order to ensure cure" [46].

One-third of a chronic Lyme disease population responded to intramuscular benzathine penicillin (1.2 to 2.4 million units per week) [16–18]. Benzathine penicillin has mainly been used in patients who have had multiple relapses while receiving oral or intravenous antibiotic therapy or who are intolerant of oral or intravenous antibiotics.

26. Combination antibiotic treatment

Combination therapy with two or more antibiotics is now increasingly used for refractory Lyme disease [11,41,45,46–49] and has also been given as initial therapy for some chronic presentations.

This approach is already used for another tickborne illness, babesiosis [50]. Oral amoxicillin, cefuroxime or (more recently) cefdinir combined with a macrolide (azithromycin or clarithromycin) are examples of combination regimens that have proven successful in clinical practice, although controlled clinical trials are lacking in persistent, recurrent and refractory Lyme disease.

Combination therapy in patients with Lyme disease raises the risk of adverse events. This risk must be weighed against the improved response to combination therapy in Lyme disease patients failing single agents [47–49].

27. Sequential treatment

Clinicians increasingly use the sequence of an intravenous antibiotic followed by an oral or intramuscular antibiotic [19,37,101,47,48]. In two recent case series that employed combination therapy and sequential therapy, most patients were successfully treated [19,47]. A logical and attractive sequence would be to use intravenous therapy first (e.g., intravenous ceftriaxone), at least until disease progression is arrested and then follow with oral therapy for persistent and recurrent Lyme disease.

28. Dosage

Increasingly, clinicians recommend that certain drugs used for Lyme disease be given at higher daily doses: for example, 3000–6000 mg of amoxicillin, 300–400 mg doxycycline and 500–600 mg of azithromycin. Some clinicians prescribe antibiotics using blood levels to guide higher doses. Close monitoring of complete blood counts and chemistries are also required with this approach.

With higher doses, there may be an increase in adverse events in general and gastrointestinal problems in particular. Acidophilus has reportedly reduced the incidence of *C. difficile* colitis and non-*C. difficile* antibiotic-related diarrhea.

Serious adverse effects of antibiotics, however, were less common than previous estimates. In a recent clinical trial of chronic Lyme disease, the overall serious adverse event rate was 3% after three months of antibiotics, including 1 month of intravenous antibiotics [23]. Clinicians who have experience with higher-dose antibiotic therapy must balance the benefit of higher drug levels achieved with this therapy against the modest risk of gastrointestinal and other side effects.

Research is needed to determine the added benefits of higher doses of antibiotics in chronic Lyme disease.

29. Duration of therapy

Because of the disappointing long-term outcome with shorter courses of antibiotics, the practice of stopping antibiotics to allow for a delayed recovery is no longer recommended for patients with persistent, recurrent and refractory Lyme disease. Reports show failure rates of 30–62% within 3 years of short-course treatment using antibiotics thought to be effective for Lyme disease [3,4,12]. Conversely for neurologic complications of Lyme disease, doubling the length of intravenous ceftriaxone treatment from 2 to 4 weeks improved the success rate from 66 to 80% [12,51].

The management of chronic Lyme disease must be individualized, since patients will vary according to severity of presentation and response to previous treatment.

Concurrent risk factors (i.e., coinfections, previous treatment failures, frequent relapses, neurologic involvement, or previous use of corticosteroids) or evidence of unusually severe Lyme disease should lead to the initiation of prolonged and/or intravenous antibiotic treatment. Physicians should always assess the patient's response to treatment before deciding on appropriate duration of therapy (i.e., weeks versus months).

30. Empiric treatment

The importance of establishing the diagnosis of Lyme disease is heightened in light of increasing concern about antibiotic overuse. After an appropriate history, physical examination and laboratory testing are completed, empiric antimicrobial therapy should be initiated on the basis of clinical clues, the severity of the patient's acute illness, underlying disease and the likelihood of *B. burgdorferi* infection. The ILADS working group recommends that empiric treatment be considered routine for patients with a likely diagnosis of Lyme disease.

31. Persistent Lyme disease

Persistent Lyme disease is more resistant to treatment and more likely to produce a relapse. Although persistent Lyme disease may resolve without additional therapy, many experts believe that this condition should be treated with repeated and prolonged antibiotics. Physicians should extend the duration of antibiotics to prevent or delay recurrent and refractory Lyme disease.

32. Recurrent Lyme disease

Despite previous antibiotic treatment, Lyme disease has a propensity for relapse and requires careful follow-up for years. The data suggest that failure to eradicate the organism may be the reason for a recurrence of symptoms [12]. Early and aggressive treatment with antibiotics is indicated for recurrent Lyme disease. The ultimate impact from retreating each episode of recurrent Lyme disease is currently unclear.

33. Refractory Lyme disease

Refractory Lyme disease is a devastating condition that usually affects patients with persistent symptomatology and long-term disability. Prompt and aggressive institution of antibiotic therapy may be essential to prevent refractory disease. Increasing evidence shows that antibiotics have a beneficial effect on the course of refractory Lyme disease even in cases where the patient is intolerant of antibiotics or when a previous regimen has failed. Several months of therapy are often required to produce clear evidence of improvement. During this time, symptomatic treatment may be combined with antibiotic treatment.

34. Treatment failure

When patients fail to respond or their conditions deteriorate after initiation of empiric therapy, a number of possibilities should be considered other than Jarisch-Herxheimer reaction. These include adverse events that limit treatment, allergic history to medication, inappropriate or inadequate dosing regimen, compliance problems, incorrect medication, immune sequelae and sequestering of the organism (e.g., in the central nervous system). An alternative diagnosis or coinfection should also be considered.

35. Symptomatic treatment

Although there may be a potential role for symptomatic treatment in chronic Lyme disease, this approach has little support due to the strong possibility of persistent infection. Owing to the potential hazard of immunosuppression and the poor outcome in one study, steroid therapy is not recommended [52]. Surgical synovectomy is associated with significant morbidity and does not address neurologic presentations; it should be reserved for knee pain failing antibiotic treatment [53]. Intra-articular steroid injection may be useful as a temporizing procedure in patients with persistent knee pain but this runs the risk of masking persistent infection.

Symptomatic therapy (particularly anti-inflammatory medications, tricyclic antidepressants, selective serotonin re-uptake inhibitors and hydroxychloroquine) may be useful in concert with antibiotics and in individuals failing antibiotics.

Hyperbaric oxygen therapy (HBOT) is under study but is not recommended for routine therapeutic use [25,54]. Other treatments, including cholestyramine (CSM), antifungal therapy and antiviral agents require further study.

Since patients are becoming more interested in alternative therapies (e.g., traditional Chinese medicine, anti-oxidants, hyperthermia, bee venom, naturopathy and homeopathy), physicians should be prepared to address questions regarding these topics.

36. Fibromyalgia

The outcome of treating fibromyalgia secondary to Lyme disease with nonantibiotic regimens has been poor. The most encouraging clinical trial showed success in only one of 15 patients and only modest improvement in 6 of 15 individuals with fibromyalgia despite 2 years of treatment [24].

Antibiotic therapy has been much more effective than supportive therapy in symptomatic patients with fibromyalgia secondary to Lyme disease.

Fibromyalgia treatment alone without antibiotics raises the risk of conversion to refractory chronic Lyme disease and/or exacerbation of an undiagnosed persistent infection and is not recommended. Increasingly, clinicians do not feel comfortable treating fibromyalgia in Lyme disease without antibiotics.

37. Decision to stop antibiotics

Several studies of patients with Lyme disease have recommended that antibiotics be discontinued after 30 days of treatment. Complicating the decision to stop antibiotics is the fact that some patients present with disease recurrence after the resolution of their initial Lyme disease symptoms. This is consistent with incomplete antibiotic therapy. Although the optimal time to discontinue antibiotics is unknown, it appears to be dependent on the extent of symptomatology, the patient's previous response to antibiotics and the overall response to therapy (see below).

Rather than an arbitrary 30-day treatment course, the patient's clinical response should guide duration of therapy. Patients must therefore be carefully evaluated for persistent infection before a decision is made to withhold therapy.

The decision to discontinue antibiotics should be made in consultation with the patient and should take into account such factors as the frequency and duration of persistent infection, frequency of recurrence, probability of refractory Lyme disease, gains with antibiotics, the importance to the patient of discontinuing antibiotics and potential for careful follow-up.

The ideal approach would be to continue therapy for Lyme disease until the Lyme spirochete is eradicated. Unfortunately there is currently no test available to determine this point [25]. Therefore, the clinician must rely on the factors outlined above to decide on the length of antibiotic therapy for chronic Lyme disease.

38. Alternative antibiotics

There is compelling evidence that Lyme disease can result in serious and potentially refractory illness. Use of alternative antibiotics to treat early Lyme disease with erythema migrans is generally not indicated unless coinfection is suspected.

The ILADS Working Group believes that the risk of alternative antibiotics is acceptable in selected Lyme disease patients presenting with chronic Lyme disease. Alternative antibiotics include less commonly used oral antibiotics (cefixime, cefdinir, metronidazole) and intravenous antibiotics (imipenem, azithromycin). The role of alternative antibiotics in low-risk patients is less certain and there is less consensus within the Working Group as to whether the potential benefits outweigh the risks.

39. Therapy for coinfection

Therapy for polymicrobial infection in Lyme disease is a rapidly changing area of clinical practice [25]. Uncomplicated Lyme disease may be managed without addressing coinfection by means of standard oral or parenteral antibiotic therapy. Some but not all experts recommend therapy for subclinical or chronic coinfection with *Ehrlichia*, *Babesia* or *Bartonella* on the basis of their belief that responses are more prompt with this approach.

The dose, duration and type of treatment for coinfections have not been defined. Published reports of coinfection are limited to a small number of patients treated in open-label, nonrandomized studies. Doxycycline has been indicated for *Ehrlichia*. A recently published randomized trial determined that treatment of severe *Babesia microti* with the combination of atovaquone and azithromycin was as effective as the use of standard oral therapy with clindamycin and quinine [55].

The decision to use alternative antibiotics should be based on the individual case, including a careful assessment of the patient's risk factors and personal preferences. Patients managed in this way must be carefully selected and considered reliable for follow-up. Further controlled studies are needed to address the optimal antimicrobial agents for coinfections and the optimal duration of therapy.

Additional research is needed to determine which antibiotics work best for *Bartonella,* but fluoroquinolones, azithromycin, doxycycline and rifampin have good *in vitro* activity.

Section V: Research needs

The ILADS Working Group encourages centers that treat large numbers of Lyme disease patients symptomatically using IDSA treatment guidelines to perform a formal evaluation of their own programs. This will allow researchers to compare the results of treatment guidelines that use more antibiotics with those that do not.

40. Ongoing development of treatment guidelines

The IDSA guidelines recommending one-time short-term antibiotic therapy have not been successful. Physician demands for better outcomes have led to the development of the ILADS guidelines, and the continued evolution of an evidence-based approach is critical for the treatment of persistent, recurrent and refractory Lyme disease.

41. Validation of guidelines

Most studies of Lyme disease were retrospective, unblinded and uncontrolled. Furthermore, the antibiotic dose and duration of therapy were not standardized.

The first double-blind clinical trial found that weekly benzathine penicillin for 3 weeks was more effective than placebo for Lyme arthritis [56]. At the other end of the spectrum, a recently completed randomized clinical trial failed to demonstrate any efficacy of 90 days of antibiotic therapy in previously treated patients with neurologic Lyme disease [23].

Two additional randomized trials are examining the practice of retreating chronic Lyme disease patients with antibiotics, and these results should be available shortly [57,58]. The retreatment approach is being validated using a single-center, prospective surveillance database.

42. Comparative studies

The IDSA and ILADS Guidelines differ substantially, revealing the wide variation in diagnosis and treatment (TABLE 1) [59,60]. This variation suggests that physicians do not use a uniform strategy to diagnose and treat Lyme disease. Physicians often treat for Lyme disease longer than 4 weeks and also retreat [8,19,47,48,57–62]. These decisions are made despite warnings against overdiagnosis and overtreatment [63–65].

Community-based clinicians and academic centers often have different criteria for diagnosis and divergent goals of care [8]. The guidelines and standards of practice used for diagnosis of Lyme disease in academic research settings may not be applicable or appropriate for community-based settings. Moreover, the clinical manifestations of Lyme disease are often subtle or atypical in the community.

Because important data concerning the treatment of chronic Lyme disease was not considered by the IDSA expert panel, ILADS introduced an evidence-based review to determine which recommendations warranted revision. This evidence-based review gave rise to the current guidelines.

Section VI: Periodic review of guidelines

New data on treatment of Lyme disease is emerging, and randomized controlled trials that address various unresolved issues in Lyme disease are ongoing. The ILADS Working Group has therefore developed a mechanism for routinely and periodically reviewing this information and for updating the guidelines on a regular basis. The most recent information will be available from the ILADS website at www.ILADS.org.

43. Grading system for evidence-based guidelines

The ILADS system for grading recommendations is similar to that used by the expert panel of the IDSA. However, the ILADS panel includes primary care clinicians, researchers and international leaders in the treatment of Lyme disease. Thus, the ILADS group is more inclusive and clinically oriented than the IDSA panel, and the ILADS guidelines reflect this diversity.

44. Table 1. Comparison of key IDSA and ILADS guidelines.

Condition	IDSA	ILADS
Lyme arthritis	B - II	A - II
Encephalopathy	A - II	A - II
Retreatment	None	A - II
Prolonged antibiotics	None	A - II
Benzathine penicillin	D - III	B - III
Intra-articular steroid	B - III	D - III
Arthroscopic Synovectomy	B - II	D - II
Coinfection	B - III	B - III
Seronegative Lyme disease	None	A - III
Combination treatment	None	B - III
Empiric treatment	None	B - III

45. Criteria for evidence-based guidelines

The ILADS recommendations are based on two criteria [10]:

- The strength of the evidence (denoted by categories A–E)
- The quality of the data (denoted by Roman numerals I–III)

Recommendations rated 'A' are considered good evidence to support the recommendation. Those rated 'B' have moderate evidence to support the recommendation. Those rated 'C' are considered optional. Measures designated 'D' generally should not be offered; those designated 'E' are contraindicated.

A rating of I indicates that at least one randomized controlled trial supports the recommendation; II, evidence from at least one well-designed clinical trial without randomization supports the recommendation; and III, 'expert opinion'.

Sources

Our data sources are English-language articles published from 1975 to 2003. The selection panel synthesized the recommendations from published and expert opinion. Human studies of Lyme disease were identified from MEDLINE (1975 to 2003) and from references in pertinent articles and reviews. Also included are abstracts and material presented at professional meetings and the collective experience of the ILADS Working Group treating tens of thousands of Lyme disease patients.

The International Lyme and Associated Diseases Society

References

1 Goldoft MJ, Schulze TL, Parkin WE, Gunn RA. Lyme disease in New Jersey. *NJ Med.* 87, 579–584 (1990).

2 CDC. Lyme disease-United States, 2000. *MMWR* 51, 29–31 (2002).

3 Shadick NA, Phillips CB, Logigian EL *et al.* The long-term clinical outcomes of Lyme disease. A population-based retrospective cohort study. *Ann. Intern. Med.* 121, 560–567 (1994).

4 Asch ES, Bujak DI, Weiss M, Peterson MGE, Weinstein A. Lyme disease: an infectious and postinfectious syndrome. *J. Rheumatol.* 21, 454–456 (1994).

5 Parola P, Raoult D. Ticks and tickborne bacterial diseases in humans: an emerging infectious threat. *Clin. Infect. Dis.* 32, 897–928 (2001).

6 Wormser GP, Nadelman RB, Dattwyler RJ *et al.* Practice guidelines for the treatment of Lyme disease. The Infectious Diseases Society of America. *Clin. Infect. Dis.* 31(Suppl. 1), 1–14 (2000).

7 Rahn DW, Malawista SE. Lyme disease: recommendations for diagnosis and treatment. *Ann. Intern. Med.* 114, 472–481 (1991).

8 Feder HM Jr. Differences are voiced by two Lyme camps at a Connecticut public hearing on insurance coverage of Lyme disease. *Pediatrics* 105(4 Pt 1), 855–857 (2000).

9 Burrascano JJ. Lyme disease. In: *Conn's Current Therapy.* WB Saunders Company, PA, USA 140–143 (1997).

10 Kish MA. Guide to development of practice guidelines. *Clin. Infect. Dis.* 32, 851–854 (2001).

11 Steere AC, Malawista SE, Snydman DR, Shope RE, Andiman WA, Ross MR, Steele FM. Lyme arthritis: an epidemic of oligoarticular arthritis in children and adults in three Connecticut communities. *Arthritis Rheum.* 20, 7–17 (1977).

12 Logigian EL, Kaplan RF, Steere AC. Chronic neurologic manifestations of Lyme disease. *N. Engl. J. Med.* 323, 1438–1444 (1990).

13 Fallon BA, Nields JA. Lyme disease: a neuropsychiatric illness. *Am. J. Psychiatry* 151, 1571–1583 (1994).

14 Tylewska-Wierzbanowska S, Chmielewski T. Limitation of serological testing for Lyme borreliosis: evaluation of ELISA and western blot in comparison with PCR and culture methods. *Wien Klin Wochenschr.* 114, 601–605 (2002).

15 Halperin JJ. Neuroborreliosis. *Am. J. Med.* 98(4A), 52S–59S (1995).

16 Battaglia HR, Alvarez G, Mercau A, Fay M, Campodónico M. Psychiatric symptomatology associated with presumptive Lyme disease: Clinical evidence. *J. Spiro Tick Dis.* 7, 22–25 (2000).

17 Corsaro L Intramuscular Bicillin for persistent pediatric Lyme disease. Proceedings of the 9th International Conference on Lyme Borreliosis & Other Tick-borne Disorders (1999).

18 Cimmino MA, Accardo S. Long-term treatment of chronic Lyme arthritis with benzathine penicillin. *Ann. Rheum. Dis.* 51, 1007–1008 (1992).

19 Fallon BA, Tager F, Keilp J, Weiss N, Liebowitz MR, Fein L, Liegner K. Repeated antibiotic treatment in chronic Lyme disease. *J. Spiro Tick Dis.* 6, 94–102 (1999).

20 Lawrence C, Lipton RB, Lowy FD, Coyle PK. Seronegative chronic relapsing neuroborreliosis. *Eur. Neurol.* 35,113–117 (1995).

21 Cameron DJ. Monitoring Lyme disease in the community – First surveillance database sentinel health site. Proceedings of the 12th Annual International Scientific Conference on Lyme Disease and Other Spirochetal and Tick-Borne Disorders (1999).

22 Fallon BA, Kochevar JM, Gaito A, Nields JA. The underdiagnosis of neuropsychiatric Lyme disease in children and adults. *Psychiatr. Clin. North Am.* 21, 693–703 (1998).

23 Klempner MS, Hu LT, Evans J *et al.* Two controlled trials of antibiotic treatment in patients with persistent symptoms and a history of Lyme disease. *N. Engl. J. Med.* 345, 85–92 (2001).

24 Dinerman H, Steere AC. Lyme disease associated with fibromyalgia. *Ann. Intern. Med.* 117, 281–285 (1992).

25 Stricker RB, Lautin A. The Lyme wars: time to listen. *Expert Opin. Investig. Drugs* 12, 1609–1614 (2003).

26 Nadelman RB, Wormser GP. Erythema migrans and early Lyme disease. *Am. J. Med.* 98(4A), S15–S24 (1995).

27 Nowakowski J, McKenna D, Nadelman RB et al. Failure of treatment with cephalexin for Lyme disease. *Arch. Fam. Med.* 9, 563–567 (2000).

28 Steere AC, Broderick TF, Malawista SE. Erythema chronicum migrans and Lyme arthritis: epidemiologic evidence for a tick vector. *Am. J. Epidemiol.* 108, 312–321 (1978).

29 Petrovic M, Vogelaers D, Van Renterghem L, Carton D, De Reuck J, Afschrift M. Lyme borreliosis – a review of the late stages and treatment of four cases. *Acta Clin. Belg.* 53, 178–183 (1998).

30 Tilton RC, Sand MN, Manak M. The Western immunoblot for Lyme disease: determination of sensitivity, specificity and interpretive criteria with use of commercially available performance panels. *Clin. Infect. Dis.* 25(Suppl. 1), S31–S34 (1997).

31 CDC. Recommendations for test performance and interpretation from the second national conference on serologic diagnosis of Lyme disease. *MMWR* 44, 590–591 (1995).

32 Trevejo RT, Krause PJ, Sikand VK, Schriefer ME, Ryan R, Lepore T, Porter W, Dennis DT. Evaluation of two-test serodiagnostic method for early Lyme disease in clinical practice. *J. Infect. Dis.* 179, 931–938 (1999).

33 Aguero-Rosenfeld ME, Nowakowski J, McKenna DF, Carbonaro CA, Wormser GP. Serodiagnosis in early Lyme disease. *J. Clin. Microbiol.* 31, 3090–3095 (1993).

34 Harris N. An understanding of laboratory testing for Lyme disease. *J. Spiro Tick Dis.* 5, 16–26 (1998).

35 Ma B, Christen B, Leung D, Vigo-Pelfrey C. Serodiagnosis of Lyme borreliosis by Western immunoblot: reactivity of various significant antibodies against *Borrelia burgdorferi*. *J. Clin. Microbiol.* 30, 370–376 (1992).

36 Engstrom SM, Shoop E, Johnson RC. Immunoblot interpretation criteria for serodiagnosis of early Lyme disease. *J. Clin. Microbiol.* 33, 419–427 (1995).

37 Magnarelli LA. Laboratory analyses for Lyme disease. *Conn. Med.* 53, 331–334 (1989).

38 Krause PJ, Telford S, Spielman A, Sikand VJ, Ryan R, Christianson D, Burke G, Brassard P, Pollack R, Peck J, Persing DH. Concurrent Lyme disease and Babesiosis: Evidence for increased severity and duration of illness. *JAMA* 275, 1657–1660 (1996).

39 Luft BJ, Dattwyler RJ, Johnson RC *et al.* Azithromycin compared with amoxicillin in the treatment of erythema migrans: a double-blind, randomized, controlled trial. *Ann. Intern. Med.* 124, 785–791 (1996).

40 Dattwyler RJ, Luft BJ, Kunkel M *et al.* Ceftriaxone compared with doxycycline for the treatment of acute disseminated Lyme disease. *N. Engl. J. Med.* 337, 289–294 (1997).

41 Barsic B, Maretic T, Majerus L, Strugar J. Comparison of azithromycin and doxycycline in the treatment of erythema migrans. *Infection* 28, 153–156 (2000).

42 Scott LJ, Ormrod D, Goa KL. Cefuroxime axetil: an updated review of its use in the management of bacterial infections. *Drugs* 61, 1455–1500 (2001).

43 Dattwyler RJ, Grunwaldt E, Luft BJ. Clarithromycin in treatment of early Lyme disease: a pilot study. *Antimicrob. Agents Chemother.* 40, 468–469 (1996).

44 Karlsson M, Hammers-Berggren S, Lindquist L *et al.* Comparison of iv. penicillin G and oral doxycycline for treatment of Lyme neuroborreliosis. *Neurology* 44, 1203–1207 (1994).

45 Dotevall L, Hagberg L. Successful oral doxycycline treatment of Lyme disease-associated facial palsy and meningitis. *Clin. Infect. Dis.* 28, 569–574 (1999).

46 Luft BJ, Volkman DJ, Halperin JJ, Dattwyler RJ. New chemotherapeutic approaches in the treatment of Lyme borreliosis. *Ann. NY Acad. Sci.* 539, 352–361 (1988).

47 Battaglia HR, Alvarez G, Mercau A, Fay M, Campodónico M. Psychiatric symptomatology associated with presumptive Lyme disease: clinical evidence. *J. Spirol. Tick Dis.* 7, 22–25 (2000).

48 Ziska MH, Donta ST, Demarest FC. Physician preferences in the diagnosis and treatment of Lyme disease in the United States. *Infection* 24, 182–186 (1996).

49 Culp RW, Eichenfield AH, Davidson RS, Drummond DS, Christofersen MR, Goldsmith DP. Lyme arthritis in children. An orthopedic perspective. *J. Bone Joint Surg. Am.* 69, 96–99 (1987).

50 Weiss LM. Babesiosis in humans: a treatment review. *Expert Opin. Pharmacother.* 3, 1109–1115 (2002).

51 Logigian EL, Kaplan RF, Steere AC. Successful treatment of Lyme encephalopathy with iv. ceftriaxone. *J. Infect. Dis.* 180, 377–383 (1999).

52 Dattwyler RJ, Halperin JJ, Volkman DJ, Luft BJ. Treatment of late Lyme borreliosis – randomized comparison of ceftriaxone and penicillin. *Lancet* 1191–1194 (1988).

53 Schoen RT, Aversa JM, Rahn DW, Steere AC. Treatment of refractory chronic Lyme arthritis with arthroscopic synovectomy. *Arthritis Rheum.* 34, 1056–1060 (1991).

54 Pavia CS. Current and novel therapies for Lyme disease. *Expert Opin. Investig. Drugs* 12, 1003–1016 (2003).

55 Krause PJ, Lepore T, Sikand VK *et al.* Atovaquone and azithromycin for the treatment of babesiosis. *N. Engl. J. Med.* 343, 1454–1458 (2000).

56 Steere AC, Green J, Schoen RT *et al.* Successful parenteral penicillin therapy of established Lyme arthritis. *N. Engl. J. Med.* 312, 869–874 (1985).

57 Fallon BA. Chronic Lyme Disease Research Study. A double-blind placebo-controlled randomized clinical trial evaluating the efficacy of ten weeks of iv. ceftriaxone and effects on brain imaging. Enrollment since 2000.

58 Cameron DJ. Lyme Disease Retreatment Study. A double-blind placebo-controlled randomized clinical trial evaluating the efficacy of oral amoxicillin for seropositive and seronegative Lyme disease. Enrollment since 2001.

59 Eppes SC, Klein JD, Caputo G, Rose CD. Physician beliefs, attitudes and approaches toward Lyme disease in an endemic area. *Clin. Pediatr.* 33, 130–134 (1994).

60 Peña CA, Mathews AA, Siddiqi NH, Strickland GT. Antibiotic therapy for Lyme disease in a population-based cohort. *Clin. Infect. Dis.* 29, 694–695 (1999).

61 Wahlberg P, Granlund H, Nyman D, Panelius J, Seppala I. Treatment of late Lyme borreliosis. *J. Infect.* 29, 255–261 (1994).

62 Donta ST. Tetracycline therapy for chronic Lyme disease. *Clin. Infect. Dis.* 25(Suppl. 1), S52–S56 (1997).

63 Reid MC, Schoen RT, Evans J, Rosenberg JC, Horwitz RI. The consequences of overdiagnosis and overtreatment of Lyme disease: an observational study. *Ann. Intern. Med.* 128, 354–362 (1998).

64 Steere AC, Taylor E, McHugh GL, Logigian EL. The overdiagnosis of Lyme disease. *JAMA* 269, 1812–1816 (1993).

65 Sigal LH. Anxiety and persistence of Lyme disease. *Am. J. Med.* 98(4A), 74S–78S (1995).

Website

101 Burrascano JJ Jr. Managing Lyme disease: diagnostic hints and treatment guidelines for Lyme borreliosis, 2003. Accessed at www.ILADS.org on November 1, 2003.

The Need for Clinical Judgment in the Diagnosis and Treatment of Lyme Disease

Elizabeth L. Maloney, M.D.

ABSTRACT

Clinical practice guidelines are increasing in number. Unfortunately, when scientific evidence is uncertain, limited, or evolving, as is often the case, conflict often arises between guideline committees and practicing physicians, who bear the direct responsibility for the care of individual patients. The 2006 Infectious Diseases Society of America guidelines for Lyme disease, which have limited scientific support, could, if implemented, limit the clinical discretion of treating physicians and the treatment options available to patients.

Introduction

Clinical practice guidelines are now ubiquitous throughout the United States. The National Guidelines Clearing House, under the category "diseases," currently lists 2,126 separate guidelines on its website.[1] Clinical guidelines are intended to assist physicians in patient care by clearly communicating the results of the guideline committees' evaluation of available therapeutic options. However, the processes by which individual guidelines are constructed may be less clear, leading to disagreements between the issuing committee and the physicians who treat patients—physicians who may well be as experienced and knowledgeable as the guideline committee.

The 2006 Infectious Diseases Society of America (IDSA) guidelines for Lyme disease were released in the fall of that year and were soon the focus of an antitrust suit brought by Connecticut's attorney general.[2] A settlement between the two sides was announced on May 1, 2008; it called for the seating of a new panel and a comprehensive review of the evidence, including a hearing to allow for presentation of divergent medical points of view.[3] This article reviews the 2006 IDSA Lyme guidelines regarding the impact various recommendations may have on the use of clinical judgment in the diagnosis and treatment of patients with Lyme disease.

Clinical Judgment in the Diagnosis of Lyme Disease

The IDSA in its 2006 Lyme disease guidelines states:

> Clinical findings are sufficient for the diagnosis of erythema migrans, but clinical findings alone are not sufficient for diagnosis of extracutaneous manifestations of Lyme disease or for diagnosis of [human granulocyctic anaplasmosis] HGA or babesiosis. Diagnostic testing performed in laboratories with excellent quality-control procedures is required for confirmation of extra cutaneous Lyme disease, HGA, and babesiosis.[4]

Initially, the statement appears innocuous; laboratory confirmation of any diagnosis is always reassuring. But here the guidelines panel goes a step further. By requiring lab confirmation, it sets up a diagnostic hierarchy in which testing supersedes clinical judgment, negative results on indirect laboratory assessments of infection overrule carefully constructed clinical assessments, and tests are deemed infallible.

Yet, this diagnostic scheme is fallible. Consider the situation in which 100 patients with undiagnosed Lyme disease seek medical attention for evaluation of fever, headache, fatigue, and body aches occurring at the end of June. Recall that CDC data indicate that erythema migrans (EM) rashes are reported in 68% of patients meeting the surveillance case definition, and that the guidelines recommend two-tier serologic testing of patients lacking the diagnostic rash.[4,5] In the two-tier scheme, patients are first tested with an enzyme-linked immunoabsorbant assay (ELISA) or indirect fluorescent antibody (IFA) test, and those with positive or equivocal results are then tested with Western blotting; patients who are negative on ELISA are not tested further. Trevejo et al.[6] found the sensitivity of two-tier testing in early Lyme disease to be 29%-32%; Bacon et al.[7] found it to be 38%. As Table 1 demonstrates, the laboratory confirmation requirement is problematic; as many as 22% of early Lyme disease patients would go untreated.

Clearly, this is unacceptable; patients would be left untreated at the stage when therapy is most efficacious. Owing to the potential for false negative results in these circumstances, Steere et al.[8] suggested that physicians consider treating patients with "summertime flu" symptoms. The need for such a suggestion emphasizes the principal reason for this challenge—laboratory confirmation requirements undermine the value and primacy of clinical data and may impede care, as would be the case in this very common clinical scenario.

The same problem with laboratory confirmation holds true for late neurologic Lyme disease. Starting again with 100 patients who have undiagnosed Lyme disease and objective, non-EM findings, 43%-56% would be misdiagnosed because of deficits in laboratory capabilities, as shown in Table 2. In late Lyme, sensitivity of the testing procedure was found to be 44% by Ledue et al.[9], and 57% by Dressler et al.[10]

The low sensitivity of two-tier testing in late neurologic Lyme disease can be traced back to the original paper by Dressler et al.,[10] from which the Centers for Disease Control and Prevention (CDC)

Table 1. Outcomes for 100 Patients with Early Lyme Disease, Following IDSA Recommendations

Description	Number	Positive two-tier	Negative two-tier	Outcome
EM positive	68	NA	NA	Treat
EM absent	32	10-12	20-22	10 treated; **22 untreated**

Table 2. Outcomes for 100 Patients with Late Neurologic Lyme Disease, Following IDSA Recommendations

Description	Positive two-tier	Negative two-tier	Outcome
Late disease, objective positive	44-57	43-56	**Roughly half would go untreated**

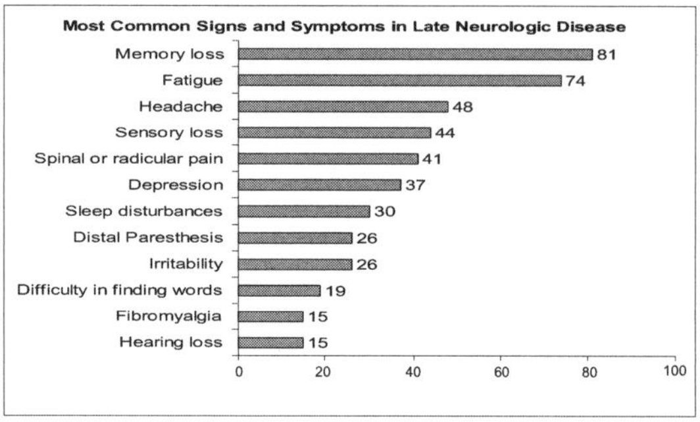

Figure 1. Frequency of Various Signs and Symptoms in Late Neurologic Lyme Disease

took its IgG Western blot criteria. After identifying the 10 bands on Western blotting that yielded the highest specificity in a retrospective study, Dressler et al. then tested the criteria in a prospective study. In that study, the paper reports that 21 of 29 patients with neuroborreliosis had positive IgG Western blot results, yielding a sensitivity of 72%.[10] The ELISA used by Dressler et al. had a sensitivity of 79%. Performing the tests sequentially, as is done in two-tier testing, results in an overall sensitivity of 57% (79% x 72%). With the two-tier sensitivity for late Lyme disease roughly 50%, a negative result does not inform physicians, but may easily lead them astray.

Other studies on the two-tier strategy yield different and higher values for sensitivity.[6,10-13] Some studies speak of the "relative sensitivity" of a test rather than the true sensitivity.[13] The disagreement between studies investigating the sensitivity of various testing methodologies for Lyme disease indicates a problem with test reliability, which has been the subject of other papers.[14,15] If the serologic tests for Lyme disease were equally reliable, sensitivity would be nearly identical across studies of similar, and appropriate, design. (A full discussion on the limitations of serologic testing is beyond the scope of this paper.)

Other methods available to support or confirm a clinical diagnosis of Lyme disease in the absence of an EM have low sensitivity (polymerase chain reaction [PCR] of cerebrospinal fluid and blood), may be invasive, or are not clinically available.[16-20]

With serologic testing being insensitive, clinical data—the history and physical examination—become even more important. Relying on clinical data to make a diagnosis is not unique to Lyme disease. One study on the relative values of history, physical examination, and diagnostic studies found that internists used history alone to establish the correct diagnosis in 76% of test cases.[21] Another found that in distributing a 100% total relative value between these three types of data, clinical faculty valued history at 63.3%, physical examination at 19.2%, and laboratory/imaging data at 17.5%.[22] Such evidence establishes that the diagnostic hierarchy proposed by the guidelines is inconsistent with the way medicine is practiced.

A Lyme disease history begins with the potential for exposure. This history, while a key element, is not always enlightening. Patients may be unaware of whether they live/work/recreate in a Lyme-endemic area; they may forget about vacations in endemic areas. Questions regarding tick bites may lead to inappropriately ruling out Lyme disease; in one study on erythema migrans, only 14% of the patients recalled being bitten by a tick.[23]

Clinically, and in keeping with its multisystemic nature, Lyme disease has been described as being "symptom rich, exam poor." Symptoms may be specific or nonspecific, mundane or unusual, acute or chronic; some are prognostic. Some physicians have been criticized for "seeing Lyme everywhere" in that they recognize scores of symptoms beyond EM rashes, Bell's palsy, and arthritis as being associated with Lyme disease.[24,25] Yet, early researchers also noted these symptoms. In a treatment trial on early Lyme disease, Massarotti et al. found that subjects reported the following symptoms: 56% had headache; 42%, stiff neck, with 19% having pain with neck flexion; 14%, dysesthesias; 11%, photophobia; and 4%, facial palsy.[26] Consider these symptoms from Logigian et al., shown in Figure 1.[27]

The wide array of Lyme disease symptoms is consistent with *Borrelia burgdorferi's* ability to infect multiple organ systems; nervous system involvement creates the potential for varied and atypical symptoms.[28-35] Common symptoms include: EM rash, fever, fatigue, headache, neck pain, joint or muscle pain, paresthesias, memory impairment, weakness of facial muscles, mood disorders, neuropathic pain.[8,16,23,26-41] A compendium of manifestations by system is given in Table 3.

Table 3. Lyme Disease Manifestations[16,27,35,42-89]

General	Gastrointestinal and Genitourinary Systems	Psychological
Fever Night sweats Fatigue, lack of endurance Unexplained weight gain/loss Generalized, unprovoked pain Migratory pain	Nausea/pain/gastroesophageal reflux Recurrent vomiting Diarrhea/constipation Irritable bladder or interstitial cystitis Testicular or pelvic pain Decreased libido Unexplained menstrual irregularity Unexplained galactorrhea	Mood swings, irritability Patient feels as "if losing my mind" Overly emotional reactions, cries easily Depression Bipolar disorder Panic attacks, anxiety Obsessive-compulsive disorder Psychosis
Head, Face, Neck Headache, mild or severe Facial flushing Pressure in head Jaw pain or stiffness Unexplained hair loss Dental problems/pain (unexplained) Facial muscle fasciculations Stiff or painful neck Facial paralysis (Bell's Palsy) Sore throat, hoarseness Tingling of nose, tongue, cheek	**Musculoskeletal System** Bone pain, joint pain or swelling Carpal tunnel syndrome Stiffness of joints, back, or neck Frequent tendonitis, lateral epicondylitis Myalgia or cramps, muscle spasms Sore soles, especially in morning	**Mental Capability** Memory loss (short or long-term) Disorientation (getting or feeling lost Confusion, difficulty in thinking Apraxia Difficulty concentrating or reading Dementia
Eyes/Vision and Ears/Hearing Diplopia or blurry vision Difficulty with night vision Increased floating spots Pain in eyes, or swelling around eyes Photophobia Flashing lights/Peripheral waves/phantom images Change in color vision Decreased hearing in one or both ears Tinnitus Pain in ears, hyperacusis Auditory hallucinations	**Respiratory and Circulatory Systems** Shortness of breath, cough Endocarditis, myocarditis, heart failure Peripheral vascular abnormalities Rhythm disturbances—PVCs, PACs, SVTs, palpitations, heart block	**Nervous System** Burning, stabbing, aching, or shock sensations Lightheadedness, syncope Paresthesias Increased motion sickness Peripheral neuropathies Abnormalities of vision, hearing, taste, smell, or touch Muscle weakness Muscle atrophy Muscle fasciculations Speech difficulty (slurred or slow) Stammering speech Word searching, misspeaking Poor balance Dizziness Difficulty walking, gait problems Tremors Seizures Sleep problems (excessive sleep, insomnia, sleep apnea, narcolepsy, unusual sleep behaviors)

It is the multisystemic nature of the illness that provides physicians with useful diagnostic information. In fact, with the exception of an isolated EM rash or swollen joint, patients with symptoms restricted to a single system are unlikely to have Lyme disease. Recognizing the potential for disease is different from "seeing it everywhere." Failure to recognize Lyme disease may lead to serious harm, as antibiotics are delayed and the infection is unchecked.[90]

The nonspecific nature of many Lyme disease symptoms leads some to suggest that such symptoms hold no diagnostic value.[91] Lyme disease is like many other illnesses that present with nonspecific and often subtle symptoms—symptoms that may go unrecognized by physicians. Examples include hypothyroidism, ovarian cancer, and acute subendocardial myocardial infarction. What gives the individual symptoms of Lyme disease value is their occurrence in clusters; a single symptom means little but four or five may, for all practical purposes, make the case. Just as abdominal bloating, urinary urgency, and pelvic pain raise "red flags" for gynecologists, the combination of fatigue, paresthesias, arthralgias, and memory complaints presenting in a single patient commands the attention of physicians aware of these potential Lyme disease symptoms.

Steere et al. noted that patients with early Lyme disease who lacked an EM rash presented with an average of four or more symptoms.[8] Fever, chills, malaise, and myalgia, all nonspecific, were present in 46%-71% of the patients with definite Lyme disease alone. In this group, it was the clustering of nonspecific symptoms in the appropriate setting that led to the correct diagnosis of Lyme disease. Logigian et al. also noted the nonspecific nature of identi-fying symptoms: "The most common form of chronic central nervous system involvement in our patients was subacute encephalopathy affecting memory, mood, and sleep, sometimes with subtle disturbances in language. *Diagnosis of this condition may be difficult because the typical symptoms are nonspecific*" [emphasis added].[27] To provide a clinical level of diagnostic sensitivity higher than two-tier testing, physicians need to recognize the symptom clusters and maintain a high index of suspicion for Lyme disease.

Symptoms not only form the basis of disease identification, they may also inform on prognosis. Dysesthesias,[26] paresthesias,[36] multiple EM lesions,[36,38] increased irritability, [37] persistent fatigue,[38] headache,[38] stiff neck,[38] and increased severity of the initial illness[38] were associated by various investigators in the early Lyme disease treatment trials with an increased risk of treatment failure. Symptoms were also used in the trials as indicators that a strategy was working or needed to be altered.[26,36,38,39]

Findings on physical exam are usually subtle and limited; they may be variably present.[29,32] The more common findings include: solitary or multiple EM lesions,[23,26,33,36-41] manifestations of cranial neuritis (such as extraocular palsies, ptosis, decreased facial sensation, facial nerve palsy, decreased hearing),[4,28,29,32,33] swollen and tender joints,[4,27,33] diminished sensation, and motor weakness. [27,29,30,32,35] Cognitive deficits are usually not readily apparent on mental status testing, but patients may be disorganized or slow to respond to questions.[16,17,27,34] A lack of physical findings does not necessarily indicate that the symptoms in those cases cannot be corroborated with objective evidence. Halperin et al. studied 14 patients with complaints of distal paresthesias;[35] 10 had completely normal sensory, motor and reflex findings on examination, three had only mild sensory loss, and one had moderate sensory and motor loss coupled with decreased reflexes. All underwent EMG testing; 13 of the 14 had "significant neurophysiologic findings." Logigian et al. also found that detailed neuropsychometric testing could reveal cognitive deficits that were not apparent on routine mental status testing.[16,27,34] Cost and time constraints do not allow for such complete testing in a community setting, but the studies suggests that with sufficiently detailed testing, objective evidence may be discovered and the subjective data supported. The absence of findings does not equal absence of disease.

Even the EM rash has a variable presentation that may cause less informed physicians to miss it. An EM lesion may have one or more of the following characteristics: homogeneously erythematous color, prominent central clearing, target-like appearance, central vesicles or pustules, partially purpuric, and not scaly, unless topical corticosteroid creams have been applied or the rash is old and fading.[4,23,33] An EM rash must be distinguished from: tick bite hypersensitivity reactions, insect or spider bites, contact dermatitis, bacterial cellulitis, and tinea.[4,33] An interesting study in *JAMA* compared responses from physicians in endemic and nonendemic areas with regard to what percentage of EM rashes in their practices had central clearing.[41] Physicians from endemic areas thought it only 19%, while those from nonendemic estimated 80%. The authors did not give a reason for the disparity; possibilities include *B. burgdorferi* strain variation or physician experience. The variable presentation of the EM rash, coupled with the fact that it does not manifest in 32% of patients,[5] makes it unwise to rely on EM as the only manifestation of Lyme disease that has clinical diagnostic utility.

Physicians use pattern recognition as a common diagnostic heuristic.[92] These cognitive "shortcuts," when used properly, allow physicians to move quickly to the correct diagnosis. Pattern recognition transforms exposure, individual symptoms, and the course of illness into a unified diagnosis; it is why some physicians specifically see "Lyme disease" when colleagues see only a generalized "positive review of systems." For physicians unfamiliar with the pattern of Lyme disease, serologic testing, combined with clinical data, offers the potential for reaching the correct diagnosis. However, serology alone cannot confirm or deny presence of infection.[93] In Lyme disease, there is no testing shortcut.

Furthermore, diagnostic criteria are situational. Clinical criteria are constructed to diagnose and treat ill patients. Research criteria are constructed to test a hypothesis in a uniform group of subjects; researchers have no duty to those excluded from the trial. Surveillance criteria are much the same, the goal being selection of a homogeneous patient subset that can be observed over time and treatment. The difference between these situations is an important consideration. This distinction is highlighted by these comments from CDC epidemiologist Dr. Paul Mead:

> A clinical diagnosis is made for the purpose of treating an individual patient and should consider the many details associated with that patient's illness. Surveillance case definitions are created for the purpose of standardization, not patient care; they exist so that health officials can reasonably compare the number and distribution of "cases" over space and time. Whereas physicians appropriately err on the side of over-diagnosis, thereby assuring they don't miss a case,

surveillance case definitions appropriately err on the side of specificity, thereby assuring that they do not inadvertently capture illnesses due to other conditions.[94]

Recognition of the differing goals allows knowledgeable physicians the discretion to diagnose Lyme disease in patients lacking the five of 10 bands required for admittance into the surveillance group.[95] Failure to acknowledge the distinction results in many patients with Lyme disease remaining undiagnosed and untreated.

Mandatory laboratory confirmation of clinical diagnoses, as advanced in the 2006 IDSA guidelines, reverses the roles of clinical and laboratory data in the diagnostic process and hierarchy. Substituting laboratory tests for physician judgment is not clinically sound, particularly when laboratory tests lack sensitivity. This recommendation is a change from the 2000 IDSA guidelines on Lyme disease, but the 2006 panel did not discuss the reasons for this change nor cite any references from the literature to support it.[4,96] Guideline developers have identified the need for reconciliation between new and former versions of the same disease guidelines;[97] the IDSA, itself, endorsed the reconciliation process, yet it did not occur in this instance.

Correctly diagnosing extracutaneous Lyme disease can be difficult. The importance of clinically derived data has been demonstrated repeatedly, as have the weaknesses of serologic testing. At this time, Lyme disease should remain a clinical diagnosis, with testing playing a supportive role.

Clinical Judgment in Management of Patients with Lyme Disease

Clinical judgment is required to appropriately manage patient care. Patient management is an evolutionary process, not a static state; ongoing assessment allows for refinement of the original diagnosis or the search for new one. Lyme disease is no exception to this rule; yet the 2006 IDSA guidelines reduce clinical management to a one-size-fits-all approach quickly chosen from a table.[4] Clinical judgment is especially important when the clinical picture is unclear and laboratory data unhelpful. After careful investigation of other potential diagnoses, physicians may need to perform an empiric treatment trial as a diagnostic modality. The use of such trials extends well beyond Lyme disease. For example, patients with nonspecific epigastric pain may be offered "GI cocktails" as a means to both diagnose and treat the condition.

Clinical decision-making in Lyme disease requires ongoing information; the longitudinal treatment trials on Lyme disease demonstrated the value of this data. Historical and physical examination data were gathered at defined points; on some occasions the information was used to alter the treatment protocol (investigators withdrew or re-treated some subjects).[26,34,36,38] Follow-up visits in many of the studies on Lyme disease demonstrated a positive correlation between reported symptomatic changes and subsequent physical findings or test results.[27,35] Long-term follow-up extending beyond the active treatment phase provides researchers, as well as physicians in clinical practice, the ability to discern the difference between placebo and treatment effects.[27]

Clinical judgment in Lyme disease requires physicians to weigh risk-benefit concerns with individual patients.[98] Treatment risks for the patient include potential adverse effects from antibiotic therapy (including risks associated with medication administration), costs associated with therapy, and lifestyle changes to accommodate treatment.[99-101] Patient benefits include improved health with attendant improvement in quality of life and lower medical costs following recovery. Antibiotic therapy, including long-term oral antibiotics, is generally safe and well tolerated.[101,102] A meta-analysis on the risks associated with intravenous (IV) access of various types found that peripheral intravenous catheters cause 0.5 bloodstream infections per 1,000 intravascular device (IVD) days while surgically implanted long-term central venous devices—cuffed and tunneled catheters—cause 1.6 infections per 1,000 IVD-days.[103] Data from Lyme disease treatment trials can inform on the risk of IV antibiotic therapy in this patient population. Table 4 reports the complication rates in the treatment groups of Lyme disease studies which used IV ceftriaxone for a minimum of 30 days.[34,104-106] Significant adverse events included medication-related events (severe allergic reactions, gall bladder toxicity, *Clostridium difficile* enterocolitis, renal failure) and catheter-related events (skin infiltration, infection, and thrombosis).

Table 4. Medication and IV Device Complications in Studies of Lyme Disease

Study	N	Days of IV antibiotic	IVD Days	Significant Adverse Events (%)	Adverse Event Rate/ 1,000 IVD Days
Logigian1999[34]	18	30	540	0	0
Klempner 2001[104]	64	30	1920	2 (3.1%)	1.0
Krupp 2003[105]	28	30	840	1 (3.6%)	1.2
Fallon 2008[106]	23	70	1610	6 (26.1%)	4.3
Total	133		4910	9 (6.8%)	1.83

Adverse events in the Fallon study[106] are considerably higher than in the others; reasons are unknown, and the small sample size makes it difficult to draw conclusions. There were three cases of ceftriaxone allergy in the 23 patients; this 13% allergic rate is higher than expected.[107] Thrombi developed in two patients, but the paper does not provide details of the site of the peripherally inserted central catheter (PICC) or its specific type. Additional studies are needed to delineate the risk of IV antibiotic therapy extending beyond 30 days in better detail, and to determine whether there would be opportunities to minimize those factors contributing to the total risk.

There are also risks to the patient associated with failure to treat a continuing infection.[108] These include declining health, decreased productivity, a potential for increased costs as more health-related services are required, and costs related to palliative medications (including their potential adverse effects).[99-101]

The IDSA guidelines raise concerns about the impact longer treatment regimens may have on society.[4] While these concerns should not sway treating physicians who are entrusted with the care of individual patients, the concerns merit some comments. The guidelines authors focus attention on treatment risks to society, citing additional costs and the potential for increased bacterial resistance in the community.[4] However, the authors ignored potential benefits to society from such treatment regimens. These benefits include improved health in the community, increased production from previously ill patients, and potential for success in this patient population to inform treatment decisions in other groups.[109]

Additionally, there are societal risks from not treating; these include ever increasing expenses for a chronically ill subpopulation and lost productivity from ill workers.[109]

In the individual patient, the decision to treat or to prolong treatment may depend on the length of time between onset of illness and diagnosis; severity of the patient's presenting symptoms; presence of neurological symptoms; whether the course of the illness is progressive; whether the illness significantly affects the patient's quality of life or functional abilities; presence of untreated co-infections; the patient's immune system status; whether diagnostic tests, symptoms or treatment response suggest ongoing infection; the patient's response to treatment; which medications the patient can tolerate; the specifics of prior treatment regarding antibiotic type, dose, and duration; whether the patient relapses when treatment is withdrawn; the risks/benefits of the treatment approach under consideration; and availability of any alternative treatment approaches and their attendant risks balanced against the risks associated with failing to treat. These highly individualized decisions are best made by the treating physician and the patient.

The controversy over antibiotic treatment duration for patients with Lyme disease exists because there is no test of cure, and individual patient responses to specific therapeutic approaches have been highly variable. Lyme disease, in many patients, is marked by periods when the illness is relatively quiescent.[26,28] Lacking a test of cure, physicians who do not rely on arbitrary cut-off points are faced with a difficult decision when attempting to determine an appropriate stopping point. Mixed results from the treatment trials add to the uncertainty.

The variable response to treatment has been well documented;[16,26,27,29,30,32,34,36-40] the causes remain unclear, as scientific evidence in this area is still evolving. Early hypotheses of autoimmune processes have not been substantiated;[110,111] persistent infection, however, has been demonstrated in case reports and animal studies.[18-20,112,113] Patients with Lyme disease are a heterogeneous group. Genetic variation may play a role in pathogenesis and treatment response. Just as HLA status may be related to treatment response in Lyme arthritis,[114] the response in patients with other types of Lyme disease pathology may be based on some yet to be discovered genetic subtype.

Variation in infecting strains of *B. burgdorferi* certainly is a factor.[115-117] More than 100 strains of *B. burgdorferi* have been identified. Certain strains are more virulent and pathogenic than others;[115,116] instances of antibiotic susceptibility varying between strains is well documented.[117] Coinfections and comorbidities also contribute to the heterogeneity of treatment response seen in Lyme disease.[118] *Ixodes scapularis* is able to carry multiple known bacterial, viral, and parasitic pathogens, and evidence for additional tick-borne pathogens continues to emerge.[119] Different combinations of pathogens require different treatment regimens; failure to identify and treat the specific pathogens causing an illness may partially explain variations in treatment responses.

As explained by Kravitz et al., "[h]eterogeneity of treatment effects reflects patient diversity to risk of disease, responsiveness to treatment, vulnerability to adverse effects, and utility for different outcomes."[108] Kravitz et al. discuss the application of generalized, or averaged, results from treatment trials to the care of an individual patient, and pitfalls inherent in applying them too strictly, noting that "misapplying averages can cause harm, by either giving patients treatments which do not help or denying patients treatments that would help them."[108] The individual patient is not a numeric average but, rather, falls somewhere on the continuum of the bell curve and, hence, requires individualized care.

Clinical guidelines should not supplant the judgment of treating physicians. Quality patient care requires the physician to consider management decisions in light of the details unique to each patient. When guideline recommendations are substituted for carefully derived, individualized decisions, there is a potential for harm.[120] The American Academy of Pediatrics policy statement on guideline development recognizes this principle.[121] The document outlines how evidentiary strength and risk-benefit analyses are integrated to yield a specific recommendation level. For example, strongly positive recommendations require benefits to clearly exceed risks, and supporting evidence must be of excellent quality.

In this scheme, strong recommendations are not made based on low-quality evidence or expert opinion. Options identify treatment alternatives. Options recognize patient preferences and respect the clinician's decision-making process. The U.S. Preventive Services Task Force also recognizes scenarios in which the certainty of the evidence is low.[122] In those situations, no recommendation is made, regardless of the perceived net magnitude of benefit or harm. Additionally, the Task Force advocates shared decision-making between individual patients and their physicians, instead of population-based recommendations, when issues under consideration are highly sensitive to patient utilities.[122]

Guideline committees are not in a position to perform risk-benefit analyses for specific patients.[121,122] Patient-specific risk-benefit analyses are the essence of clinical judgment. Such judgments are the domain of individual treating physicians; guideline committees may inform judgments through their evaluation of therapeutic options, but they may not substitute their judgments for those of the treating physicians. A recent *JAMA* editorial by Shaneyfelt and Centor said as much: "Guidelines are not patient-specific enough to be useful and rarely allow for individualization of care. Most guidelines have a one-size-fits-all mentality and do not build flexibility or contextualization into the recommendations."[123] While the 2006 IDSA guidelines contain the typical legal disclaimer that "they are not intended to supplant physician judgment with respect to particular patients or special clinical situations," formulaic disclaimers cannot overcome the failure of the guidelines to provide treatment options and to recognize the role of clinical judgment in individualized care. These shortcomings cannot be addressed in boilerplate disclaimers; they can only be addressed in the substance of the guidelines.

Available laboratory tests for Lyme disease have poor sensitivity.[5-14] Treatment trials cited in the guidelines for early Lyme disease were dissimilar, making it hard to compare outcomes;[26,36-40,124-126] those for late neurologic Lyme disease involved only 96 patients whose treatment responses can be analyzed.[27,34,127,128] Both the early and late treatment trials yielded poor outcome rates for complete recovery. The prophylaxis recommendation is based on a single study performed under conditions unlikely to be reproduced in community practices, and the list of "not recommended" therapeutic modalities is apparently based on panel opinion.[4,129] Given the limits of guidelines in general, and the specific shortcomings of the 2006 IDSA guidelines on Lyme disease, patients and their physicians should be free to act without interference; many may justifiably decide to decide for themselves which strategy to embrace.

Elizabeth L. Maloney, M.D., is a family physician from a Lyme disease endemic area in Minnesota. Contact: P.O. Box 84, Wyoming, MN 55092, tel. (651) 462-0192; email bettymal2003@yahoo.com.

Acknowledgments: The author would like to acknowledge Lorraine B. Johnson, J.D., M.B.A., and Dr. Bea Szantyr for their input and thoughtful editorial comments.

Potential Conflicts of interest: The author receive speaker's fees for creating and presenting continuing education courses on Lyme disease. She submitted six challenges to the IDSA Lyme disease guideline review panel and is a member of the International Lyme and Associated Disease Society (ILADS).

REFERENCES

[1] U.S. Department of Health and Human Services. National Guideline Clearinghouse. Available at: sww.guideline.gov/browse/browsemode.aspx?node=29255&type=1. Accessed Aug 18, 2009.

[2] Landers SJ. Lyme disease debate provokes treatment divide, legal action. *AM News*, Dec 25, 2006. Available at: www.ama-assn.org/amednews/2006/12/25/hlsa1225.htm. Accessed Aug 19, 2009.

[3] State of Connecticut Attorney General's Office. Press release, May 1, 2008. Available at www.ct.gov/ag/cwp/view.asp?Q=414284&A=2795. Accessed Jul 15, 2008.

[4] Wormser GP, Dattwyler RJ, Shapiro ED, et al. The clinical assessment, treatment, and prevention of Lyme disease, human granulocytic anaplasmosis, and babesiosis: clinical practice guidelines by the Infectious Diseases Society of America. *Clin Infect Dis* 2006;43:1089-1134.

[5] CDC. Lyme disease—United States 2001-2002. *MMWR* 2004;53(17):365-369.

[6] Trevejo RT, Krause PJ, Sikand VK, et al. Evaluation of two-test serodiagnostic method for early Lyme disease in clinical practice. *J Infect Dis* 1999;179:931-938.

[7] Bacon RM, Bickerstaff BJ, Schreifer ME, et al. Serodiagnosis of Lyme disease by kinetic enzyme-linked immunosorbent assay using recombinant VlsE1 or peptide antigens of *Borrelia burgdorferi* compared with two-tiered testing using whole cell lysates. *J Infect Dis* 2003;187:1187-1199.

[8] Steere A, Dhar A, Hernandez J, et al. Systemic symptoms without erythema migrans as the presenting picture of early Lyme disease. *Am J Med* 2003;114:58-62.

[9] Ledue TB, Collins MF, Craig WY. New laboratory guidelines for serologic diagnosis of Lyme disease: evaluation of the two-test protocol. *J Clin Microbiol* 1996;34:2343-50.

[10] Dressler F, Whalen JA, Reinhardt BN, Steere AC. Western blotting in the serodiagnosis of Lyme disease. *J Infect Dis* 1993;167:392-400.

[11] Steere AC, McHugh G, Damle N, Sikand VK. Prospective study of serologic tests for Lyme disease. *Clin Infect Dis* 2008;47:188-195.

[12] Tilton RC, Sand MN, Manak M. The Western immunoblot for Lyme disease: determination of sensitivity, specificity, and interpretive criteria with use of commercially available performance panels. *Clin Infect Dis* 1997;25(Jul Suppl 1):S31-S34.

[13] Mogilyansky E, Loa CC, Adelson ME, Mordechai E, Tilton RC. Comparison of Western immunoblotting and the C6 Lyme antibody test for laboratory detection of Lyme disease. *Clin Diagn Lab Immunol* 2004;11:924-929.

[14] Bakken LL, Callister SM, Wand PJ, Schell RF. Intralaboratory comparison of test results for detection of Lyme disease by 516 participants in the Wisconsin State Laboratory of Hygiene/College of American Pathologists Proficiency Testing Program. *J Clin Microbiol* 1997;35:537-543.

[15] Hunfeld KP, Stanek G, Straube E, et al. Quality of Lyme disease serology. Lessons from the German Proficiency Testing Program 1999-2001. a preliminary report. *Wien Klin Wochenschr* 2002;114(13-14):591-600.

[16] Logigian EL. Reversible cerebral hypoperfusion in Lyme encephalopathy. *Neurology* 1997;49:1661-1670.

[17] Fallon BA, Das S, Plutchok JJ, et al. Functional brain imaging and neuropsychological testing in Lyme disease. *Clin Infect Dis* 1997;25(Suppl 1):S57-S63.

[18] Oksi J, Uksila J, Marjamäki M, Nikoskelainen J, Viljanen MK. Antibodies against whole sonicated Borrelia burgdorferi spirochetes, 41-kilodalton flagellin, and P39 protein in patients with PCR- or culture-proven late Lyme borreliosis. *J Clin Microbiol* 1995;33:2260-2264.

[19] Nocton JJ, Dressler F, Rutledge BJ, et al. Detection of *Borrelia burgdorferi* DNA by polymerase chain reaction in synovial fluid from patients with Lyme arthritis. *N Engl J Med* 1994;330:229-234.

[20] Nocton JJ, Bloom BJ, Rutledge BJ, et al. Detection of *Borrelia burgdorferi* DNA by polymerase chain reaction in cerebrospinal fluid in Lyme neuroborreliosis. *J Infect Dis* 1996;174:623-627.

[21] Peterson MC, Holbrook JH, Hales D, Smith NL, Von Staker LV. Contributions of the history, physical examination, and laboratory investigation in making medical diagnoses. *West J Med* 1992;156:163-165.

[22] Markert RJ, Haist SA, Hillson HD, et al. Comparative value of clinical information in making a diagnosis. *Med Gen Med* 2004;6:64.

[23] Berger BW. Dermatologic manifestations of Lyme disease. *Rev Infect Dis* 1989;11(Suppl 6):6:S1475-S1481.

[24] Sigal LH. Summary of the first 100 patients seen at a Lyme disease referral center. *Am J Med* 1990;88:577-581.

[25] Steere AC, Taylor E, McHugh GL, et al. The overdiagnosis of Lyme disease. *JAMA* 1993;269:1812-1816.

[26] Massarotti EM, Luger SW, Rahn DW, et al. Treatment of early Lyme disease. *Am J Med* 1992;92:396-403.

[27] Logigian EL, Kaplan RF, Steere AC. Chronic neurologic manifestations of Lyme disease. *N Engl J Med* 1990;323:1438-1444.

[28] Cook SP, Macartney KK, et al. Lyme disease and seventh nerve paralysis in children. *Am J Otolaryngol* 1997;18:320-323.

[29] Coyle PK. Neurologic aspects of Lyme disease. *Med Clin North Am* 2002;86:261-284.

[30] Halperin JJ. Lyme disease and the peripheral nervous system. *Muscle Nerve* 2003;28:133-143.

[31] Dotevall L. Pain as presenting symptom in Lyme neuroborreliosis. *Eur J Pain* 2003;7:235-239.

[32] Fallon, BA. Lyme borreliosis: neuropsychiatric aspects and neuropathology. *Psychiatric Ann* 2006;36:120-128.

[33] Hengge UR. Lyme Borreliosis. *Lancet Infect Dis* 2003;3:489-500.

[34] Logigian EL, Kaplan RF, Steere AC. Successful treatment of Lyme encephalopathy with intravenous ceftriaxone. *J Infect Dis* 1999; 180:377-383.

[35] Halperin JJ, Little BW, Coyle PK, Dattwyler RJ. Lyme disease: cause of a treatable peripheral neuropathy. *Neurology* 1987;37:1700-1706.

[36] Nadelman RB, Luger SW, Frank E, et al. Comparison of cefuroxime axetil and doxycycline in the treatment of early Lyme disease. *Ann Intern Med* 1992;117:273-280.

[37] Luger SW, Paparone P, Wormser GP, et al. Comparison of cefuroxime axetil and doxycycline in treatment of patients with early Lyme disease associated with erythema migrans. *Antimicrob Agents Chemother* 1995;39:661-667.

[38] Steere AC, Hutchinson GJ, Rahn DW, et al. Treatment of early manifestations of Lyme disease. *Ann Intern Med* 1983;99:22-26.

[39] Luft BJ, Dattwyler RJ, Johnson RC, et al. Azithromycin compared with amoxicillin in the treatment of erythema migrans: a double blind, randomized, controlled trial. *Ann Intern Med* 1996;124:785-791.

[40] Dattwyler RJ, Volkman DJ, Conaty SM, Platkin SP, Luft BJ. Amoxicillin plus probenecid versus doxycycline for treatment of erythema migrans borreliosis. *Lancet* 1990;336:1404-1406.

[41] Tibbles CD, Edlow JA. Does this patient have erythema migrans? *JAMA* 2007;297:2617-2627.

[42] Ackermann R, Rehse-Kupper B, Gollmer E, Schmidt R. Chronic neurologic manifestations of erythema migrans borreliosis. *Ann NY Acad Sci* 1988;539:16-23.

[43] Arav-Boger R, Crawford T, Steere AC, Halsey NA. Cerebellar ataxia as the presenting manifestation of Lyme disease. *Pediatr Infect Dis J* 2002;21:353-356.

[44] Bhambhani N, Disla E, Cuppari G. Lyme disease presenting with sequential episodes of ruptured baker cysts. *J Clin Rheumatol* 2006;12:160-162.

[45] Bloom BJ, Wyckoff PM, Meissner HC, Steere AC. Neurocognitive abnormalities in children after classic manifestations of Lyme disease. *Pediatr Infect Dis J* 1998;17:189-196.

[46] Cassarino DS, Quezado MM, Ghatak NR, Duray PH. Lyme-associated parkinsonism: a neuropathologic case study and review of the literature. *Arch Pathol Lab Med* 2003;127:1204-1206.

[47] Chancellor MB, McGinnis DE, Shenot PJ, Kiilholma P, Hirsch IH. Urinary dysfunction in Lyme disease. *J Urol* 1993;149:26-30.

[48] Dinerman H, Steere AC. Lyme disease associated with fibromyalgia. *Ann Intern Med* 1992;117:281-285.

[49] Duray PH, Steere AC. Clinical pathologic correlations of Lyme disease by stage. *Ann NY Acad Sci* 1988;539:65-79.

[50] Faller J, Thompson F, Hamilton W. Foot and ankle disorders resulting from Lyme disease. *Foot Ankle* 1991;11:236-238.

[51] Fallon BA, Kochevar JM, Gaito A, Nields J. The underdiagnosis of neuropsychiatric Lyme disease in children and adults. *Psychiatr Clin N Am* 1998;21:693-703.

[52] Fallon BA, Nields JA. Lyme disease: a neuropsychiatric illness. *Am J Psychiat* 1994;151:1571-1583.

[53] Fallon BA, Nields JA, Liegner K, DelBene D, Liebowtitz MR. The neuropsychiatric manifestations of Lyme borreliosis. *Psychiatr Q* 1992;63:95-117.

[54] Gasser R, Horn S, Reisinger E, et al. First description of recurrent pericardial effusion associated with *Borrelia burgdorferi* infection. *Int J Cardiol* 1998;64:309-310.

[55] Halperin JJ. Neuroborreliosis. *Am J Med* 1995;98(4A):52S-56S.

[56] Halperin JJ, Kaplan GP, Brazinsky S, et al. Immunologic reactivity against *Borrelia burgdorferi* in patients with motor neuron disease. *Arch Neurol* 1990;47:586-594.

[57] Halperin JJ, Volkman DJ, Luft BJ, Dattwyler RJ. Carpal tunnel syndrome in Lyme borreliosis. *Muscle Nerve* 1989;12:397-400.

[58] Haupl T, Hahn G, Rittig M, et al. Persistence of *Borrelia burgdorferi* in ligamentous tissue from a patient with chronic Lyme borreliosis. *Arthritis Rheum* 1993;36:1621-1626.

[59] Horowitz HW, Sanghera K, Goldberg N, et al. Dermatomyositis associated with Lyme disease: case report and review of Lyme myositis. *Clin Infect Dis* 1994;18:166-171.

[60] Karma A, Seppala I, Mikkila H, et al. Diagnosis and clinical characteristics of ocular Lyme borreliosis. *Am J Ophthalmol* 1995;119:127-135.

[61] Kirsch M, Ruben FL, Steere AC, et al. Fatal adult respiratory distress syndrome in a patient with Lyme disease. *JAMA* 1988;259:2737-2739.

[62] Krupp LB, Masur D, Schwartz J, et al. Cognitive functioning in late Lyme borreliosis. *Arch Neurol* 1991;48:1125-1129.

[63] Lader E. Lyme disease misdiagnosed as a temporomandibular joint disorder. *J Prosthet Dent* 1990;63:82-85.

[64] Lo R, Menzies DJ, Archer H, Cohen TJ. Complete heart block due to Lyme carditis. *J Invasive Cardiol* 2003;15:367-369.

[65] MacDonald AB. Concurrent neocortical borreliosis and Alzheimer's disease: Demonstration of a spirochetal cyst form. *Ann NY Acad Sci* 1988;539:468-470.

[66] Mikkila HO, Seppala IJ, Viljanen MK, Peltomaa MP, Karma A. The expanding clinical spectrum of ocular Lyme borreliosis. *Ophthalmology* 2000;107:581-587.

[67] Mormont E, Esselinckx W, De Ronde T, et al. Abdominal wall weakness and lumboabdominal pain revealing neuroborreliosis: a report of three cases. *Clin Rheumatol* 2001;20:447-450.

[68] Moscatello AL, Worden DL, Nadelman RB, Wormser G, Lucente F. Otolaryngologic aspects of Lyme disease. *Laryngoscope* 1991;101(6 Pt 1):592-595.

[69] Nord JA, Karter D. Lyme disease complicated with pseudotumor cerebri. *Clin Infect Dis* 2003;37:E25-E26.

[70] Oksi J, Marjamaki M, Nikoskelainen J, Viljanen MK. *Borrelia burgdorferi* detected by culture and PCR in clinical relapse of disseminated Lyme borreliosis. *Ann Med* 1999;31:225-232.

[71] Oksi J, Voipio-Pulkki L-M, Uksila J, et al. *Borrelia burgdorferi* infection in patients with suspected acute myocardial infarction. *Lancet* 1997;350:1447-1448.

[72] Pachner AR, Steere AC. The triad of neurological manifestations of Lyme disease: meningitis, cranial neuritis, and radiculoneuritis. *Neurology* 1985;35:47-53.

[73] Pachner AR, Steiner I. Lyme neuroborreliosis: infection, immunity, and inflammation. *Lancet Neurol* 2007;6:544-552.

[74] Reik L, Steere AC, Bartenhagen NH, Shope RE, Malawista SE. Neurologic abnormalities of Lyme disease. *Medicine* 1979;58:281-294.

[75] Richardson H, Birchall JP, Hill J, McMaster T. Should we routinely screen for Lyme disease in patients with asymmetrical hearing loss? *Br J Audiol* 1994;28:59-61.

[76] Riedel M, Straube A, Schwarz MJ, Wilske BM, Muller N. Lyme disease presenting as Tourette's syndrome. *Lancet* 1998;351:418-419.

[77] Rosenhall U, Hanner P, Kaijser B. Borrelia infection and vertigo. *Acta Otolaryngol* 1988;106:111-116.

[78] Shadick NA, Phillips CB, Logigian EL, et al. The long-term clinical outcomes of Lyme disease. *Ann Intern Med* 1994;121:560-567.

[79] Shamim EA, Shamim SA, Liss G, et al. Constipation heralding neuroborreliosis: an atypical tale of 2 patients. *Arch Neurol* 2005;62:671-673.

[80] Sigal L. Clinical manifestations of Lyme disease. *N J Med* 1990;87:549-555.

[81] Sigler S, Kershaw P, Scheuch R, Sklarek H, Halperin J. Respiratory failure due to Lyme meningopolyradiculitis. *Am J Med* 1997;103:544-547.

[82] Siwula JM, Mathieu G. Acute onset of facial nerve palsy associated with Lyme disease in a 6-year-old child. *Pediatr Dent* 2002;24:572-574.

[83] Smith JL, Winward KE, Nicholson DF, Albert DW. Retinal vasculitis in Lyme borreliosis. *J Clin Neuroophthalmol* 1991;11(1):7-15.

[84] Steere AC. Lyme disease. *N Engl J Med* 1989;321:586-596.

[85] Steere AC, Bartenhagen NH, Craft JE, et al. The early clinical manifestations of Lyme disease. *Ann Intern Med* 1983;99:76-82.

[86] Steere AC, Malawista SE, Hardin JA, et al. Erythema chronicum migrans and Lyme arthritis: the enlarging clinical spectrum. *Ann Intern Med* 1977;86:685-698.

[87] Steere AC, Malawista SE et al. The clinical spectrum and treatment of Lyme disease. *Yale J Biol Med* 1984;57:453-464.

[88] Tager FA, Fallon BA, Keilp J, et al. A controlled study of cognitive deficits in children with chronic Lyme disease. *J Neuropsychiatry Clin Neurosci* 2001;13:500-507.

[89] Weissenbacher S, Ring J, Hofmann H. Gabapentin for the symptomatic treatment of chronic neuropathic pain in patients with late-stage Lyme borreliosis: a pilot study. *Dermatology* 2005;211:123-127.

[90] Cameron DJ. Consequences of treatment delay in Lyme disease. *J Eval Clin Pract* 2007;13:470-472.

[91] Feder HM Jr, Johnson BJ, O'Connell S, et al. A critical appraisal of "chronic Lyme disease." *N Engl J Med* 2007;357:1422-1430.

[92] Groopman J. *How Doctors Think*. New York, N.Y.: Houghton Mifflin; 2007.

[93] Brown SL, Hansen SL, Langone JJ. Role of serology in the diagnosis of Lyme disease. *JAMA* 1999;282:62-66.

[94] Mead P. Statement by Paul Mead M.D., M.P.H., on Hearing: CDC's Lyme Disease Prevention and Control Activities before the Connecticut Department of Public Health and the Connecticut Attorney General's Office; Jan 29, 2004. Available at: www.hhs.gov/asl/testify/t040129.html. Accessed Aug 19, 2009.

[95] Reed K. Laboratory testing for Lyme disease: possibilities and practicalities. *J Clin Microbiol* 2002;40:319-324.

[96] Wormser GP, Nadelman RB, Dattwyler RJ, et al. Practice guidelines for the treatment of Lyme disease. *Clin Infect Dis* 2000;31(Suppl 1):S1-S14.

[97] Kish M. Guide to development of practice guidelines. *Clin Infect Dis* 2001;32:851-854.

[98] AMA Principles of Medical Ethics. E-8.08 Informed Consent. Available at: www.ama-assn.org. Accessed Feb 20, 2009.

[99] Zhang X, Meltzer MI, Peña CA, et al. Economic impact of Lyme disease. *Emerg Infect Dis* 2006;12:653-660.

[100] Meltzer MI, Dennis DT, Orloski KA. The cost effectiveness of vaccinating against Lyme disease. *Emerg Infect Dis* 1999;5:321-328.

[101] Maes E, Lecomte P, Ray N. A cost-of-illness study of Lyme disease in the United States. *Clin Ther* 1998;20:993-1008.

[102] Cooper C. Safety of long-term therapy with penicillin and penicillin derivatives. U.S. Food and Drug Administration; Apr 30, 2009. Available at: http://www.fda.gov/Drugs/EmergencyPreparedness/Bioterrorism andDrug Preparedness/ucm072755.htm. Accessed Aug 19, 2009.

[103] Maki DG, Kluger DM, Crnich CJ. The risk of bloodstream infection in adults with different intravascular devices: a systematic review of 200 published prospective studies. *Mayo Clin Proc* 2006;81:1159-1171.

[104] Klempner MS, Hu LT, Evans J, et al. Two controlled trials of antibiotic treatment in patients with persistent symptoms and a history of Lyme disease. *N Engl J Med* 2001;345:85-92.

[105] Krupp LB, Hyman LG, Grimson R, et al. Study and treatment of post Lyme disease (STOP-LD): a randomized double masked clinical trial. *Neurology* 2003;60:1923-1930.

[106] Fallon BA, Keilp JG, Corbera KM, et al. A randomized, placebo-controlled trial of repeated IV antibiotic therapy for Lyme encephalopathy. *Neurology* 2008;70:992-1003.

[107] Pichichero ME. Cephalosporins can be prescribed safely for penicillin-allergic patients. *J Fam Pract* 2006;55(2):106-112.

[108] Kravitz RL, Duan N, Braslow J. Evidenced-based medicine, heterogeneity of treatment effects, and the trouble with averages. *Milbank Q* 2004;82:661-687.

[109] Joss AW, Davidson MM, Ho-Yen DO, Ludbrook A. Lyme disease—what is the cost for Scotland? *Public Health* 2003;117(4):264-273.

[110] Steere AC, Malawista SE, Newman JH, Spieler PN, Bartenhagen NH. Antibiotic therapy in Lyme disease. *Ann Intern Med* 1980;93:1-8.

[111] Stricker RB, Johnson L. Searching for autoimmunity in "antibiotic-refractory" Lyme arthritis. *Mol Immunol*. 2008;45:3023-3024.

[112] Oksi J, Marjamäki M, Nikoskelainen J, Viljanen MK. *Borrelia burgdorferi* detected by culture and PCR in clinical relapse of disseminated Lyme borreliosis. *Ann Med* 1999;31:225-332.

[113] Hodzic E, Feng S, Holden K, Freet KJ, Barthold SW. Persistence of *Borrelia burgdorferi* following antibiotic treatment in mice. *Antimicrob Agents Chemother* 2008;52:1728-1736.

[114] Steere AC, Dwyer E, Winchester R. Association of chronic Lyme arthritis with HLA-DR4 and HLA-DR2 alleles. *N Engl J Med* 1990;323:219-223.

[115] Seinost G., Dykhuizen DE, Dattwyler RJ, et al. Four clones of *Borrelia burgdorferi* sensu stricto cause invasive infection in humans. *Infect Immun* 1999;67:3518-3524.

[116] Wormser G. P., Liveris D., Nowakowski J., et al. Association of specific subtypes of *Borrelia burgdorferi* with hematogenous dissemination in early Lyme disease. *J Infect Dis* 1999;180:720-725.

[117] Preac Mursic V, Marget W, Busch U, Pleterski Rigler D, Hagl S. Kill kinetics of *Borrelia burgdorferi* and bacterial findings in relation to the treatment of Lyme borreliosis. *Infection*. 1996;24(1):9-16. Erratum in: *Infection* 1996;24(2):169.

[118] Krause PJ, Telford SR III, Spielman A, et al. Concurrent Lyme disease and babesiosis: evidence for increased severity and duration of illness. *JAMA* 1996;275:1657-60.

[119] Billeter SA. Levy MG, Chomel BB, Breitschwerdt EB. Vector transmission of Bartonella species with emphasis on the potential for tick transmission. *Med Vet Entomol* 2008;22:1-15.

[120] Tobin M. Counterpoint: Evidence-based medicine lacks a sound scientific base. *Chest* 2008;133:1071-1974.

[121] American Academy of Pediatrics Steering Committee on Quality Improvement and Management. Classifying recommendations for clinical practice guidelines. *Pediatrics* 2004;114:874-877.

[122] U.S. Preventive Services Task Force Procedure Manual, AHRQ Publication No. 08-05118-EF; July 2008:46.

[123] Shaneyfelt TM, Centor RM. Reassessment of clinical practice guidelines: go gently into that good night. *JAMA* 2009;301:868-869.

[124] Dattwyler RJ, Luft BJ, Kunkel M, et al.. Ceftriaxone compared with doxycycline for the treatment of acute disseminated Lyme disease. *N Engl J Med* 1997;337:289-294.

[125] Eppes SC, Childs JA. Comparative study of cefuroxime axetil versus amoxicillin in children with early Lyme disease. *Pediatrics* 2002;109:1173-1177.

[126] Wormser GP, Ramanathan R, Nowakowski J, et al.. Duration of antibiotic therapy for early Lyme disease: a randomized, double-blind, placebo-controlled trial. *Ann Intern Med* 2003;138:697-704.

[127] Dattwyler RJ, Halperin JJ, Pass H, Luft BJ. Ceftriaxone as effective therapy for refractory Lyme disease. *J Infect Dis* 1987;155:1322-1325.

[128] Dattwyler RJ, Halperin JJ, Volkman DJ, Luft BJ. Treatment of late Lyme borreliosis—randomized comparison of ceftriaxone and penicillin. *Lancet* 1988;1(8596):1191-1194.

[129] Nadelman RB, Nowakowski J, Fish D, et al.. Prophylaxis with single-dose doxycycline for the prevention of Lyme disease after an *Ixodes scapularis* tick bite. *N Engl J Med* 2001; 345:79-84.

ADVANCED TOPICS IN LYME DISEASE

DIAGNOSTIC HINTS AND TREATMENT GUIDELINES FOR LYME AND OTHER TICK BORNE ILLNESSES

Sixteenth Edition
Copyright October, 2008

JOSEPH J. BURRASCANO JR., M.D.

Board Member,
International Lyme and Associated Diseases Society

DISCLAIMER: The information contained in this monograph is meant for informational purposes only. The management of tick-borne illnesses in any given patient must be approached on an individual basis using the practitioner's best judgment.

TABLE OF CONTENTS

WELCOME!

Welcome to the sixteenth edition of the "Guidelines".
Amazingly, this edition is not only the sixteenth in the series, but as the first edition appeared in 1984, this reflects *twenty four years of effort!*

Since the last edition, enough new information has become available to justify this revision. New insights regarding co-infections, tests and treatment regimens are included. Nearly every item has been revised, but despite great effort to condense the information, the huge amount of new information included here has resulted in more pages than ever. Information included here is based on the literature, presentations at scientific meetings, the many valuable observations noted by my colleagues, plus experience from caring for my own patients. I have tried to make this information as up-to-date as possible and as inclusive as is practical. Please use the information presented in this document as an information resource and guide. It can never replace your own experience and clinical judgment.

I once again extend my best wishes to the many Lyme patients and their caregivers whose wisdom I deeply appreciate, and a sincere thank you to my colleagues whose endless contributions have helped me shape my approach to tick borne illnesses. I hope that this new edition proves to be useful. Happy reading!

BACKGROUND INFORMATION

WHAT IS LYME DISEASE?

I take a broad view of what Lyme Disease actually is. Traditionally, Lyme is defined an infectious illness caused by the spirochete, *Borrelia burgdorferi* (Bb). While this is certainly technically correct, clinically the illness often is much more than that, especially in the disseminated and chronic forms.

Instead, I think of Lyme as the illness that results from the bite of an infected tick. This includes infection not only with *B. burgdorferi*, but the many co-infections that may also result. Furthermore, in the chronic form of Lyme, other factors can take on an ever more significant role- immune dysfunction, opportunistic infections, co-infections, biological toxins, metabolic and hormonal imbalances, deconditioning, etc. I will refer to infection with *B. burgdorferi* as "Lyme Borreliosis" (LB), and use the designation "Lyme" and "Lyme Disease" to refer to the more broad definition I described above.

GENERAL PRINCIPLES

In general, you can think of LB as having three categories: acute, early disseminated, and chronic. The sooner treatment is begun after the start of the infection, the higher the success rate. However, since it is easiest to cure early disease, this category of LB must be taken VERY seriously. Undertreated infections will inevitably resurface, usually as chronic Lyme, with its tremendous problems of morbidity and difficulty with diagnosis and treatment and high cost in every sense of the word. So, while the bulk of this document focuses of the more problematic chronic patient, strong emphasis is also placed on earlier stages of this illness where closest attention and care must be made.

A very important issue is the definition of **"Chronic Lyme Disease".** Based on my clinical data and the latest published information, I offer the following definition. To be said to have chronic LB, these three criteria must be present:

1. Illness present for at least one year (this is approximately when immune breakdown attains clinically significant levels).
2. Have persistent major neurologic involvement (such as encephalitis/encephalopathy, meningitis, etc.) or active arthritic manifestations (active synovitis).
3. Still have active infection with B. burgdorferi (Bb), regardless of prior antibiotic therapy (if any).

Chronic Lyme is an altogether different illness than earlier stages, mainly because of the inhibitory effect on the immune system (Bb has been demonstrated *in vitro* to both inhibit and kill B- and T-cells, and will decrease the count of the CD-57 subset of the natural killer cells). As a result, not only is the infection with Bb perpetuated and allowed to advance, but the entire issue of co-infections arises. Ticks may contain and transmit to the host a multitude of potential pathogens. The clinical presentation of Lyme therefore reflects which pathogens are present and in what proportion. Apparently, in early infections, before extensive damage to the immune system has occurred, if the germ load of the co-infectors is low, and the Lyme is treated, many of the other tick-transmitted microbes can be contained and eliminated by the immune system. However, in the chronic patient, because of the inhibited defenses, the individual components of the co-infection are now active enough so that they too add to features of the illness and must be treated. In addition, many latent infections which may have pre-dated the tick bite, for example herpes viruses, can reactivate, thus adding to the illness.

An unfortunate corollary is that serologic tests can become *less* sensitive as the infections progress, obviously because of the decreased immune response upon which these tests are based. In addition, immune complexes form, trapping Bb antibodies. These complexed antibodies are not detected by serologic testing. Not surprisingly the seronegative patient will convert to seropositive 36% of the time after antibiotic treatment has begun and a recovery is underway. Similarly, the antibody titer may rise, and the number of bands on the western blot may increase as treatment progresses and the patient recovers. Only years after a successfully treated infection will the serologic response begin to diminish.

The severity of the clinical illness is directly proportional to the spirochete load, the duration of infection, and the presence of co-infections. These factors also are proportional to the intensity and duration of treatment needed for recovery. More severe illness also results from other causes of weakened defenses, such as from severe stress, immunosuppressant medications, and severe intercurrent illnesses. **This is why steroids and other immunosuppressive medications are absolutely contraindicated in Lyme. This also includes intra-articular steroids.**

Many collateral conditions result in those who have been chronically ill so it is not surprising that damage to virtually all bodily systems can result. Therefore to fully recover not only do all of the active infections have to be treated, but all of these other issues must be addressed in a thorough and systematic manner. ***No single treatment or medication will result in full recovery of the more ill patient. Only by addressing all of these issues and engineering treatments and solutions for all of them will we be able to restore full health to our patients.*** Likewise, a patient will not recover unless they are completely compliant with every single aspect of the treatment plan. This must be emphasized to the patient, often on repeated occasions.

It is clear that in the great majority of patients, chronic Lyme is a disease affecting predominantly the nervous system. Thus, careful evaluation may include neuropsychiatric testing, SPECT and MRI brain scans, CSF analysis when appropriate, regular input from Lyme-aware neurologists and psychiatrists, pain clinics, and occasionally specialists in psychopharmacology.

HYPOTHALAMIC-PITUITARY AXIS

As an extension of the effect of chronic Lyme Disease on the central nervous system, there often is a deleterious effect on the hypothalamic-pituitary axis. Varying degrees of pituitary insufficiency are being seen in these patients, the correction of which has resulted in restoration of energy, stamina and libido, and resolution of persistent hypotension. Unfortunately, not all specialists recognize pituitary insufficiency, partly because of the difficulty in making the laboratory diagnosis. However, the potential benefits of diagnosing and treating this justify the effort needed for full evaluation. Interestingly, in a significant number of these patients, successful treatment of the infections can result in a reversal of the hormonal dysfunction, and hormone replacement therapies can be tapered off!

CO-INFECTION

A huge body of research and clinical experience has demonstrated the nearly universal phenomenon in chronic Lyme patients of co-infection with multiple tick-borne pathogens. These patients have been shown to potentially carry Babesia species, Bartonella-like organisms, Ehrlichia, Anaplasma, Mycoplasma, and viruses. Rarely, yeast forms have been detected in peripheral blood. At one point even nematodes were said to be a tick-borne pathogen. Studies have shown that co-infection results in a more severe clinical presentation, with more organ damage, and the pathogens become more difficult to eradicate. In addition, it is known that Babesia infections, like Lyme Borreliosis, are immunosuppressive.

There are changes in the clinical presentation of the co-infected patient as compared to when each infection is present individually. There may be different symptoms and atypical signs. There may be decreased reliability of standard diagnostic tests, and most importantly, there is recognition that chronic, persistent forms of each of these infections do indeed exist. As time goes by, I am convinced that even more pathogens will be found.

Therefore, real, clinical Lyme as we have come to know it, especially the later and more severe presentations, probably represents a mixed infection with many complicating factors. I will leave to the reader the implications of how this may explain the discrepancy between laboratory study of pure Borrelia infections, and what front line physicians have been seeing for years in real patients.

I must very strongly emphasize that all diagnoses of tick-borne infections remains a clinical one. Clinical clues will be presented later in this monograph, but testing information is briefly summarized below.

In **Lyme Borreliosis**, western blot is the preferred serologic test. Antigen detection tests (antigen capture and PCR), although insensitive, are very specific and are especially helpful in evaluating the seronegative patient and those still ill or relapsing after therapy. Often, these antigen detection tests are the only positive markers of Bb infection, as seronegativity has been reported to occur in as many as 30% to 50% of cases. Nevertheless, active LB can be present even if all of these tests are non-reactive! Clinical diagnosis is therefore required.

In **Babesiosis**, no single test is reliable enough to be used alone. Only in early infections (less than two weeks duration) can the standard blood smear be helpful. In later stages, one can use serology, PCR, and fluorescent in-situ hybridization ("FISH") assay. Unfortunately, many other protozoans can be found in ticks, most likely representing species other than *B. microti*, yet commercial tests for only B. microti and B duncani (Formerly known as WA-1) are available at this time! In other words, the patient may have an infection that cannot be tested for. Here, as in Borrelia, clinical assessment is the primary diagnostic tool.

In **Ehrlichiosis and Anaplasmosis**, by definition you must test for both the monocytic and granulocytic forms. This may be accomplished by blood smear, PCR and serology. Many presently uncharacterized Ehrlichia-like organisms can be found in ticks and may not be picked up by currently available assays, so in this illness too, these tests are only an adjunct in making the diagnosis. Rarely, Rocky Mountain Spotted Fever can coexist, and even be chronic. Fortunately, treatment regimens are similar for all agents in this group.

In **Bartonella**, use both serology and PCR. PCR can be performed not only on blood and CSF, but as in LB, can be performed on biopsy specimens. Unfortunately, in my experience, these tests, even when both types are done, will presently miss over half the cases diagnosed clinically.

Frequent exposures to **Mycoplasmas** are common, resulting in a high prevalence of seropositivity, so the best way to confirm active infection is by PCR.

Chronic viral infections may be active in the chronic patient, due to their weakened immune response. PCR testing, and not serologies, should be used for diagnosis. Commonly seen viruses include HHV-6, CMV, and EBV.

COLLATERAL CONDITIONS

Experience has shown that collateral conditions exist in those who have been ill a long time. The evaluation should include testing both for differential diagnosis and for uncovering other subtle abnormalities that may coexist.

Test **B12 levels**, and be prepared to aggressively treat with parenteral formulations. If neurologic involvement is severe, then consideration should be given to treatment with methylcobalamin (as outlined below in the section on nutritional support).

Magnesium deficiency is very often present and quite severe. Hyperreflexia, muscle twitches, myocardial irritability, poor stamina and recurrent tight muscle spasms are clues to this deficiency. Magnesium is predominantly an intracellular ion, so blood level testing is of little value. Oral preparations are acceptable for maintenance, but those with severe deficiencies need additional, parenteral dosing: 1 gram IV or IM at least once a week until neuromuscular irritability has cleared.

Pituitary and other endocrine abnormalities are far more common than generally realized. Evaluate fully, including growth hormone levels. Quite often, a full battery of provocative tests is in order to fully define the problem. When testing the thyroid, measure free T3 and free T4 levels and TSH, and nuclear scanning and testing for autoantibodies may be necessary.

Activation of the **inflammatory cascade** has been implicated in blockade of cellular hormone receptors. One example of this is insulin resistance; clinical hypothyroidism can result from receptor blockade and thus hypothyroidism can exist despite normal serum hormone levels. These may partly account for the dyslipidemia and weight gain that is noted in 80% of chronic Lyme patients. In addition to measuring free T3 and T4 levels, check basal A.M. body temperatures. If hypothyroidism is found, you may need to treat with both T3 and T4 preparations until blood levels of both are normalized. To ensure sustained levels, when T3 is prescribed, have it compounded in a time-release form.

Neurally mediated hypotension (NMH) is not uncommon. Symptoms can include palpitations, lightheadedness and shakiness especially after exertion and prolonged standing, heat intolerance, dizziness, fainting (or near fainting), *and an unavoidable need to sit or lie down.* It is often confused with hypoglycemia, which it mimics. NMH can result from autonomic neuropathy and endocrine dyscrasias. If NMH is present, treatment can dramatically lessen fatigue, palpitations and wooziness, and increase stamina. NMH is diagnosed by tilt table testing. This test should be done by a cardiologist and include Isuprel challenge. This will demonstrate not only if NMH is present, but also the relative contributions of hypovolemia and sympathetic dysfunction. Immediate supportive therapy is based on blood volume expansion (increased sodium and fluid intake and possibly Florinef plus potassium). If not sufficient, beta blockade may be added based on response to the Isuprel challenge. The long term solution involves restoring proper hormone levels and treating the Lyme to address this and the autonomic dysfunction.

SPECT scanning of the brain- Unlike MRI and CT scans, which show structure, SPECT scans show function. Therefore SPECT scans give us information unattainable through X-rays, CT scans, MRI's, or even spinal taps. In the majority of chronic Lyme Borreliosis patients, these scans are abnormal. Although not diagnostic of Lyme specifically, if the scan is abnormal, the scan can not only quantify the abnormalities, but the pattern can help to differentiate medical from psychiatric causes of these changes. Furthermore, repeat scans after a course of treatment can be used to assess treatment efficacy. Note that improvement in scans lag behind clinical improvement by many months.

If done by knowledgeable radiologists using high-resolution equipment, scanning will show characteristic abnormalities in Lyme encephalopathy- global hypoperfusion (may be homogenous or heterogeneous). What these scans demonstrate is neuronal dysfunction and/or varying degrees of cerebrolvascular insufficiency. If necessary, to assess the relative contributions of these two processes, the SPECT scan can be done before and after acetazolamide. If the post acetazolamide scan shows significant reversibility of the abnormalities, then vasoconstriction is present, and can be treated with vasodilators, which may clear some cognitive symptoms. Therapy can include acetazolamide, serotonin agonists and even Ginkgo biloba, provided it is of pharmaceutical quality. Therapeutic trials of these may be needed.

Acetazolamide should not be given if there is severe kidney/liver disease, electrolyte abnormalities, pregnancy, sulfa allergy, recent stroke, or if the patient is taking high dose aspirin treatment

LYME BORRELIOSIS

DIAGNOSTIC HINTS

Lyme Borreliosis (LB) is diagnosed clinically, as no currently available test, no matter the source or type, is definitive in ruling in or ruling out infection with these pathogens, or whether these infections are responsible for the patient's symptoms. The entire clinical picture must be taken into account, including a search for concurrent conditions and alternate diagnoses, and other reasons for some of the presenting complaints. Often, much of the diagnostic process in late, disseminated Lyme involves ruling out other illnesses and defining the extent of damage that might require separate evaluation and treatment.

Consideration should be given to tick exposure, rashes (even atypical ones), evolution of typical symptoms in a previously asymptomatic individual, and results of tests for tick-borne pathogens. Another very important factor is response to treatment- presence or absence of Jarisch Herxheimer-like reactions, the classic four-week cycle of waxing and waning of symptoms, and improvement with therapy.

ERYTHEMA MIGRANS

Erythema migrans (EM) is diagnostic of Bb infection, but is present in *fewer than half.* Even if present, it may go unnoticed by the patient. It is an erythematous, centrifugally expanding lesion that is raised and may be warm. Rarely there is mild stinging or pruritus. The EM rash will begin four days to several weeks after the bite, and may be associated with constitutional symptoms. Multiple lesions are present less than 10% of the time, but do represent disseminated disease. Some lesions have an atypical appearance and skin biopsy specimens may be helpful. When an ulcerated or vesicular center is seen, this may represent a mixed infection, involving other organisms besides B. burgdorferi.

After a tick bite, serologic tests (ELISA. IFA, western blots, etc.) are not expected to become positive until several weeks have passed. Therefore, if EM is present, treatment must begin immediately, and one should not wait for results of Borrelia tests. You should not miss the chance to treat early disease, for this is when the success rate is the highest. Indeed, many knowledgeable clinicians will not even order a Borrelia test in this circumstance.

DIAGNOSING LATER DISEASE

When reactive, serologies indicate exposure only and do not directly indicate whether the spirochete is now currently present. Because Bb serologies often give inconsistent results, test at well-known reference laboratories. The suggestion that two-tiered testing, utilizing an ELISA as a screening tool, followed, if positive, by a confirmatory western blot, is illogical in this illness. The ELISA is not sensitive enough to serve as an adequate screen, and there are many patients with Lyme who test negative by ELISA yet have fully diagnostic western blots. I therefore recommend against using the ELISA. Order IgM and IgG western blots- but be aware that in late disease there may be repeatedly peaking IgM's and therefore a reactive IgM may not differentiate early from late disease, but it does suggest an active infection. When late cases of LB are seronegative, 36% will transiently become seropositive at the completion of successful therapy. In chronic Lyme Borreliosis, the CD-57 count is both useful and important (see below).

Western blots are reported by showing which bands are reactive. 41KD bands appear the earliest but can cross react with other spirochetes. The 18KD, 23-25KD (Osp C), 31KD (Osp A), 34KD (Osp B), 37KD, 39KD, 83KD and the 93KD bands are the species-specific ones, but appear later or may not appear at all. You should see at least the 41KD and one of the specific bands. 55KD, 60KD, 66KD, and 73KD are nonspecific and nondiagnostic.

PCR tests are now available, and although they are very specific, sensitivity remains poor, possibly less than 30%. This is because Bb causes a deep tissue infection and is only transiently found in body humors. Therefore, just as in routine blood culturing, multiple specimens must be collected to increase yield; a negative result does not rule out infection, but a positive one is significant. You can test whole blood, buffy coat, serum, urine, spinal and other body fluids, and tissue biopsies. Several blood PCRs can be done, or you can run PCRs on whole blood, serum and urine simultaneously at a time of active symptoms. The patient should be antibiotic-free for at least six weeks before testing to obtain the highest yield.

Antigen capture is becoming more widely available, and can be done on urine, CSF, and synovial fluid. Sensitivity is still low (on the order of 30%), but specificity is high (greater than 90%).

Spinal taps are not routinely recommended, as a negative tap does not rule out Lyme. Antibodies to Bb are mostly found in Lyme meningitis, and are rarely seen in non-meningitic CNS infection, including advanced encephalopathy. Even in meningitis, antibodies are detected in the CSF in less than 13% of patients with late disease! Therefore, spinal taps are only performed on patients with pronounced neurological manifestations in whom the diagnosis is uncertain, if they are seronegative, or are still significantly symptomatic after completion of treatment. When done, the goal is to rule out other conditions, and to determine if Bb (and Bartonella) antigens or nucleic acids are present. It is especially important to look for elevated protein and white cells, which would dictate the need for more aggressive therapy, as well as the opening pressure, which can be elevated and add to headaches, especially in children.

I strongly urge you to **biopsy** all unexplained skin lesions/rashes and perform PCR and careful histology. You will need to alert the pathologist to look for spirochetes.

THE CD-57 TEST

Our ability to measure CD-57 counts represents a breakthrough in LB diagnosis and treatment.

Chronic LB infections are known to suppress the immune system and can decrease the quantity of the CD-57 subset of the natural killer cells. As in HIV infection, where abnormally low T-cell counts are routinely used as a marker of how active that infection is, in LB we can use the degree of decrease of the CD-57 count to indicate how active the Lyme infection is and whether, after treatment ends, a relapse is likely to occur. It can even be used as a simple, inexpensive screening test, because at this point we believe that only Borrelia will depress the CD-57. Thus, a sick patient with a high CD-57 is probably ill with something other than Lyme, such as a co-infection.

When this test is run by LabCorp (the currently preferred lab, as published studies were based on their assays), we want our Lyme patients to measure above 60; a normal count is above 200. There generally is some degree of fluctuation of this count over time, and the number does not progressively increase as treatment proceeds. Instead, it remains low until the LB infection is controlled, and then it will jump. If the CD-57 count is not in the normal range when a course of antibiotics is ended, then a relapse will almost certainly occur.

CHECK LIST OF ***CURRENT*** SYMPTOMS: This is not meant to be used as a diagnostic scheme, but is provided to streamline the office interview. Note the format- complaints referable to specific organ systems and specific co-infections are clustered to clarify diagnoses and to better display multisystem involvement.

Have you had any of the following in relation to this illness? (CIRCLE "NO" OR "YES")

Tick bite	*N Y*	*"EM" rash (discrete circle)*	*N Y*
Spotted rash over large area	*N Y*	*Linear, red streaks*	*N Y*

	CURRENT SEVERITY				CURRENT FREQUENCY				
SYMPTOM OR SIGN	**NONE**	**MILD**	**MODERATE**	**SEVERE**	**NA**	**NEVER**	**OCCASIONAL**	**OFTEN**	**CONSTANT**
Persistent swollen glands									
Sore throat									
Fevers									
Sore soles, esp. in the AM									
Joint pain									
Fingers, toes									
Ankles, wrists									
Knees, elbows									
Hips, shoulders									
Joint swelling									
Fingers, toes									
Ankles, wrists									
Knees, elbows									
Hips, shoulders									
Unexplained back pain									
Stiffness of the joints or back									
Muscle pain or cramps									
Obvious muscle weakness									
Twitching of the face or other muscles									
Confusion, difficulty thinking									
Difficulty with concentration, reading, problem absorbing new information									
Word search, name block									
Forgetfulness, poor short term memory, poor attention									
Disorientation: getting lost, going to wrong places									
Speech errors- wrong word, misspeaking									
Mood swings, irritability, depression									
Anxiety, panic attacks									
Psychosis (hallucinations, delusions, paranoia, bipolar)									
Tremor									
Seizures									
Headache									
Light sensitivity									
Sound sensitivity									

Vision: double, blurry, floaters									
Ear pain									
	CURRENT SEVERITY				CURRENT FREQUENCY				
SYMPTOM OR SIGN	NONE	MILD	MODERATE	SEVERE	NA	NEVER	OCCASIONAL	OFTEN	CONSTANT
Hearing: buzzing, ringing, decreased hearing									
Increased motion sickness, vertigo, spinning									
Off balance, "tippy" feeling									
Lightheadedness, wooziness, unavoidable need to sit or lie									
Tingling, numbness, burning or stabbing sensations, shooting pains, skin hypersensitivity									
Facial paralysis-Bell's Palsy									
Dental pain									
Neck creaks and cracks, stiffness, neck pain									
Fatigue, tired, poor stamina									
Insomnia, fractionated sleep, early awakening									
Excessive night time sleep									
Napping during the day									
Unexplained weight gain									
Unexplained weight loss									
Unexplained hair loss									
Pain in genital area									
Unexplained menstrual irregularity									
Unexplained milk production; breast pain									
Irritable bladder or bladder dysfunction									
Erectile dysfunction									
Loss of libido									
Queasy stomach or nausea									
Heartburn, stomach pain									
Constipation									
Diarrhea									
Low abdominal pain, cramps									
Heart murmur or valve prolapse?									
Heart palpitations or skips									
"Heart block" on EKG									
Chest wall pain or ribs sore									
Head congestion									
Breathlessness, "air hunger", unexplained chronic cough									
Night sweats									

Exaggerated symptoms or worse hangover from alcohol									
Symptom flares every 4 wks.									
Degree of disability									

DIAGNOSTIC CHECKLIST

To aid the clinician, a workable set of diagnostic criteria were developed with the input of dozens of front line physicians. The resultant document, refined over the years, has proven to be extremely useful not only to the clinician, but it also can help clarify the diagnosis for third party payers and utilization review committees. **It is important to note that the CDC's published reporting criteria are for surveillance only, not for diagnosis. They should not be misused in an effort to diagnose Lyme or set guidelines for insurance company acceptance of the diagnosis, nor be used to determine eligibility for coverage.**

LYME BORRELIOSIS DIAGNOSTIC CRITERIA	RELATIVE VALUE
Tick exposure in an endemic region	1
Historical facts and evolution of symptoms over time consistent with Lyme	2
Systemic signs & symptoms consistent with Bb infection (other potential diagnoses excluded):	
Single system, e.g., monoarthritis	1
Two or more systems, e.g., monoarthritis and facial palsy	2
Erythema migrans, physician confirmed	7
Acrodermatitis Chronica Atrophicans, biopsy confirmed	7
Seropositivity	3
Seroconversion on paired sera	4
Tissue microscopy, silver stain	3
Tissue microscopy, monoclonal immunofluorescence	4
Culture positivity	4
B. burgdorferi antigen recovery	4
B. burgdorferi DNA/RNA recovery	4

DIAGNOSIS

Lyme Borreliosis Highly Likely	7 or above
Lyme Borreliosis Possible	5-6
Lyme Borreliosis Unlikely	4 or below

I suggest that when using these criteria, you state Lyme Borreliosis is "unlikely", "possible", or "highly likely" based upon the following criteria"- then list the criteria.

LYME DISEASE TREATMENT GUIDELINES

LYME BORRELIOSIS:

GENERAL INFORMATION

After a tick bite, Bb undergoes rapid hematogenous dissemination, and for example, can be found within the central nervous system as soon as *twelve hours* after entering the bloodstream. This is why even early infections require full dose antibiotic therapy with an agent able to penetrate all tissues in concentrations known to be bactericidal to the organism.

It has been shown that the longer a patient had been ill with LB prior to first definitive therapy, the longer the duration of treatment must be, and the need for more aggressive treatment increases.

More evidence has accumulated indicating the severe detrimental effects of the concurrent use of immunosuppressants including steroids in the patient with active B. burgdorferi infection. **Never give steroids or any other immunosuppressant to any patient who may even remotely be suffering from Lyme, or serious, permanent damage may result, especially if given for anything greater than a short course.** If immunosuppressive therapy is absolutely necessary, then potent antibiotic treatment should begin at least 48 hours prior to the immunosuppressants.

TREATMENT RESISTANCE

Bb contains beta lactamases and cephalosporinases, which, with some strains, may confer resistance to cephalosporins and penicillins. This is apparently a slowly acting enzyme system, and may be overcome by higher or more continuous drug levels especially when maintained by continuous infusions (cefotaxime) and by depot preparations (benzathine penicillin). Nevertheless, some penicillin and cephalosporin treatment failures do occur and have responded to sulbactam/ampicillin, imipenem, and vancomycin, which act through different cell wall mechanisms than the penicillins and the cephalosporins.

Vegetative endocarditis has been associated with Borrelia burgdorferi, but the vegetations may be too small to detect with echocardiography. Keep this in mind when evaluating patients with murmurs, as this may explain why some patients seem to continually relapse after even long courses of antibiotics.

COMBINATION THERAPY

Treatment of chronic Lyme usually requires combinations of antibiotics. There are four reasons for this:

1. TWO COMPARTMENTS- Bb can be found in both the fluid and the tissue compartments, yet no single antibiotic currently used to treat Bb infections will be effective in both compartments. This is one reason for the need to use combination therapy in the more ill patient. A logical combination might use, for example, azithromycin plus a penicillin.
2. INTRACELLULAR NICHE- Another reason, discussed below, is the fact that Bb can penetrate and remain viable within cells and evade the effects of extracellular agents. Typical combinations include an extracellular antibiotic, plus an intracellular agent such as an erythromycin derivative or metronidazole. Note that some experts discourage the co-administration of bactericidal plus bacteriostatic agents, thus the recommendation to avoid a cell wall drug combined with a tetracycline.
3. L-FORMS (SPHEROPLAST)- It has been recognized that B. burgdorferi can exist in at least two, and possibly three different morphologic forms: spirochete, spheroplast (or l-form), and the recently discovered cystic form (presently, there is controversy whether the cyst is different from the l-form). L-forms and cystic forms do not contain cell walls, and thus beta lactam antibiotics will not affect them. Spheroplasts seem to be susceptible to tetracyclines and the advanced erythromycin derivatives. Apparently, Bb can shift among the three forms during the course of the infection. Because of this, it may be necessary to cycle different classes of antibiotics and/or prescribe a combination of dissimilar agents.

4. CYSTIC FORM- When present in a hostile environment, such as growth medium lacking some nutrients, spinal fluid, or serum with certain antibiotics added, Bb can change from the spiral form ("spirochete") into a cyst form. This cyst seems to be able to remain dormant, but when placed into an environment more favorable to its growth, Bb can revert into the spirochete form. The antibiotics commonly used for Lyme do not kill the cystic form of Bb. However, there is laboratory evidence that metronidazole and tinidazole will disrupt it. Therefore, the chronically infected patient who has resistant disease may need to have metronidazole (or tinidazole) added to the regimen. More details are provided in the section on treatment options.

BORRELIA NEUROTOXIN (With thanks to Dr. Shoemaker)
Two groups have reported evidence that Borrelia, like several other bacteria, produce neurotoxins. These compounds reportedly can cause many of the symptoms of encephalopathy, cause an ongoing inflammatory reaction manifested as some of the virus-like symptoms common in late Lyme, and also potentially interfere with hormone action by blocking hormone receptors. At this time, there is no assay available to detect whether this compound is present, nor can the amount of toxin be quantified. Indirect measures are currently employed, such as measures of cytokine activation and hormone resistance. A visual contrast sensitivity test (VCS test) reportedly is quite useful in documenting CNS effects of the neurotoxin, and to follow effects of treatment. This test is available at some centers and on the internet.

It has been said that the longer one is ill with Lyme, the more neurotoxin is present in the body. It probably is stored in fatty tissues, and once present, persists for a very long time. This may be because of enterohepatic circulation, where the toxin is excreted via the bile into the intestinal tract, but then is reabsorbed from the intestinal tract back into the blood stream. This forms the basis for treatment.

Two prescription medications that can bind these toxins include cholestyramine resin and Welchol pills. When take orally in generous amounts, the neurotoxin present in the intestinal tract binds to the resin, is trapped, and then excreted. Thus, over several weeks, the level of neurotoxin is depleted and clinical improvement can be seen. Current experience is that improvement is first seen in three weeks, and treatment can continue for a month or more. Retreatment is always possible.

These medications may bind not only toxins but also many drugs and vitamin supplements. Therefore no other oral medications or supplements should be taken from a half hour before, to two hours after a dose of one of these fiber agents.

Cholestyramine should be taken two to four times daily, and Welchol is prescribed at three pills twice daily. While the latter is obviously much simpler to use, it is less effective than cholestyramine. The main side effects are bloating and constipation, best handled with increased fluid intake and gentle laxatives.

TREATING LYME BORRELIOSIS

LYME DISEASE TREATMENT INFORMATION
There is no universally effective antibiotic for treating LB. The choice of medication used and the dosage prescribed will vary for different people based on multiple factors. These include duration and severity of illness, presence of co-infections, immune deficiencies, prior significant immunosuppressant use while infected, age, weight, gastrointestinal function, blood levels achieved, and patient tolerance. Doses found to be effective clinically are often higher than those recommended in older texts. This is due to deep tissue penetration by Bb, its presence in the CNS including the eye, within cells, within tendons, and because very few of the many strains of this organism now known to exist have been studied for antibiotic susceptibility. In addition, all animal studies of susceptibility to date have only addressed early disease in models that behave differently than human hosts. Therefore, begin with a regimen appropriate to the setting, and if necessary, modify it over time based upon antibiotic blood level measurements and clinical response.

ANTIBIOTICS

There are four types of antibiotics in general use for Bb treatment. The TETRACYCLINES, including doxycycline and minocycline, are bacteriostatic unless given in high doses. If high blood levels are not attained, treatment failures in early and late disease are common. However, these high doses can be difficult to tolerate. For example, doxycycline can be very effective but only if adequate blood levels are achieved either by high oral doses (300 to 600 mg daily) or by parenteral administration. Kill kinetics indicate that a large spike in blood and tissue levels is more effective than sustained levels, which is why with doxycycline, oral doses of 200 mg bid is more effective than 100 mg qid. Likewise, this is why IV doses of 400 mg once a day is more effective than any oral regimen.

PENICILLINS are bactericidal. As would be expected in managing an infection with a gram negative organism such as Bb, amoxicillin has been shown to be more effective than oral penicillin V. With cell wall agents such as the penicillins, kill kinetics indicate that sustained bactericidal levels are needed for 72 hours to be effective. Thus the goal is to try to achieve sustained blood and tissue levels. However, since blood levels are extremely variable among patients, peak and trough levels should be measured (for details, refer to the antibiotic dosage table). Because of its short half-life and need for high levels, amoxicillin is usually administered along with probenecid. An extended release formulation of amoxicillin+clavulanate ("Augmentin XR") may also be considered if adequate trough levels are difficult to attain. An attractive alternative is benzathine penicillin ("Bicillin-LA"- see below). This is an intramuscular depot injection, and although doses are relatively small, the sustained blood and tissue levels are what make this preparation so effective.

CEPHALOSPORINS must be of advanced generation: first generation drugs are rarely effective and second generation drugs are comparable to amoxicillin and doxycycline both in-vitro and in-vivo. Third generation agents are currently the most effective of the cephalosporins because of their very low MBC's (0.06 for ceftriaxone), and relatively long half-life. Cephalosporins have been shown to be effective in penicillin and tetracycline failures. Cefuroxime axetil (Ceftin), a second generation agent, is also effective against staph and thus is useful in treating atypical erythema migrans that may represent a mixed infection that contains some of the more common skin pathogens in addition to Bb. Because this agent's G.I. side effects and high cost, it is not often used as first line drug. As with the penicillins, try to achieve high, sustained blood and tissue levels by frequent dosing and/or the use of probenecid. Measure peak and trough blood levels when possible.

When choosing a third generation cephalosporin, there are several points to remember: Ceftriaxone is administered twice daily (an advantage for home therapy), but has 95% biliary excretion and can crystallize in the biliary tree with resultant colic and possible cholecystitis. GI excretion results in a large impact on gut flora. Biliary and superinfection problems with ceftriaxone can be lessened if this drug is given in interrupted courses (known commonly as "pulse therapy"- refer to chapter on this on page 20), so the current recommendation is to administer it four days in a row each week. Cefotaxime, which must be given at least every eight hours or as a continuous infusion, is less convenient, but as it has only 5% biliary excretion, it never causes biliary concretions, and may have less impact on gut flora.

ERYTHROMYCIN has been shown to be almost ineffective as monotherapy. The azalide azithromycin is somewhat more effective but only minimally so when given orally. As an IV drug, much better results are seen. Clarithromycin is more effective as an oral agent than azithromycin, but can be difficult to tolerate due to its tendency to promote yeast overgrowth, bad aftertaste, and poor GI tolerance at the high doses needed. These problems are much less severe with the ketolide telithromycin, which is generally well tolerated.

Erythromycins (and the advanced generation derivatives mentioned above) have impressively low MBCs and they do concentrate in tissues and penetrate cells, so they theoretically should be ideal agents. So why is it that erythromycin ineffective, and why have initial clinical results with azithromycin (and to a lesser degree, clarithromycin) have been disappointing? It has been suggested that when Bb is within a cell, it is held within a vacuole and bathed in fluid of low pH, and this acidity may inactivate azithromycin and clarithromycin. Therefore, they are administered concurrently with hydroxychloroquine or amantadine, which raise vacuolar pH, rendering these antibiotics more effective. It is not known whether this same technique will make erythromycin a more effective antibiotic in LB. Another alternative is to administer azithromycin parenterally. Results are excellent, but expect to see abrupt Jarisch-Herxheimer reactions.

Telithromycin, on the other hand, is stable in the intracellular acid environment, which may be why this is currently by far the most effective drug of this class, and may replace the others in the majority of patients with LB. Likewise, there is no need to co-administer amantadine or hydroxychloroquine. This antibiotic has other advantages- it has been engineered to prevent drug resistance, has almost no negative impact on E. coli in the intestinal tract (hopefully minimizing the risk for diarrhea), and it can be taken with or without food.

However, there are disadvantages:

1. May interact with a wide variety of medications because it is an inhibitor of the cytochrome CYP3A4. It is vital that this be taken into account as many Lyme patients take a variety of medications concurrently, and often from several practitioners.
2. May lengthen the QT interval. This should be measured prior to prescribing this drug, and if borderline, rechecked after it is begun.
3. Can transiently cause blurry vision, delayed accommodation, and even double vision.
4. Liver enzymes may become elevated. Blood tests should be done regularly to monitor this.
5. The usual precautions of any antibiotic also still apply- risk for allergy, stomach upset, Herxheimer reactions, etc.

QTc INTERVAL

- QTc is the QT corrected for heart rate
- Measure the precordial lead that has the best T wave (usually V-2 or V-5)
- Measure from the start of the Q wave to the end of the T wave
- QT interval is inversely related to the heart rate (slow pulse results in a longer QT)
- $QTc = QT \div \sqrt{RR}$ interval
- Normals: Females <450 ms, Males < 470 ms
- Want K+ > 4.0, Mg++ > 2.0; avoid hypocalcemia

METRONIDAZOLE (Flagyl) When present in a hostile environment, such as growth medium lacking some nutrients, spinal fluid, or serum with certain antibiotics added, Bb can change into a cyst form. This cyst seems to be able to remain dormant, but when placed into an environment more favorable to its growth, the cyst can revert into the spirochete form. The conventional antibiotics used for Lyme, such as the penicillins, cephalosporins, etc do not kill the cystic form of Bb, yet there is laboratory evidence that metronidazole will kill it. Therefore, the trend now is to treat the chronically infected patient who has resistant disease by combining metronidazole with one or two other antibiotics to target all forms of Bb. Because there is laboratory evidence that tetracyclines may inhibit the effect of Flagyl, this class of medication should not be used in these two- and three-drug regimens. Some clinicians favor tinidazole as this may be equally effective but result in fewer side effects. However, this has yet to be documented.

Important precautions:

1. Pregnancy while on Flagyl is not advised, as there is a risk of birth defects.
2. No alcohol consumption! A severe, "Antabuse" reaction will occur, consisting of severe nausea, flushing, headache, and other symptoms.
3. Yeast overgrowth is especially common. A strict anti-yeast regimen must be followed.
4. Flagyl can be irritative to the nervous system- in the short term, it may cause irritability, "spacey" feelings, etc. Longer term, it can affect the peripheral nerves, causing tingles, numbness, etc. If mild, a change in dose may be required. Often, extra vitamin B can clear these symptoms. If the nerve symptoms persist or are strong, then metronidazole must be discontinued or these symptoms may become very long lasting.
5. Strong Herxheimer-like reactions are seen in almost everyone.

RIFAMPIN is a well-known antibiotic that has been in use for many decades. It is primarily used to treat tuberculosis, but also has been used in other conditions, such as prevention of meningitis in those exposed, for treating resistant Staph, etc. Potentially, rifampin may be effective in treating Bartonella, Ehrlichia, Mycoplasma, and Borrelia. There are as yet no formal clinical studies on the use of this medication in these illnesses, but many patients have been treated with rifampin and have had favorable results. When used, regular blood tests (CBC, liver enzymes) are usually performed to monitor for side effects. Rifampin can also discolor urine, tears and sweat (brownish-orange). It may also stain some types of water-permeable contact lenses. Taking rifampin during pregnancy is not advised. Finally, because this drug is an inducer of cytochromes (CYP3A4), co-administration with other medications may result in lower and more brief blood levels of the co-administered drug. Thus, be aware of these potential drug interactions.

BENZATHINE PENICILLIN Comparative studies published by Fallon et. al. at Columbia University have shown that parenteral therapy is superior to oral therapy in chronic patients. Options include intramuscular long acting penicillin G (benzathine penicillin, or "Bicillin-LA") or intravenous antibiotics.

For an antibiotic in the penicillin class to be effective, time-killing curves show that significant levels of antibiotic must be sustained for 72 hours. Bicillin LA is a sustained release formulation that meets these criteria.

Published studies in children and adults, combined with over a decade of experience with this therapy by front line, Lyme-treating physicians have established the efficacy, safety and usefulness of this medication. In many patients it is more effective than oral antibiotics for treating Lyme, and compares closely to intravenous therapy in terms of efficacy if the dose is high enough.

It is usually administered three or four times weekly for six to twelve months. It has the advantage of being relatively inexpensive, free of gastrointestinal side effects, unlikely to promote the overgrowth of yeast, and has an excellent safety record spanning many decades.

Finally, an added plus is that family members can be trained to administer this treatment at home.

CEFTRIAXONE TREATMENT A subset of patients who have severe, longstanding illness due to Borrelia burgdorferi carry persistent infection despite having previously received antibiotic treatments which have eliminated the disease in less ill individuals. The mechanism for such persistence has been the subject of many peer reviewed articles. They include persistence of B. burgdorferi in protective niches, inhibition and lysis of lymphocytes, survival in phagocytic vacuoles, antigenic shifts, slow growth, shifting into alternate forms, and dormancy and latency.

One successful approach in the more ill patient, published in the early 1990s, is to use higher doses of ceftriaxone in a pulsed-dose regimen. Since then, clinical experience has expanded upon this concept, and at the MLDA Lyme Congress in September, 2002, Cichon presented data on a pulsed, high dose regimen which supports and refines this concept. This regimen is now considered the current standard of care in the use of ceftriaxone.

Treatment with ceftriaxone is dosed at 4 grams daily- given either as 2 grams IV twice daily, or 4 grams slowly once a day, four days in a row each week, usually for 14 or more weeks. Such a regimen is not only more effective in the Chronic Lyme patient, but regular interruptions in treatment lessen the potential complications of intensive antibiotic therapy with ceftriaxone, such as biliary sludging and colitis. Hence a more effective, safer regimen that by virtue of the treatment breaks, is less costly and affords the patient a more acceptable lifestyle. IV access with a heparin lock becomes possible (and preferred).

COURSE DURING THERAPY

As the spirochete has a very long generation time (12 to 24 hours *in vitro* and possibly much longer in living systems) and may have periods of dormancy, during which time antibiotics will not kill the organism, treatment has to be continued for a long period of time to eradicate all the active symptoms and prevent a relapse, especially in late infections. If treatment is discontinued before all symptoms of active infection have cleared, the patient will remain ill and possibly relapse further. In general, early LB is treated for four to six weeks, and late LB usually requires a minimum of four to six months of continuous treatment. All patients respond differently and therapy must be individualized. It is not uncommon for a patient who has been ill for many years to require open ended treatment regimens; indeed, some patients will require ongoing maintenance therapy for years to remain well.

Several days after the onset of appropriate antibiotic therapy, symptoms often flare due to lysis of the spirochetes with release of increased amount of antigenic material and possibly bacterial toxins. This is referred to as a Jarisch Herxheimer-like reaction. Because it takes 48 to 72 hours of therapy to initiate bacterial killing, the Herxheimer reaction is therefore delayed. This is unlike syphilis, in which these reactions can occur within hours.

It has been observed that symptoms will flare in cycles every four weeks. It is thought that this reflects the organism's cell cycle, with the growth phase occurring once per month (intermittent growth is common in Borrelia species). As antibiotics will only kill bacteria during their growth phase, therapy is designed to bracket at least one whole generation cycle. This is why the minimum treatment duration should be at least four weeks. If the antibiotics are working, over time these flares will lessen in severity and duration. The very occurrence of ongoing monthly cycles indicates that living organisms are still present and that antibiotics should be continued.

With treatment, these monthly symptom flares are exaggerated and presumably represent recurrent Herxheimer-like reactions as Bb enters its vulnerable growth phase and then are lysed. For unknown reasons, the worst occurs at the fourth week of treatment. Observation suggest that the more severe this reaction, the higher the germ load, and the more ill the patient. In those with long-standing highly symptomatic disease who are on I.V. therapy, the week-four flare can be very severe, similar to a serum sickness reaction, and be associated with transient leucopenia and/or elevations in liver enzymes. If this happens, decrease the dose temporarily, or interrupt treatment for several days, then resume with a lower dose. If you are able to continue or resume therapy, then patients continue to improve. Those whose treatment is stopped and not restarted at this point usually will need retreatment in the future due to ongoing or recurrent symptoms because the infection was not eradicated. Patients on I.V. therapy who have a strong reaction at the fourth week will need to continue parenteral antibiotics for several months, for when this monthly reaction finally lessens in severity, then oral or IM medications can be substituted. Indeed, it is just this observation that guides the clinician in determining the endpoint of I.V. treatment. In general, I.V. therapy is given until there is a clear positive response, and then treatment is changed to IM or po until free of signs of active infection for 4 to 8 weeks. Some patients, however, will not respond to IM or po treatment and I.V. therapy will have to be used throughout. As mentioned earlier, leucopenia may be a sign of persistent Ehrlichiosis, so be sure to look into this.

Repeated treatment failures should alert the clinician to the possibility of an otherwise inapparent immune deficiency, and a workup for this may be advised. Obviously, evaluation for co-infection should be performed, and a search for other or concurrent diagnoses needs to be entertained.

There are three things that will predict treatment failure regardless of which regimen is chosen: Non-compliance, alcohol use, and sleep deprivation. Advise them to take a break when (or ideally before) the inevitable mid afternoon fatigue sets in (napping is encouraged).

All patients must keep a carefully detailed daily diary of their symptoms to help us document the presence of the classic four week cycle, judge the effects of treatment, and determine treatment endpoint. One must follow such diaries, temperature readings in late afternoon, physical findings, notes from physical therapists, and cognitive testing to best judge when to change or end antibiotics.

Remember- there currently is no test for cure, so this clinical follow-up assumes a major role in Lyme Disease care.

ANTIBIOTIC CHOICES AND DOSES

ORAL THERAPY: Always check blood levels when using agents marked with an *, and adjust dose to achieve a peak level above ten and a trough greater than three. Because of this, the doses listed below may have to be raised. Consider Doxycycline first in early Lyme due to concern for Ehrlichia co-infections.

*Amoxicillin- Adults: 1g q8h plus probenecid 500mg q8h; doses up to 6 grams daily are often needed
Pregnancy: 1g q6h and adjust.
Children: 50 mg/kg/day divided into q8h doses.
*Doxycycline- Adults: 200 mg bid with food; doses of up to 600 mg daily are often needed, as doxycycline is only effective at high blood levels. Not for children or in pregnancy.
If levels are too low at tolerated doses, give parenterally or change to another drug.
*Cefuroxime axetil- Oral alternative that may be effective in amoxicillin and doxycycline failures. Useful in EM rashes co-infected with common skin pathogens.
Adults and pregnancy: 1g q12h and adjust. Children: 125 to 500 mg q12h based on weight.
Tetracycline- Adults only, and not in pregnancy. 500 mg tid to qid
Erythromycin- Poor response and not recommended.
Azithromycin- Adults: 500 to 1200 mg/d. Adolescents: 250 to 500 mg/d
Add hydroxychloroquine, 200-400 mg/d, or amantadine 100-200 mg/d
Cannot be used in pregnancy or in younger children.
Overall, poor results when administered orally
Clarithromycin- Adults: 250 to 500 mg q6h plus hydroxychloroquine, 200-400 mg/d, or amantadine 100-200 mg/d. Cannot be used in pregnancy or in younger children.
Clinically more effective than azithromycin
Telithromycin- Adolescents and adults: 800 mg once daily
Do not need to use amantadine or hydroxychloroquine
So far, the most effective drug of this class, and possibly the best oral agent if tolerated. Expect strong and quite prolonged Herxheimer reactions.
Must watch for drug interactions (CYP3A-4 inhibitor), check the QTc interval, and monitor liver enzymes.
Not to be used in pregnancy.
*Augmentin- Standard Augmentin cannot exceed three tablets daily due to the clavulanate, thus is given with amoxicillin, so that the total dose of the amoxicillin component is as listed above for amoxicillin. This combination can be effective when Bb beta lactamase is felt to be significant.
*Augmentin XR 1000- This is a time-release formulation and thus is a better choice than standard Augmentin.
Dose- 1000 mg q 8 h, to 2000 mg q 12 h based on blood levels.
Chloramphenicol- Not recommended as not proven and potentially toxic.
Metronidazole: 500 to 1500 mg daily in divided doses. Non-pregnant adults only.

PARENTERAL THERAPY
Ceftriaxone- Risk of biliary sludging (therefore often Actigall is co-administered- one to three tablets daily).
Adults and pregnancy: 2g q12 h, 4 days in a row each week

Children: 75 mg/kg/day up to 2g/day

Cefotaxime- Comparable efficacy to ceftriaxone; no biliary complications.

Adults and pregnancy: 6g to 12g daily. Can be given q 8 h as divided doses, but a continuous infusion may be more efficacious. When exceeding 6 g daily, use pulsed-dose schedule

Children: 90 to 180 mg/kg/day dosed q6h (preferred) or q8h, not to exceed 12 g daily.

*Doxycycline- Requires central line as is caustic.

Surprisingly effective, probably because blood levels are higher when given parenterally and single large daily doses optimize kinetics of killing with this drug.

Always measure blood levels.

Adults: Start at 400 mg q24h and adjust based on levels.

Cannot be used in pregnancy or in younger children.

Azithromycin- Requires central line as is caustic.

Dose: 500 to 1000 mg daily in adolescents and adults.

Penicillin G- IV penicillin G is minimally effective and not recommended.

Benzathine penicillin- Surprisingly effective IM alternative to oral therapy. May need to begin at lower doses as strong, prolonged (6 or more week) Herxheimer-like reactions have been observed.

Adults: 1.2 million U- three to four doses weekly.

Adolescents: 1.2 to 3.6 million U weekly.

May be used in pregnancy.

Vancomycin- observed to be one of the best drugs in treating Lyme, but potential toxicity limits its use.

It is a perfect candidate for pulse therapy to minimize these concerns. Use standard doses and confirm levels.

Primaxin and Unisyn- similar in efficacy to cefotaxime, but often work when cephalosporins have failed.

Must be given q6 to q8 hours.

Cefuroxime- useful but not demonstrably better than ceftriaxone or cefotaxime.

*Ampicillin IV- more effective than penicillin G. Must be given q6 hours.

TREATMENT CATEGORIES

PROPHYLAXIS of high risk groups- education and preventive measures. Antibiotics are not given.

TICK BITES - Embedded Deer Tick With No Signs or Symptoms of Lyme (see appendix):

Decide to treat based on the type of tick, whether it came from an endemic area, how it was removed, and length of attachment (anecdotally, as little as four hours of attachment can transmit pathogens). The risk of transmission is greater if the tick is engorged, or of it was removed improperly allowing the tick's contents to spill into the bite wound. High-risk bites are treated as follows (remember the possibility of co-infection!):

1) Adults: Oral therapy for 28 days.
2) Pregnancy: Amoxicillin 1000 mg q6h for 6 weeks. Test for Babesia, Bartonella and Ehrlichia.
   Alternative: Cefuroxime axetil 1000 mg q12h for 6 weeks.
3) Young Children: Oral therapy for 28 days.

EARLY LOCALIZED - Single erythema migrans with no constitutional symptoms:

1) Adults: oral therapy- must continue until symptom and sign free for at least one month, with a 6 week minimum.
2) Pregnancy: 1st and 2nd trimesters: I.V. X 30 days then oral X 6 weeks
   3rd trimester: Oral therapy X 6+ weeks as above.
   Any trimester- test for Babesia and Ehrlichia
3) Children: oral therapy for 6+ weeks.

DISSEMINATED DISEASE - Multiple lesions, constitutional symptoms, lymphadenopathy, or any other manifestations of dissemination.

EARLY DISSEMINATED: Milder symptoms present for less than one year and not complicated by immune deficiency or prior steroid treatment:

1) Adults: oral therapy until no active disease for 4 to 8 weeks (4-6 months typical)
2) Pregnancy: As in localized disease, but treat throughout pregnancy.
3) Children: Oral therapy with duration based upon clinical response.

PARENTERAL ALTERNATIVES for more ill patients and those unresponsive to or intolerant of oral medications:

1) Adults and children: I.V. therapy until clearly improved, with a 6 week minimum. Follow with oral therapy or IM benzathine penicillin until no active disease for 6-8 weeks. I.V. may have to be resumed if oral or IM therapy fails.
2) Pregnancy: IV then oral therapy as above.

LATE DISSEMINATED: present greater than one year, more severely ill patients, and those with prior significant steroid therapy or any other cause of impaired immunity:

1) Adults and pregnancy: extended I.V. therapy (14 or more weeks), then oral or IM, if effective, to same endpoint. Combination therapy with at least two dissimilar antibiotics almost always needed.
2) Children: IV therapy for 6 or more weeks, then oral or IM follow up as above. Combination therapy usually needed.

CHRONIC LYME DISEASE (PERSISTENT/RECURRENT INFECTION)

By definition, this category consists of patients with active infection, of a more prolonged duration, who are more likely have higher spirochete loads, weaker defense mechanisms, possibly more virulent or resistant strains, and probably are significantly co-infected. Neurotoxins may also be significant in these patients. Search for and treat for all of these, and search for concurrent infections including viruses, chlamydias, and mycoplasmas. Be sure to do an endocrine workup if indicated. These patients require a full evaluation for all of these problems, and each abnormality must be addressed.

This group will most likely need parenteral therapy, especially high dose, pulsed therapy, and antibiotic combinations, including metronidazole. Antibiotic therapy will need to continue for many months, and the antibiotics may have to be changed periodically to break plateaus in recovery. Be vigilant for treatment-related problems such as antibiotic-associated colitis, yeast overgrowth, intravenous catheter complications, and abnormalities in blood counts and chemistries.

If treatment can be continued long term, then a remarkable degree of recovery is possible. However, attention must be paid to all treatment modalities for such a recovery- not only antibiotics, but rehab and exercise programs, nutritional supplements, enforced rest, low carbohydrate, high fiber diets, attention to food sensitivities, avoidance of stress, abstinence from caffeine and alcohol, and absolutely no immunosuppressants, even local doses of steroids (intra-articular injections, for example).

Unfortunately, not all patients with chronic Lyme disease will fully recover and treatment may not eradicate the active Borrelia infection. Such individuals may have to be maintained on open-ended, ongoing antibiotic therapy, for they repeatedly relapse after antibiotics are stopped. Maintenance antibiotic therapy in this select group is thus mandatory.

In patients who have chronic Lyme, who do not fully respond to antibiotics, one must search for an explanation. In many cases, these patients are found to have pituitary insufficiency of varying degrees. The abnormalities may be extremely subtle, and provocative testing must be done for full diagnosis. Persistent fatigue, limited stamina, hypotension, and loss of libido suggest this possibility.

Similarly, a small but significant number of these patients harbor toxic levels of heavy metals. Challenge testing by knowledgeable, experienced clinicians is necessary for evaluation. Treatment must be directed toward correcting the specific abnormalities found, and post-treatment retesting to assess efficacy of treatment and endpoint of therapy should be done. Suspect this when poor immune responsiveness and persistent neuropathic signs and symptoms are present.

INDICATORS FOR PARENTERAL THERAPY

(The following are guidelines only and are not meant to be absolute. It is based on retrospective study of over 600 patients with late Lyme disease.)

- Illness for greater than one year
- Prior immunosuppressive therapy while infected with Bb.
- Major neurological involvement
- Active synovitis with high sedimentation rate
- Elevated protein or cells in the CSF

ADVANCED TREATMENT OPTIONS

PULSE THERAPY consists of administering antibiotics (usually parenteral ones) two to four days in a row per week. This allows for several advantages:

* Dosages are doubled (ie: cefotaxime, 12 g daily), increasing efficacy
* More toxic medications can be used with increased safety (ie: vancomycin)
* May be effective when conventional, daily regimens have failed.
* IV access may be easier or more tolerable
* More agreeable lifestyle for the patient
* Often less costly than daily regimens

Note that this type of treatment is expected to continue for a minimum of ten weeks, and often must continue beyond twenty weeks. The efficacy of this regimen is based on the fact that it takes 48 to 72 hours of continuous bactericidal antibiotic levels to kill the spirochete, yet it will take longer than the four to five days between pulses for the spirochetes to recover. As with all Lyme treatments, specific dosing and scheduling must be tailored to the individual patient's clinical picture based upon the treating physician's best clinical judgment.

COMBINATION THERAPY (see page 12)

This consists of using two or more dissimilar antibiotics simultaneously for antibiotic synergism, to better compensate for differing killing profiles and sites of action of the individual medications, and to cover the three known forms of Bb. A typical combination is the use of a cell wall agent plus a protein inhibitor (ie: amoxicillin plus clarithromycin). Note that GI intolerance and yeast superinfections are the biggest drawbacks to this type of treatment. However, these complications can often be prevented or easily treated, and the clinically observed benefits of this type of regimen clearly have outweighed these problems in selected patients.

LYME DISEASE AND PREGNANCY

It is well known that B. burgdorferi can cross the placenta and infect the fetus. In addition, breast milk from infected mothers has been shown to harbor spirochetes that can be detected by PCR and grown in culture.

The Lyme Disease Foundation in Hartford, CT had kept a pregnancy registry for eleven years beginning in the late 1980s. They found that if patients were maintained on adequate doses of antibiotic therapy during gestation, then no babies were born with Lyme. My own experience over the last twenty years agrees with this.

The options for treating the mother include oral, intramuscular, and intravenous therapy as outlined above. It is vital that peak and trough antibiotic levels be measured if possible at the start of gestation and at least once more during treatment.

During pregnancy, symptoms generally are mild as the hormonal changes seem to mask many symptoms. However, post-partum, mothers have a rough time, with a sudden return of all their Lyme symptoms including profound fatigue. Post partum depression can be particularly severe. I always advise help in the home for at least the first month, so adequate rest and time for needed treatments are assured.

I also advise against breast feeding for obvious reasons as mentioned above.

MONITORING THERAPY

Drug levels are measured, where possible, to confirm adequate dosing. Often, the regimen may have to be modified to optimize the dose. This may have to be repeated again at any time major changes in the treatment regimen occur, and serially during pregnancy. With parenteral therapy, CBC and chem/liver panels are done at least twice each month, especially during symptom flares, with urinalysis and pro-time monitored less frequently.

SAFETY

Over two decades of experience in treating thousands of patients with Lyme has proven that therapy as described above, although intense, is generally well tolerated. The most common adverse reaction seen is allergy to probenecid. In addition, yeast superinfections are seen, but these are generally easily recognized and managed. The induction of Clostridium difficile toxin production is seen most commonly with ceftriaxone, but can occur with any of the antibiotic regimens mentioned in this document. However, pulsed dose therapy and regular use of the lactobacillus preparations seems to be helpful in controlling yeast and antibiotic related colitis, as the number of cases of C. difficile in Lyme patients is low when these guidelines are followed. Be sure to test stool for both toxin A and toxin B when evaluating for C. difficile colitis.

When using central intravenous lines including PICC lines (peripherally inserted central catheters), if ANY line problems arise, it is recommended that the line be pulled for patient safety. Salvage attempts (urokinase, repairing holes) are often ineffective and may not be safe.

Please advise all patients who take the tetracyclines of skin and eye sensitivity to sunlight and the proper precautions, and advise birth control if appropriate. When doxycycline is given parenterally, do not refreeze the solution prior to use!

Remember, years of experience with chronic antibiotic therapy in other conditions, including rheumatic fever, acne, gingivitis, recurrent otitis, recurrent cystitis, COPD, bronchiectasis, and others have not revealed any consistent dire consequences as a result of such medication use. Indeed, the very real consequences of untreated, chronic persistent infection by B. burgdorferi can be far worse than the potential consequences of this treatment.

CO-INFECTIONS IN LYME

PIROPLASMOSIS (Babesiosis)

GENERAL INFORMATION

It had been thought that Babesia microti is the only significant piroplasm affecting humans. Now it is believed that many of the over two dozen known species of piroplasms can be carried by ticks and potentially be transmitted to the human. Unfortunately, we have no widely available tests for these non-microti species. That is why, again, a clinical diagnosis is required.

Piroplasms are not bacteria, they are protozoans. Therefore, they will not be eradicated by any of the currently used Lyme treatment regimens. Therein lies the significance of co-infections- if a Lyme patient has been extensively treated yet is still ill, and especially if they are experiencing atypical symptoms, suspect a co-infection. From the literature:

- "Co-infection generally results in more intense acute illness, a greater array of symptoms, and a more prolonged convalescence than accompany either infection alone."
- "Spirochete DNA was evident more often and remained in the circulation longer in co-infected subjects than in those experiencing either infection alone."
- "Co-infection might also synergize spirochete-induced lesions in human joints, heart and nerves."
- "Babesia infections may impair human host defense mechanisms..."
- "The possibility of concomitant Babesia infection should be considered when moderate to severe Lyme Disease has been diagnosed."

Babesia infection is becoming more commonly recognized, especially in patients who already have Lyme Disease. It has been published that as many as 66% of Lyme patients show serologic evidence of co-infection with Babesia microti. It has also been reported that Babesia infections can range in severity from mild, subclinical infection, to fulminant, potentially life threatening illness. Subclinical infection is often missed because the symptoms are incorrectly ascribed to Lyme. Babesia infections, even mild ones, may recur even after treatment and cause severe illness. This phenomenon has been reported to occur at any time, including up to several years after the initial infection! Furthermore, such Babesia carriers pose a risk to the blood supply as this infection has been reported to be passed on by blood transfusion.

SYMPTOMS
Clues to the presence of Babesiosis include a more acute initial illness- patients often recall a high fever and chills at the onset of their Lyme. Over time, they can note night sweats, air hunger, an occasional cough, persistent migraine-like headache, a vague sense of imbalance without true vertigo, encephalopathy and fatigue. The fulminant presentations are seen in those who are immunosuppressed, especially if asplenic, and in advanced ages. They include high fevers, shaking chills and hemolysis, and can be fatal.

DIAGNOSTIC TESTS
Diagnostic tests are insensitive and problematic. There are at least thirteen, and possibly as many as two dozen Babesia forms found in ticks, yet we can currently only test for B. microti and WA-1 with our serologic and nuclear tests. Standard blood smears reportedly are reliable for only the first two weeks of infection, thus are not useful for diagnosing later infections and milder ones including carrier states where the germ load is too low to be detected. Therefore, multiple diagnostic test methods are available and each have their own benefits and limitations and often several tests must be done. Be prepared to treat based on clinical presentation, even with negative tests.

- SEROLOGY- Unlike Lyme, Babesia titers can reflect infection status. Thus, persistently positive titers or western blots suggest persistent infection.
- PCR- This is more sensitive than smears for B. microti, but will not detect other species.
- ENHANCED SMEAR- This utilizes buffy coat, prolonged scanning (up to three hours per sample!) and digital photography through custom-made microscopes. Although more sensitive than standard smears, infections can still be missed. The big advantage is that it will display multiple species, not just B. microti.
- FLUORESCENT IN-SITU HYBRIDIZATION ASSAY (FISH)- This technique is also a form of blood smear. It is said to be 100-fold more sensitive than standard smears for B. microti, because instead of utilizing standard, ink-based stains, it uses a fluorescent-linked RNA probe and ultraviolet light. The Babesia organisms are then much easier to spot when the slides are scanned. The disadvantage is that currently only B. microti is detected.

TREATMENT
Treating Babesia infections had always been difficult, because the therapy that had been recommended until 1998 consisted of a combination of clindamycin plus quinine. Published reports and clinical experience have shown this regimen to be unacceptable, as nearly half of patients so treated have had to abandon treatment due to serious side effects, many of which were disabling. Furthermore, even in patients who could tolerate these drugs, there was a failure rate approaching 50%.

Because of these dismal statistics, the current regimen of choice for Babesiosis is the combination of atovaquone (Mepron, Malarone), 750 mg bid, plus an erythromycin-type drug, such as azithromycin (Zithromax), clarithromycin (Biaxin), or telithromycin (Ketek) in standard doses. This combination was initially studied in animals, and then applied to Humans with good success. Fewer than 5% of patients have to halt treatment due to side effects, and the success rate is clearly better than that of clindamycin plus quinine.

The duration of treatment with atovaquone combinations for Babesiosis varies depending on the degree of infection, duration of illness before diagnosis, the health and immune status of the patient, and whether the patient is co-infected with Borrelia burgdorferi. Typically, a three-week course is prescribed for acute cases, while chronic, longstanding infections with significant morbidity and co-infection will require a minimum of four months of therapy. Relapses have occurred, and retreatment is occasionally needed.

Problems during therapy include diarrhea, mild nausea, the expense of atovaquone (over $600.00 per bottle-enough for three weeks of treatment), and rarely, a temporary yellowish discoloration of the vision. Blood counts, liver panels and amylase levels are recommended every three weeks during any prolonged course of therapy as liver enzymes may elevate. Treatment failures usually are related to inadequate atovaquone levels. Therefore, patients who are not cured with this regimen can be retreated with higher doses (and atovaquone blood levels can be checked), as this has proven effective in many of my patients. Artemesia (a non-prescription herb) should be added in all cases. Metronidazole or Bactrim can also be added to increase efficacy, but there is minimal clinical data on how much more effective this will be.

BARTONELLA-LIKE ORGANISMS

It has been said that Bartonella is the most common of all tick-borne pathogens. Indeed, there seems to be a fairly distinct clinical syndrome when this type of organism is present in the chronic Lyme patient. However, several aspects of this infection seem to indicate that this tick-associated strain of Bartonella is different from that described as "cat scratch disease". For example, in patients who fit the clinical picture, standard Bartonella blood testing is commonly non-reactive. Furthermore, the usual Bartonella medications do not work for this- they suppress the symptoms but do not permanently clear them. For these reasons I like to refer to this as a "Bartonella-like organism" (BLO), rather than assume it is a more common species.

Indicators of BLO infection include CNS symptoms out of proportion to the other systemic symptoms of chronic Lyme. There seems to be an increased irritability to the CNS, with agitation, anxiety, insomnia, and even seizures, in addition to other unusually strong symptoms of encephalitis, such as cognitive deficits and confusion. Other key symptoms may include gastritis, lower abdominal pain (mesenteric adenitis), sore soles, especially in the AM, tender subcutaneous nodules along the extremities, and red rashes. These rashes may have the appearance of red streaks like stretch marks that do not follow skin planes, spider veins, or red papular eruptions. Lymph nodes may be enlarged and the throat can be sore.

Because standard Bartonella testing, either by serology or PCR, may not pick up this BLO, the blood test is very insensitive. Therefore, the diagnosis is a clinical one, based on the above points. Also, suspect infection with BLO in extensively treated Lyme patients who still are encephalitic, and who never had been treated with a significant course of specific treatment.

The drug of choice to treat BLO is levofloxacin. Levofloxacin is usually never used for Lyme or Babesia, so many patients who have tick-borne diseases, and who have been treated for them but remain ill, may in fact be infected with BLO. Treatment consist of 500 mg daily (may be adjusted based on body weight) for at least one month. Treat for three months or longer in the more ill patient. It has been suggested that levofloxacin may be more effective in treating this infection if a proton pump inhibitor is added in standard doses.

Another subtlety is that certain antibiotic combinations seem to inhibit the action of levofloxacin, while others seem to be neutral. I advise against using an erythromycin-like drug, as clinically such patients do poorly. On the other hand, combinations with cephalosporins, penicillins and tetracyclines are okay. Alternatives to levofloxacin include rifampin, gentamicin and possibly streptomycin. A very recent article suggests that prior use of quinine-like drugs including atovaquone (Mepron, Malarone) may render Levaquin less effective. Therefore, in a co-infected patient, treat the BLO before you address Babesia species.

Levofloxacin is generally well tolerated, with almost no stomach upset. Very rarely, it can cause confusion- this is temporary (clears in a few days) and may be relieved by lowering the dose. There is, however, one side effect that would require it to be stopped- it may cause a painful tendonitis, usually of the largest tendons. If this happens, then the levofloxacin must be stopped or tendon rupture may occur. It has been suggested that loading the patient with magnesium may prevent this problem, and if the tendons do become affected, parenteral high dose vitamin C (plus parenteral magnesium) may afford rapid relief.

Unfortunately, levofloxacin and drugs in this family cannot be given to those under the age of 18, so other alternatives, such as azithromycin, are used in children.

Incidentally, animal studies show that Bartonella may be transmitted across the placenta. No human studies have been done.

EHRLICHIA (AND ANAPLASMA)

GENERAL INFORMATION

While it is true that this illness can have a fulminant presentation, and may even become fatal if not treated, milder forms do exist, as does chronic low-grade infection, especially when other tick-borne organisms are present. The potential transmission of Ehrlichia during tick bites is the main reason why doxycycline is now the first choice in treating tick bites and early Lyme, before serologies can become positive. When present alone or co-infecting with B. burgdorferi, persistent leukopenia is an important clue. Thrombocytopenia and elevated liver enzymes, common in acute infection, are less often seen in those who are chronically infected, but likewise should not be ignored. Headaches, myalgias, and ongoing fatigue suggest this illness, but are extremely difficult to separate from symptoms caused by Bb.

DIAGNOSTIC TESTING

Testing is problematic with Ehrlichia, similar to the situation with Babesiosis. More species are known to be present in ticks than can be tested for with clinically available serologies and PCRs. In addition, serologies and PCRs are of unknown sensitivity and specificity. Standard blood smears for direct visualization of organisms in leukocytes are of low yield. Enhanced smears using buffy coats significantly raise sensitivity and can detect a wider variety of species. Despite this, infection can be missed, so clinical diagnosis remains the primary diagnostic tool. Again, consider this diagnosis in a Lyme Borreliosis (LB) patient not responding well to Lyme therapy who has symptoms suggestive of Ehrlichia.

TREATMENT

Standard treatment consists of Doxycycline, 200 mg daily for two to four weeks. Higher doses, parenteral therapy, and longer treatment durations may be needed based on the duration and severity of illness, and whether immune defects or extreme age is present. However, there are reports of treatment failure even when higher doses and long duration treatment with doxycycline is given. In such cases, consideration may be given for adding rifampin, 600 mg daily, to the regimen.

SORTING OUT THE CO-INFECTIONS

In addition to *Borrelia burgdorferi* (Bb), ticks may carry and transmit other infections. Furthermore, patients with disseminated Lyme complicated by these co-infections are usually immunocompromized and may also manifest signs and symptoms of reactivated latent infections and opportunists. All can add to morbidity and may need to be treated.

Because of the large number of these other infections, the cost of reliably testing for all of them as a matter of routine is prohibitive. Also, as in the case with Bb infection, laboratory tests for them are often insensitive. Thus there is a need to sort it all out clinically to provide guidance in testing and treatment. Here are some clues:

CLASSIC LYME (Bb infection)-

- Gradual onset of initial (viral-like) symptoms- this often makes it difficult to pinpoint when the infection began.
- Multisystem- almost always, in disseminated stages, involves more than one part or system (i.e. joint pain plus cognitive dysfunction).
- Migratory- first a knee will hurt, then over time this may lessen and the elbow or shoulder acts up, and later the joints calm down but headaches worsen.
- Stiff joints and loud joint crepitus, especially the neck ("Lyme shrug").
- Headaches are often nuchal and associated with stiff, painful and crepitant neck.
- Afternoon fevers, often unnoticed- most Lyme patients have subnormal temperatures in the AM but rise to 99+ by early to mid-afternoon. No obvious sweats.
- Tiredness and limited stamina- often is a strong need to rest or even nap in the afternoon, especially when the flushed face and elevated temperature appears.
- 4-week cycles- Bb activity, and thus symptoms, wax and wane in a cycle that repeats roughly every four weeks. This cycle, if clear, can guide your treatments.
- Slow response to treatment, with an initial symptom flare in most ("Herxheimer-like reaction") then improvement over weeks, punctuated by the monthly symptom flares. Likewise, if treatment is ended too soon, an initial period of well-being will gradually, over a few weeks, be replaced by a return of symptoms.
- EM rash in 25% to 50%

BARTONELLA & "BARTONELLA-LIKE ORGANISMS"-

- Gradual onset of initial illness.
- CNS symptoms are out of proportion to the musculoskeletal ones- if a patient has no or minimal joint complaints but is severely encephalopathic (see below), then think of Bartonella/BLO.
- Obvious signs of CNS irritability can include muscle twitches, tremors, insomnia, seizures, agitation, anxiety, severe mood swings, outbursts and antisocial behavior.
- GI involvement may present as gastritis or abdominal pain (mesenteric adenitis).
- Sore soles, especially in the morning.
- Tender sub-cutaneous nodules along the extremities, especially outer thigh, shins, and occasionally along the triceps.
- Occasional lymphadenopathy.
- Morning fevers, usually around 99. Occasionally light sweats are noted.
- Elevated vascular endothelial growth factor (VEGF) occurs in a minority, but the degree of elevation correlates with activity of the infection and may be used to monitor treatment.
- Rapid response to treatment changes- often symptoms improve within days after antibiotics are begun, but relapses occur also within days if medication is withdrawn early.
- May have papular or linear red rashes (like stretch marks that do not always follow skin planes), especially in those with GI involvement.

BABESIA SPECIES-

- Rapid onset of initial illness, often with sudden onset of high fever, severe headaches, sweats and fatigue, thus it is easy to know when infection began.
- Obvious sweats, usually at night, but can be day sweats as well.
- Air hunger, need to sigh and take a deep breath; dry cough without apparent reason.
- Headaches can be severe - dull, global (involves the whole head, described like the head is in a vise).
- Fatigue is prominent, does not clear with rest, and is made worse with exercise.
- Mental dullness and slowing of reactions and responses.
- Dizziness- more like a tippy feeling, and not vertigo or purely orthostasis.
- Symptoms cycle rapidly, with flares every four to six days.
- Hypercoaguable states are often associated with *Babesia* infections.
- Rarely, splenomegaly

- Very severe Lyme Disease can be a clue to *Babesia* infection, as it will make Lyme symptoms worse and Lyme treatments less effective.

EHRLICHIA/ANAPLASMA-

- Rapid onset of initial illness with fever, headache, prostration.
- Headaches are sharp, knife-like, and often behind the eyes.
- Muscle pain, not joint pain, and can be mild or severe.
- Low WBC count, elevated liver enzymes, and (rarely) inclusions seen in the WBCs.
- Rarely see diffuse vasculitic rash, including palms and soles (less than 10%).
- Rapid response to treatment.

DNA VIRUSES (HHV-6, EBV, CMV)

- Persistent fatigue, made worse with exercise.
- Sore throat, lymphadenopathy, and other viral-like complaints.
- May see elevated liver enzymes and low WBC counts.
- Autonomic dysfunction.

SUPPORTIVE THERAPY

CERTAIN **ABSOLUTE RULES** MUST BE FOLLOWED IF LYME SYMPTOMS ARE TO BE PERMANENTLY CLEARED:

1. Not allowed to get behind in sleep, or become overtired.
2. No caffeine or other stimulants that may affect depth or duration of sleep, or reduce or eliminate naps.
3. Absolutely no alcohol!
4. No smoking at all.
5. Aggressive exercises are required and should be initiated as soon as possible.
6. Diet must contain generous quantities of high quality protein and be high in fiber and low in fat and carbohydrates- no simple carbohydrates are allowed. Instead, use those with low glycemic index.
7. Certain key nutritional supplements should be added.
8. COMPLIANCE!

NUTRITIONAL SUPPLEMENTS IN DISSEMINATED LYME DISEASE

BACKGROUND INFORMATION

Studies on patients with chronic illnesses such as Lyme and Chronic Fatigue have demonstrated that some of the late symptoms are related to cellular damage and deficiencies in certain essential nutrients. Double blinded, placebo controlled studies, and in one case direct assay of biopsy specimens have proven the value of some of the supplements listed. Some are required, while others are optional -see below. They are listed in order of importance.

I suggest patients use a pill organizer. These are multi-compartment boxes that you pre-fill with your pills once a week. This makes the task of taking a large number of tablets much, much simpler and can markedly minimize missed doses. The Vitamin Shop sells a variety of good organizers.

I have found that the quality of supplements used is often more important than the dose. In fact, I do not recommend "mega doses". Instead, seek out, if possible, pharmaceutical grade products, especially if USP certified. I recommend, among others, Pharmanex, Researched Nutritionals and Nature Made products because they fit these criteria. In the list below, it is indicated whether the products should be gotten from Pharmanex, Researched Nutritionals, a different specific manufacturer, or even if a generic substitute is OK.

To order products from Pharmanex, users need to register as a customer with a referral from another registered customer. You may use my referral number (US9256681) to get started. Call 1-800-487-1000.
To order products from Researched Nutritionals, patients will need a physician's referral. If you do not have your own account, you may use my name when ordering. Call 1-800-755-3402.
Nature Made products are widely available in vitamin stores and pharmacies.

BASIC DAILY REGIMEN (in order of importance)

1. PROBIOTICS (required when on antibiotics)
Kefir: This is a yogurt-like drink that is said to more permanently replenish beneficial flora. It is only necessary to drink 2 to 4 ounces a day.
Acidophilus: the best kinds are frozen or refrigerated to ensure potency. Usual dose is two with each meal. Plan to mix together several different brands to broaden the spectrum. Acidophilus can be gotten from most vitamin stores but some generic brands are of unknown freshness and potency. An alternative that does not need refrigeration and can be taken only once a day is a high potency, patented product called "**Pro Bio**" from Pharmanex. The ultimate mix of pre- and probiotics with soil based organisms is a product called "**Prescript-Assist Pro**" from Researched Nutritionals. This too does not need refrigeration.
In addition, have 4 ounces of sugar-free **yogurt** on occasion.

2. MULTI-VITAMIN (required)
I recommend the **Life Pack** family of multivitamins available through Pharmanex. These are unique supplements- pharmaceutical grade and USP certified, they are the only products clinically proven in double blinded, placebo controlled crossover studies to quench free radicals and raise antioxidant levels in the blood and lipids. Choose LifePak for males under 40, LifePak Women for hormonally active women, LifePak Prenatal when pregnant, and LifePak Prime for postmenopausal women and for men over 40. LifePak Teen is also available. Continue long term.

3. CO-Q10- ***required, but do not use while taking the prescription drug atovaquone (Mepron, Malarone).***
Deficiencies have been related to poor function of the heart, limitations of stamina, gum disease, and poor resistance to infections. Heart biopsy studies in Lyme patients indicated that they should take between 300 and 400mg daily. I recommend the Co Q-10 from Researched Nutritionals. One caplet contains 400 mg, so the dose is one a day with food.

4. ALPHA LIPOIC ACID (required)
This facilitates entry of CoQ-10 into mitochondria. Dose is 300 mg twice daily. Generic is OK.

5. VITAMIN B (required).
Clinical studies demonstrated the need for supplemental vitamin B in infections with Borrelia, to help clear neurological symptoms. Take one 50 mg B-complex capsule daily. If neuropathy is severe, an additional 50 mg of B-6 can be added. Generics are OK.

6. MAGNESIUM (required)
Magnesium supplementation is very helpful for the tremors, twitches, cramps, muscle soreness, heart skips and weakness. It may also help in energy level and cognition. The best source is magnesium L-lactate dehydrate ("**Mag-tab SR**", sold by Niche Pharmaceuticals: 1-800-677-0355, and available at Wal-Mart). DO NOT rely on "cal-mag", calcium plus magnesium combination tablets, as they are not well absorbed. Take at least one tablet twice daily. Higher doses increase the benefit and should be tried, but may cause diarrhea. In some cases, intramuscular or intravenous doses may be necessary.

7. ESSENTIAL FATTY ACIDS: (required)
Studies show that when EFAs are taken regularly, statistically significant improvements in fatigue, aches weakness, vertigo, dizziness, memory, concentration and depression are likely. There are two broad classes: GLA (omega-6 oils) and EPA (omega-3 oils), derived respectively from plant and fish oils. This is what to take:

Plant Oil: Use a refrigerated liquid product of mixed omega oils obtained from the local health food store (always avoid capsules as the plant oils within may be rancid and you would never know). Take one to two tablespoons of the liquid oil daily. May be mixed with food, put on salads, etc.
Fish Oil: Use "**Marine Omega**" by Pharmanex. Use four daily, taken on a full stomach (this brand is required because it is made not from fish, but from Krill and is certified to be free of any measurable amounts of heavy metals and organic toxins).

8. NT-FACTOR

This product addresses the mitochondrial damage thought to underlie the metabolic dysfunction associated with chronic diseases which, in patients with tick-borne illnesses, is manifest by fatigue and neurologic dysfunction. *It is the single most reliable agent I have found that can give noticeably increased energy levels.* When supplements known to support neurological function are added (see below), improved cognition and memory often result. Effects will be noted in two to three weeks. It also contains high quality prebiotics and probiotics. Available from Researched Nutritionals.

OPTIONAL SUPPLEMENTS FOR SPECIAL CIRCUMSTANCES

FOR NEUROLOGIC SYMPTOMS- here, the goal is three-fold- supply the metabolic needs, replenish what has become depleted, and protect the neurons and their supportive cells. The "required" supplements, above, must be taken, and the items that follow below are considered "add-ons".

ACETYL-L-CARNITINE- this is taken along with **SAM-e**. This combination can result in noticeable gains in short term memory, mood and cognition. The Acetyl Carnitine also is said to help heart and muscle function. Doses: Acetyl-L-carnitine- 1500-2000 mg daily on empty stomach; SAM-e- 400 mg daily with the acetyl carnitine. Positive results may appear as early as 3 weeks; use for 2 to 3 months, but repeat or extend this course if needed. Available in most vitamin stores; Generic acetyl carnitine is okay, but I recommend "Nature Made" brand SAM-e (also available at most vitamin stores).

METHYLCOBALAMIN (Methyl B12)

Methylcobalamin is a prescription drug derived from vitamin B12. This can help to heal problems with the central and peripheral nervous system, improve depressed immune function, and help to restore more normal sleeping patterns. Many patients note improved energy as well. Because the oral form is not absorbed when swallowed or dissolved under the tongue, Methyl B12 must be taken by injection. Dose is generally 25 mg. (1 c.c.) daily for 3 to 6 months. Long term studies have never demonstrated any side effects from this drug. However, *the urine is expected to turn red shortly after each dose*- if the urine is not red, a higher dose may be needed or the present supply may have lost potency. The injectable form of this is not available in regular drug stores. It must be manufactured (compounded) by specialty pharmacies on order.

GREEN TEA

Green, but not black or white tea contains some of the most potent antioxidants around (80-100 times more effective than vitamin C). I strongly recommend this to any patient with degenerative changes to the central nervous system. At least four cups daily are needed to reap this benefit, and the tea must be decaffeinated. A nice alternative is "**TeGreen**" capsules by Pharmanex. They contain 97% pure tea polyphenols and each capsule is the equivalent of four cups of decaffeinated green tea. Take one to three daily.

CORDYMAX

Cordyceps is a well-known herb from Tibet that has been shown in clinical studies to improve stamina, fatigue, and enhance lung and antioxidant function. It also raises superoxide dismutase levels, important to prevent lesions in the central nervous system, which is why *this (along with green tea) is essential if neurodegeneration is part of your illness.* The positive effects can be dramatic; should be used long term. USP- certified cordyceps is available from Pharmanex as "**CordyMax**".

CITICHOLINE
Many studies have shown benefits to cognition, *especially memory*. Benefits are slow to notice, so plan to use this long-term. Dose is 500 to 1000 mg twice a day.

FOR IMMUNE SUPPORT
"REISHI MAX "
This enhanced extract from cracked spores of the Reishi mushroom has been shown in clinical studies to augment function of the Natural Killer Cells as well as macrophages. Recommended in all patients who have a CD-57 count below 60. Take four a day. Available only from Pharmanex.

TRANSFER FACTORS are the body's natural signals meant to activate the pathogen-killing effects of the cellular immune system. Therapy with these agents consists of taking both a general stimulator, plus specific transfer factors for the infection you have. Personal experience made me a believer in transfer factor therapy. For Lyme patients, use **Transfer Factor Multi-Immune** as the general stimulant, and **Transfer Factor Lyme-Plus** as the specific agent. Both are exclusives from Researched Nutritionals, and I have found them to be surprisingly effective in making the very ill respond better to treatment. Take as directed on the label.

FOR JOINT SYMPTOMS
GLUCOSAMINE
Glucosamine can be of long term benefit to the joints. Do not be misled into buying a product that also contains chondroitin, as this chemical does not add anything, but it can make the product more expensive. Look for a product that contains the herb Boswellia serrata- this is a non-irritative anti-inflammatory. Although many generics exist, the Pharmanex product, "**Cartilage Formula**" has the right ingredients and is of proven efficacy. Expect improvement only over time (several weeks), but plan to use this indefinitely to maintain joint health.

VITAMIN C
Vitamin C is important to aid in maintaining healthy connective tissues. High doses are recommended- 1000 to 6000 mg a day as tolerated (if the dose is too high for you it may cause acid stomach, gas and loose stools, so therefore dose titration is necessary). Consider using **"Ester-C"** (non-acid and longer acting), or **"C-Salts"** (very well tolerated). Start with a low dose and increase slowly to find your tolerance level.

FLEX CREAM
This is an amazing liniment-like product that really works and has a money back guarantee. Use for any type of body pain- spread on a thick layer and do not rub in. It takes 30 to 60 minutes to work, then lasts many hours. A Pharmanex exclusive.

OTHER OPTIONAL SUPPLEMENTS
VITAMIN D
Surprisingly, most people in America are vitamin D deficient. In the Lyme patient, low vitamin D levels can cause diffuse body aches and cramps that are not responsive to magnesium or calcium supplements. Some also believe that vitamin D is essential for normal immune and hormone function. I strongly urge you to have a fasting blood level drawn. It is recommended that the blood levels be in the upper half or the normal range. If it is not, then 2000 to 4000 units daily are needed for several weeks to make up for the deficit, and then a lower maintenance dose may be necessary, based on results from repeated blood level monitoring. If vitamin D is needed, improvements take 2 to 3 weeks to note, but are well worth the wait.

CREATINE
Creatine has been shown to be of benefit in neuromuscular degenerative diseases such as Lou Gherig's Disease (ALS) and can be very helpful in supporting low blood pressure, as in NMH. It may also benefit strength, stamina, and heart function. Important: To use this safely, you must have an adequate fluid intake.

The creatine product should contain taurine, an amino acid needed to enhance creatine absorption, plus some carbohydrate to aid creatine entry into muscle. You will need a 20 gram daily loading dose for the first five days, then 4 to 10 grams daily maintenance. Try "**Cell Tech**" from the Vitamin Shop, and follow label directions.

MILK THISTLE
Useful to support liver function. Take 175 mg daily- use an 80% Silymarin extract. Available from many vitamin stores.

LYME DISEASE REHABILITATION

Despite antibiotic treatments, patients will NOT return to normal unless they exercise, so therefore an aggressive rehab program is absolutely necessary. It is a fact that a properly executed exercise program can actually go beyond the antibiotics in helping to clear the symptoms and to maintain a remission.

Although the scientific basis for the benefits of exercises is not known, there are several reasonable theories. It is known that Bb will die if exposed to all but the tiniest oxygen concentrations. If an aggressive exercise program can increase tissue perfusion and oxygen levels, then this may play a role in what is being seen. Also, during aggressive exercise, the core body temperature can rise above 102 degrees; it is known that B. burgdorferi is very heat sensitive. Perhaps it is the added tissue oxygenation, or higher body temperature, or the combination that weakens the Lyme Borrelia, and allows the antibiotics and our defenses to be more effective. Regular exercise-related movements can help mobilize lymph and enhance circulation. In addition, there is now evidence that a carefully structured exercise program may benefit T-cell function: this function will depress for 12 to 24+ hours after exercise, but then rebound. This T-cell depression is more pronounced after aerobics which is why aerobics are not allowed. The goal is to exercise intermittently, with exercise days separated by days of total rest, including an effort to have plenty of quality sleep. The trick is to time the exercise days to take advantage of these rebounds. For an example, begin with an exercise day followed by 3 to 5 rest days; as stamina improves, then fewer rest days will be needed in between workouts. However, because T-cell functions do fall for at least one day after aggressive exercises, be sure to never exercise two days in a row. Finally, an in intermittent exercise program, properly executed, may help to reset the HPA axis more towards normal. On the following page is an exercise prescription that details these recommendations.

This program may begin with classical physical therapy if necessary. The physical therapy should involve massage, heat, ultrasound and simple range of motion exercises to relieve discomfort and promote better sleep and flexibility. Ice (vasoconstriction) and electrical stimulation (muscle spasm and trauma) should not be used!

The program must evolve into a graded, ultimately strenuous exercise program that consists of a specific regimen of *non-aerobic* conditioning- see below. Have the patient complete a gentle hour of prescribed exercise, then go home, have a hot bath or shower, than try to take a nap. Initially, patients will need this sleep, but as they recover, the exercise will energize them and then a nap will no longer be needed.
NOTE: a cardiac stress test may be necessary prior to exercising to ensure safety.

LYME REHAB-PHYSICAL THERAPY PRESCRIPTION

NAME____

D.O.B.______________________ DATE____________________

Please enroll this patient in a program of therapy to rehabilitate him/her from the effects of chronic tick-borne diseases. If necessary, begin with classic physical therapy, then progress when appropriate to a **whole body conditioning program.**

THERAPEUTIC GOALS (to be achieved in order as the patient's ability allows):

PHYSICAL THERAPY (if needed):

1. **The role of physical therapy here is to prepare the patient for the required, preferably gym-based exercise program outlined below. Plan on several weeks of classic PT then transition to the gym.**
2. Relieve pain and muscle spasms utilizing multiple modalities as available and as indicated: massage, heat, ultrasound, and passive and active range of motion. DO NOT use ice or electrical stim unless specifically ordered by our office. Paraffin baths can be quite useful.
3. Increase mobility, tone and strength while protecting damaged and weakened joints, tendons, and ligaments, and teach these techniques to the patient. Use minimal resistance but a lot of repetitions in any exercises prescribed. At the start of the exercise program, especially if the patient is weak, avoid free weights, bands and large exercise balls, and favor machines (especially hydraulics) that can guide limbs through a prescribed arc; free weights, etc. can risk hyperextension and uncontrolled movements that may cause or add to injuries. Transition the patient slowly to the gym-based program outlined below. **Note-aerobics are not permitted.**
4. Please see the patient two or three days per week- but do not schedule two days in a row!

EXERCISE Begin with a private trainer for careful direction and education.

PATIENT EDUCATION AND MANAGEMENT (to be done during the initial one-on-one sessions and reinforced at all visits thereafter):

1. Instruct patients on **correct exercise technique**, including proper warm-up, breathing, joint protection, proper body positioning during the exercise, and how to cool-down and stretch afterwards.
2. Please work one muscle group at a time and perform extensive and extended **stretching** to each muscle group immediately after each one is exercised, before moving on to the next muscle group.
3. A careful **interview** should be performed at the start of each session to make apparent the effects, both good and bad, from the prior visit's therapy, and adjust therapy accordingly.

PROGRAM:

1. **Aerobic exercises are NOT allowed**, not even low impact variety, until the patient has recovered.
2. **Conditioning**: work to improve strength and reverse the poor conditioning that results from Lyme, through a whole-body exercise program, consisting of light calisthenics and/or resistance training, using light resistance and many repetitions. This can be accomplished in exercise classes called "stretch and tone", or "body sculpture", or can be achieved in the gym with exercise machines or carefully with free weights (see cautions above).
3. **Each session should last one hour**. A gentle hour is preferable to a strenuous half-hour. If the patient is unable to continue for the whole hour, then decrease the intensity to allow him/her to do so.
4. **Exercise no more often than every other day**. The patient may need to start by exercising every 4th or 5th day initially, and as abilities improve, work out more often, but NEVER two days in a row. The non-exercise days should be spent resting.
5. This whole-body conditioning program is what is required to achieve wellness. A simple walking program will not work, and simply placing the patient on a treadmill or an exercise bike is not acceptable (except very briefly, as part of a warm-up), as aerobics can be damaging and must be avoided.

PHYSICIAN'S SIGNATURE____

MANAGING YEAST OVERGROWTH

Many patients with weakened defenses, such as from chronic illnesses, including Lyme Disease, develop an overgrowth of yeast. This begins in the mouth and then spreads to the intestinal tract. Therefore the primary line of defense is careful oral hygiene, replenishing the beneficial bacteria by daily intake of yogurt, Kefir, and/or acidophilus, and by following a strict low carbohydrate diet.

ORAL HYGEINE:

CLEANSING

Brush the teeth, tongue, gums, inner cheeks and palate first with toothpaste, then again for 30 seconds while holding an antiseptic mouthwash in the mouth Then, rinse by scrubbing while holding plain water in the mouth.

TOOTHPASTE

Use "AP-24" toothpaste, sold by NuSkin Enterprises. Unlike conventional toothpastes that may contain alcohols, formaldehydes and abrasives, this product cleans in a unique way. It contains two "surfactants" (detergent-like cleansers) that are very effective without being harsh. This product is available in two forms- regular and whitening (both contain fluoride). Choose either one.

In addition, get from them their patented toothbrush that is designed to work with this toothpaste. It cleans better and is far gentler than regular or electric toothbrushes.

Order AP-24 products by calling 1-800-487-1000. The U.S. reference # is 9256681-R

MOUTHWASHES

Use an antiseptic mouthwash (Scope, Listerine, etc.), and brush the teeth, tongue, gums, cheeks and the roof of the mouth while holding the mouthwash in the mouth. Do this for 30 seconds, then rinse repeatedly with water.

For especially thick or resistant thrush, the most effective (and drastic) treatment, employed as a last resort, consists of using "Dakin's Solution" as a mouth rinse. Make this by mixing one teaspoon of household liquid bleach (Clorox) in four ounces of water. A small amount is held in the mouth while brushing, then spit out, and repeated until the thrush has cleared. This is usually a one-time treatment, but may have to be repeated every few weeks.

After using an antiseptic, it is necessary to immediately eat yogurt or chew an acidophilus capsule to replenish the beneficial flora in the mouth. Because the germ count, both harmful and beneficial, will be artificially reduced after such a cleaning, and because yeasts are opportunists, the yeast infection can come back. By having the yogurt or acidophilus then, the yeast will be crowded out and a more normal oral flora will result.

INTESTINAL TRACT: An overgrowth of yeast here will ferment dietary sugars and starches, forming acids, gas, alcohols and a variety of organic chemicals. Symptoms include gas, bloat, heartburn and/or pain in the stomach area, and because of the organic chemicals, there can be headaches, dizziness, lightheadedness, wooziness and post-meal fatigue. To clear intestinal yeast, first the tongue and mouth must be cleansed so yeast does not reenter the system with every swallow. Next, since yeast germs feed on sugars and starches, follow the low carbohydrate diet outlined below. Finally, to replenish the normal, beneficial microbes, eat PLAIN yogurt daily, drink Kefir, 4 ounces daily, and/or take acidophilus, 2 capsules three times daily after meals.

YEAST CONTROL DIET- restricted carbohydrate regimen

UNRESTRICTED FOODS

All protein foods, such as meat, fish, fowl, cheese, eggs, dairy, tofu

RESTRICTED FOODS

FRUITS

Fruits may be a problem because they contain a large amount of sugars. However, if the fruit contains a lot of fiber, this may make up for the sugars to some degree. Thus:

- Fruits are only allowed at the end of a meal, and never on an empty stomach
- Only high fiber fruits are allowed
- Only very small amounts!

EXAMPLES:

ALLOWED IN GENEROUS AMOUNTS
Grapefruit, lemons, limes, tomatoes, avocado
ALLOWED IN SMALL AMOUNTS ONLY! (The high fiber content in these hard, crunchy fruits partially makes up for the carbohydrates)
Pears, apples, strawberries, cantaloupe, etc.
NOT ALLOWED (These soft fruits do not have enough fiber)
Oranges, watermelons, bananas, grapes, etc.
No fruit juices either!

VEGETABLES
Green vegetables and salads are O.K. Avoid or limit starchy vegetables (potato, rice, beans, etc.) and avoid pasta.

STARCHES
None!! If it is made from flour- any kind of flour- it is not allowed. (No breads, cereals, cake, etc.)

SWEETENERS
NOT ALLOWED
No sugars at all, and no fructose or corn syrup
ALLOWED (if tolerated)
Stevia (safest), honey, and Splenda,
Aspartame (NutraSweet, Equal) may not be tolerated by some patients
Saccharin products are not recommended

DRINKS
ALLOWED
Water, seltzer, caffeine-free diet sodas, coffee and tea without sugar or caffeine, vegetable juices
NOT ALLOWED
Fruit juices, regular sodas, and any drinks sweetened with sugars or syrups
No Alcohol at all

OTHERS
Do not skip any meals. At least three regular meals daily are needed; a better option is to eat very small portions but have between meal snacks to maintain blood sugar and insulin levels. Bedtime snacks, if taken, must be totally carbohydrate free!

PATIENT INSTRUCTIONS ON TICK BITE PREVENTION AND TICK REMOVAL

HOW TO PROTECT YOURSELF FROM TICK BITES

PROPERTY Remove wood piles, rock walls, and bird feeders as these attract tick-carrying small animals and can increase the risk of acquiring Lyme.
INSECTICIDES: Property should be treated with a product designed to target the rodents that carry ticks- bait boxes and a product called "Damminix" can be used. Use these products in conjunction with liquid or granular insecticides.
LIQUID & GRANULAR PESTICIDES: Products meant for widespread application such as permethrin and its derivatives are preferred. They are available as a liquid concentrate and as granules. If liquid insecticides are used, application should be by fogging, not by coarse sprays. Apply these products in a strip a few feet wide at the perimeter of the lawn at any areas adjacent to woods and underbrush. Also treat any ornamental shrubs near the house that may serve as a habitat for small animals. The best time to apply these products is in late Spring and early Fall. In every case, professional application is recommended.

CLOTHING When wearing long pants, tuck the cuffs into the socks so any ticks that get on shoes or socks will crawl on the outside of the pants and be less likely to bite. Also, light colored clothing should be worn so the ticks will be easier to spot. Smooth materials such as windbreakers are harder for ticks to grab onto and are preferable to knits, etc.

Tick repellents that contain "permethrin" (Permanone, Permakill) are meant to be sprayed onto clothing. Spray the clothes before they're put on, and let them dry first. Do not apply this chemical directly to the skin.

Ticks are very intolerant of being dried out. After being outdoors in an infested area, place clothes in the dryer for a few minutes to kill any ticks that may still be present.

SKIN: Insect repellents that contain "DEET" are somewhat effective when applied to the arms, legs, and around the neck. Do not use any repellent over wide areas of the body as they can be absorbed causing toxicity. Also, it is inadvisable to use a product that contains more than 50% DEET, and 25% concentrations are preferred. Use repellents cautiously on small children, as they are more susceptible to their toxic effects. Be aware that this repellent evaporates quickly and must be reapplied frequently.

Check carefully for ticks not only when you get home but frequently while still outside!

HOW TO REMOVE AN ATTACHED TICK
Using a tweezer (not fingers!), grasp the tick as close to the skin as possible and pull straight out. Then apply an antiseptic. Do not try to irritate them with heat or chemicals, or grasp them by the body, as this may cause the tick to inject more germs into your skin. Tape the tick to a card and record the date and location of the bite. Remember, the sooner the tick is removed, the less likely an infection will result.

APPENDIX
RATIONALE FOR TREATING TICK BITES
Prophylactic antibiotic treatment upon a known tick bite is recommended for those who fit the following categories:

1. People at higher health risk bitten by an unknown type of tick or tick capable of transmitting Borrelia burgdorferi, e.g., pregnant women, babies and young children, people with serious health problems, and those who are immunodeficient.
2. Persons bitten in an area highly endemic for Lyme Borreliosis by an unidentified tick or tick capable of transmitting B. burgdorferi.
3. Persons bitten by a tick capable of transmitting B. burgdorferi, where the tick is engorged, or the attachment duration of the tick is greater than four hours, and/or the tick was improperly removed. This

means when the body of the tick is squeezed upon removal, irritated with toxic chemicals in an effort to get it to back out, or disrupted in such a way that its contents were allowed to contact the bite wound. Such practices increase the risk of disease transmission.

4. A patient, when bitten by a known tick, clearly requests oral prophylaxis and understands the risks. This is a case-by-case decision.

The physician cannot rely on a laboratory test or clinical finding at the time of the bite to definitely rule in or rule out Lyme Disease infection, so must use clinical judgment as to whether to use antibiotic prophylaxis. Testing the tick itself for the presence of the spirochete, even with PCR technology, is helpful but not 100% reliable.

An established infection by B. burgdorferi can have serious, long-standing or permanent, and painful medical consequences, and be expensive to treat. Since the likelihood of harm arising from prophylactically applied anti-spirochetal antibiotics is low, and since treatment is inexpensive and painless, it follows that the risk-benefit ratio favors tick bite prophylaxis.

SUGGESTED ADDITIONAL READING

Evidence Based Guidelines for the Management of Lyme Disease. The International Lyme and Associated Diseases Society. Expert Rev. Anti-infect. Ther.2(1), Suppl. (2004)

Lyme Disease: Point/Counterpoint. Stricker, Raphael B. Lautin, Andrew. Burrascano, Joseph J. Expert Rev. Anti-infect. Ther, April 2005. 3(2), 155-165

An Understanding of Laboratory Testing for Lyme Disease. Harris, Nick S. J. Spiro. and Tick-Borne Dis. Vol 5, 1998. 16-26

Gestational Lyme Borreliosis. MacDonald, Alan B. Rheumatic Diseases Clinics of North America 15 (4), Nov. 1989. 657-678

Cerebral Malaria. Newton, Charles R.et al. J. Neurol. Neurosurg. Psychiatry. 2000. Vol 69, 433-441.

RESOURCES

International Lyme and Associated Diseases Society
www.ILADS.org
P.O. Box 341461
Bethesda, MD 20827-1461

Lyme Disease Association, Inc.
P.O. Box 1438, Jackson, NJ 08527
(888) 366-6611
www.lymediseaseassociation.org

Lyme disease: A Look Beyond Antibiotics

Dietrich K.Klinghardt, MD, PhD

Bellevue WA aant@neuraltherapy.com 1/7/05 and 1/7/06
425-637-9339

In the last decade the majority of outcome-oriented physicians observed a major shift: we realized that it was neither the lack of vitamins or growth hormone that made our patients ill. We discovered that toxicity and chronic infections were most often at the core of the client's suffering. We watched the discussion, which infection may be the primary one: mycoplasma, stealth viruses, HHV-6, trichomonas, Chlamydia pneumoniae, leptospirosis, mutated strep, or what else?

The new kid on the block is Borrelia burgdorferi (Bb) and some of us have looked at it for a long time as possibly being the bug that opens the door for all the other infections to enter the system. Lyme disease has become a buzzword in the alternative medical field. Since none of the recommended treatments are specific to either one of the microbes, we can never assume that we really know what we treated once a patient has recovered.

Microbiologist Gitte Jensen, PhD had shown, that the older we get, the more foreign DNA is attached to our own DNA. Somewhere along the line pathogenic microbes invade the host's DNA and become a permanent part of it. Since we use only 2% of our DNA, it may not be a problem. In fact, it may make us who we finally become. It may also cause a number of symptoms and chronic illness. Genius Guenther Enderlein's discoveries take us off the hook: if one microbe can change into another given the right environment, why bother to find out, who we are infected with? The book "Lab 257" suggests that Bb is an escaped man-made US military bio-warfare organism (just like myoplasma incognitus and HHV 6).

Other authors suggest that different subtypes of Borrelia, which cause illness in humans, such as B. afzelii and B.garinii have probably existed longer then B.burgdorferi and occur naturally (1, 2) and have been with us for a long time, maybe centuries or much longer then that.

Neurologist Prof. J. Faust MD, PhD of the Albert-Ludwig University in Freiburg, Germany (3) related many neurological and psychiatric illnesses to spirochete infections as early as the 1960s. He was so skilled in his clinical knowledge that he could – based on clinical neurological symptoms – accurately predict which valley in the Black Forest the infected patient was from! This clearly was a time before Bb - showing that non-syphilis spirochete infections were around earlier then the famous Bb outbreak in Connecticut in the mid seventies. It also makes a strong statement to the fact how easily these creatures may mutate and adapt to local conditions. It may however validate the findings published in "Lab 257": Tuebingen, the place where German/US warfare spirochete expert Traub was continuing his spirochete experiments in the early 50s, is situated in the Black Forest also. Were these spirochetes genuine or have they escaped from a university laboratory?

Making the diagnosis

It appears that many patients with MS, ALS, Parkinson's disease, autism, joint arthritis, chronic fatigue, sarcoidosis and even cancer are infected with Borrelia burgdorferi. But is the infection causing the illness or is it an opportunistic infection simply occurring in people weakened by other illnesses.

My experience is based on:

a) using direct microscopic proof of the presence of Borrelia burgdoferi (Bb) and other spirochetes (4, 5)
b) the information many affected clients have brought to me
c) my own clinical training and experience (30 years in Medical practice, 15 years Bb cognizant)
d) ART testing (autonomic response testing), which is the most advanced and scientifically validated method of muscle testing (6)
e) regular lab parameters affected by Lyme:
    - Abnormal lipid profile (moderate cholesterol elevation with significant LDL elevation)
    - insulin resistance
    - borderline low wbc, normal SED rate and CRP
    - normal thyroid hormone tests but positive Barnes test and excellent response to giving T3
    - type 2 (high cortisol, low DHEA) or type 3 adrenal failure (low cortisol and DHEA)
    - low testosterone and DHEA
    - decreased urine concentration (low specific gravity)

complex changes in cytokines, interferones, NK cells, white blood cell indicators, etc.

Bb tends to infect the B-lymphocytes and other components of the immune system which are responsible for creating the antibodies, which are then measured by an ELISA test or Western Blot test. Since antibody production is greatly compromised in infected individuals, it makes no sense to use these tests as the gold standard or benchmark for the presence of Bb (7). We also are aware that in endemic areas in the US up to 22% of stinging flies and mosquitoes (2, 8, 9, and 10) are carriers of Bb and co-infections. In South East Germany and Eastern Europe 12 % of mosquitoes have been shown to be infected. Also many spiders, flees, lice and other stinging insects carry spirochetes and co-infections.

Making the history of a tick bite a condition for a physician to be willing to even consider the possibility of a Bb infection seems cynical and cruel. To use conventional diagnostic tests such as the Western Blot, one has to think in paradoxes: the patient has to be treated with an effective treatment modality first before the patient recovers enough to produce the antibodies, which then are looked for in the test. A positive Western Blot proves that the treatment given worked to some degree. *A negative Western Blot does not and cannot prove the absence of the infection.*

Having taken another route altogether, we have recognized that today many if not most Americans are carriers of the infection. Most infected people are symptomatic, but the severity and type of the symptoms varies greatly. The microbes often invade tissues that had been injured: your chronic neck pain or sciatica really may be a Bb infection. The same may be true for your chronic TMJ problem, your adrenal fatigue, your thyroid dysfunction, your GERD and many other seemingly unrelated symptoms. Many Bb symptoms are mistaken for problems of natural or premature aging.

In most places the diagnosis of an active Bb infection is made only if the symptoms are severe, persistent, obvious, and many non-specific and fruitless avenues of treatment have been exhausted. Acute new "typical" cases of Bb infection are rare in my practice. Symptoms tend to get stranger and more obscure every year.

Frequently, if the patient is fortunate enough to see a practitioner who is "Lyme cognizant", the diagnosis of a supposedly fresh case of symptomatic

Lyme disease is made when a significant tissue toxin level has been reached (threshold phenomenon) or when a new co-infection has occurred recently. The symptoms can mimic any other existing medical, psychological or psychiatric condition. The list of significant co-infections is limited: roundworms, tapeworms, threadworms, toxoplasmosis, giardia and amoebas, clostridia, the herpes virus family, parvovirus B 19, active measles (in the small intestine), leptospirosis, chronic strep infections and their mutations, Babesia, Brucella, Ehrlichiosis, Bartonella, mycoplasma, Rickettsia, Bartonella and a few others. Molds and fungi are always part of the picture.

The pattern of co-infections and the other preexisting conditions such as mercury toxicity determine the symptom-picture but not the severity. The severity of symptoms correlates most closely with the overall summation or body burden of coexisting conditions and with the genetically determined ability to excrete neurotoxins. The genes coding for the glutathione S-transferase and for the different alleles of apolipoprotein E (E2, E3 and E4) play a major role. E2 can carry twice as much sulfhydryl-affinitive toxins (such as mercury and lead) out of the cell as the E3 subtype, E4 carries out none. Trouble in the methylation, acetylation and sulfation pathways is also common. Other factors, such as diet and food allergies, past toxic and electromagnetic exposures, emotional factors and unhealed ancestral trauma, scar interference fields and occlusal jaw and bite problems are also important (6). The severity of symptoms is not related to the number of spirochetes in the system but rather to the individual's immune responses.

Taken all of the above into account, we do not distinguish between people who have the Bb infection and those who don't. We distinguish between people who have Lyme disease and those who don't.

a) patients who are infected with any type of Borrelia and are symptomatic have "Lyme" disease
b) healthy people who are not symptomatic often already have a spirochete infection as well. They may or may not be disasters waiting to happen. But they do not (yet) have Lyme "disease".

Most often several of the "co-infections" are already present prior to the infection with Bb or other spirochetes.

In treatment we focus on exploring the difference between symptomatic and asymptomatic carriers. We treat what the symptomatic person is missing (such as enough magnesium in the diet) or has extra (such as mercury) compared to the asymptomatic one.

The group suffering most is newborn babies and young children, who rarely are diagnosed correctly and therefore are not treated appropriately. They often carry the labels ADHD, autistic spectrum disorder (ASD), seizure disorder and others. Detoxifying these kids with transdermal DMPS and treating the chronic infections is often curative.

The 3 Components of Lyme disease

Lyme disease has three components, which should be recognized and addressed with treatment:

Component #1: The presence of spirochete **infection and co-infections**

The co-infections are bacterial, viral, fungal and parasitic. Since the spirochetes paralyze multiple aspects of the immune system, the organism is without defenses against many microbes. Many - if not most - of the co-infections are really a consequence of the spirochete infection and not truly a simultaneously occurring "co-infection".

For this aspect of treatment we use pulsed electromagnetic fields (KMT-microbial inhibition frequencies), niacin in high doses (12) herbs, minerals, bee venom (6) and - sometimes - ant parasitic medication and antibiotics. *The KMT microcurrent technology is new and revolutionary (17). The instruments are FDA approved for pain control. Designed by Japanese engineers they use four different - but simultaneously applied - high frequency superimposed biological waveforms. The interference pattern is creating thousands of harmonics which are then manipulated into the specific published microbial inhibition frequencies (against Bb, mycoplasma etc.).*

This stealthy microcurrent travels freely through the body reaching every tissue. The instrument measures the skin conductance over a 100 times/second adjusting the amperage constantly (so that the body never creates habituation/resistance against it). The microbes are inhibited in their metabolic and sexual activity and gradually die out or disappear from the body

The instrument looks not much different then a TENS unit and is applied via four electrodes to the skin or used by translating the electric field into a vector force field using signal enhancer technology. The KMT frequencies are designed to not only interfere with the reproductive mechanism of the microbes and parasites, but also to awaken the immune system, entrain the white cells to recognize the invaders and at the same time help to absorb and shuttle the effective medication to the body compartment, where the infection actually is. Otherwise, most treatment substances given never reach the target in sufficient concentration.

<u>Component #2</u>: the illness producing effect of microbial exo- and endotoxins and toxins produced by the host in response to microbial trigger

Most of these are neurotoxins, some appear to be carcinogenic as well, others block the T3 receptor on the cell wall, etc. Decreased hormonal output of the gonads and adrenals is a commonly observed toxin mediated problem in Lyme patients. Central inhibition of the pineal gland, hypothalamus and pituitary gland is almost always an issue that has to be resolved somewhat independently from treating the infection. Furthermore, biotoxins from the infectious agents have a synergistic effect with heavy metals, xenobiotics and thioethers from cavitations and NICO lesions in the jaw and from root filled teeth. My published neurotoxin elimination protocol can be downloaded for free (6).

We use toxin binding agents such as fiber rich ground up raw vegetables, chlorella (14), cholestyramine (13), beta-Sitosterol, propolis powder, apple pectin and Mucuna bean powder (14). A solid heavy metal detoxification program should be used simultaneously with the first phases of the Lyme treatment. Safe toxic metal elimination is an art unto itself. However, the information is widely available now (15).

The more difficult objective is to choose agents and methods to trigger the release of neurotoxins from their respective binding sites. Only then can they be transported to the liver, processed and enter the small intestine from where they can be carried out by the binding agents.

The toxins occupying the T3 receptor are competitively displaced by oral T3 - cycled with the Wilson protocol (*available at most compounding pharmacies*). The toxins blocking the cortisol receptor are mobilized with the herb forskolin. CGF chlorella - a sophisticated mix of chlorella and chlorella growth factor (14) - and cilantro given together with a non-irradiated Mucuna bean powder mobilize most everything else. I also use alternate day dosing of an energetically enhanced phospholipid/EDTA/Alpha-Lipoic acid mix ("PhosphoLipid Exchange") which is currently the most tolerated and effective form of phospholipids for the Lyme patient (14).

The KMT microcurrent frequencies dramatically increase the speed of toxin mobilization and access body compartments the biochemical compounds cannot (17). Psychotherapeutic intervention (15) to uncover and treat old trauma is most profoundly effective in triggering a neurotoxin release when none of the other methods appear to work anymore. After each APN session we pre-medicate the patient with CGF-chlorella. Sometimes the extraction of a devitalized tooth or the injection of one of the facial/cervical ganglia with glutathione or another detox agent can trigger a major neurotoxin release (16). Lymph drainage in combination with colon hydrotherapy accesses toxins stored in the lymphatic body-compartment. German practitioners have pioneered the combination of oral cilantro and the "Toxaway" microcurrent footbath.

Component #3: The **immune reactions** provoked by the presence of both toxins and microbes (there are three sub-possibilities, which have to be recognized and addressed)

The immune reactions are largely depending on host factors, such as genetics, prior illnesses, mental-emotional baggage, early childhood traumatization, current exposure to electromagnetic fields (sleeping location, use of cell phones, poor wiring in car or home, etc), food allergies and diet, socio-economic background, marital stress etc. A multitude of biochemical serum markers is used today to determine the status of the infection (see below). A subset of NK killer cells, CD 57+ is emerging as a valid marker for activity of the illness (lower counts indicate worsening).

1: Anergy - the absence of reaction due to the successful evasion of the host-defenses. One of the more known mechanisms the microbes use to create anergy is hyper coagulation. The microbes tend to live in the endothelium, where the food is most abundant. They trigger the host's coagulation mechanism to lay down a layer of fibrin on top of them to evade recognition by the immune system, etc. For this aspect we use three techniques:

a) the KMT-microcurrent technology and homeopathics to wake up and entrain the immune system

b) Rechtsregulat ("right rotatory fluid") which is an enzyme rich extract of fermented fruits and vegetables (14). It has outperformed the s.c. injection of heparin in our own trials and frequently leads to rapid subjedtive improvement. Lumbrokinase is far more effective then Nattokinase. Both appear weak when compared to Rechtsregulat. We also work on recognizing and eliminating those factors that block the client's system (geopathic stress, EM stress, food allergies, emotional factors, interference fields such as scars and disturbed ganglia and we substitute vitamins and minerals based on ART testing).

c) the Enderlein remedies (especially the haptens) from Pleomorphic-Sanum

2: Allergy - appropriate or exaggerated immune reactions (both cellular TH1-reaction and TH2-cytokine activation). In Lyme disease often (not always)TH-1 is overly active early in the illness and can easily be downregulated by fluconazole, later TH2 becomes overly active. Nothing works better then the APN-desensitization procedure (15): while the patient is exposed to the allergen (we use a glass-carrier fixated culture of the offending microbes) the ANS is kept in a state of equilibrium, using tapping of acupuncture-points, hypnotherapeutic trauma-recall and intervention techniques and our proprietary psycho kinesiology (muscle-biofeedback psychotherapy).

A very effective and yet simple technique to re-regulate TH1 and TH2 back is auto-urine therapy. The patient's urine concentrates the antigens (disposed cell walls and cell fragments of offending microbes which the immune system has successfully eliminated). By passing the client's urine through a micro pore filter and injecting it i.m., the lymphocytes on patrol in the connective tissue are brought in contact with the antigen and quickly mount a specific and appropriate immune response. We use 2 ml of filtered urine once weekly for 12 weeks. All other similar approaches (autohemotherapy, homeopathic autonosodes, manipulating the immune system with supplements) are far less effective.

3: Autoimmunity – the toxins and microbes often act as haptens – marking the cell, cell wall or tissue in which they are hiding as foreign and therefore for destruction . This happens especially against a back drop of pre existing heavy metal toxicity, which has to be addressed aggressively and prior to treating the microbes themselves. We use the MELISA test (memory lymphocyte immune-stimulation assay) to establish which metals the patient is reactive to. The same lab in Bremen, Germany also offers the most sensitive Bb test.

The KMT microcurrent technology is very effective in recognition entrainment, helping the immune cells to mount a specific and targeted attack on the invaders, sparing the body's own tissues. It breaks through one of the prime mechanisms the offending germs are using: molecular mimicry (the pathogens present antigens on their surface that are indistinguishable from a normal body tissue).
The technique also breaks another trick the spirochetes have developed: the molecular interaction that occurs between a specific Lyme virulence factor (OspE) and a host protein fH (factor H). Some surface antigens in the spirochete are identical to myelin. This explains why anti-myelin antibodies are often present.

The novice in the field tends to treat component #1 only. We have only rarely observed lasting improvement when course after course of antibiotics was given. Because of the defense mechanisms inherent in the Bb and co-infections, current wisdom suggests that 18 months of antibiotics would be curative in many cases (25). We have observed severe, lasting and unacceptable side effects from this approach (such as tinnitus, kidney failure, intractable immune system breakdown and others).

By using the synergistic effect between treatment-modalities which simultaneously address the three issues outlined above, lasting improvements are the norm rather than the exception. By using the synergy principle and abandoning the arrogant idea of being able to eradicate all of the microbes in the system "for good", chronic Lyme patients can often live a normal healthy life again. The use of herbs alone or in combination with antibiotics has emerged as the most important core strategy.

The Mineral Issue

To feed, fuel and perk up the cells of the immune system (especially NK cells and macrophages) numerous interventions have been attempted, mostly based on orthomolecular and herbal medicine principles. We found that amongst those approaches, abundant mineral substitution based on the red cell mineral analysis is most rewarding. Rarely should medical drugs be used.

Amazingly, the most depleted minerals in our Lyme patients are often copper, magnesium, manganese (in Lyme) and iron (in Babesiosis). Bb and Bartonella need magnesium to duplicate and deplete the host's body rapidly. Copper and iron have all but disappeared from most of our supplements based on faulty interpretation of hair analysis. The immune system uses those two metals in the process of phagocytosis. They are the main constituent of the enzymes (or "bullets") the immune cells use in the battle against the invaders.

Oxidized used-up iron and copper get displaced into the extracellular compartment and body fluids and appears in the hair and skin, as the body's most efficient way of excreting toxins without hurting the kidneys. This has led to the dangerous and in its consequence catastrophic assumption, that these metals are the enemy and need to be restricted. It is true, that oxidized metals pose a danger and have to be reduced (=substitution of electrons) or eliminated. However, when copper and iron are needed and substituted appropriately, major improvements have been observed. Appropriate antioxidant treatment can reduce these metals. Homeopathic copper and iron will lead to beneficial redistribution of these metals and makes them bio-available again.

Lithium-orotate or aspartate in low doses (15 mg/day) has been shown to protect CNS structures from neurotoxin damage. Patients almost always benefit clinically from frequent treatment with parenteral magnesium. It is most meaningfully given in a modified Meyer's cocktail. We also use a 5:2 ratio of folic acid (not folinic) and hydroxycobolamine (not methyl- or cyano-) sublingually several times/day. In addition methyl-cobolamine is given i.m. twice weekly and is important in the methylation/restoration of reduced glutathione. Hydroxy-B12 protects the brain from nitric oxide induced damage.

Many Lyme patients suffer from Pyrroluria, a metabolic illness where abnormal porphyrins carry out significant amounts of needed zinc and vitamin B6. Diagnosis is made with the appropriate test at the Pfeiffer institute in Chicago. Even though it is assumed that this illness is hereditary I have my doubts, since most Lyme sufferers have a degree of it. I suspect that the appearance of kryptopyrroles in the urine is induced by the illness. However, I am careful with excessive substitution of zinc. Zinc has a synergistic effect with mercury in the brain and also promotes the growth of the herpes viruses.

If clients show abnormal high losses of sex steroid hormones in the urine, the patient may be cobalt deficient. The urine hormone test and cobalt drops are available at the *Tahoma Clinic* Renton, WA. For a while selenium should be given in high doses to suppress viral replication and render bioavailable mercury non-reactive.

The element most critical in the Lyme patient however is iodine. A two inch square of Lugol's iodine is painted on the patient's skin and should remain visible for 24 hours. The sooner it is absorbed the more deficient the patient. An oral form of Lugol's is available under the name *Iodoral (Optimox, Torrance, Ca).*

Filling up the body's mineral reserves has always been the most essential part of our heavy metal detox program. It is also the most essential part of our Lyme treatment.

Sequencing

There is an inherent order in which the microbes should be treated. If the order is correct, gentle methods work. Treatment should always combine electromagnetic interventions, using specific microbial inhibition frequencies (KMT technology) with the appropriate herb, antibiotic or other antimicrobial strategy. It should also always be combined with a toxin elimination program, good psychotherapy and general life style hygiene.

The Lyme ABC

A. We start with **deworming** our clients. We often use a simple yet aggressive seasalt/Vit C protocol (19) which has an independent effect against the spirochetes also. The high salt concentration kills large parasites by osmotically induced dehydration (osmotic shock). High salt levels also increase the enzyme elastase which has a strong antimicrobial/anti-spirochete effect (4).

Protocol: 1.5 grams of sea salt per 20 lbs of body weight in 4 divided doses per day for 3 weeks. With each dose also give 1-4 gms of Vit C (dose has to be just below bowel tolerance). Three 3-6-week cycles with a 2 week break in-between. The blood pressure should be monitored and not elevate outside acceptable levels. Five percent of the population are salt sensitive and react with a significantly increased blood pressure. In the off weeks we give tsp of sea salt in a glass of water first thing in the morning.

Sometimes we enhance the program by using the "Arise-and-Shine" herbal program. Often I will add in a course of Albendazole (same family as metronidazole), Biltricide or ALinia in high doses and parasitic CDs for entrainment of the immune system. The frequencies of the CDs were developed by German physicists by taping the sounds of microbes in their respective live activity in an underground lab which was soundproof and electromagnetically completely shielded (6).

B. The next step is the treatment of **giardia, entamoeba histolytica and trichomonas**, which most often are overlooked. Lab detection of large parasites in most US labs is hopeless. Amoeba and giardia trophozoites can only be detected in a fresh stool for about 20 minutes. None of the labs available to us comply with this necessity. The detection rate is so substandard that only ART testing, a therapeutic trial or abdominal palpation by an experienced practitioner is capable of establishing the diagnosis.

Protocol: organic freeze dried garlic (14) treats all of the above astoundingly successfully. Sometimes we add Tinidazole 500 mg bid for 10 days always followed by long term garlic therapy (three caps tid after meals).

C. Next we attend to the chronic **strep infections**, which often coexist with the herpes viruses. No other treatment has been as successful as Pleo Not (penicillum notatum) from Pleomorphic-Sanum followed by a six month course of Pleo Sancom (antidotes for aspergillus niger and mucor racemosus).

We always look at the tonsils: if they are scarred with crypts, or lymph tissue has regrown since the tonsillectomy ("tonsillar tags"), surgical intervention is needed. Otherwise these patients (which are most of them) never get well. We recommend a procedure developed by Dr. Sergej Dorochov, MD, PhD called "regenerative cryotherapy" (20). It involves freezing the surfaces of all lymphatic tissue of the head/neck region which creates a barrage of growth factor and cytokine responses, which often lead to dramatic improvements in our Lyme patients.

Lymph drainage using the KMT technology has been superb in speeding the healing of the sinus/head/neck/region.

D. The next step is the treatment of **Babesia**. There are now at least 17 subtypes of this intracellular Malaria-like organism. Eye, brain and dental symptoms are most often caused by this mean microbe.

Protocol: Frequency #2 in the KMT 23 TENS unit inhibits the metabolic activity of Babesia and is used 3 times weekly.

I also use PC-Noni extract and Artemisinin: see the protocol below. Watch iron levels! Artemisinin provokes the intestinal wall to secrete an enzyme which destroys the medication before it can be absorbed. This process builds up over 3 weeks. After a one week pause the enzyme has disappeared and takes another 3 weeks to reemerge. Grapefruit juice prevents formation of this enzyme.

Alternatives are the Swiss Malaria drug Riamet (1 course) which is very well tolerated but only seems to work short term, and Mepron, which is forbiddingly expensive

E. The next step is to start the client on a systemic **antiviral treatment**. I use the ayurvedic herb cocktail - Indian Gooseberry, Chebulic and Beleric myrobalan (14), which has given the most profound and lasting effect on the viruses of the herpes family, which flourish in the immune suppressed Lyme patient. I also use liquid olive leaf, which shows some effect. The Japanese mushroom extracts have also been helpful. I also like the North American product "Pro Boost" (thymus extract) to help awaken the cellular immune system. As long as clients use bee venom therapy, the symptoms of herpes viral infections (seizures, brain fog, emotional ups and downs, chronic pain sysndromes especially "discogenic" back pain and sciatica, fatigue) disappear.

Virox and other chaparral- derivatives have been disappointing. The insomnia of Lyme disease is often herpes viral in nature (EBV, VZ or HSV 1, HSV II). As a diagnostic trial I often use 1000 mg of the medical antiviral drug Valtrex at bedtime. If there is a dramatic improvement, herbal antiviral treatment has to be considered for a long time.

We have designed an antiviral program for the KMT instruments (frequency #4) and an anti viral CD, which is played through a walk man or regular sound system at low volume 3 times/week. This has been extremely effective. Zinc fosters the growth of HSV I and II, copper and selenium inhibit it.

F. I simultaneously address the **fungal/yeast** component which is most often present, especially if clients had prior antibiotic treatment. Fungi and viruses seem to support each other in yet unknown ways. I use both the antifungal CD and the KMT TENS-frequencies in program #4 which contains all known anti-yeast and anti-mold frequencies (6).

With ART technology we could show that the most successful and well tolerated antifungal is either fluconazole (100 mg twice daily) which also has an anti Bb effect and seems to downregulate TH-1, the drug amphotericin B (250 mg bid) or the combination of organic freeze dried garlic (14) and oil of oregano. Substitution with microbes is important. We use "Matrix Microbes" (14) which contains over 80 lesser known beneficial microbes. Every patient is also on a more traditional acidophilus/bifidus/FOS product.

Eating a low carbohydrate diet is often a must. We monitor the fasting insulin level. If it is low, we are ok. If it is high, we restrict the carbohydrates. Do not restrict the carbohydrates if it is not necessary. We have seen dangerous mistakes in this field. In general, bacterial infections benefit from the acidic environment created by a high protein diet. Molds and fungi benefit from a high carb environment. Metabolic typing is a safeguard, but time consuming to do at home, especially if you are very ill. I use the "diet therapy software" (21) for a rapid and profound diet evaluation and recommendation. Most successful is the ART food sensitivity test for every single item in the client's diet (6). It may take 15 minutes, is more sensitive then the ELISA, MELISA and other lab tests - and it does not incur lab fees (6). The rotation diet by Sally Rockwell prevents relapses.

G. Mycoplasma responds well to enzymes, when it is treated in sequence with the other microbes as outlined here. The most effective strategy is the German product Rechtsregulat (14). This simple drink has been extremely effective in eradicating mycoplasma and other cell wall deficient microbes. It also has a heparin like anti-fibrin effect that surpasses injected heparin by far. It has just like heparin, a strong biological effect against Babesia as well.

Dosage: 1 tbs/2 times per day in a glass of water. The KMT program #4 is designed for treatment of mycoplasma (6).

H. The spirochetes and their close relatives (**Bartonella, Babesia, Rickettsia, Ehrlichiosis, and Brucella abortis**) are best treated last - with antimicrobial herbs or antibiotics. Many herbs have enormous potential in the treatment of chronic Lyme disease (see below).

Frequency #1 in the KMT TENS unit inhibits the microbial growth of spirochetes and Bartonella, # 2 is a series of anti-Babesia frequencies. This modulated microcurrent simultaneously activates specific immune responses and aids the uptake of antimicrobial herbs.

Injected bee venom has long been my favorite during this phase of the treatment (22, 23). The peptide mellitin has strong antibiotic activity against all spirochetes (24). Bee venom also contains nerve growth factor, the very substance needed for healing, when everything else has been attended to.

For the psychiatric presentations of Lyme disease I use large doses of Niacin. (Niacinamide and no-flush Niacin do not work.) 3-6 gms in 3-4 divided doses often show amazing results. It appears that Niacin has tremendous antibiotic potential against all types of Borrelia (12). I suspect that our mentor and genius in orthomolecular psychiatry, Abraham Hoffer, MD discovered a treatment for Bb long before Lyme-disease was known.

The current antibiotic protocols are discussed and listed elsewhere (10).

Often patients develop sarcoidosis, which is rarely recognized (11). The Lyme infected lymph nodes produce abnormal amounts of 1.25 di-hydroxy vitamin D. The client often develops marked osteoporosis (most often in the spine) along with other more typical Lyme symptoms. The blood test (1.25 di-OH vit D) will usually reveal the pathology (levels over 45), necessitating therapy with the Trevor Marshall protocol (18). It uses antibiotics together with the angiotensin II receptor blocker olmesartan –medoxomil. By adding the KMT lymph drainage technology twice/week results are often rapid and miraculous. We hope to find alternatives to the antibiotic regimen in the near future.

When the sequence outlined here is observed, few people have severe Herxheimer reactions, which are the rule in other approaches.

Outlook

Most clients will need some support for several years, before they have found and adapted to a new life style in which the symptoms are absent. Lyme disease is marked by cyclic rhythms and unexpected returns of the symptom from time to time. Once a patient has figured out what works for him or her best, most of my patients learn how to manage the illness with very little help - on their own, living normal healthy lives worth living.

In the course of conquering the illness there has been a lot of personal growth and a lot of learning. Many treatment modalities have been surprisingly ineffective: ozone, hyperbaric oxygen, ICHT (intracellular hyperthermia). Some treatments have been unexpectedly effective: dental splints, color therapy, Tomatis therapy and neuro sensory stimulation, elevating the body temperature with T3 supplementation, regular bee venom injections, tonsillectomies and cryotherapy and many others.

After 15 years of dealing consciously with this illness, Lyme disease is still a mystery to me. Currently its impact outweighs other important issues like heavy metal toxicity, unresolved psychological issues and nutritional deficiencies.

There has been much speculation, why Lyme disease seems to be increasingly common. The book "Lab 257"is an investigative report on the issues involved. The insects which are the vectors for these microbes thrive in warmer climates. I have no doubt, that to a large degree the greenhouse effect is responsible and will be confronting us with the onslaught of more and more aggressive microbes. The partial pressure of oxygen on the earth at sea level has decreased from 30% 150 years ago to 19% today. The oxygen producing algae in the oceans are dying.

The response of the public health system so far has been denial and anger towards those who try to uncover the puzzle and help the afflicted patients. This will certainly change in the near future. I expect that by the time the institutions discover Lyme disease as a far more important factor in chronic illness then is currently acknowledged, we will be confronted with new, far more dangerous microbes. Antibiotics have disappointed in the treatment of Lyme disease as a single modality. Antibiotics alone will not help us to cope with the coming plagues.

All of us as practitioners have to start looking beyond antibiotics for help and for hope. The microbes have always been with us. They are not the enemy. It is us who have altered the environment so severely and in a way which facilitates the growth of lower evolved species like cell wall deficient microbes and viruses - and ends the life for many more evolved species. Extinction may be forever.

Lyme disease is a messenger. If we don't change, we may be on the endangered species list someday not too far from now.

Helpful References

1. Borrelia burgdorferi group: in-vitro antibiotic sensitivity: Orv Hetil, 2002 May 26; 143(21): 1195-8 (article in Hungarian), JP Henneberg, U Neubert –department of dermatology, Ludwig-Maximillian University, Munich, Germany
2. Erythema chronicum migrans (Afzelii) associated with mosquito bite: acta Derm Venereol (Stockholm) 46, 473-476
3. Personal experience while doing a residency rotation in neurology at the Albert Ludwig-University, Freiburg, Germany under Prof.Faust (1976)
4. www.BradfordResearchInst.org
5. www.Bowen.org
6. www.neuraltherapy.com
7. www.vcu.edu/ Journal of Immunology Dec 2004
8. The etiologic agent of Lyme disease in deer flies, horse flies and mosquitoes, J Infect Dis 154 (1986), 355-358, LA Magnarelli, JF Anderson, AG Barbour
9. Klinik der Lyme-Borreliose: Hans Huber Verlag, Bern, CH (2002). 39-40, Norbert Satz
10. www.Lymenet.org
11. Borrelia Burgdorferi infection may be the cause of sarcoidosis, Hua B, Li QD: Chin Med J (Engl) 1992 Jul; 105(7): 560-3
12. www.vorsoft.com/medical/niacin/index.htm
13. www.chronicneurotoxins.com
14. www.biopureUS.com also: biopure@aol.com
15. www.neuraltherapy.com applied neurobiology (APN) manual/video
16. www.neuraltherapy.com neuraltherapy papers
17. www.neuraltherapy.com Klinghardt Matrix Therapy (KMT)
18. marshallprotocoll@yahoogroups.com
19. www.lymephotos.com

20. www.kryopraxis.com
21. nurse@andreannavaughan.com
22. Bee Venom Therapy for Chronic Pain: D Klinghardt, J. of Neurol and Orthop. Med and Surg., Vol. 11, Issue 9, Oct 1990, pp. 195-197
23. The Treatment of Lyme Disease with Bee Venom: D Klinghardt, M.D., Ph.D., 1999
24. Bee Stings as Lyme Inhibitor: L. L. Lubke and C. F. Garon, J. Clin. Infect. Diseases, July 1997, 25 Suppl. 1, pp. 48-51
25. Lyme disease, potential plague of the 21st century: R Bradford and H Allen, Townsend Letter for Doctors and Patients, Jan 2005, 70-79

Brief introduction to the cast of characters:

Borrelia:
One of eight genera of spirochetes. Hundreds of species in these eight genera. "Borrelia" is the genus, "Burgdorferi" the species. Other famous spirochets: treponema pallidum (syphilis), leptospira (leptopspirosos from animal feces contaminated drinking water, common in Maui, New Mexico, etc). Bb sensu lato includes B. Afzelii, B. garinii, B.lonstari, B.andersonii and many others. Bb sensu stricto refers only to Bb, but includes many species that cause identical symptoms. In Europe, five strains of Bb sensu lato, in Japan 61 strains.

Also be aware that microbes constantly exchange via plamids DNA with each other and we found Bb microbes with properties usually only found in Babesia or mycoplasma, etc. There are no fixed boundaries between many of these microbes.

6 major sites of infection:

1. Large joints (Bb sensu stricto) and connective tissue: onset 4.3 months after insect bite, often self limited (4 years). Flare ups during Herxheimer reactions very common.

Bb has recently been found by us as one of the causes of spinal osteoporosis, disc degeneration and many other "orthopedic" problems.

2. Skin and connective tissue (B. afzelii):
acrodermatitis chronica atrophicans

general collagen breakdown (premature aging)
collagen diseases

3. CNS (B.garinii), PHS and ANS: after insect bite it only takes a few hours before spirochetes are found in CNS even though it takes on average 2 years before symptoms are established. Most common symptom: brain fog and short term memory loss. Later stages demyelination. Severe early changes in SPECT scan (functional), MRI changes much later (physical)

CNS problems:

- Physical: epileptic seizures, insomnia, tremor, ataxia, movement disorders (torticollis, etc.)
- Emotional: irritability (key symptom in children), depression, bi-phasic behavior (manic depression), bouts of anger, listlessness;
- Mental: confusion, **difficulty thinking**, poor short term **memory**, increasingly messy household and desk, difficulty finding the right word, feeling of information overload;
- Mixed pictures:
  can resemble or imitate any known psychiatric illness.
  Chronic Fatigue (more severe in the early afternoon);
  Lack of endurance;
  Non-healing infections in the jaw bone, devitalized teeth, dental pain;
  Fibromyalgia;
  Multiple Chemical Sensitivity;
  loss of zest for life,
  sensitivity to electric appliances.

Peripheral Nervous System problems:
Paraesthesia
Burning
vibration
numbness
shooting pains

Cranial Nerve Problems:
Facial nerve: Bell's palsy (60 % are caused by Lyme disease, 30 % by one of six common viruses from the herpes family, such as EBV, Herpes simplex type I, type II, type 6 etc);

Trigeminal nerve: sense of vibration in the face, TMJ and facial pain, headache, tension and cramps in the face/skull/jaw;
Ears (VII, VIII): tinnitus, vertigo, and hypersensitivity to noise;
Eyes (II, III, IV, VI): decreasing and changing eye sight (fluctuates during the day), light sensitivity, floaters;
Vagus (X), Glossopharyngeal nerve (IX) and Hypoglossus (XII): difficulty swallowing, faulty swallowing, reflux, hiatus hernia, heart palpitations, supraventricular arrythmias.

4. **Heart:** Lyme carditis is difficult to diagnose with current methods (PET scan positive early on) and has multiple symptoms from arrhythmia to angina. Has to be taken serious with first symptoms.

5. **Kidney/bladder**: the highest concentration of tissue spirochetes has been found in kidney and bladder. Symptoms often include:

- interstitial cystitis
- prostatitis (Babesia often also involved)
- sexual dysfunction
- loss of libido
- pelvic pain
- menstrual disorders
- filtration problems in the kidney (low specific weight of urine)
- urethritis after intercourse (the spirochetes are attracted during intercourse to the urethra and cause acute inflammation).

6. **Immune system infection** (white blood cells, thymus, brain, lymphnodes, adrenals, etc)

- Non-healing infections in the jaw bone (also Babesia, Bartonella)
- devitalized teeth
- dental pain;
- Immune system failure: with all known secondary illnesses such as herpes virus infection, intestinal parasites, malaise, : hair loss

Babesia:
intra-cellular Malaria like protozoal organism. Infects red-cells. 2/3rds of Lyme clients also have Babesia, which is hard to diagnose: over 17 antigen-different subspecies. Most common: B.microti, WA-1 strain in Western States and B. divergens and others in Europe

Diagnosis: best is long term observation of blood under darkfield microscope. Babesia tends to leave dying cells while under darkfield observation.

Vertigo
headache fatigue
dental problems: accelerated tooth decay and cavitation formation
TMJ problems
eye problems (floaters and blurry vision)
weight loss and abdominal problems (GERD)
fibromyalgia,
shortness of breath
malaise
drenching night sweats and fever/chills during Herxheimer reactions.

Therapy: think Mepron or Noni, Artemisinin and Oxo

Bartonella

B.henselae is the most commonly found intra-cellular co-infection today found in rbc's, endothelial cells, bone marrow and macrophages. 70% of the cats in Italy are infected with it (cat scratch disease), cat–to-human transfer is common. B.quintana brough down Napoleon's troups in Russia, the true cause for his defeat. The microbes are found today in his troup's teeth in the mass graves.

Other types are found on a regular basis.

Symptoms:

swollen lymph glands
endocardits
hepatitis
neovacularization
fatigue
low grade fever
jaw bone cavitations
devitalized teeth
often co-infection in ALS
fibromyalgia and joint pain

Therapy: think Zithro, Doxy and Rifampin together or: Polygonum and Stephania root

Ehrlichiosis

Human granulocytic Ehrlichiosis (HGE) is caused by Anaplasma phagocytophila. Human monocytic Ehrlichiosis (HME) is caused by Ehrlichia chaffeensis. Often found in clients that have contact with horses and farm animals.

Symptoms:

- Fever (only after initial infection)
- Myalgia and arthralgia
- Headcache
- Lycopenia and thrombocytopenia
- Hyponatremia
- Mental confusion
- Skin rashes, genital and oral ulcers
- Severe pain syndromes
- Nausea and vomiting (acute flare-ups)

Therapy: think astragalus (elevates interferon gamma) and colchicine (read papers by Michael Rask – not to be used during dental surgery or pregnancy)

General Guidelines for the Biological Treatment of Lyme Disease

Bee Venom Therapy

The most influential pioneer of this work was the beekeeper Charles Mraz from Middlebury, Vermont to whom I owe my health and understanding.

The pain relieving effect of bee venom in the treatment of clinical conditions similar to Lyme disease has been established a long time ago. Bee venom contains a number of potent peptides which are responsible for its healing effect ("Bee Venom Therapy for Chronic Pain, Dietrich Klinghardt, J. of Neurol and Orthop. Med and Surg., Vol. 11, Issue 9, Oct 1990, pp. 195-197).

Recent research proved that one of the peptides in bee venom, melittin, has a strong inhibitory effect on the Lyme spirochete at very low doses ("Bee Stings as Lyme Inhibitor" by L. L. Lubke and C. F. Garon, J. Clin. Infect. Diseases, July 1997, 25 Suppl. 1, pp. 48-51). When the spirochete is inhibited it does not multiply and is vulnerable to the host's own immune system and to medication.

The dosage and frequency of treatment is determined by the patient's clinical response. Patients with Babesia or Mycoplasma infections require higher dosages then those with only B. burgdorferi infections.

Different bee venoms are on the market. I use the product VeneX, which comes in two different strengths: VeneX-10 and VeneX-20 (Table 1.). VeneX-20 is twice as concentrated as VeneX-10. VeneX-10 contains 1.0 mg of bee venom per 1.0 ml. A 0.1 ml of this solution delivers approximately the same amount of bee venom as a natural bee sting. The venom is harvested and purified by Michael Simics who is worldwide considered the genius and master of this process, in which the bees are not harmed. VeneX Forte has added homeopathic dilutions of bee venom which has been most helpful in preventing allergic reactions.

The content of melittin in bee venom is dependent on where it is collected on the hive; the season and the pollen source the bees have access to at the time. Generally between one third and one half of the venom is melittin. Because of these variables the symptoms seen on administration of the venom can also vary. Bee venom is used for desensitization and is approved with the FDA for this purpose. There is an official monograph in the

Homeopathic Pharmacopoea of the United States (HPUS), also recognized by the FDA.

Product	Vial Size	DVSE* /	DVSE* /	DVSE* /	DVSE* /
VeneX-	9.0	90	10	1	0.5
VeneX-	12.5	250	20	2	1
* Dried Venom Sac Equivalent (DVSE): 0.1 mg bee venom					

Table 1. Comparison of Venom Solutions.

The average maintenance dosage is 1.0 ml of VeneX-10 (or 0.5 ml of VeneX-20) mixed with 2.0 ml preservative free buffered procaine (available from ApotheCure in Dallas, TX) injected subcutaneously, given between one and three times weekly for 6-12 months. Even though much of the venom's effect is systemic, independent of the location where it is given, additional benefits are observed by injecting the venom in specific target areas.

These areas include:

1. All tender areas in the body, transition areas in the body, where soft tissue meets bone, the occipital nuchal line, above and below the zygoma, around the mastoid and jaw bone, the para-sternal area, the spinous processes of the vertebrae;

2. The kidney and adrenal area (often palpation reveals significantly tender areas); tends to lessen allergic reactions, if treatment is started in this area for first few sessions

3. The thymus (upper end of the sternum);

4. Painful joints (in the most tender areas);

5. Acupuncture points (Bladder 23 for stimulating the adrenals, Gallbladder 1 to improve Lyme related problems with vision, Bladder 10 and Gallbladder 20 to stimulate melittin uptake into the brainstem (cranial nerve problems), Kidney 3 to improve Lyme related kidney dysfunction, etc.);

6. Neural therapy points: over the mastoid to improve Lyme related hearing and balance problems

7. Over the vagus nerve: to treat Lyme related dental and jaw problems (infected jaw bone, cavitations, Lyme related chronic pulpitis/sensitive teeth);

8. Frankenhauser points: to treat Lyme related bladder problems, pelvic/prostate/sexual dysfunction.

Procedure:

Distribute the 2.5 -3.0 ml bee venom and procaine mix over 10 areas, using 0.25 ml to 0.3 ml per injection. The injection is given with a 30 g " needle. The needle is advanced just deep enough for the needle tip to barely reach beyond the sensory skin nerves. Procaine does not lessen the bee venom effect as some practitioners falsely assume. However, lidocaine and marcaine disturb the sensitive peptides in bee venom. Bee venom should be kept in the fridge most the time but not frozen and protected from uv-rays and electromagnetic fields (like very living substance should).

If it burns, the needle is not deep enough. If it never burns, most likely the injections are given too deep, where the medication will be quickly flushed away by the blood stream and lymphatics, without having the much-desired local effect. For a "long needle this means that the needle is inserted into the skin less than half way.

These injections should be painless and well tolerated. There is a welling up, itchiness and aching after 10 minutes or so, which becomes less with an increasing number of treatments. The discomfort may increase during the first four or five treatments and then lessen over time. The initial response determines the treatment frequency. The first injection often triggers an increase in well-being and a decrease of pain levels after a few hours; sometimes as late as 24 hours after the injection.

It may take several weeks of treatment before the first positive results are observed. The initial improvement may last between 12 hours and several days. This determines if the patient needs to be treated once a day or as little as once/week. If the improvement is less than desired a higher dose of bee venom may be needed.

I start with a low initial dose of 0.1 ml VeneX-10 or 0.05 ml VeneX-20 to ride out the often strong initial reactions. Over the next treatments I increase the dose, depending on the response, rather rapidly to the full treatment dose (Table 2. and Table 3.). It is wise to wait with injecting around the head until the patient no longer has strong local reactions (redness, swelling).

For the first 4-6 months the injections have to be given every other day, after that time, when the client and symptoms are stabilized, twice weekly until the patient is lastingly stable and well. Bee venom has a positive synergistic effect with most herbs but seems weakened by the concomitant use of antibiotics. I stop bee venom during courses of antibiotics but resume immediately afterwards.

The Herbs

Always take the herbs together with **Matrix Electrolyte** or ME (BioPure) for better absorption and transport of the active ingredients through the matrix to the cell membrane. ME also activates all functions of the ANS and improves trans-cell-membrane communication. **Freeze dried garlic** has a profound stabilizing effect in most symptomatic patients. It should either be taken immediately after meals on a full stomach (2-3 cap 3-4 times/day) or 2 caps should be dissolved in 1-2oz of water and taken away from meals.

1. BioPure PC Samento

(pentacyclic TOA-reduced energetically modified, ethically wild-crafted Amazon Cat's Claw):

In my work this product has shown the most consistent action against Borrelia, Bartonella, Ehrlichiosis, Rickettsia, mycoplasma and other co-infefctions. Herxheimer reactions are expected and may occur at any stage of the treatment (on the first day of use or after many months) and repeatedly. During the "Herxes"I recommend colon hydrotherapy, KMT lymphatic drainage, raw food diet, moderate exercise, drinking more water then usual, a massage and a nurturing environment.

Dosage: start with 4 drops twice daily (or 8 dr/day). Wait one week before increasing. If condition worsens, reduce dose. Sometimes patients initially tolerate only 1 drop/day (rare). Final dose: 2 dropperful/day

Contraindication: organ transplant immunotherapy. Don't use if trying to become pregnant. May interfere with blood thinning treatment

2. PC-Noni
(a concentrated energy-enhanced extract of Noni where the ingredients are made bio-available with a unique proprietary process)
It is in our experience the most reliable remedy to treat and eliminate intracellular microbes over time. This process is slow (months) and very rewarding. Several German practitioners have found this amazing property mostly with darkfield microscopy. I am not aware of unbiased published studies to confirm this. However, it is consistent with our ART findings and clinical observation.

Dosage: start with 6 drops twice daily and increase to a total of 3 dropper full/day for 1 year.

I suggest the each person makes a 1 liter glass bottle of filtered water in the morning and add the herbs for the day one by one into the bottle. Since PC Samento and PC Noni are also carriers for sophisticated anti-Lyme frequencies, the bottle should be sucussed 50 times after introducing PC Samento and again after introducing PC Noni. If other herbs are added to the bottle both should be added last. The content should then be taken throughout the day and used up by bedtime. It is best to take our herbs away from food. PC Samento has to be activated by acid. Either add the daily dose of Rechtsregulat (acidic ph) into the bottle or take on empty stomach, when stomach-ph is low.

3. Artemisinin
has disappointed in our experience in the treatment of Babesia, unless given in very high doses: 1200-1500 mg/day given 3 days in a row, repeat after a 2 week break. This is the way the drug is used in China for treatment of Malaria. After the initial 2 courses a 2-3 day course should be given once/month

Contraindication: early pregnancy

The expanded herbal Lyme PDR

4. Andrographis paniculata:

Science:

rapid excretion via kidneys

anti-spirochetal

crosses blood brain barrier

protects heart muscle
anti-inflammatory
calming
potent modulating effect on mast cell and neutrophil activity: turns off inappropriate mast-cell allergic reactions in tissue
enhances liver function
significant **protective** effects against inflammation-mediated **neurodegeneration** of brain, spinal chord and CSF

Other published positive effects:
filaria
leptospirosis
malaria (suggesting strong effect against Babesia)
decreases heart muscle damage after MI
Hepatitis A and B
tuberculosis
tonsillitis
pneumonia
snake bites
e.coli
herpes viruses
mumps
periodontal bacteria (gum disease)
AIDS
cancers: prostate breast colon anal stomach skin melanoma
leukemia

Dosage: 400 mg capsules standardized to 10% androgrpholides
Start with 1 cap 4 times/day. Slowly increase to 3 caps 4 times/day. Stay on this dose till Lyme sx significantly decreased, then slowly decrease dose. Stop during severe Herxheimer reactions. 1 year

Contraindications: andrograpis lowers progesterone (natural contraceptive), pregnancy, acute gallbladder disease

5. Polygonum cuspidatum (Japanese Knotweed)
Peer review literature/Science
Effective against:
Leptospirosis
Treponema denticola (spirochets in oral flora)

Bartonella (Buhner)
Many gram neg and gram pos bacteria
Anti-viral
Hepatitis B (and C?)

Other published positive effects:
Crosses blood brain barrier: anti-inflammatory, antimicrobial, protects against microbial endotoxins
High content of resveratrol increases microcirculation (vasodilation and inhibits platelet aggregation: pos effect on eye, heart, skin (ideal synergist)
Lowers cholesterol and lipids
Increases wound healing
Angiogenesis modulator
Ischemic heart disease
Potent antioxidant
Inhibits lipoxygenase (anti-inflammatory)
Inhibition prostaglandin E
Inhibits nuclear factor kappa B (NF kB) which upregulated in Lyme causing a cascade of immune mediated cellular responses
Leukemia
Stimulates fibroblasts (proliferative effect)
Rheumatoid arthritis
Psoriasis
Increases bone mass
Anti-aging
Reduces auto-immunity
Strongly neuroprotective
Effects against: ALS, Alzheimer, Parkinson MS cerebral ischemia
Stimulates microcirculation in brain

Dosage: Whole herb (Hu Zhang) standardized to 8% total resveratrols and 10 mg resveratrol. Source Naturals 500 mg tablet.
Use 3-4 caps 3-4 times/day. Work up slowly to this dose

Contraindications: Pregnancy, Consider carefully when giving with blood thinners (synergistic effect)

Overdose: GI-symptoms

6. Smilax glabra (Sarsaparilla)

Peer review literature/Science:
effective against:

- Leptospirosis
- Treponema pallidum (syphilis)
- liver flukes (clonorchis sinensis)
- trypanosome
- shigella and salmonella (common in chromnic Lyme)
- leprosy and TB
- fungal skin infections

Other published results:

- Lyme endotoxin binding
- Lessens Herxheimer reactions
- Improvement in **mental and psychological** parameters in chronic syphilis
- Modulates immune responses
- **Arthritis** anti-inflammatory
- **Psoriasis** and eczema
- Neuroprotective (crosses blood brain barrier)
- Reduces skin breakdown
- Pain relief
- Improves liver function
- Lessens **fatigue**
- Increases libido
- Asthma, hay fever, rhinitis
- **Cervical spondylosis** (Lyme related disc degeneration and facet joint arthritis)
- Chronic liver disease (dramatic) including Hepatitis C
- Reversal of cognitive impairment
- Autoimmune dysregulation
- Protects from anti-androgenic substances in Lyme (ie gossypol)

Dosage: 425-500 mg caps 1-3 caps 3-4 times/day. Increase slowly to full dosage, stay on it for 2 months, then slowly reduce to amintainance dose of 1 caps 3 times/day. At least 1 year

Contraindications: Increased digitalis and Bismuth absorbtion (careful with Am. Biologics Lyme protocol), increased elimination of hypnotic drugs

7. Stephania Root (Stephania tetrandra and S.cepharantha)

Peer review literature/Science:
effective against:

- Potent anti-inflammatory
- Alopecia
- Radiation injury (leukemia)
- Asthma
- Induces IL-1 beta, IL-alpha, TNF-a, IL-6, IL-8 (especially in CNS and joints)
- Reduces NF-kappa B and IL-6 during neuroborreliosis
- Modulates HLA-DR expression (Lyme arthritis connected to CD3 generated HLA-DR alleles)
- Treatment of silicosis (also breast implant immune complications)
- Protects endothelium form endotoxin damage
- Reduces vascular permeability
- Bell's palsy
- Free radical scavenger
- Inhibits toxic glutamate levels in brain
- Ca-channel blocker
- Asthma and heart disease
- Retinopathy (modulates formation of new blood vessels and improvement of vision)
- Malaria (and Babesia)
- Inhibits cancer cell proliferation
- Anti-fibrotic/anti-scar formation
- Blocks abnormal histamine release/stabilizes mast cells

Dosage: 1:5 tincture of both forms of Stepania, -1 tsp t.i.d.

Contraindication: use judgement when using together with Ca-channel blockers. Constipation. May potentiate the effect of other drugs.

8. Other important herbs:

Teasel Root: give high doses over 3 months (1-2 tsp 3-4 times/day)

Has been shown first by German ethno-botanist Stoerl to be highly effective against Bb.

Good for **arthritis** and Lyme related insomnia

Turmeric, nettle and devils claw also good for Lyme-arthritis

Poke Root and Red Root for lymphatic drainage

Colchicum autumnale: effective against Ehrlichiosis. Best used iv (Eli Lilly). Give 1 amp (=1 mg) twice weekly for 6 weeks. Has to be given strictly i.v. with 25 g butterfly, otherwise causes severe long lasting burn. Alternative: oral tincure: 15 -20 drops daily for 7 days. Repeat after 2 week pause. 4-6 courses

Astragalus: potent anti-viral. Good synergistic effects with the other herbs. Elevates interferon gamma which is depressed in Ehrlichiosis, MS and many of the more severe Lyme related illnesses

Practical Considerations and Recipes:

Neuroborreliosis:

- read and understand the "Klinghardt Neurotoxin Elimination Protocol"
- bee venom therapy is superior
- most patients have a degree of kryptopyrroluria (excretion of abnormal hemoglobin breakdown products) which leads to a loss of excessive amounts of zinc, B6, and Omega 6 fatty acids. It is recognized by either ART testing or by finding a low or low normal alkaline phosphatase (below 50). Replace zinc, copper, Magnesium, B6 (I ask the client to increase the amount until he/she has vivid dreams regularly) Niacin (work up to 3000 mg/day) and Udo's oil.
- Do not give zinc without copper in Lyme!
- Use KMT to vagus, spheno-palatine ganglion and superior cervical ganglion. Always use Rechtsregulat to reach microcirculation.
- Always use BioPure "Phospholipid Exchange".
- In Bell's palsy use Stephania root.1 tsp t.i.d.
- At least 2/3rds of clients with Bb also have a Babesia co-infection which has to be treated early.
- Use polygonum, smilax and andrographis early on
- Use neural therapy, especially in the ganglia together with glutathione or DMPS

Considerations in connective tissue/lyme **arthritis**:

- Bee venom therapy is most effective in the long run

- antioxidants (especially polygonum/resveratrol), cetyl-meristoleate, intra-articular ozone injections)
- para-joint neural therapy
- APN desensitization
- L-carnosine and growth hormone for premature tissue aging (collagen breakdown).
- KMT therapy directly to involved joint
- Consider high dose enzyme therapy
- Use Stephania root tsp t.i.d.

Ocular borreliosis:

- Bee venom therapy very effective (sting Gb-1 and SI-3 regularly)
- high doses B2 (700-1000 mg/day) for a few months
- eyebright tincture 2 dropperfull 2-3 times/day
- gingko extract
- KMT microcurrent directly to the eye
- Manual lymph/fluid drainage to eye (Klinghardt method)
- Use Stephania root 1 tsp t.i.d.and Polygonum! Valuable especially for macular degeneration

Lyme **carditis**:

- Systemic bee venom therapy 3 times/week for 3 months, then 2 times/week till resolved (years)
- always use antibiotics early on in high doses
- Use KMT over stellate ganglia and right vagus
- APN desensitization
- Use neural therapy over the heart with Enderlein remedies (Pleo SanBruc, San Strep, Nig and Muc, Lat)
- Always use "Phospholipid Exchange" from BioPure
- Turn off excessive immune activity with auto-urine therapy
- Use the herbs: andrographis, polygonum and hawthorne.

Ehrlichiosis:

- include Colchicine injections (or Colchicum drops) and astragalus

Bartonella:

- include Polygonum/ Resveratrol

References in: "Healing Lyme – Naturtal Healing and Prevention of Lyme Borreliosis and its Co-Infections" Stephen Buhner Raven Press 2005

Treatment should always keep in mind that our immune-system is in a never- ending training and adaptation program. We are evolving. The same is true for the microbes. We are seeking a peaceful inner state - in which microbes are welcome as long as they contribute to the greater whole.

We do not yet understand Lyme disease in this way, but our unconscious and our immune-system does. Plant adaptogens have far greater potential in helping us in this necessary process of evolution then any man-made chemical compound. Plant medicines are intelligent, human medications are usually quite dumb. Antibiotics have their place, but it is limited.

LYME DISEASE
Overview and Laboratory Testing

Dr. Jyotsna S. Shah
Laboratory Director
IGeneX, Inc

May 18, 2008

1

WHAT IS LYME DISEASE?

Lyme disease is the illness caused by the bacteria B. burgdorferi (Bb) and related co-infections that result from the bite of an infected deer tick.

2

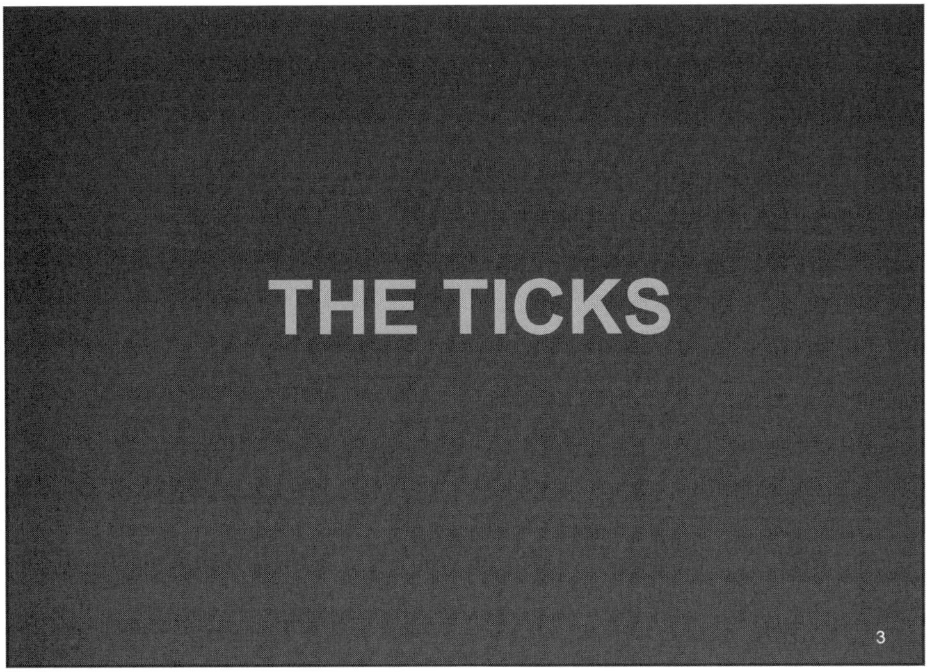
THE TICKS
3

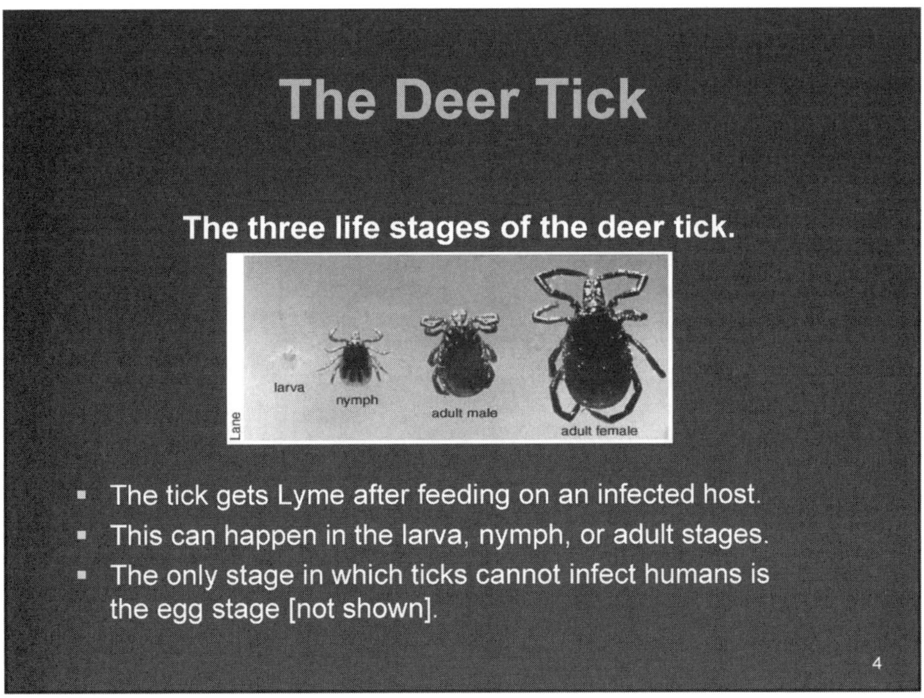
The Deer Tick
The three life stages of the deer tick.
larva
nymph
adult male
adult female
Lane
▪ The tick gets Lyme after feeding on an infected host.
▪ This can happen in the larva, nymph, or adult stages.
▪ The only stage in which ticks cannot infect humans is the egg stage [not shown].
4

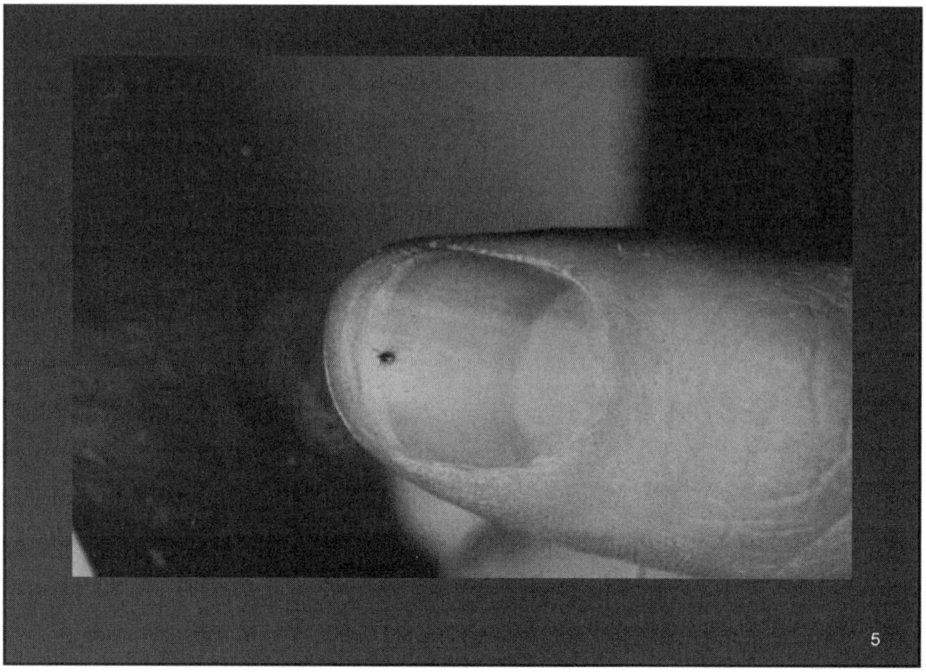
5

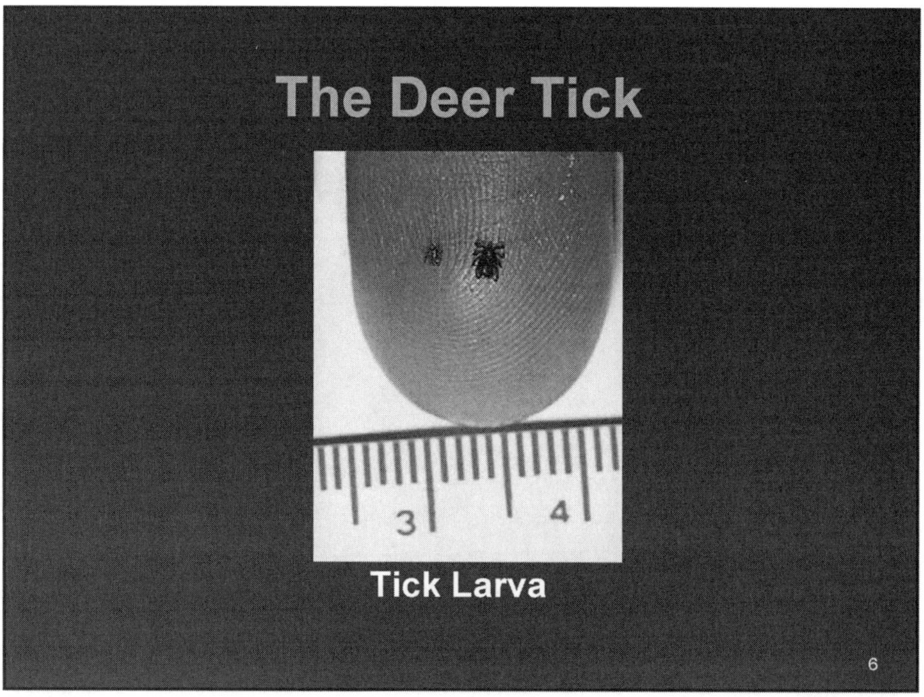
The Deer Tick
3
4
Tick Larva
6

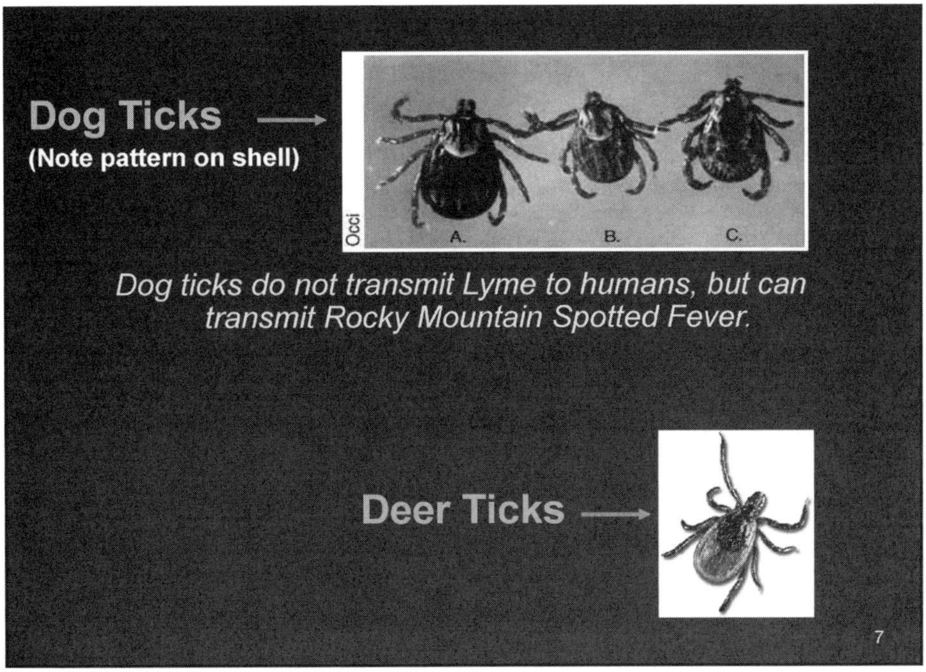
Dog Ticks
(Note pattern on shell)
Occi
A.
B.
C.
Dog ticks do not transmit Lyme to humans, but can transmit Rocky Mountain Spotted Fever.
Deer Ticks
7

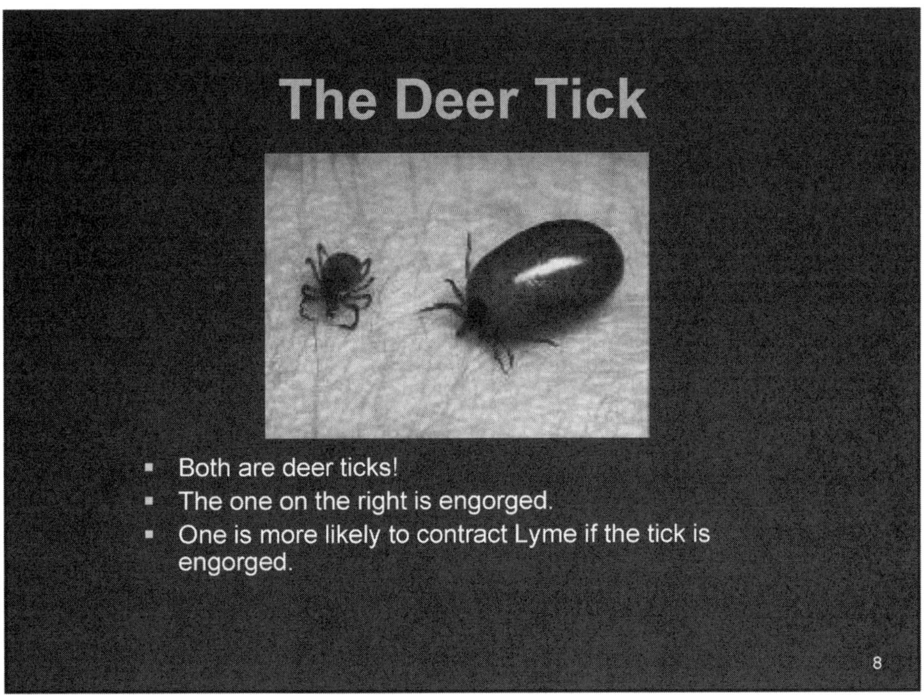
The Deer Tick
Both are deer ticks!
The one on the right is engorged.
One is more likely to contract Lyme if the tick is engorged.
8

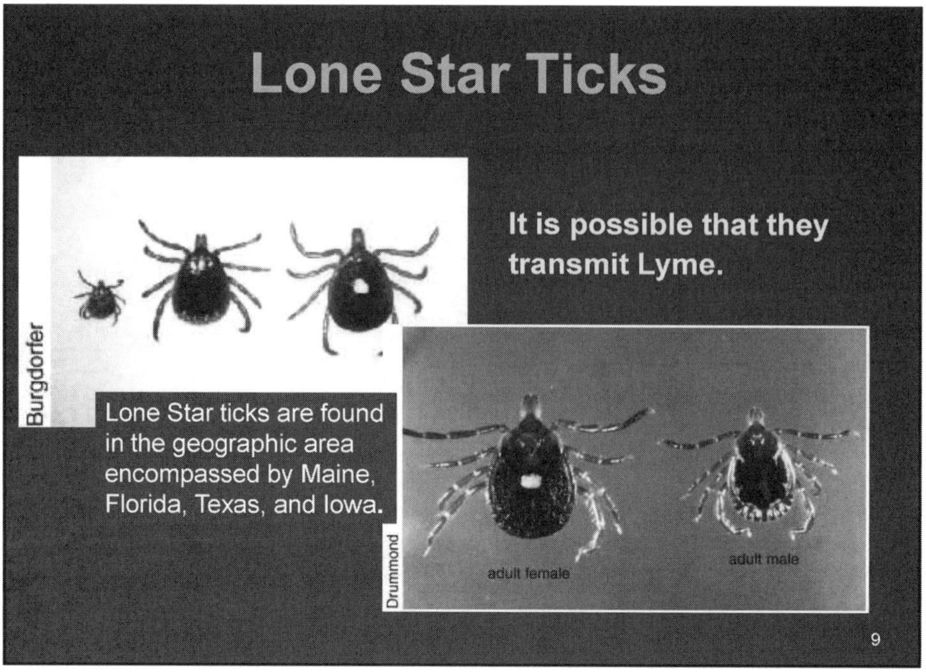
Lone Star Ticks
It is possible that they transmit Lyme.
Burgdorfer
Lone Star ticks are found in the geographic area encompassed by Maine, Florida, Texas, and Iowa.
Drummond
adult female
adult male
9

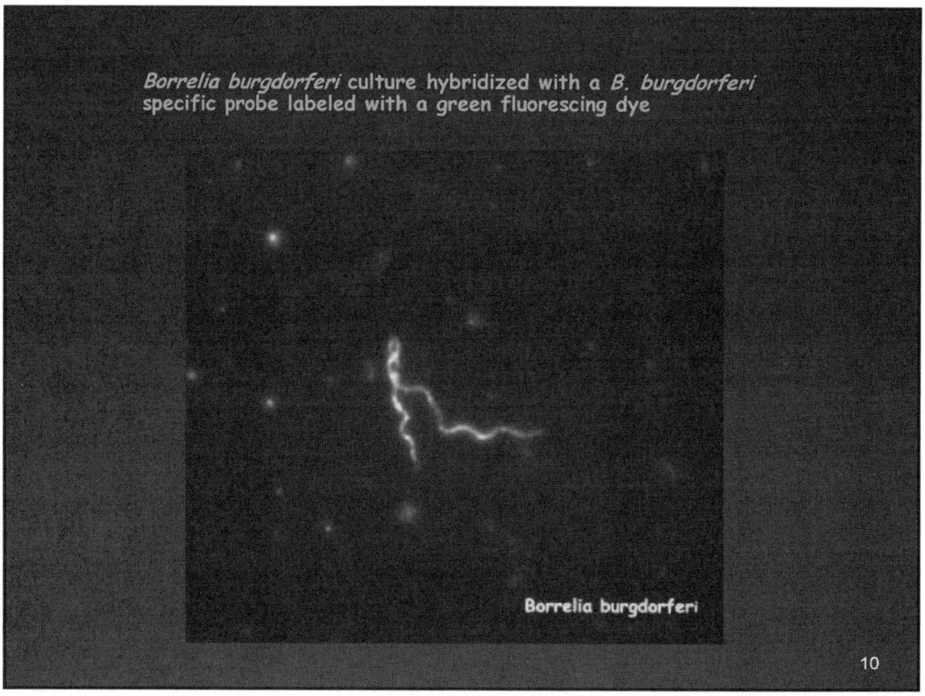
Borrelia burgdorferi culture hybridized with a *B. burgdorferi* specific probe labeled with a green fluorescing dye
Borrelia burgdorferi
10

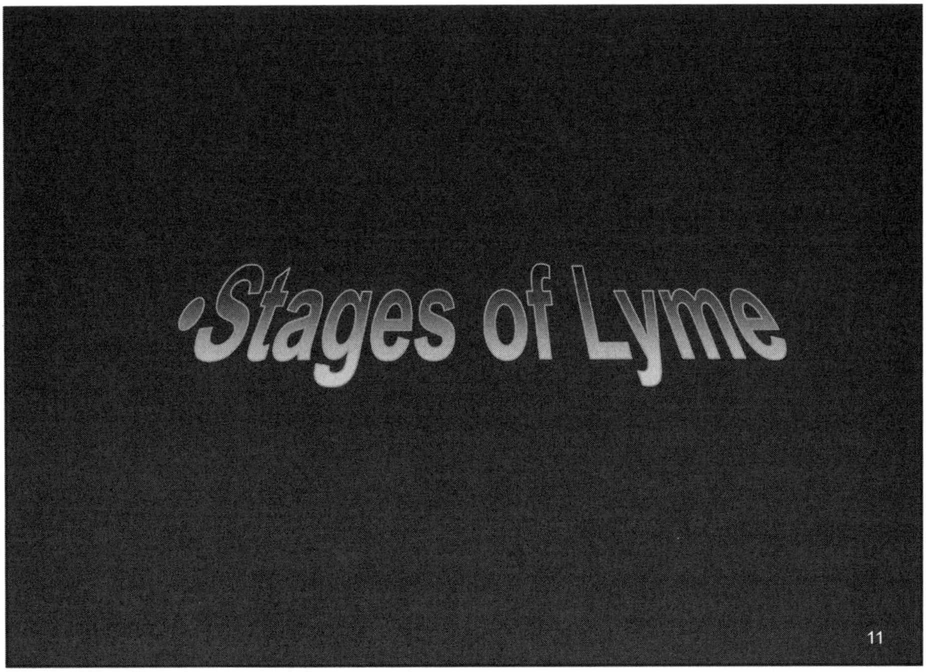
Stages of Lyme
11

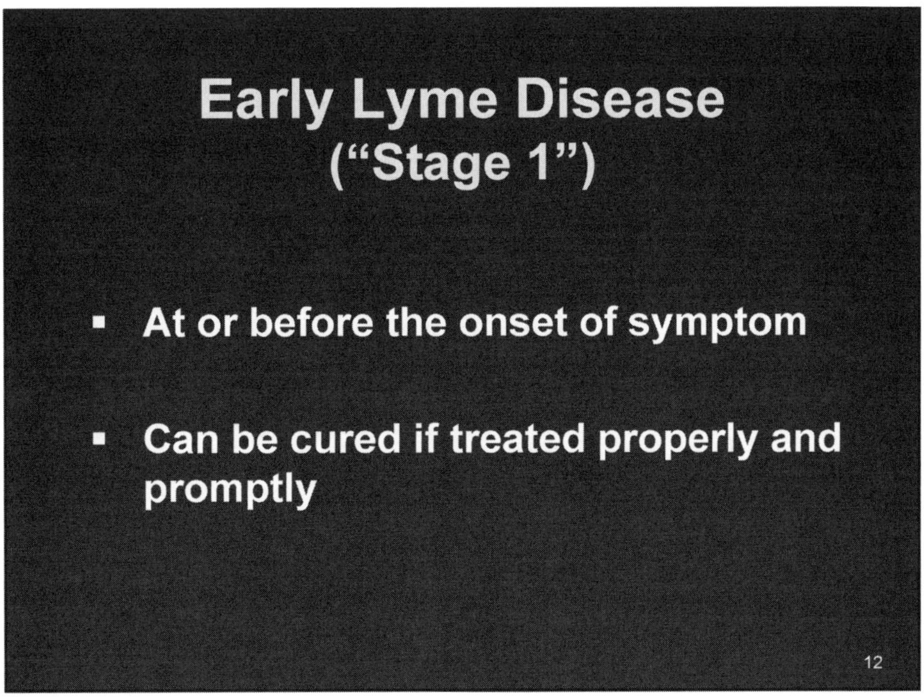
Early Lyme Disease
("Stage 1")
▪ At or before the onset of symptom
▪ Can be cured if treated properly and promptly
12

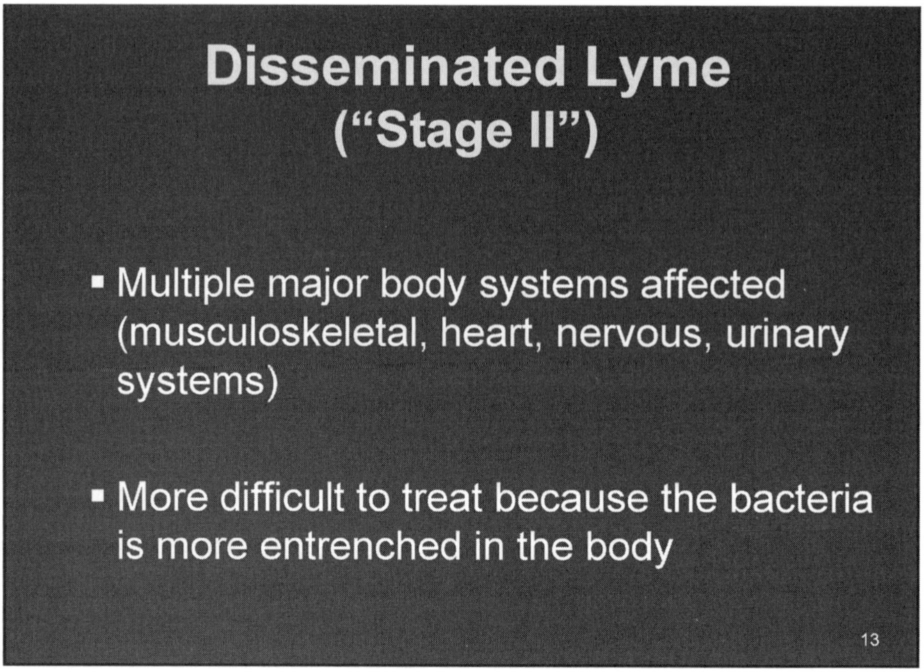
Disseminated Lyme
("Stage II")
▪ Multiple major body systems affected (musculoskeletal, heart, nervous, urinary systems)
▪ More difficult to treat because the bacteria is more entrenched in the body
13

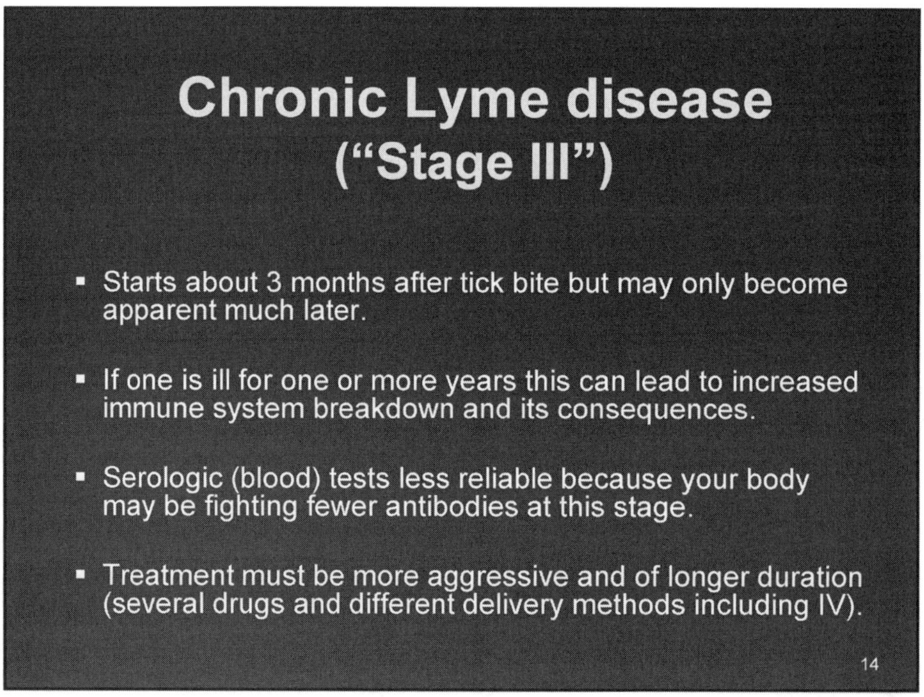
Chronic Lyme disease
("Stage III")
▪ Starts about 3 months after tick bite but may only become apparent much later.
▪ If one is ill for one or more years this can lead to increased immune system breakdown and its consequences.
▪ Serologic (blood) tests less reliable because your body may be fighting fewer antibodies at this stage.
▪ Treatment must be more aggressive and of longer duration (several drugs and different delivery methods including IV).
14

DIAGNOSING LYME

Lyme is a "clinical diagnosis"

- A clinical diagnosis is based on a patient's history and symptoms but is not definitive the way a laboratory test is. Tests can be insensitive or provide false positives so it is difficult to tell for sure if a patient does or does not have Lyme.
- Only 17% of people with Lyme recall a bite (Texas Dept. of Health; Dutchess Co. Dept. of Health).
- Only 36% recall a rash [typical symptom of Lyme] (Texas Dept. of Health).
- Only 50% to 70% have a positive ELISA or Western Blot [2 most common blood tests]

15

EARLY LYME
("Stage I")

- *Rapid diagnosis is critical- fully curable at this stage*
  - Start treatment at first sign of rash- do not wait for blood tests, which take weeks to become positive
  - May NEVER get a positive test!
  - If no rash, but high suspicion, treat, observe clinically, and wait for tests.
- *Symptoms*
  - Tiredness, body and head aches, stiff neck, abdominal pain, swollen glands, even pink eye.

16

Identifying Erythema Migrans

Lyme disease-induced rashes

- TYPICAL "BULLSEYE" RASH
- Several concentric circles
- Expands over time
- Painless
- Raised
- May be warm

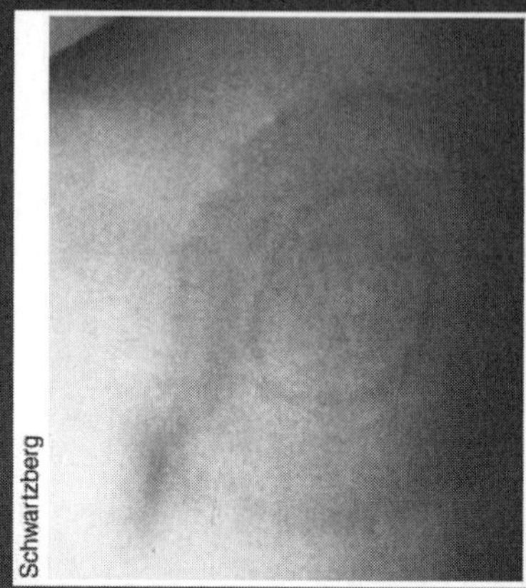

17

EARLY LYME IS STILL DANGEROUS

- At Stage I, early Lyme may already be disseminated and patients are symptomatic.
- A patient can think it's a minor problem, but it may have already spread throughout the body.
- You don't necessarily have to wait six weeks to see Lyme disseminate.

18

DISSEMINATED LYME ("Stage II")

- Clinical diagnosis (always is!)
- Lyme may be present despite negative blood tests.
- Look for multisystem involvement with symptoms that move and vary over time.
  - Example: You may have a sore elbow for a time that disappears, but then you have a sore knee. That goes away and then you have headaches. That goes away. Then you have confusion. This makes it obvious that something is moving around in your body. Some weeks are bad and other weeks are fine. These symptoms can lead to patients being diagnosed as hypochondriacs instead of having Lyme.
- Will need antibiotic therapy for at least several months.

19

Why Do We Test?

- To Confirm Clinical Diagnosis, since Lyme Disease symptoms are often confused with MS, Chronic Fatigue, osteo-arthritis, etc.
- To ensure patient that he or she is getting the right treatment.

20

Who Do You Test With?

- CLIA Certified
- Medicare Approved
- New York State Approved
- California Approved

FDA Approval NOT Required

21

Lyme Disease Testing

Indirect Tests: Detection of Patient's Immune responses to Borrelia burgdorferi, causative agent of Lyme Disease.

Serology (C6, ELISA), Western blots, Immunofluorescence

Direct Tests: Detection of the Borrelia burgdorferi, specific proteins (antigens), DNA and RNA, in patient clinical specimen (blood, serum, urine, CSF, etc.)

Culture, Lyme Urine Antigen (LDA), PCR, Reverse Western blot (for Confirmation of LDA Positive, PCR Negative Samples)

IgX

22

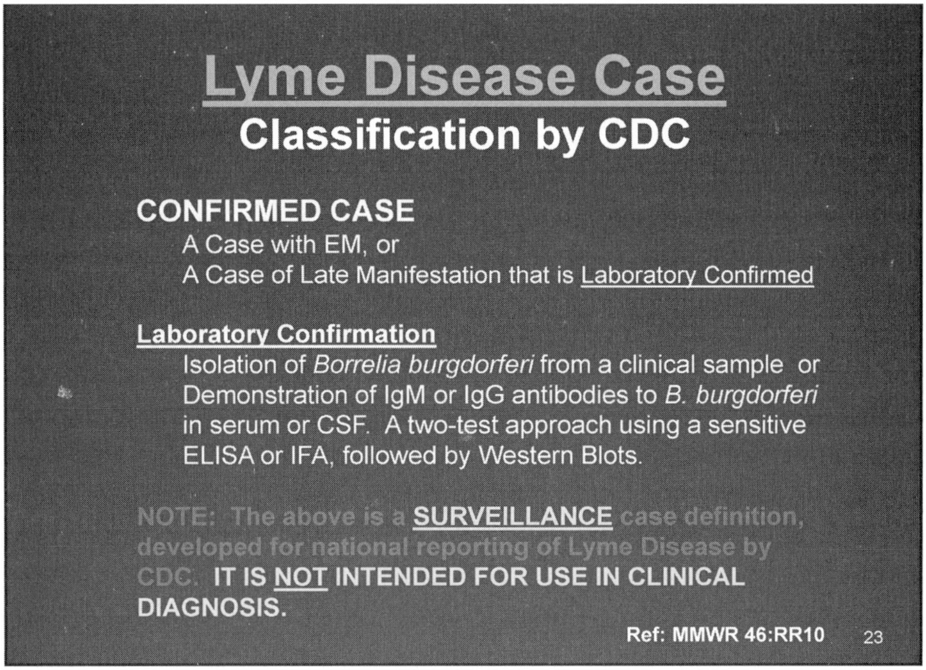
Lyme Disease Case
Classification by CDC
CONFIRMED CASE
A Case with EM, or
A Case of Late Manifestation that is Laboratory Confirmed
Laboratory Confirmation
Isolation of *Borrelia burgdorferi* from a clinical sample or
Demonstration of IgM or IgG antibodies to *B. burgdorferi*
in serum or CSF. A two-test approach using a sensitive
ELISA or IFA, followed by Western Blots.
NOTE: The above is a SURVEILLANCE case definition,
developed for national reporting of Lyme Disease by
CDC. IT IS NOT INTENDED FOR USE IN CLINICAL
DIAGNOSIS.
Ref: MMWR 46:RR10
23

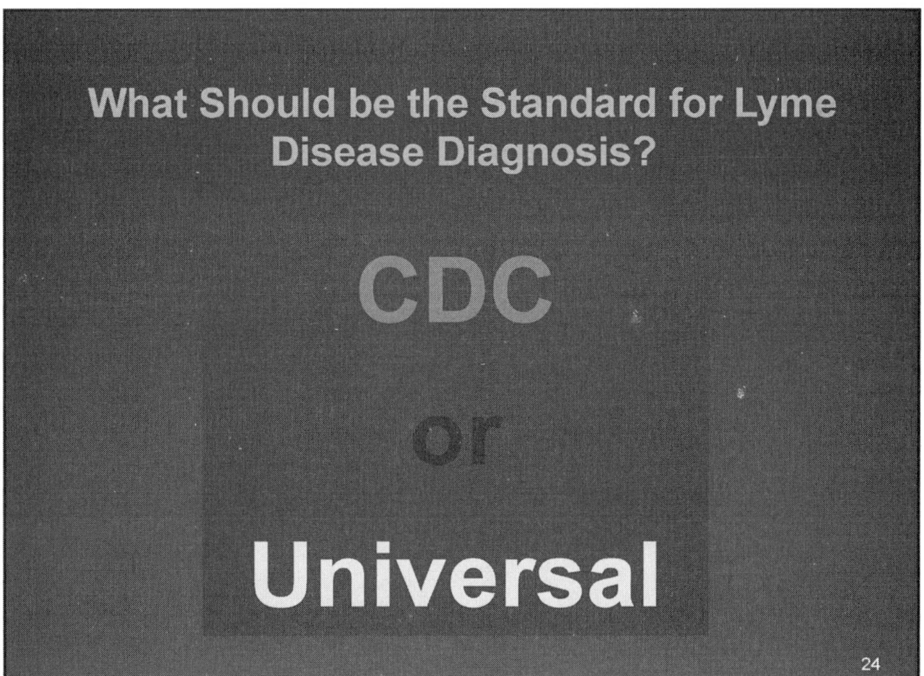
What Should be the Standard for Lyme
Disease Diagnosis?
CDC
or
Universal
24

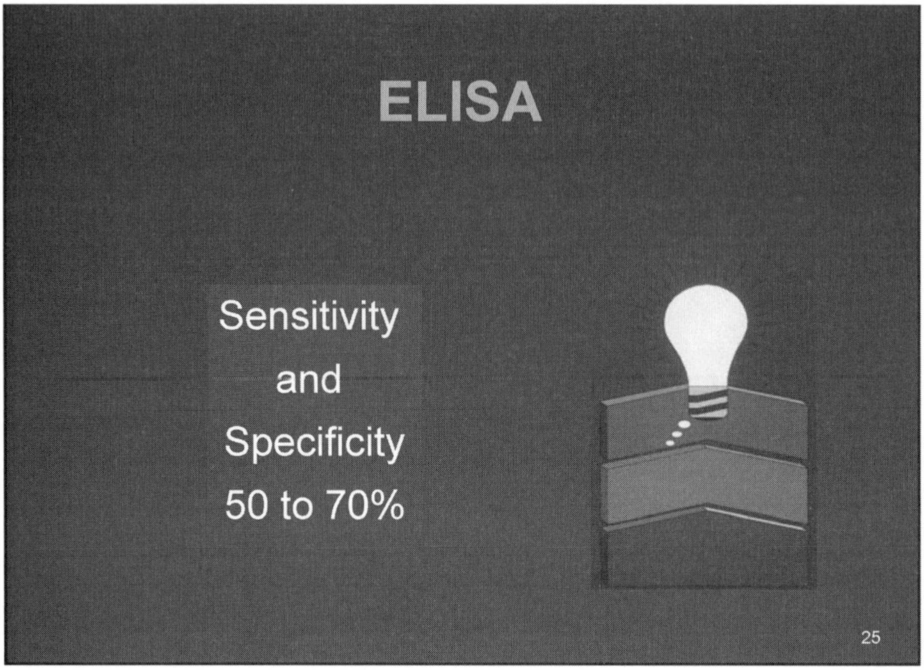
ELISA
Sensitivity
and
Specificity
50 to 70%
25

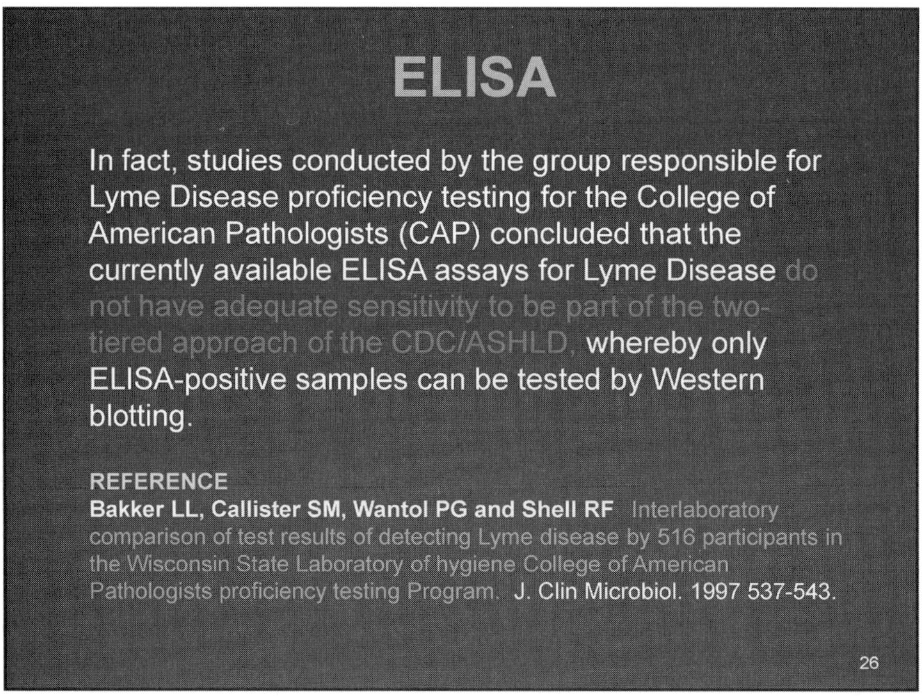
ELISA
In fact, studies conducted by the group responsible for Lyme Disease proficiency testing for the College of American Pathologists (CAP) concluded that the currently available ELISA assays for Lyme Disease do not have adequate sensitivity to be part of the two-tiered approach of the CDC/ASHLD, whereby only ELISA-positive samples can be tested by Western blotting.
REFERENCE
Bakker LL, Callister SM, Wantol PG and Shell RF Interlaboratory comparison of test results of detecting Lyme disease by 516 participants in the Wisconsin State Laboratory of hygiene College of American Pathologists proficiency testing Program. J. Clin Microbiol. 1997 537-543.
26

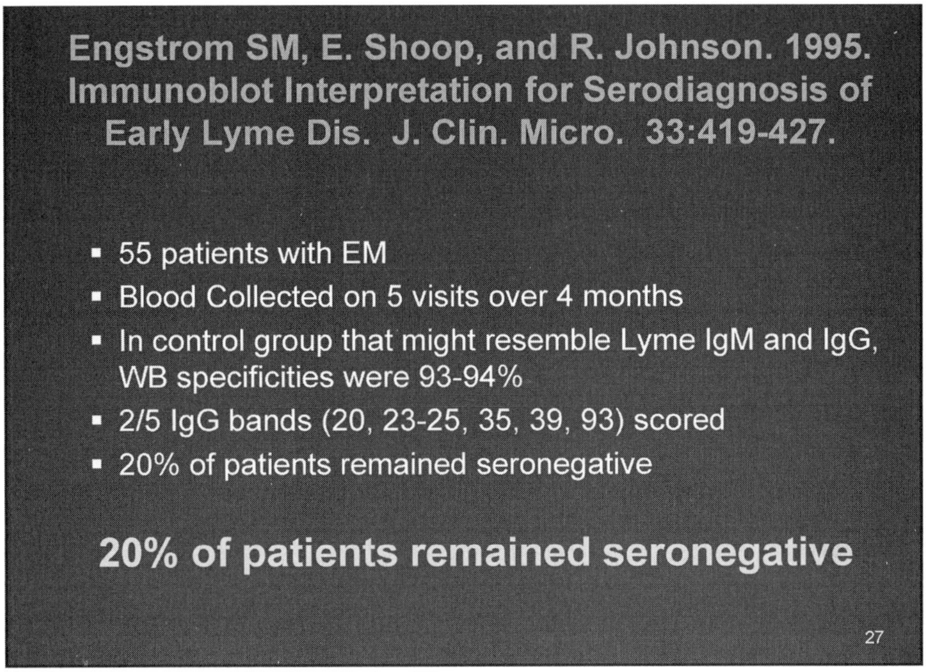
Engstrom SM, E. Shoop, and R. Johnson. 1995. Immunoblot Interpretation for Serodiagnosis of Early Lyme Dis. J. Clin. Micro. 33:419-427.
▪ 55 patients with EM
▪ Blood Collected on 5 visits over 4 months
▪ In control group that might resemble Lyme IgM and IgG, WB specificities were 93-94%
▪ 2/5 IgG bands (20, 23-25, 35, 39, 93) scored
▪ 20% of patients remained seronegative
20% of patients remained seronegative
27

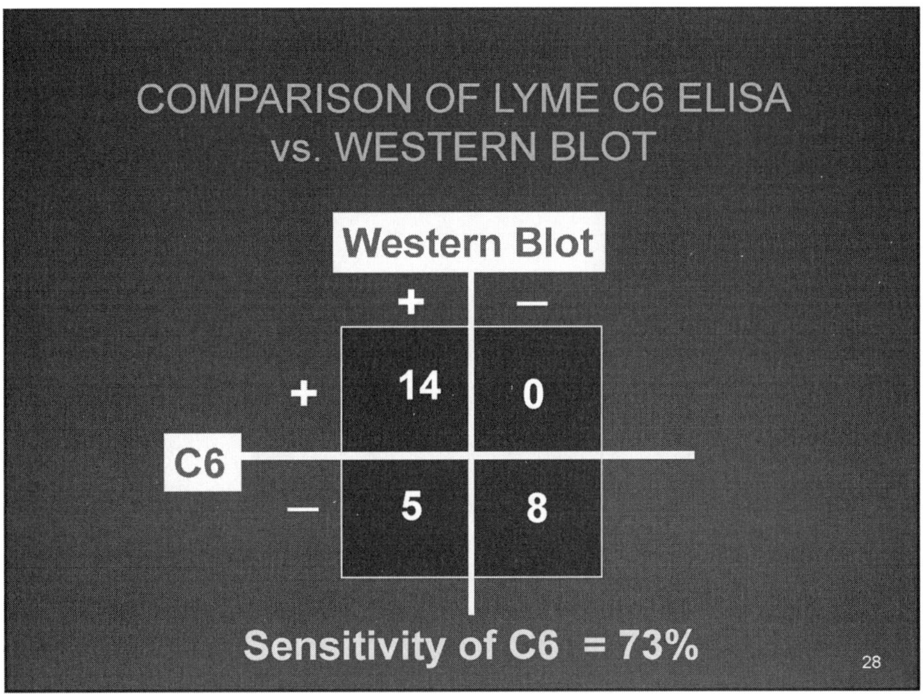
COMPARISON OF LYME C6 ELISA vs. WESTERN BLOT
Western Blot
+
—
C6
+
—
14
0
5
8
Sensitivity of C6 = 73%
28

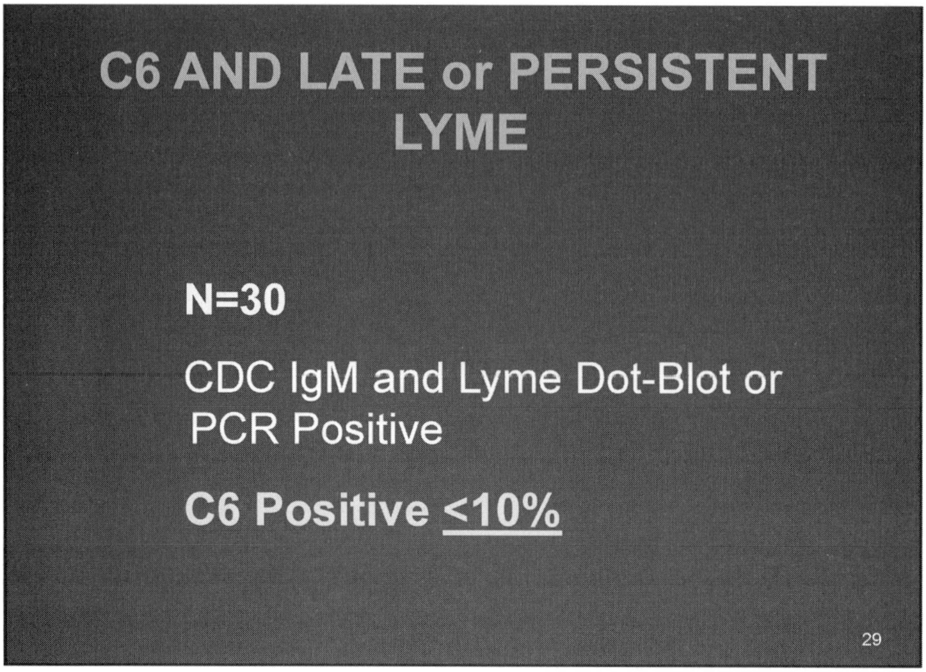
C6 AND LATE or PERSISTENT LYME
N=30
CDC IgM and Lyme Dot-Blot or PCR Positive
C6 Positive <10%
29

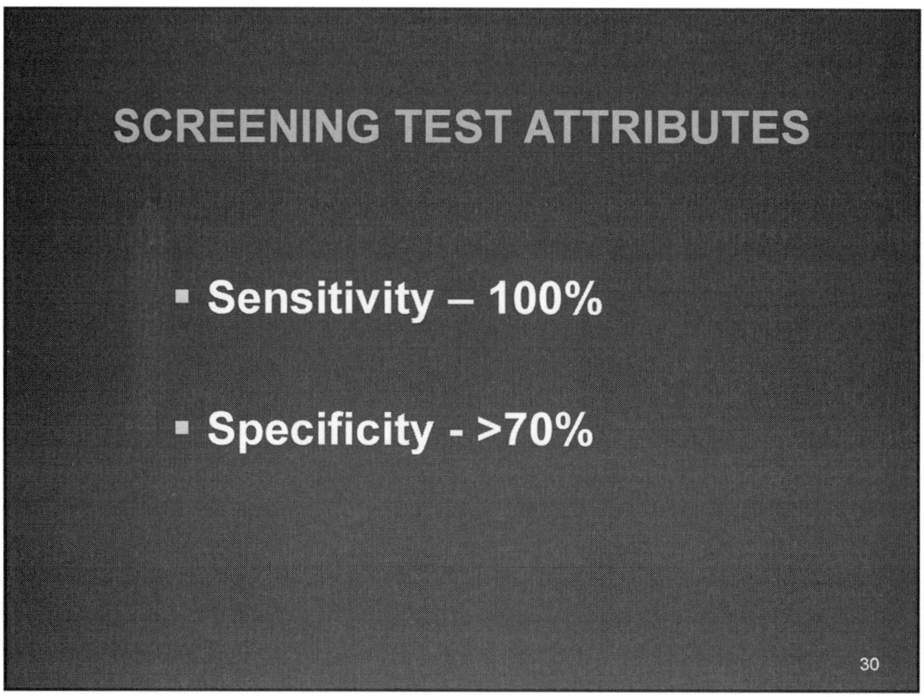
SCREENING TEST ATTRIBUTES
Sensitivity – 100%
Specificity - >70%
30

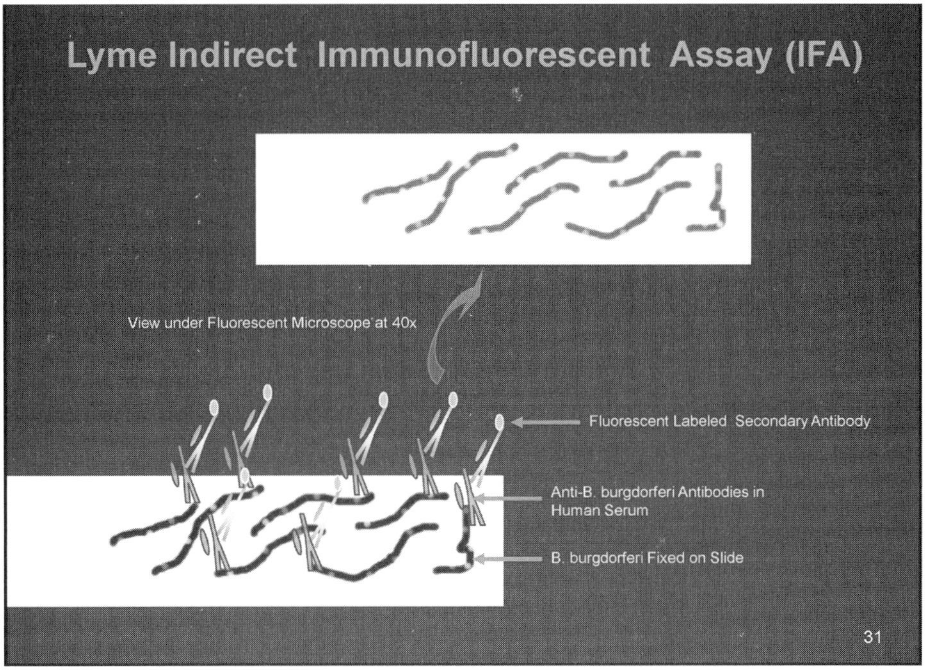
Lyme Indirect Immunofluorescent Assay (IFA)
View under Fluorescent Microscope at 40x
Fluorescent Labeled Secondary Antibody
Anti-B. burgdorferi Antibodies in Human Serum
B. burgdorferi Fixed on Slide
31

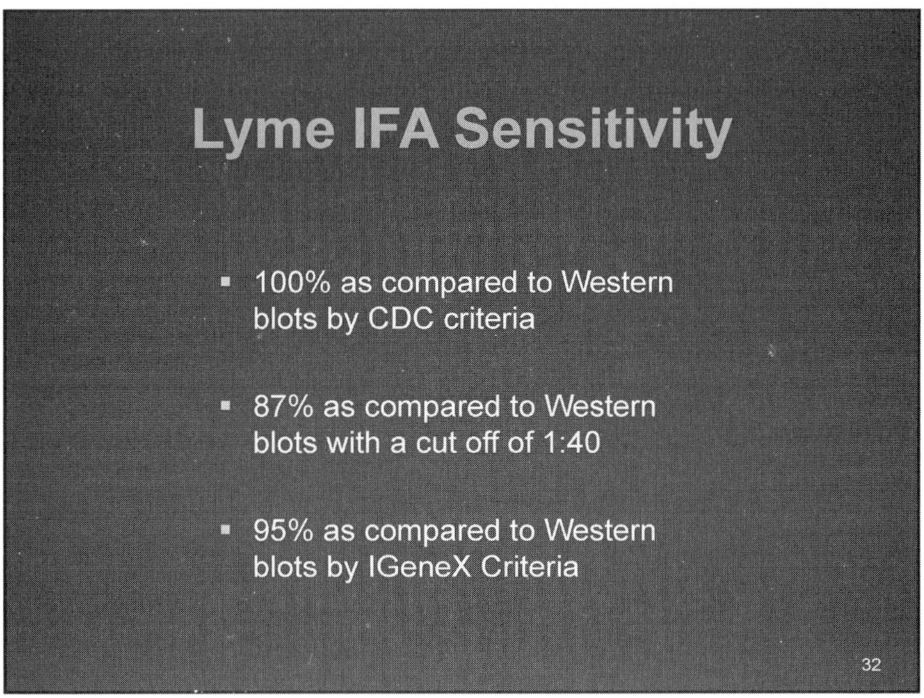
Lyme IFA Sensitivity
▪ 100% as compared to Western blots by CDC criteria
▪ 87% as compared to Western blots with a cut off of 1:40
▪ 95% as compared to Western blots by IGeneX Criteria
32

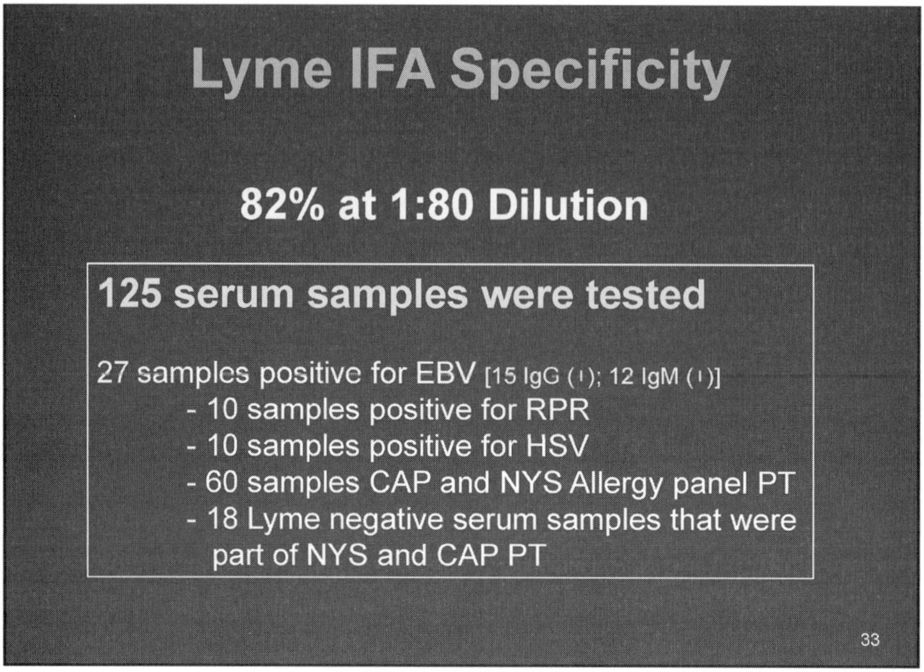
Lyme IFA Specificity
82% at 1:80 Dilution
125 serum samples were tested
27 samples positive for EBV [15 IgG (+); 12 IgM (+)]
- 10 samples positive for RPR
- 10 samples positive for HSV
- 60 samples CAP and NYS Allergy panel PT
- 18 Lyme negative serum samples that were part of NYS and CAP PT
33

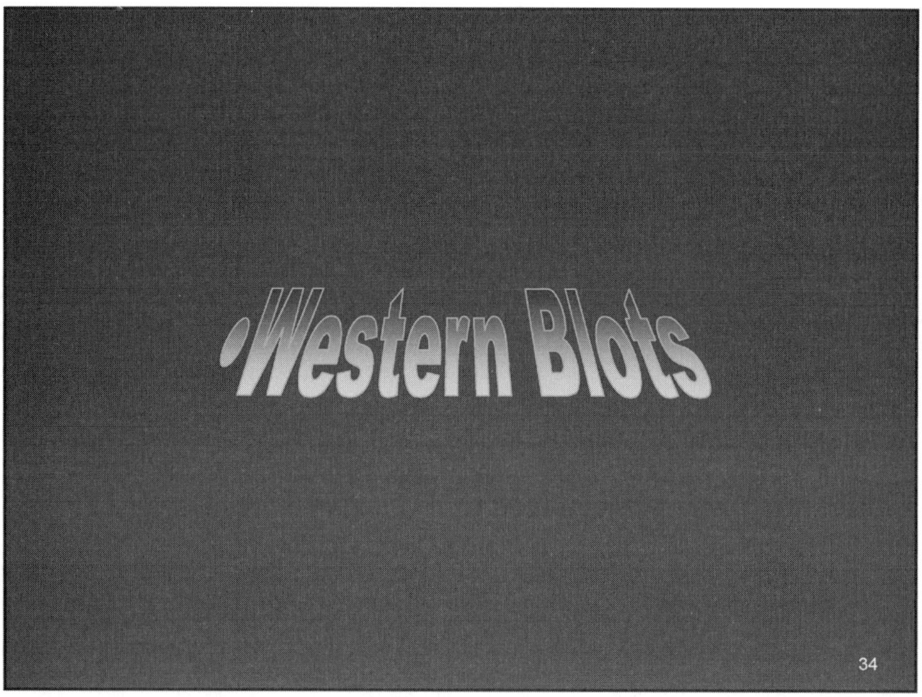
•Western Blots
34

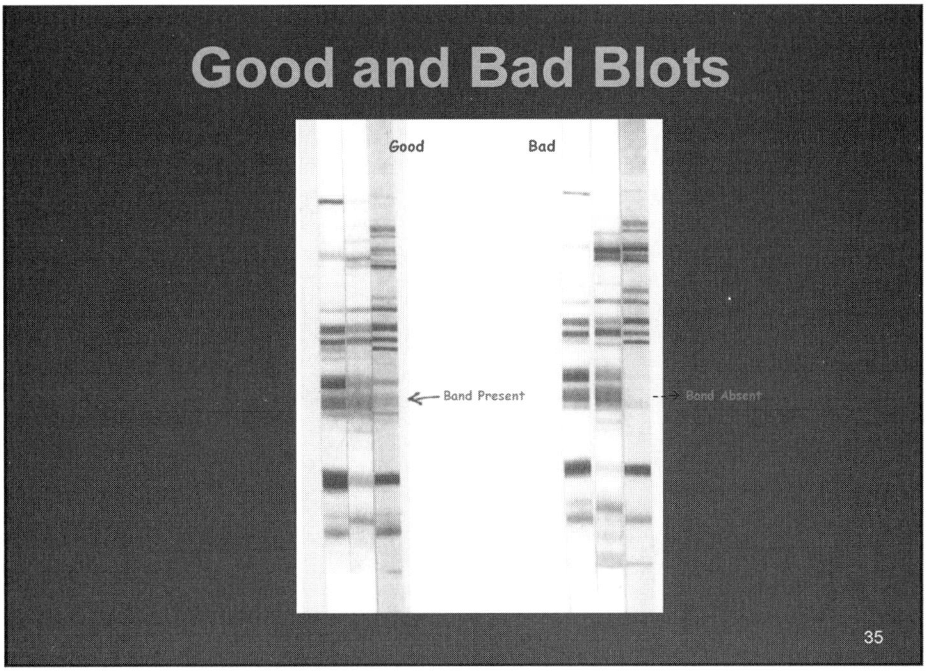
Good and Bad Blots
Good
Bad
Band Present
Band Absent
35

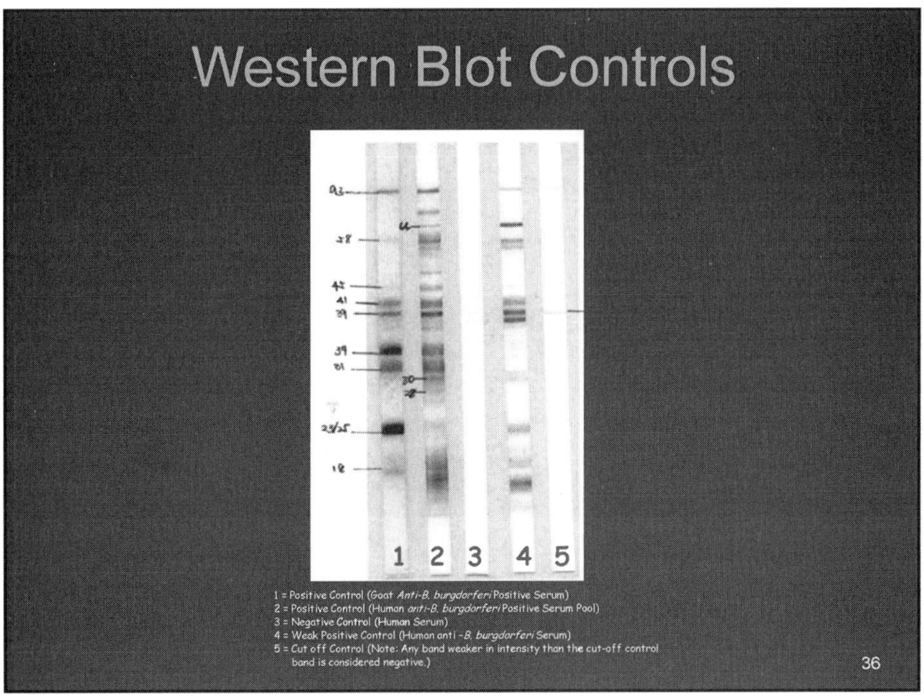
Western Blot Controls
1 2 3 4 5
1 = Positive Control (Goat *Anti-B. burgdorferi* Positive Serum)
2 = Positive Control (Human *anti-B. burgdorferi* Positive Serum Pool)
3 = Negative Control (Human Serum)
4 = Weak Positive Control (Human anti -*B. burgdorferi* Serum)
5 = Cut off Control (Note: Any band weaker in intensity than the cut-off control band is considered negative.)
36

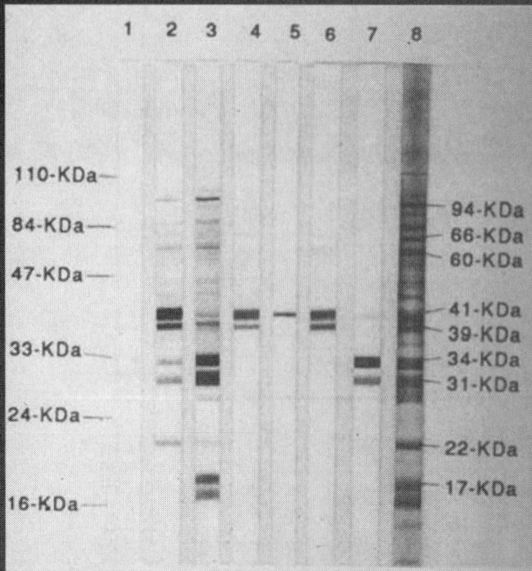

Western Blots

Variations in Antibodies to B. burgdorferi in Lyme Positive Patients (#2-#6)

37

Western Blot Band Specificity

- IgG Western Blot
  - Group A (Highly Specific): 23-25, 31, 34, 39 and 83-93 kDA
  - Group B (Tick-borne Disease Specific): 18, 41 and 58 kDA
  - Group C (non-Specific): 28, 30, 45 and 66 kDA
- IgM Western Blot
  - Group A (Highly Specific): 23-25, 31, 34, 39 and 83-93 kDA
  - Group B (Tick-borne Disease Specific): 41 kDA

IGeneX Criteria for IgG and IGM Western Blots

Positive if 2 of the following bands are present
23-25, 31, 34, 39, 41 and 83-93 kDA

38

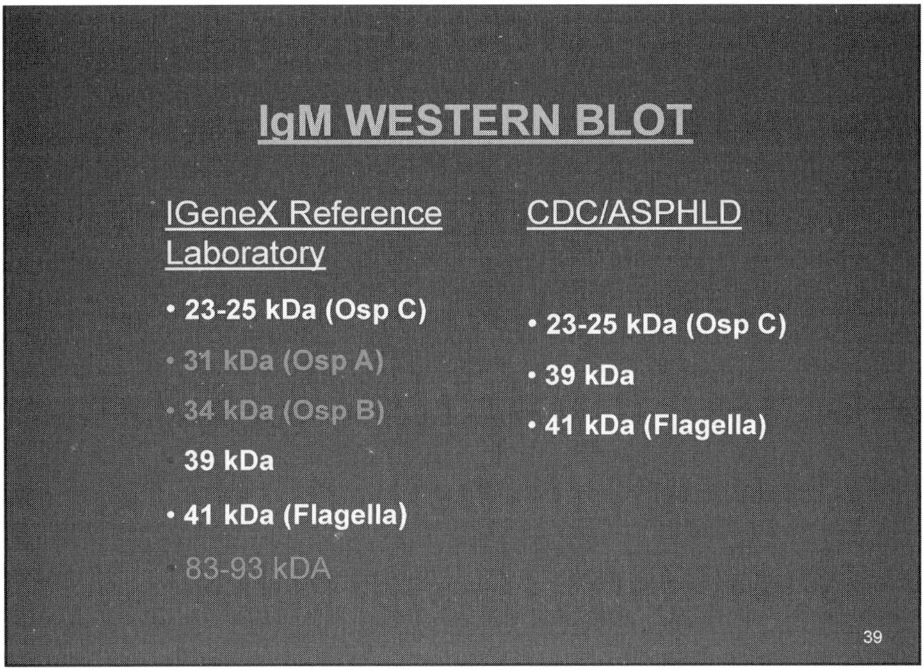
IgM WESTERN BLOT
IGeneX Reference Laboratory
• 23-25 kDa (Osp C)
• 31 kDa (Osp A)
• 34 kDa (Osp B)
• 39 kDa
• 41 kDa (Flagella)
• 83-93 kDA
CDC/ASPHLD
• 23-25 kDa (Osp C)
• 39 kDa
• 41 kDa (Flagella)
39

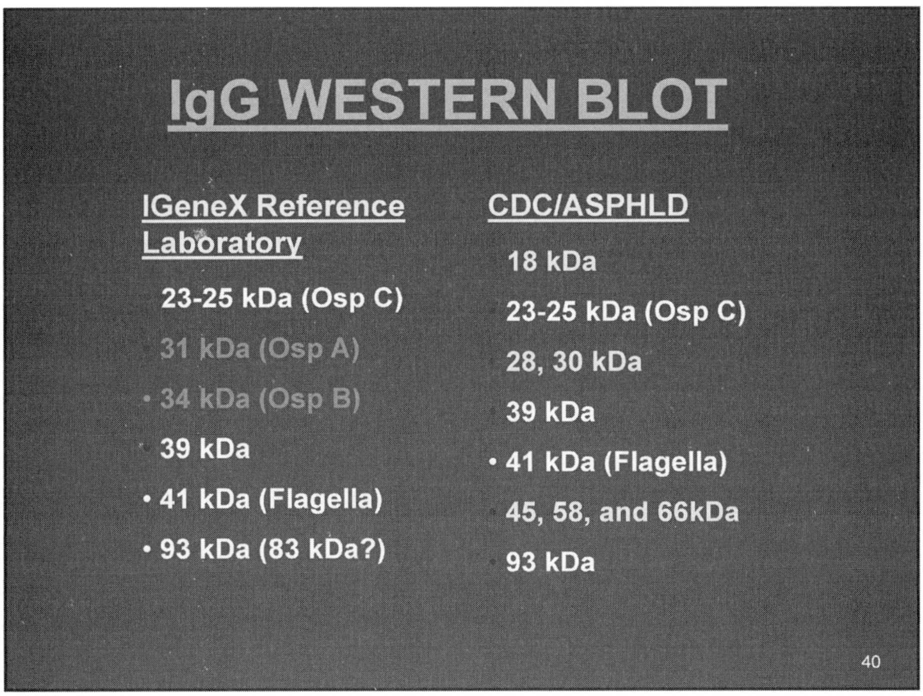
IgG WESTERN BLOT
IGeneX Reference Laboratory
• 23-25 kDa (Osp C)
• 31 kDa (Osp A)
• 34 kDa (Osp B)
• 39 kDa
• 41 kDa (Flagella)
• 93 kDa (83 kDa?)
CDC/ASPHLD
• 18 kDa
• 23-25 kDa (Osp C)
• 28, 30 kDa
• 39 kDa
• 41 kDa (Flagella)
• 45, 58, and 66kDa
• 93 kDa
40

Lyme Western Blot Assay (n=343)

Western Blots	CDC Criteria	IGeneX Criteria
IgG		
Specificity	100%	96%
Sensitivity	67%	81%
IgM		
Specificity	99%	96%
Sensitivity	69%	78%
IgG+ IgM		
Specificity	99%	96%
Sensitivity	70%	88%

Serum Sample Types
37 Lyme positive patients (CDC LD Panel)
30 Lyme positive patients with neurological symptoms
231* Tick-borne disease negative patients
45 Lyme negative, other tick-borne disease positive patients

Tick-borne Negative Samples
- 71 PT samples
- 5 Provided by CDC
- 10 provided by Dr. fallon
- 49 Positive for Autoimmune Ab.
- 94 Positive for viral antibodies

41

CONCLUSION

A positive Western Blot, IgG or IgM using IGeneX criteria confirms exposure to *B. burgdorferi*.

42

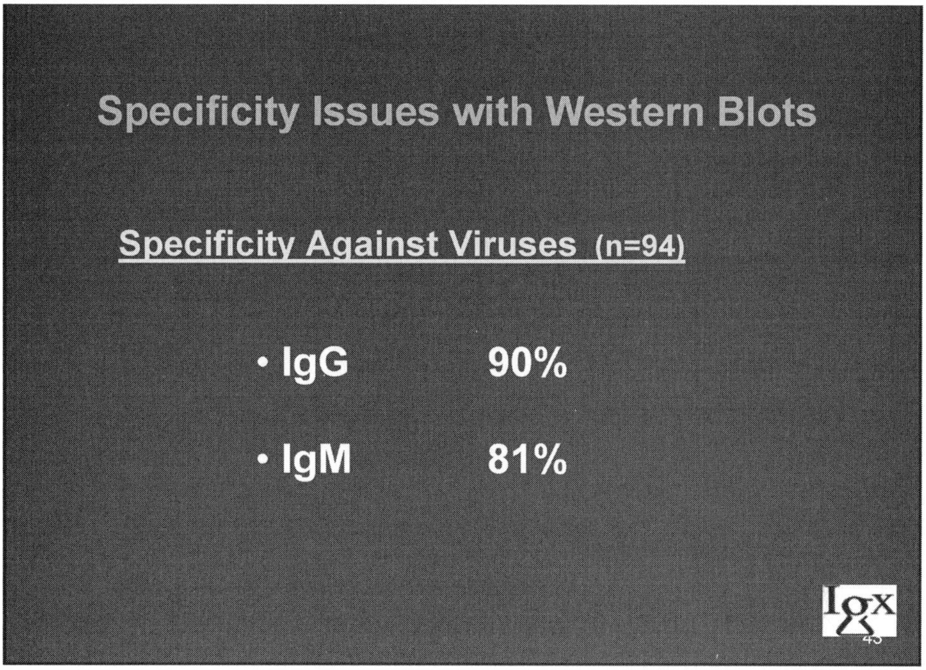
Specificity Issues with Western Blots
Specificity Against Viruses (n=94)
• IgG 90%
• IgM 81%
Igx

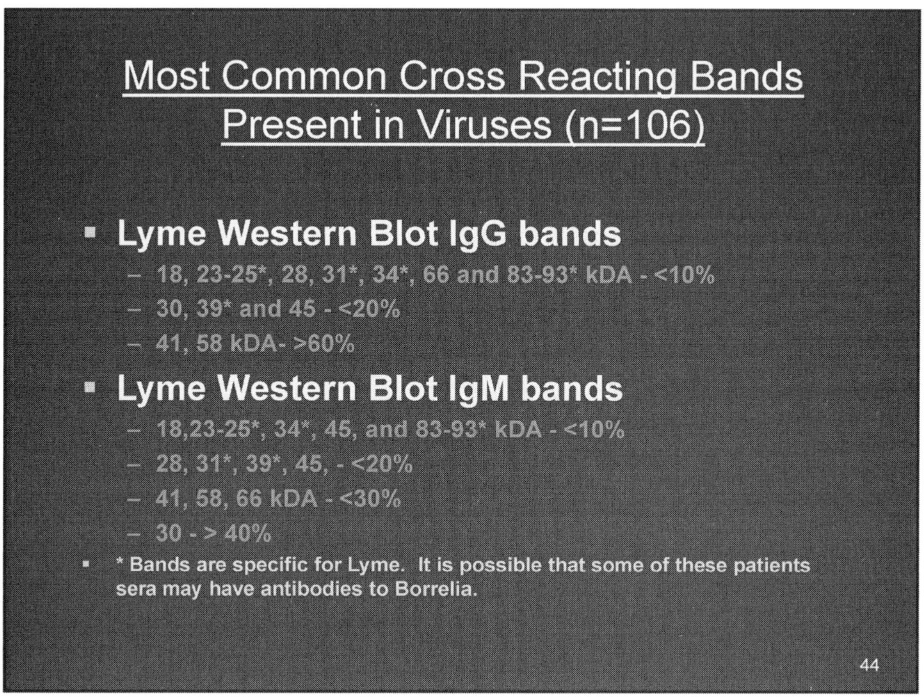
Most Common Cross Reacting Bands Present in Viruses (n=106)
Lyme Western Blot IgG bands
– 18, 23-25*, 28, 31*, 34*, 66 and 83-93* kDA - <10%
– 30, 39* and 45 - <20%
– 41, 58 kDA- >60%
Lyme Western Blot IgM bands
– 18,23-25*, 34*, 45, and 83-93* kDA - <10%
– 28, 31*, 39*, 45, - <20%
– 41, 58, 66 kDA - <30%
– 30 - > 40%
* Bands are specific for Lyme. It is possible that some of these patients sera may have antibodies to Borrelia.
44

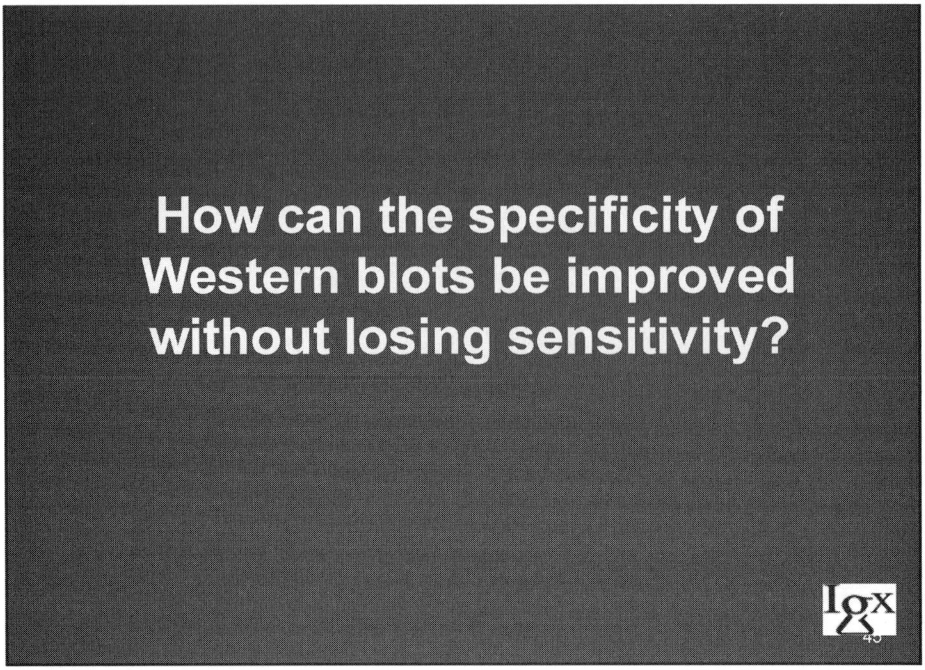
How can the specificity of Western blots be improved without losing sensitivity?

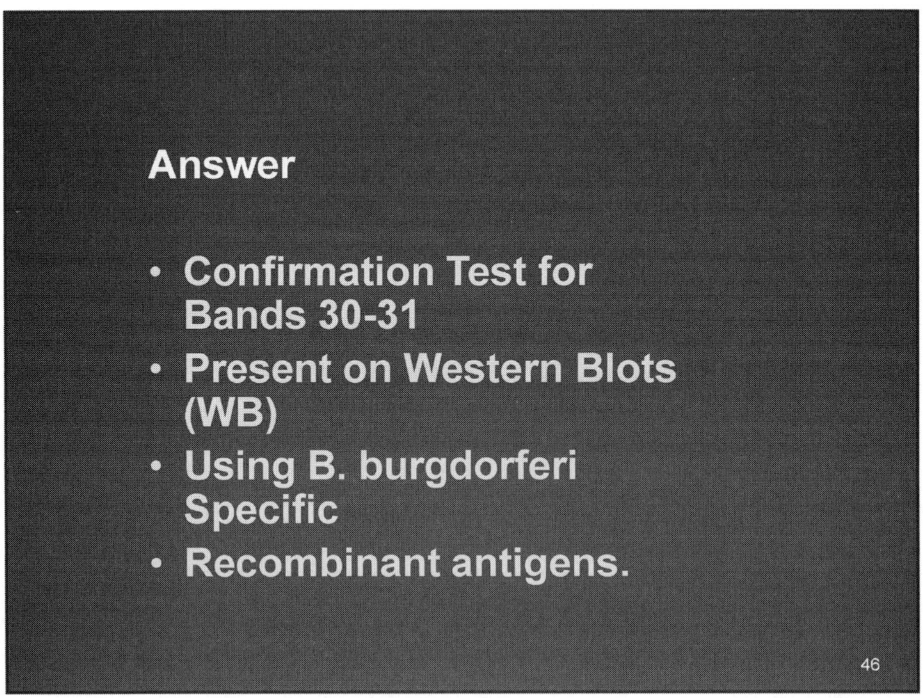
Answer
• Confirmation Test for Bands 30-31
• Present on Western Blots (WB)
• Using B. burgdorferi Specific
• Recombinant antigens.
46

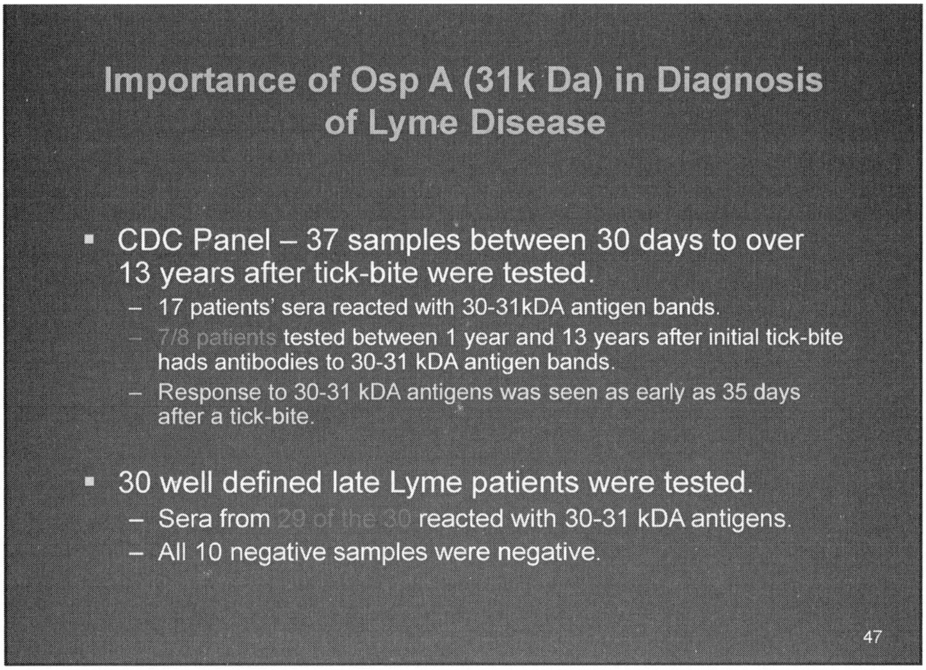
Importance of Osp A (31k Da) in Diagnosis of Lyme Disease
CDC Panel – 37 samples between 30 days to over 13 years after tick-bite were tested.
– 17 patients' sera reacted with 30-31kDA antigen bands.
– 7/8 patients tested between 1 year and 13 years after initial tick-bite hads antibodies to 30-31 kDA antigen bands.
– Response to 30-31 kDA antigens was seen as early as 35 days after a tick-bite.
30 well defined late Lyme patients were tested.
– Sera from 29 of the 30 reacted with 30-31 kDA antigens.
– All 10 negative samples were negative.
47

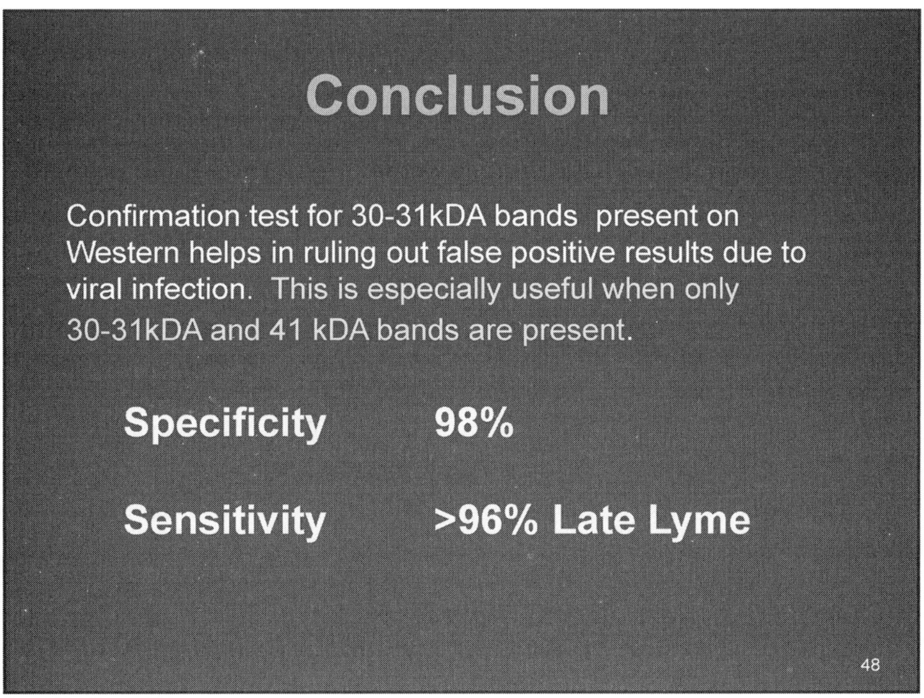
Conclusion
Confirmation test for 30-31kDA bands present on Western helps in ruling out false positive results due to viral infection. This is especially useful when only 30-31kDA and 41 kDA bands are present.
Specificity 98%
Sensitivity >96% Late Lyme
48

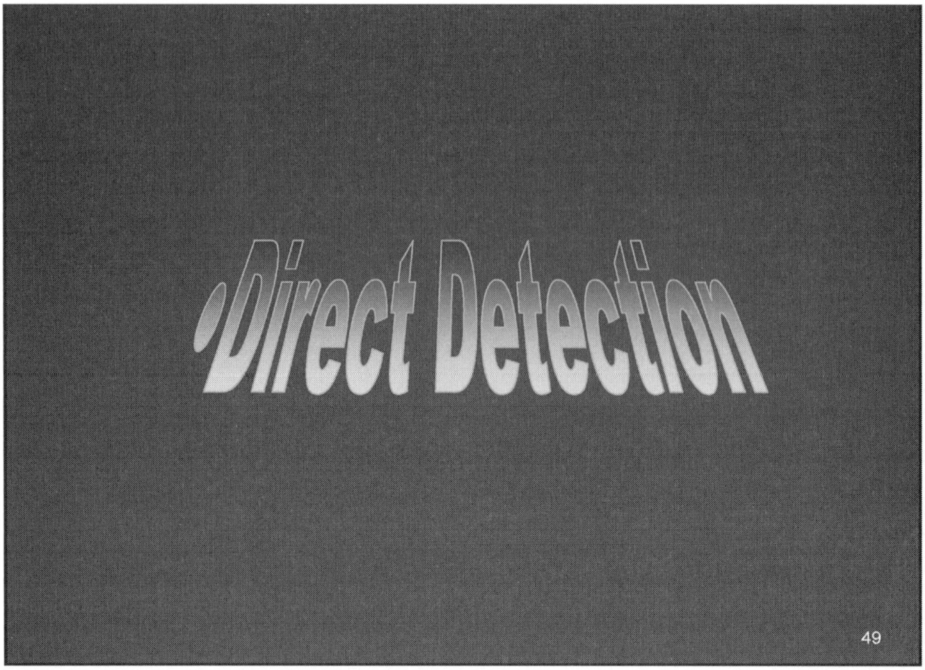

Direct Detection
49

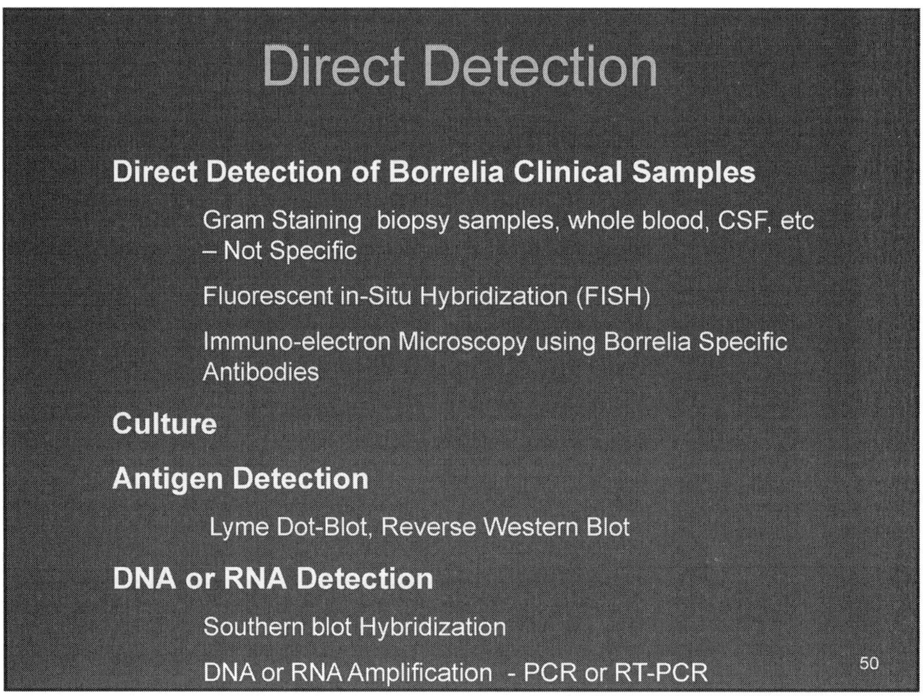

Direct Detection
Direct Detection of Borrelia Clinical Samples
Gram Staining biopsy samples, whole blood, CSF, etc – Not Specific
Fluorescent in-Situ Hybridization (FISH)
Immuno-electron Microscopy using Borrelia Specific Antibodies
Culture
Antigen Detection
Lyme Dot-Blot, Reverse Western Blot
DNA or RNA Detection
Southern blot Hybridization
DNA or RNA Amplification - PCR or RT-PCR
50

Giemsa Stained Tissue showing *Borrelia burgdorferi*

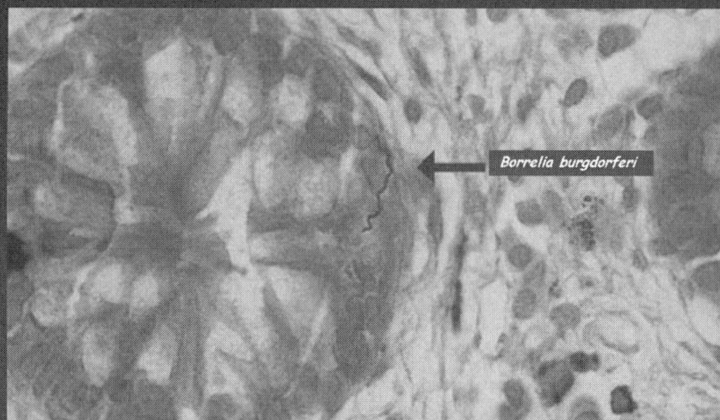

51

Culture

- Schwan TG, Burgdorfer W, Schrumpf ME, Karstens RH. 1988. The urinary bladder, a consistent source of *B. burgdoferi* in experimentally infected white-footed mice. J Clin Microbiology 26: 893-895.
- Spirochetes more frequently isolated from the bladder (94%) followed by kidney (75%), spleen (61%), blood (13%), urine (0%).

52

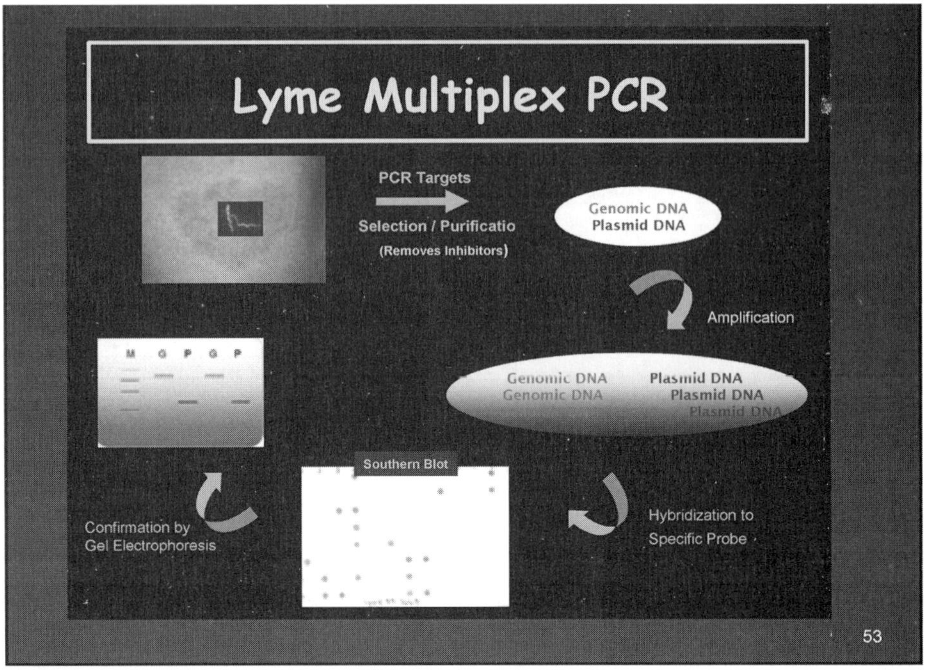
Lyme Multiplex PCR
PCR Targets
Selection / Purificatio
(Removes Inhibitors)
Genomic DNA
Plasmid DNA
Amplification
M G P G P
Genomic DNA
Genomic DNA
Plasmid DNA
Plasmid DNA
Plasmid DNA
Southern Blot
Confirmation by
Gel Electrophoresis
Hybridization to
Specific Probe
53

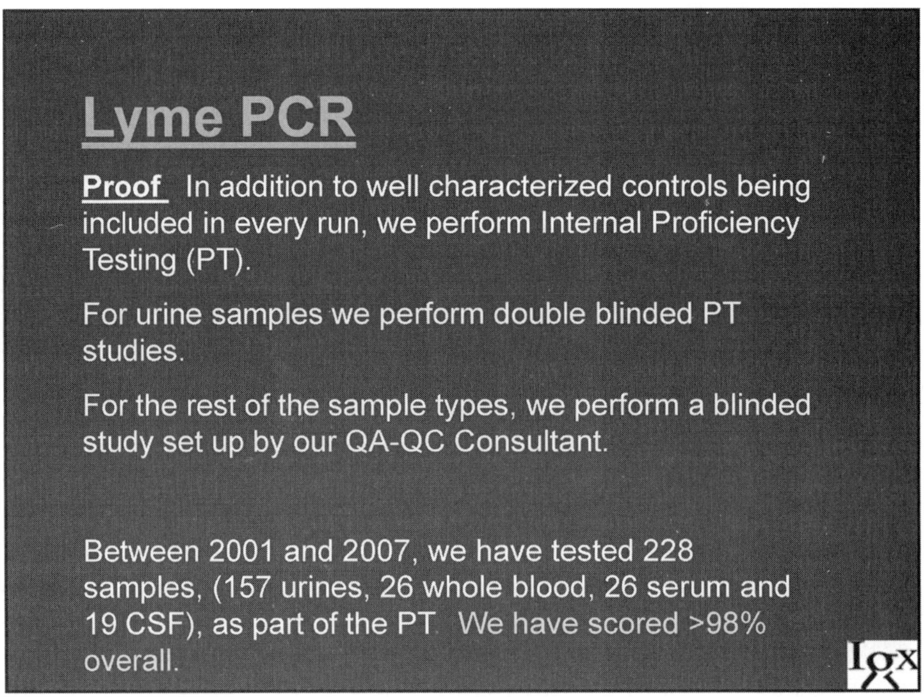
Lyme PCR
Proof In addition to well characterized controls being included in every run, we perform Internal Proficiency Testing (PT).
For urine samples we perform double blinded PT studies.
For the rest of the sample types, we perform a blinded study set up by our QA-QC Consultant.
Between 2001 and 2007, we have tested 228 samples, (157 urines, 26 whole blood, 26 serum and 19 CSF), as part of the PT. We have scored >98% overall.
IGX

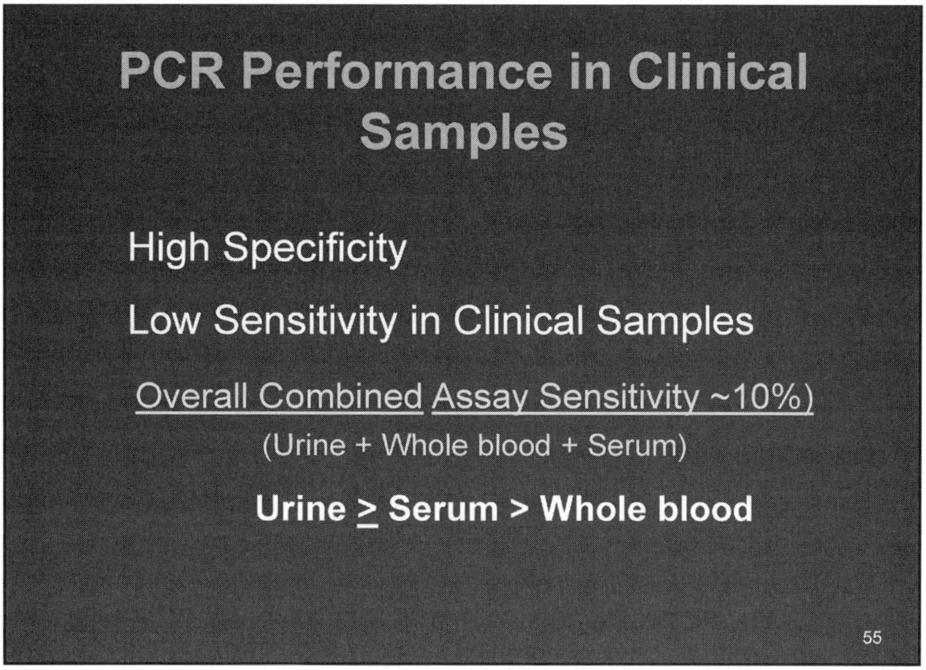
PCR Performance in Clinical Samples
High Specificity
Low Sensitivity in Clinical Samples
Overall Combined Assay Sensitivity ~10%)
(Urine + Whole blood + Serum)
Urine ≥ Serum > Whole blood
55

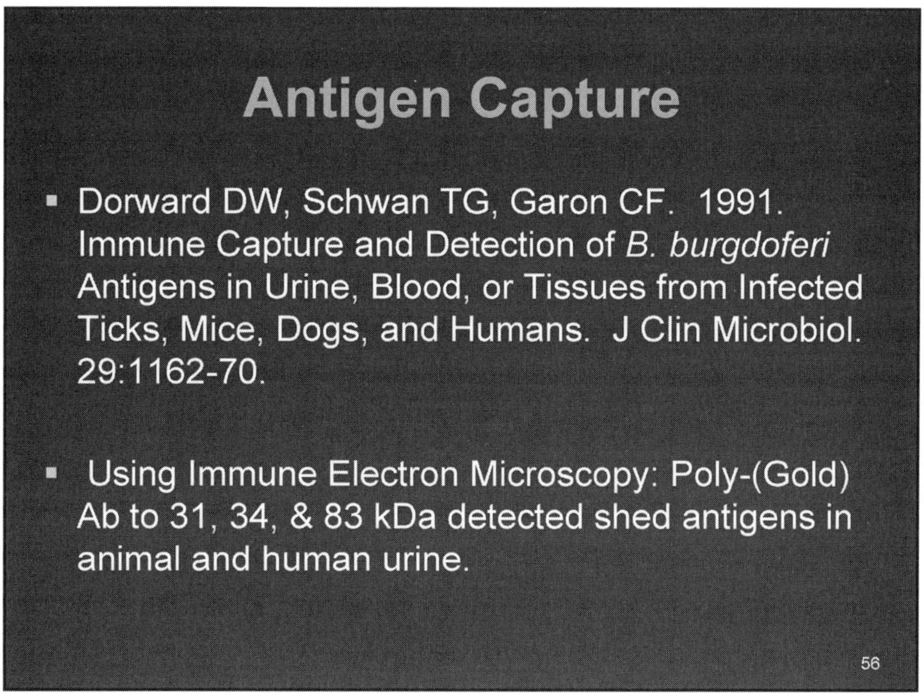
Antigen Capture
Dorward DW, Schwan TG, Garon CF. 1991. Immune Capture and Detection of *B. burgdoferi* Antigens in Urine, Blood, or Tissues from Infected Ticks, Mice, Dogs, and Humans. J Clin Microbiol. 29:1162-70.
Using Immune Electron Microscopy: Poly-(Gold) Ab to 31, 34, & 83 kDa detected shed antigens in animal and human urine.
56

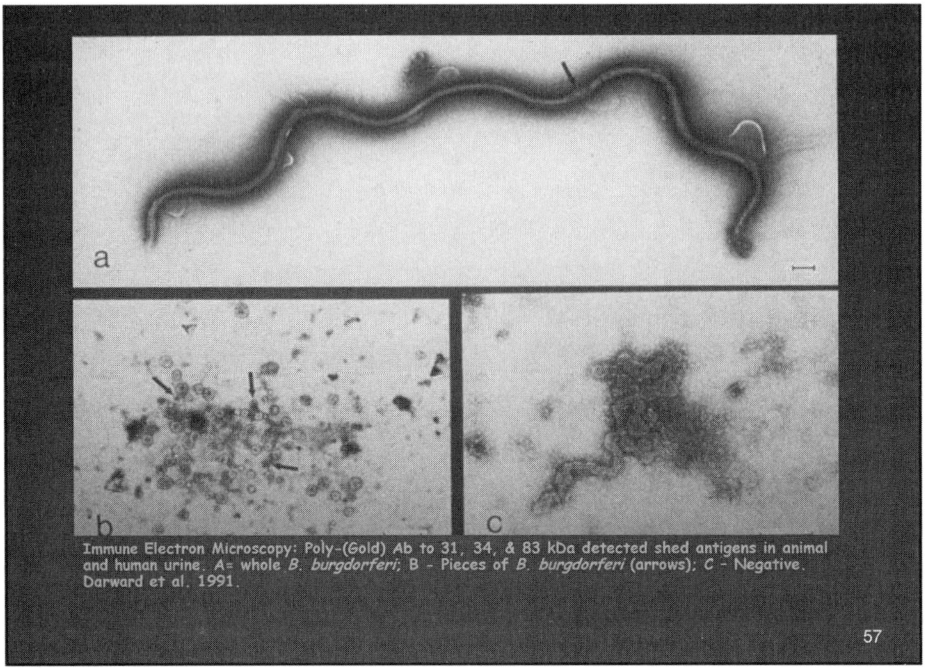
a
b
c
Immune Electron Microscopy: Poly-(Gold) Ab to 31, 34, & 83 kDa detected shed antigens in animal and human urine. A= whole *B. burgdorferi*; B - Pieces of *B. burgdorferi* (arrows); C - Negative. Darward et al. 1991.
57

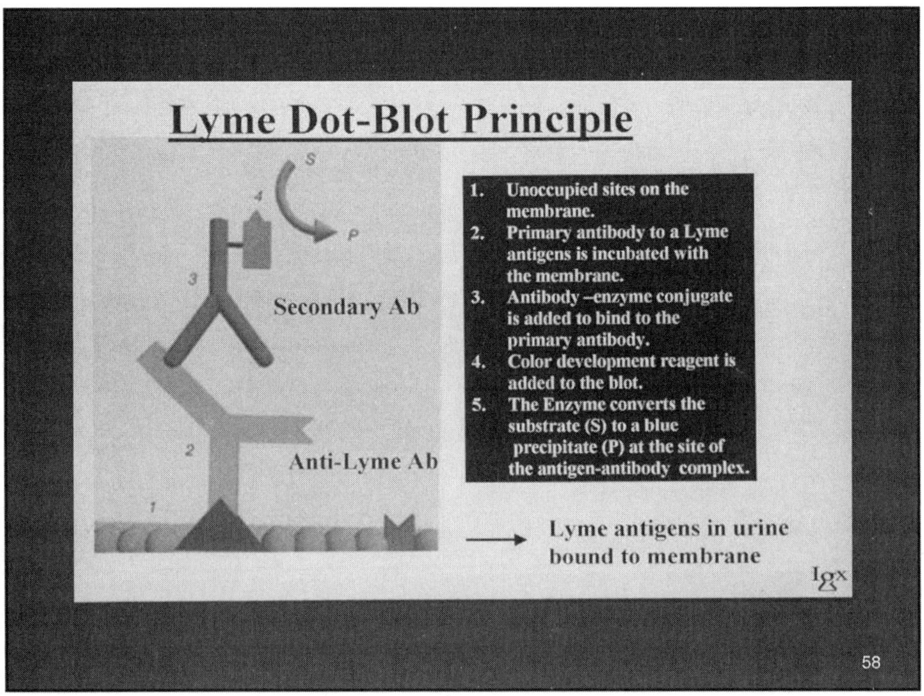
Lyme Dot-Blot Principle
S
P
4
3
Secondary Ab
2
Anti-Lyme Ab
1
1. Unoccupied sites on the membrane.
2. Primary antibody to a Lyme antigens is incubated with the membrane.
3. Antibody –enzyme conjugate is added to bind to the primary antibody.
4. Color development reagent is added to the blot.
5. The Enzyme converts the substrate (S) to a blue precipitate (P) at the site of the antigen-antibody complex.
Lyme antigens in urine bound to membrane
58

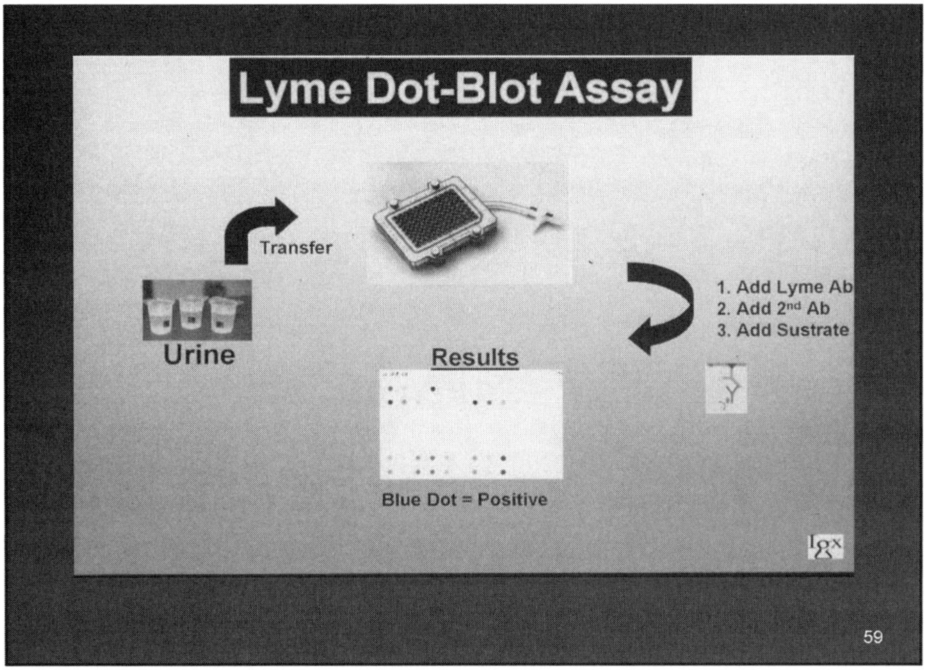
Lyme Dot-Blot Assay
Transfer
Urine
1. Add Lyme Ab
2. Add 2nd Ab
3. Add Sustrate
Results
Blue Dot = Positive
59

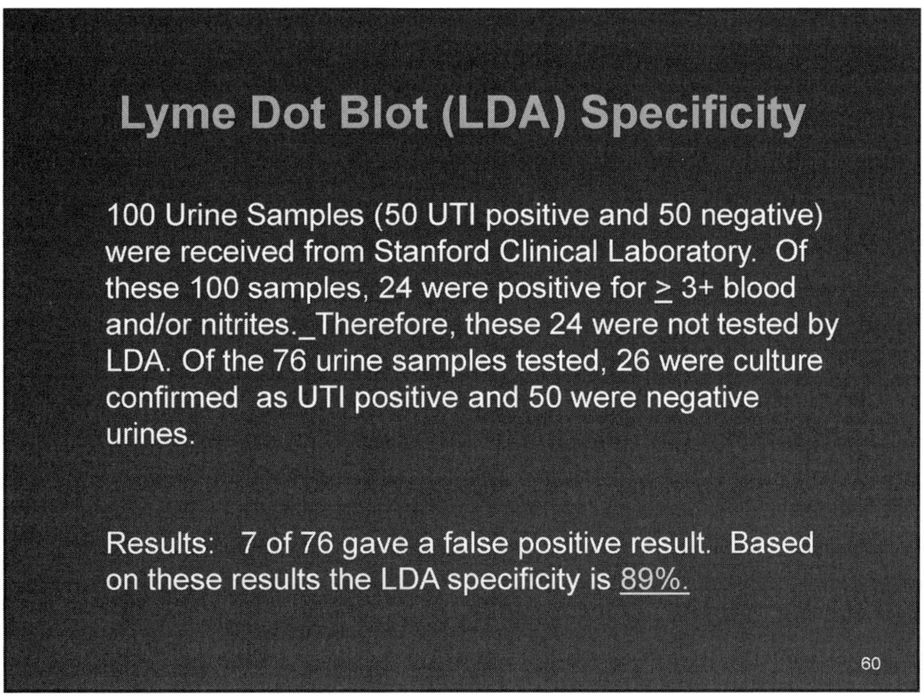
Lyme Dot Blot (LDA) Specificity
100 Urine Samples (50 UTI positive and 50 negative) were received from Stanford Clinical Laboratory. Of these 100 samples, 24 were positive for ≥ 3+ blood and/or nitrites._Therefore, these 24 were not tested by LDA. Of the 76 urine samples tested, 26 were culture confirmed as UTI positive and 50 were negative urines.
Results: 7 of 76 gave a false positive result. Based on these results the LDA specificity is 89%.
60

LDA Positive Patients and Co-Infections

33 Patients Positive for Co-infections were tested for Western blots (WB), PCR, and Lyme Dot blot Assay (LDA)

30 Positive by Western Blot (WB)

14 Positive by LDA (13 WB Positive)

LDA Assay Sensitivity = 42%

- All 14 LDA Positive Patients had Co-infections
  - 1 Babesia and Ehrlichia
  - 3 Babesia
  - 10 Ehrlichia

61

2nd Generation LDA

- Highly specific polyclonal antibody developed using recombinant proteins specific for B. burgdorferi antigens – 23-25kDa, 31kDa, 39kDa and 83-93kDa.

Sensitivity – 2.6x of current LDA test

Specificity – 95% (50 normal controls and 28 patients with UTI like symptoms)

62

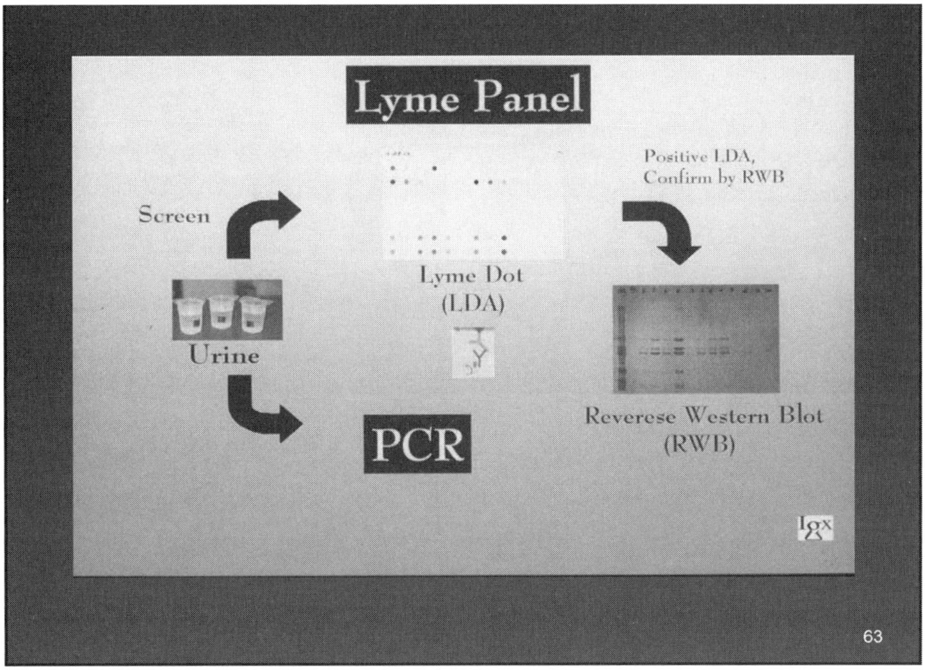
Lyme Panel
Positive LDA,
Confirm by RWB
Screen
Lyme Dot
(LDA)
Urine
PCR
Reverese Western Blot
(RWB)
Igx
63

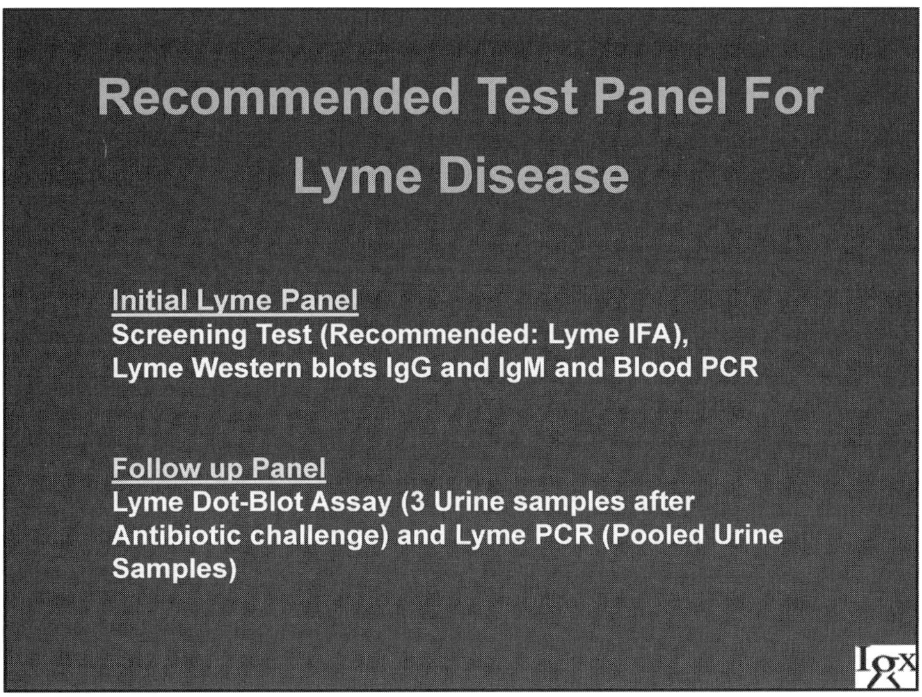
Recommended Test Panel For
Lyme Disease
Initial Lyme Panel
Screening Test (Recommended: Lyme IFA),
Lyme Western blots IgG and IgM and Blood PCR
Follow up Panel
Lyme Dot-Blot Assay (3 Urine samples after
Antibiotic challenge) and Lyme PCR (Pooled Urine
Samples)
Igx

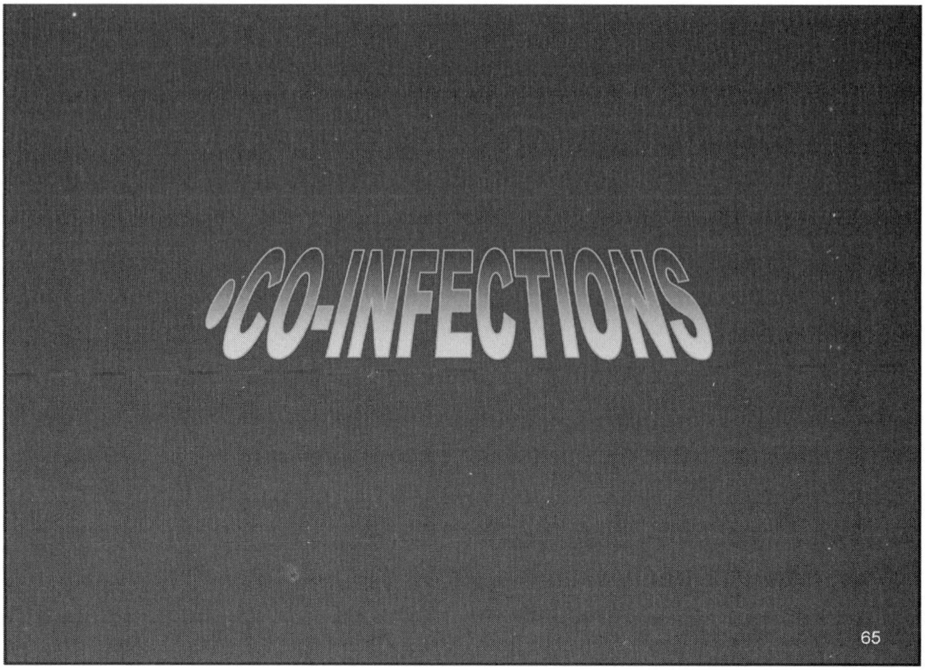
•CO-INFECTIONS
65

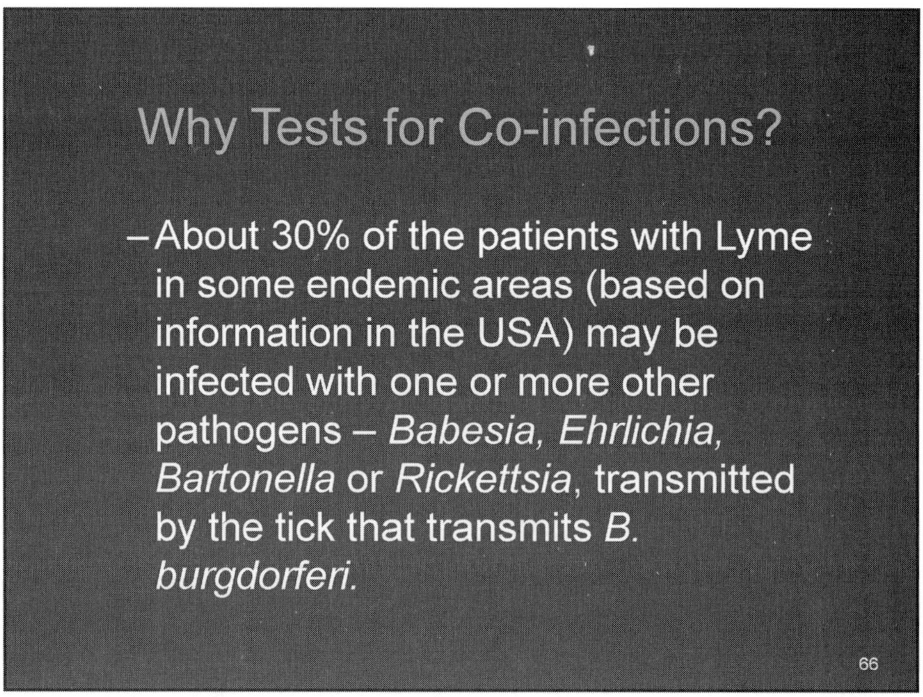
Why Tests for Co-infections?
–About 30% of the patients with Lyme in some endemic areas (based on information in the USA) may be infected with one or more other pathogens – *Babesia, Ehrlichia, Bartonella* or *Rickettsia*, transmitted by the tick that transmits *B. burgdorferi.*
66

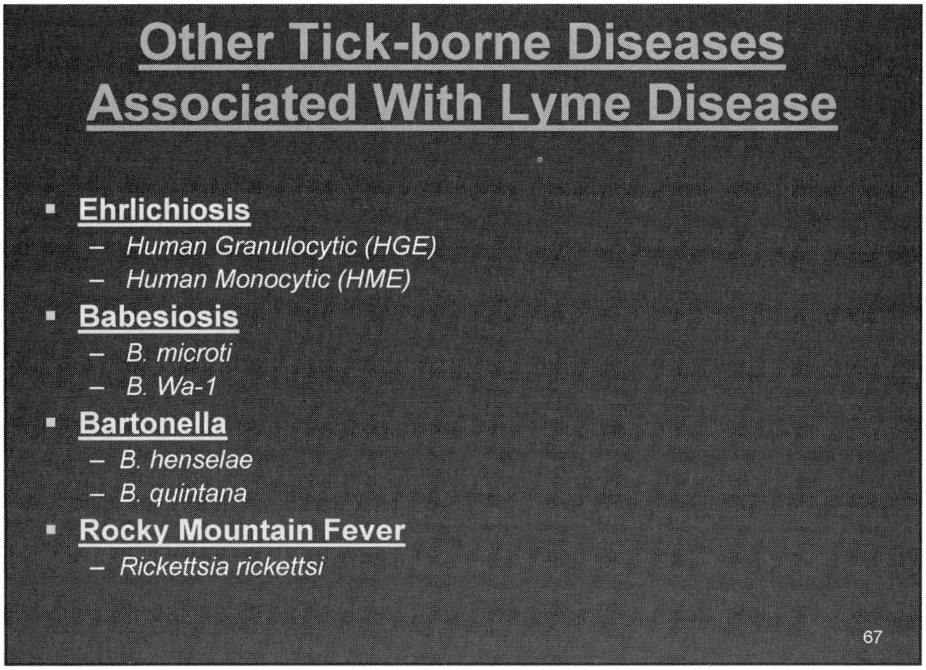
Other Tick-borne Diseases Associated With Lyme Disease
Ehrlichiosis
– Human Granulocytic (HGE)
– Human Monocytic (HME)
Babesiosis
– B. microti
– B. Wa-1
Bartonella
– B. henselae
– B. quintana
Rocky Mountain Fever
– Rickettsia rickettsi
67

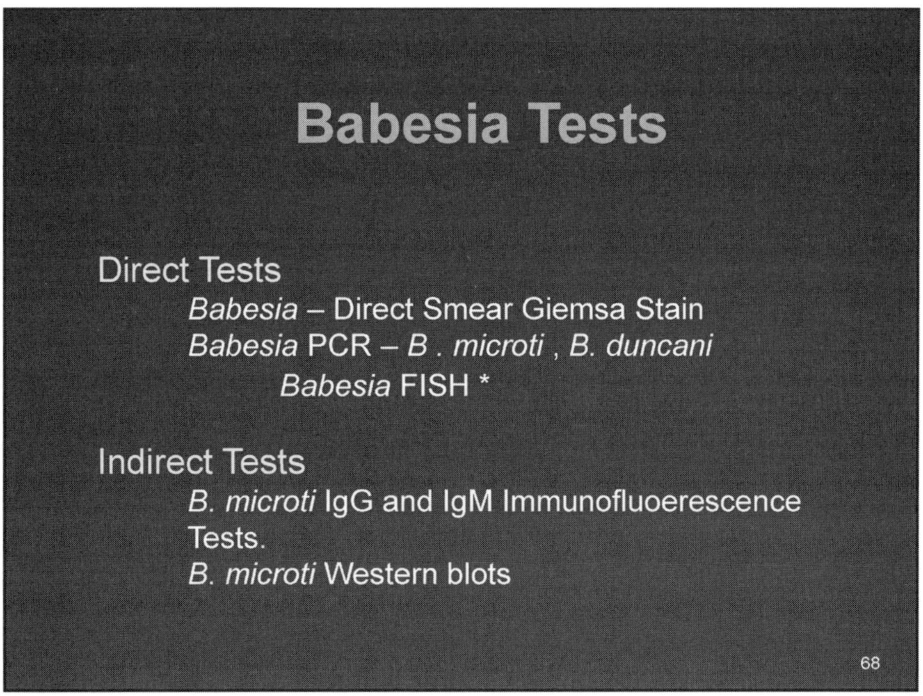
Babesia Tests
Direct Tests
Babesia – Direct Smear Giemsa Stain
Babesia PCR – B . microti , B. duncani
Babesia FISH *
Indirect Tests
B. microti IgG and IgM Immunofluoerescence Tests.
B. microti Western blots
68

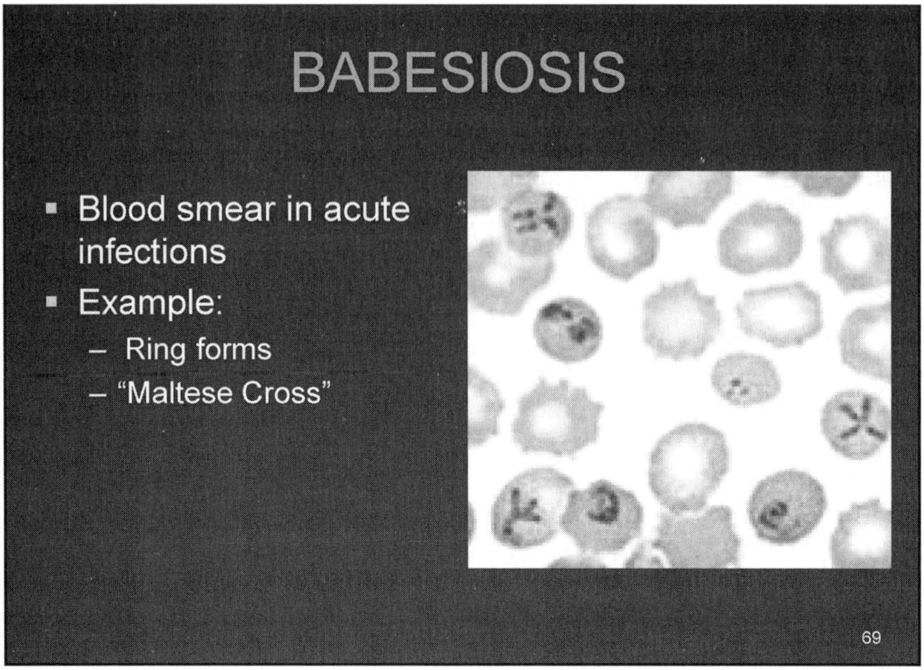
BABESIOSIS
▪ Blood smear in acute infections
▪ Example:
– Ring forms
– "Maltese Cross"
69

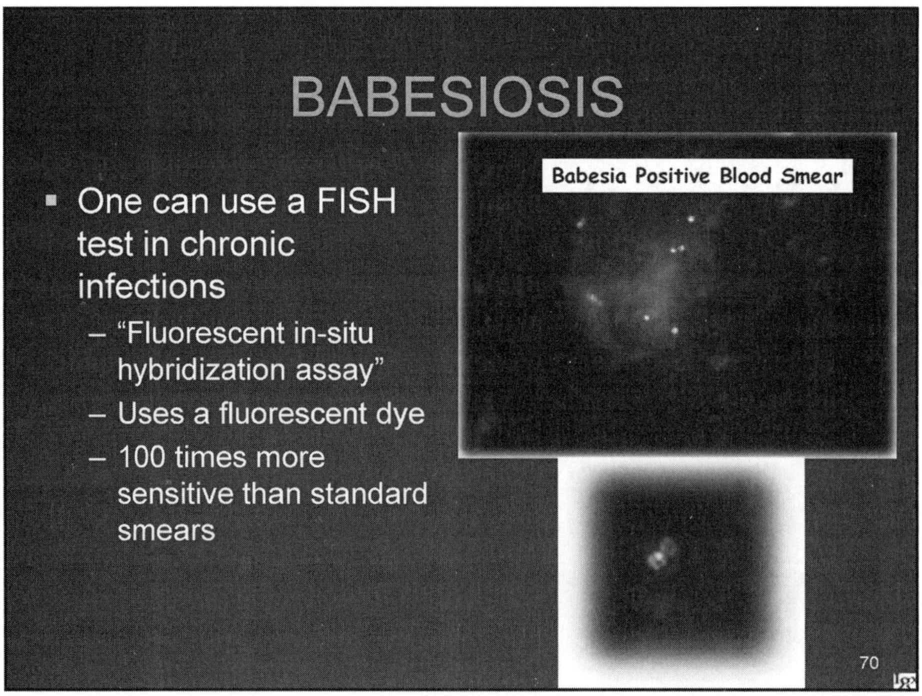
BABESIOSIS
▪ One can use a FISH test in chronic infections
– "Fluorescent in-situ hybridization assay"
– Uses a fluorescent dye
– 100 times more sensitive than standard smears
Babesia Positive Blood Smear
70

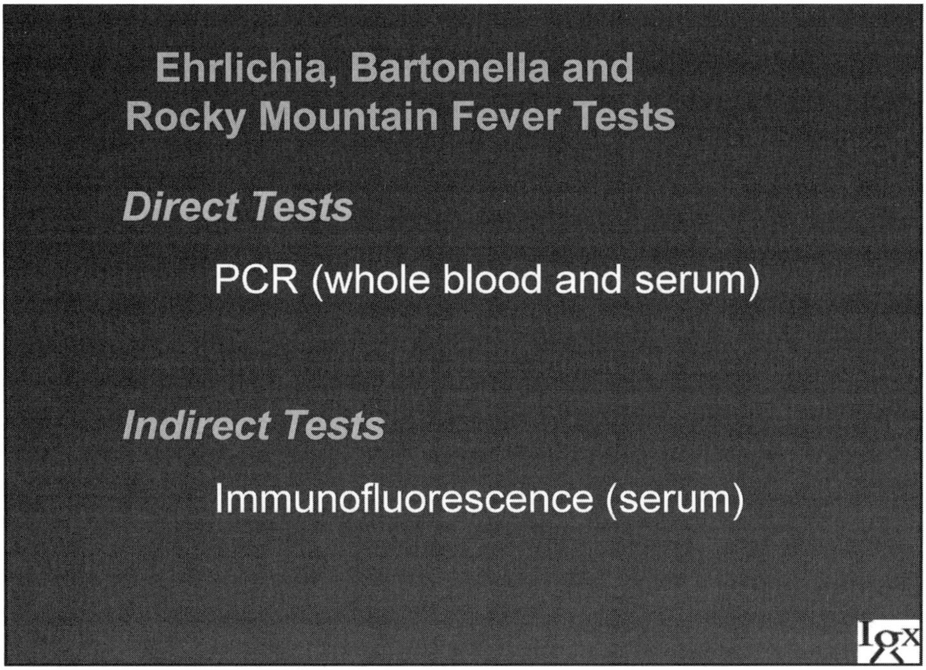
Ehrlichia, Bartonella and
Rocky Mountain Fever Tests
Direct Tests
PCR (whole blood and serum)
Indirect Tests
Immunofluorescence (serum)

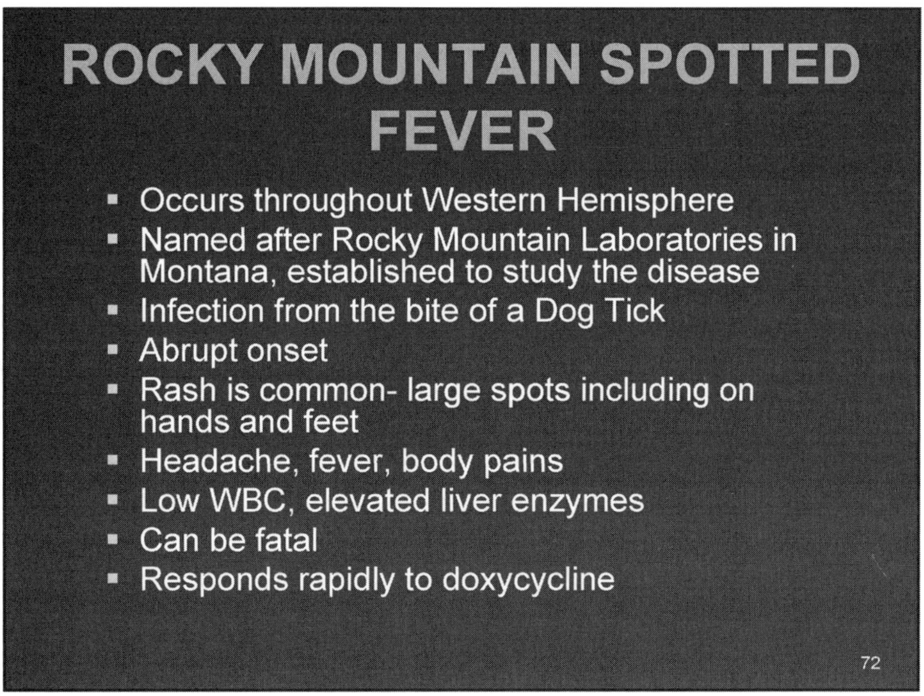
ROCKY MOUNTAIN SPOTTED FEVER
▪ Occurs throughout Western Hemisphere
▪ Named after Rocky Mountain Laboratories in Montana, established to study the disease
▪ Infection from the bite of a Dog Tick
▪ Abrupt onset
▪ Rash is common- large spots including on hands and feet
▪ Headache, fever, body pains
▪ Low WBC, elevated liver enzymes
▪ Can be fatal
▪ Responds rapidly to doxycycline
72

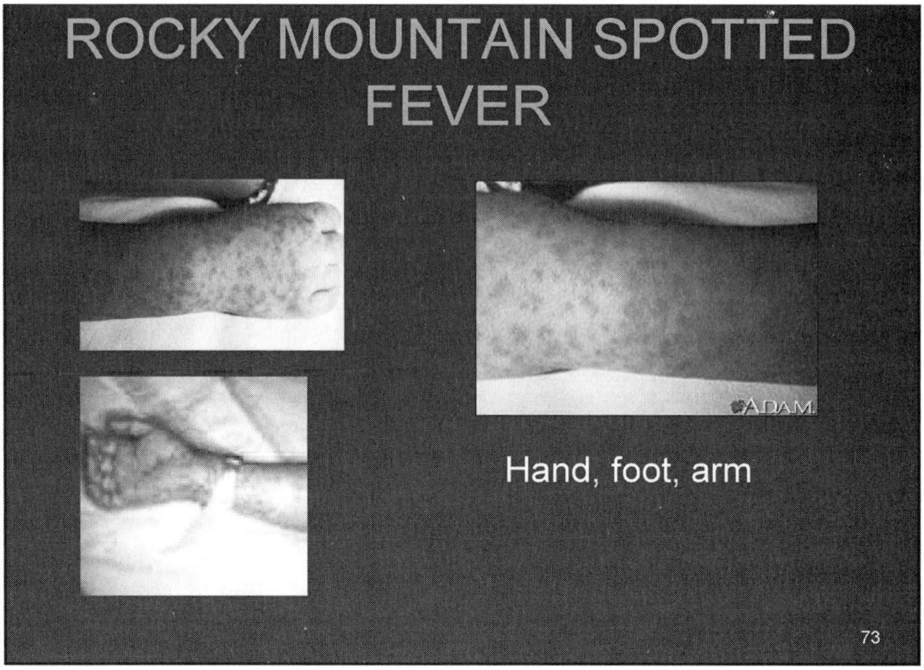
ROCKY MOUNTAIN SPOTTED FEVER
©A.D.A.M.
Hand, foot, arm
73

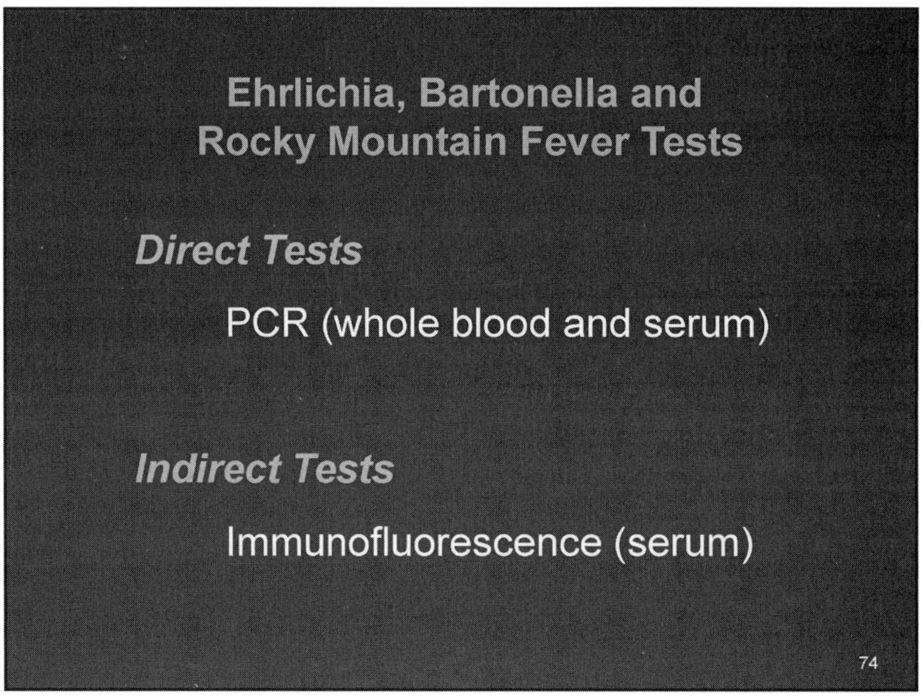
Ehrlichia, Bartonella and
Rocky Mountain Fever Tests
Direct Tests
PCR (whole blood and serum)
Indirect Tests
Immunofluorescence (serum)
74

MYCOPLASMA

- "Chronic fatigue" germ – immune system is fighting something
- Test for Mycoplasma with a blood PCR test. If it's positive, that means that Mycoplasma infection is active.
- Its origin or source is unclear
- Very difficult to detect
- More often seen in the immunosuppressed
- Test with serial PCRs (still insensitive)
- Treat with doxycycline and/or a fluoroquinolone, and add hydroxychloroquine (Plaquenil)
- Erythromycins & rifampin, with added hydroxychloroquine OK but less effective
- Treat for months to years

75

OTHER CO-INFECTIONS

Especially in the chronic Lyme and immunosuppressed patients

- Chlamydia – Recent tests show that ticks can carry Chlamydia. This is a different form of the illness which occurs in the eye and is different from the one that causes genital infections.
- Viruses
  - HHV-6, CMV, other herpes
- Yeasts
- Q-fever
- Others exist, but are unknown

76

RESOURCES FOR PATIENTS & RECOMMENDED READING

www.CanLyme.ca for Lyme-literate doctors, Canadian data on Lyme, treatment, political action, insurance issues, scientific literature, and more

www.ILADS.org for Lyme-literate doctors practicing in North America, information on training doctors can take to become Lyme-literate, research resources, legal resources

www.lymediseaseassociation.org for Lyme-literate doctors practicing in North America, up-to-date information on political action for Lyme patients

http://LymeActionGroup.blogspot.com for information on Lyme issues in Ontario; this blog is run by the Lyme Action Group of Ontario, the group that is the source of this book and financed its publication. Financial support of this non-profit organization goes wholly towards making the Lyme disease epidemic widely known, for providing support to Lyme patients looking for treatment, and providing information to those who wish to join the ongoing political activism work of LAG and similar grass-roots organizations in Canada. Having Lyme disease also entails becoming politically active.

www.lymeontario.org provides information for patients and physicians as well as support to patients and their families. The Lyme Disease Association of Ontario supports research into the causal organisms of Lyme disease and publishes a newsletter four times a year. The scientific advisor is John Scott, author of chapter 2; his work, supported by scientists in B.C., started the awareness of Lyme-carrying ticks in Canada and began to be published in the *Canadian Medical Association Journal* in the lat 1990s. Contact lymeont@hotmail.com

www.breathineasy.net Tel. 519-599-1111 breathingeasy@bellnet.ca for information on how to eliminate electro-magnetic field injury and other environmental toxins that impair the immune system

Documentary film on Lyme disease: *Under Our Skin*, 2008, DVD available through www.underourskin.com

For reliable testing for Lyme and other tick-borne diseases iGenix Inc. laboratories: www.igenixinc.com or Tel.: 1-800-538-9820 or 206-388-2372 or info@igenixinc.com

For treatment options other than antibiotics www.xpressnet.com.

On Lyme and Infectious Disease

M.C. Carroll, ***Lab 257 The Disturbing Story of the Government's Secret Germ Laboratory***, Harper Collins, 2005

J. Hall, ***Colloidal Silver—Medical Uses, Toxicology & Manufacture***, 3rd ed., 2009, self-published, available on amazon.com

H. Johnson, ***Osler's Web—Inside the Labyrinth of the Chronic Fatigue Syndrome Epidemic***, Penguin, 1996

B. Rosner, ed. ***The Top 10 Lyme Disease Treatments***, BM Printing Group, 2007

B. Rosner, When Antibiotics Fail: Lyme Disease and Rife Machines, 2004, order through www.lymebook.com/resources

K.B. Singleton, MD, ***The Lyme Disease Solution***, 2008, www.booksurge.com

C. Strasheim, ed. ***Insights into Lyme Disease Treatment—13 Lyme-literate Health Care Practitioners Share Their Healing Strategies***, BM Printing Group, 2009

P. Weintraub, ***Cure Unknown—Inside the Lyme Epidemic***, St. Martin's Press, 2008 (the paperback with an updating postscript appeared 2009).

The Townsend Letter for Doctors and Patients, see the February/March 2006 and the April 2007 issues: both dedicated to Lyme Disease

On the Current State of Corruption in Medical Science and Regulatory Authorities

H. Brody, MD, ***Hooked—Ethics, the Medical Profession and the Pharmaceutical Industry***, Rowman & Littlefield, 2007

S. Chopra, ***Corrupt to the Core—Memoirs of A Health Canada Scientists***, KOS, 2009

D. Haely, MD, ***Let Them Eat Prozac***, Lorimer, 2003

J. P. Kassirer MD, ***On the Take—How Medicine's Complicity with Big Business Can Endanger your Health***, Oxford University Press,2005

D. Michaels, ***Doubt is Their Product—How Industry's Assault on Science Threatens Your Health***, Oxford University Press, 2008

R. Smith, ***The Trouble With Medical Journals***, Royal Society of Medicine, 2007

W. Wagner & R. Steinzor eds. ***Rescuing Science from Politics—Regulation and the Distortion of Scientific Research***, Cambridge University Press, 2006

T. Young, ***Death by Prescription***, Key Porter, 2009 (the author is the Conservative Member of Parliament for Okaville, Ontario)

On the Persecution of Good Doctors and Medical Research in Canada

Canadian Association of University Teachers, ***The Olivieri Report***, Lorimer, 2001

H. Ferrie, ***Dispatches from the War Zone of Environmental Health***, KOS Publishing Inc., 2004—now available for free on the internet at www.kospublishing.com

H. Ferrie, ***What Part of No! Don't They Understand? Rescuing Medicine and Food from Government Abuse—A Manifesto***, KOS Publishing Inc., 2008—now available for free on the internet at www.kospublishing.com

D. Haley, ***Politics in Healing—The Suppression and Manipulation of American Medicine***, Potomac Valley Press, 2000

J. Krop MD, ***Healing the Planet One Patient At A Time***, KOS, 3rd edition 2008

The Glasnost Report 2001 on the persecution of medicine in Ontario (available on many websites—search by title on Google)

What Good Medicine Looks Like

M. Bliss, ***William Osler—A Life In Medicine***, University of Toronto Press, 1999

A. Hoffer MD & A. W. Saul MD, ***Orthomolecular Medicine for Everyone—Megavitamin Therapeutics for Families and Physicians***, Basic Health, 2008

S. Johnson, ***The Ghost Map—The Story of London's Most Terrifying Epidemic and How It Changed Science, Cities and the Modern World***, Riverhead Books, 2006

T. Randolph MD, ***Environmental Medicine—Beginnings and Bibliographies of Clinical Ecology***, Clinical Ecology Publications, Fort Collins, 1987

H. D. Riordan MD, ***Medical Mavericks***, Volume 3, Bio-Communications Press, 2005

H. Strauss, ***Dr. Max Gerson—Healing the Hopeless***, (1959) Quarry Press, 2002

ABOUT THE AUTHORS

Jo Burrascano, Jr. M.D. is a graduate of New York University School of Medicine. Dr. Burrascano is a leading authority in the diagnosis and treatment of tick-borne diseases. During his 25 years as an internist in East Hampton, N.Y.—an area hyper endemic for Lyme disease—he treated more than 11,000 patients from 46 states and 16 countries. He is the author of the ILADS *Lyme Diagnosis and Treatment Guidelines* and has published numerous papers in medical journals. Dr. Burrascano has trained many doctors in the treatment and diagnostic methods for Chronic Lyme disease. Currently, he is heading an ongoing research project developing a universal Lyme and associated diseases database. He is currently working with ILADS on the creation of a comprehensive database system to improve treatment and outcomes for people with persistent Lyme and other tick-borne diseases. He has spoken before the US House of Representatives and the military on tick-borne diseases and testified before the Rhode Island Governor's Commission. Dr. Burrascano's work and personal experience with Chronic Lyme disease are described in the award-winning book *Cure Unknown—Inside the Lyme Disease Epidemic,* St. Martin's Press, 2008

David Cubberley is a former MLA and civic councillor in Saanich, B.C. who served for 18 months as provincial health critic. A long-time public-health activist, he's a vocal proponent of the redesign of cities to enable more walking, cycling and transit use. He volunteers as a director of the Canadian Lyme Disease Foundation and works as a public policy consultant.

Helke Ferrie M.A., was born in Germany to Nazi resistance fighters who survived to work for the newly independent Indian government. She was raised and educated in an international American school in the foothills of the Himalayas in India and went to university in Switzerland and in India in the 1960s where she met Robert Ferrie, a Canadian physician who practiced urology for about twenty years and then trained to become a psychotherapist who specializes on post traumatic stress disorder. They have been married for 40 years and raised a family of three biological and eleven adopted children of international and Canadian origin. They now have many grandchildren and live in Alton, Ontario. In the 1970s, Robert and Helke ran an international child-welfare agency devoted to the needs of handicapped and older children. In the 1980s, Helke earned a masters degree in physical anthropology from the University of Toronto; her special area of interest was the evolution of disease. Through a serious illness caused by mercury amalgam dental fillings and exposure to pesticides, Helke became aware of the destructive political presence in modern medicine. Upon recovering her health, she began writing and in 2003 opened KOS Publishing Inc. Her monthly articles on the politics of medicine have been published in Toronto's *Vitality* Magazine for over ten years. She frequently contributes to *StraightGoods*, the *Canadian Center for Policy Alternatives' Monitor*, *CorporateWatch, Medical Veritas,* and others. She is the author of *Dispatches from the War Zone of Environmental Health* (KOS 2004), and *What Part of No! Don't They Understand—Rescuing Food and Medicine from Government Abuse* (KOS 2008)—both available for free on her website www.kospublishing.com. Helke is the editor of the present volume.

Paul Haefling, M.A., LL.B, is a labour relations Arbitrator and Mediator and an Ontario lawyer. His interest in and curiosity about Lyme disease arose after a family member was diagnosed with "Chronic Lyme disease," the most serious form of the disease, but a condition that is still not being acknowledged and recognized formally and officially by public health agencies in Canada. That situation prompted his continuing research and study into known manifestations of Lyme disease and his drive to continue to pressure provincial and federal government public health bodies in Canada to take action, to recognize the need, and to create and undertake newer and better policies, practices and programs, as well as needed and new leading-edge research on Lyme disease. All of those steps are now necessary in the face of growing numbers of Canadians being diagnosed with Lyme disease who, to this point, try their best to live with but all too often are being left to suffer in silence the effects of this terrible and debilitating (but treatable) illness.

Karin Klouman was born and grew up in Norway and spent some of her teenage years in Tanzania, East Africa. She met her Canadian husband at the foot of Mount Kilimanjaro in 1972 and immigrated to Canada in 1976. Karin is a graduate with

Honours from a Norwegian Agricultural College with a major in Animal Science. She has also completed several undergraduate bio-science courses, from the University of Guelph. As a self-employed business owner, Karin operate a large boarding and breeding kennel (www.kyonkennels.com) on the family farm, where she has also been raising a large family of 6 children, with her husband of 36 years. Karin is actively involved in the purebred dog industry and shows, trials and trains dogs. She has also written articles for various national and international dog magazines. Karin became ill with Lyme disease in 1993, but remained unaware of this until 2002, at which point she had fallen severely ill to a complex multi-system illness; with severe neurological, reproductive, joint, cardiac and gastro-intestinal involvement. Once diagnosed Karin started on aggressive antibiotic and intravenous therapy, prescribed by a doctor who is trained and certified by the International Lyme and Associated Disease Society (ILADS). Karin no longer suffers from any Lyme symptoms, is no longer on any medication and has remained in a fully sustained remission, since late 2006.

Jozef Krop, M.D. received his medical degree from the Jagellonian University in Krakow, Poland and was a paediatrician before emigrating to Canada in 1972. Introduced to Orthomolecular Medicine in Saskatoon in 1975 by Dr. Abram Hoffer, he integrated these concepts into his medical practice in 1977 and those of Environmental Medicine since 1979. Since 2001 he has been interested in the subject of Chronic Lyme Disease and is one of the few doctors in Canada treating this condition. Dr. Krop has published peer-reviewed research in nutritional and environmental medicine, chemical sensitivity and treatment of food sensitivities. His book, *Healing the Planet One Patient at a Time: A Primer in Environmental Medicine (KOS Publishing, 2002)* offers strategies of prevention and treatment for the toxic effects of environmental hazards and pathogens in our food, air, and water on human physiology and behaviour. It has been translated into French and Polish. Dr. Krop has been involved in teaching environmental medicine principles at conferences in European universities. He has a private medical practice in Mississauga, Ontario, and has been an advocate for his patients for over 30 years. Dr. Krop is a fellow of the American Academy of Environmental Medicine, a founding member of the Canadian Society for Environmental Medicine, a member of the American College for Advancement in Medicine, the Ontario Society of Physicians for Complementary Medicine, and the International Lyme and Associated Diseases Society.

Linda Laidlaw, PhD, when she is not spending time with her two young daughters, is an associate professor in language and literacy in the Department of Elementary Education in the Faculty of Education at the University of Alberta. She is the author of *Reinventing Curriculum: A Complex Perspective on Language and Writing*, and is currently completing research for a book on diversity and schools. As a result of her daughter Xian's experiences with Lyme disease, she is investigating possibilities for a future research project looking at the impact of paediatric Lyme disease on learning and school experience.

John D. Scott was born at the end of WW II, and raised on an Oxford County dairy farm where daily chores, constant repairs, and problem-solving were an ongoing fact of life. He went to Paris District High School, and then attended the University of Guelph where he completed a 4-year honours science degree in agriculture in 1970. He obtained his M.Sc. while working as a professional agrologist and biology researcher. To date, he has published 12 peer-reviewed scientific papers on ticks and Lyme disease in Canada. In 1973, he married Catherine "Kit" Hunt, and has two children, David and Janet, and a granddaughter, Alicia. For 23 years of their married life, he has battled with the fallout of persistent, Chronic Lyme disease—a living nightmare from hell. He has worked to find the source of Lyme disease across Canada, and to uncover why patients are contracting this spirochetal zoonosis nationwide.

Felix Sperling (PhD 1991 Cornell University) is a Professor of Biological Sciences and Curator of the Strickland Museum of Entomology at the University of Alberta. His research encompasses patterns and processes of arthropod biodiversity. He has provided training for numerous insect taxonomists who now occupy faculty or research scientist positions around the world. A major focus of his work is the development of DNA based diagnostics and delimitation of insect species. **Janet Sperling** is a board member of the Canadian Lyme Disease Foundation. Trained as an entomologist at the University of Alberta (MSc 1988), she and her husband Felix spent two years navigating the complexities of the diagnosis and effective treatment of Lyme borreliosis for their oldest son. The unresolved nature of this experience has persuaded Janet to contribute her energies toward developing and establishing a made-in-Canada policy for Lyme disease that both increases awareness of the disease and reduces the suffering of Lyme patients. Together Janet and Felix have recently written a review of 'Lyme borreliosis in Canada: biological diversity and diagnostic complexity from an entomological perspective' for The Canadian Entomologist.

Jim M. Wilson A.I.I.C. is the father of four children who began his career in the insurance industry in 1974. Investigating insurance claims over the years, including medical malpractice gave him a unique glimpse into the far from perfect world of medicine and science. He became infected with Lyme disease in 1991 in Dartmouth, Nova Scotia. Years of illness followed, but finally with a diagnosis and long-term antibiotic treatment he was able to regain his health. In 2001, living back in British Columbia, two of his children were diagnosed with Lyme disease, this allegedly rare disease in Canada. It was going through the battle of getting his children's diagnoses confirmed, and finding a doctor who had the knowledge to treat them that prompted him to start the Canadian Lyme Disease Foundation (CanLyme.com). When the CanLyme website hit the internet in 2003, CanLyme quickly revealed that Lyme disease is not rare in Canada, it is the diagnosis that is rare.

Terence Young is the Member of Parliament (Conservative) for Oakville, Ontario, having been elected in 2008. Previously, from 1995 to 1999, he was a Progressive Conservative member for the provincial legislature of Ontario. He is the author of the book *Death by Prescription—A Father Takes On His Daughter's Killer: The Multibillion Dollar Pharmaceutical Industry*, published by Key Porter in April 2009. He became an outspoken health advocate following the death of his teenage daughter Vanessa who died in 2000 as a result of taking the Johnson & Johnson prescription drug Cisapride (also known as Prepulsid). The drug was taken off the market by Health Canada in August 2000, due to reports of "serious cardiac arrhythmias" causing death. In April, 2009, he placed a Private Member's Motion on the order papers of the parliament of Canada which, if passed, would create an independent drug agency for Canada focusing on drug safety, similar to the Nuclear Safety Agency or Transportation Safety Board.

ACKNOWLEDGEMENTS

This book was written over a period of a year by people who are highly experienced in matters pertaining to the politics, medicine, and personal experience with Lyme disease. Some still suffered from its worst symptoms while working on this book. Getting this done, occasionally seemed to be endangered by their illness, Herxheimer reactions, overwhelming fatigue, and the time-consuming treatments. In the end, those among the authors who were sick, or taking care of family members with Lyme, managed to get their contributions completed. Their work expands the meaning of the term "a labor of love."

We are especially grateful to Rosanna Magnotta for her determined work for Lyme disease research and awareness, and share in her grief for the loss of her husband Gabe, who died from the complications of Chronic Lyme disease, and to whom this book is dedicated together with Dr. Joe Kucan. Without Joe the Lyme Action Group might not have come into being; his sudden and unexpected death we all still feel keenly, and we miss his wisdom, advice and understanding. We hope this book does some justice to the hopes and vision of both Gabe and Joe.

The Lyme Action Group, which some of the authors helped to bring into existence, raised the money for the publication costs of this book, which is published on a non-profit basis. LAG will oversee its distribution in close and continuing companionship with the national Lyme disease group, CanLyme. Jim Wilson's CanLyme organization has been working for Lyme patients for many years, and our very recently founded group has benefitted from CanLyme's experience and guidance more than we can describe.

The LAG fundraising events, initiated most of the time by Rob Manten of LAG, served also to increase Lyme awareness in Ontario through the many events at which he showed the documentary film, *Under Our Skin* in churches and to private organizations. Julia Woodford, the editor of *Vitality* Magazine and the host of the annual While Life Expo, and Helen McLellan, host of the annual Total Health Show, generously supported our efforts with free booths and the opportunity to talk about Lyme disease to hundreds upon hundreds of people at their events.

Without the frequent support of Pat Smith, the indefatigable president of the enormously successful Lyme Disease Association in the US, we would not have been blessed with so much information, helpful leads, and key documentation.

A very special thanks is offered to Drs. Joe Burrescano, Eva Sapi, R. Stricker, Dr. J. S. Shah of IGeneX and to lawyer Elaine Johnson—all Lyme disease warriors par excellence—who allowed us to publish their treatment and testing protocols, provided key references from the medical literature, and educational DVDs to guide us through a crash course on Lyme research, epidemiology, diagnostic and treatment methods as they evolved and are continuing to be developed.

We cannot mention by name the few Canadian doctors who, in defiance of the political rot underlying the Lyme disease medicine, continue to treat these unfortunate patients, despite the attending danger to themselves, but we appreciate them more than they will ever know. Dr. Krop kindly agreed to join the Lyme Action Group's project for this book, and we are very honored and most thankful to have his excellent, though tragic, story in this book.

Behind every great doctor stands a great and determined wife who not only loves him but also loves medicine. Elizabeth Krop not only supports her husband's pioneering work in medicine, but makes life possible for him—and thus by extension for his patients—by understanding the stress he chooses make the characteristic flavor of his professional life. Those of us who worked with Dr. Krop through the MCS ordeal as well as the Lyme disease drama, often refer to her as "Saint Elizabeth."

Eleanor Johnston is endowed with a unique capability of attention to detail that quite possibly outstrips the powers of a computer (she does not own one, and probably does not need one). No detail escapes her, and no effort is too great for her to hunt down correct governmental designations and related published materials, construct perfect phrases that are correctly informed and useful, and to provide insights into historical material pertaining to government, regulatory institutions, and technical literature, the details and significance of which escapes most of us with less experience. This project would not have been possible without her.

Among politicians we had helpful and understanding support from all parties and often in unexpected ways, for which we thank them most heartily. We are counting on their continued involvement. In Ontario we thank Christine Elliott (Conservative MPP), France Gelinas (NDP MPP), Elizabeth Witmer (Conservative MPP), Sophia Aggelonitis (Liberal MPP) and Monte Kwinter (Liberal MPP) who helped start our public campaign for Lyme disease. Federally, we are especially grateful to MP Judy Wasylycia-Leis (NDP Winnipeg North) for helping to increase Lyme disease awareness, to NDP Leader, Jack Layton, who provided us with support, information, and encouragement, to Liberal MP Dr. Caroline Bennett for her strong support of our concerns about the safety of the blood supply, and to (Conservative MP) Terrence Young for writing a preface to this book.

Our families helped in countless ways, as they are integrally part of the Lyme disease battle. For me, the editor of this book, the companionship of my cats Tuxido or Kubla Khan, who spend much of their days snoozing next to my computer, I am grateful because they reduce my stress hormone production while I work.

Helke Ferrie,
KOS Publishing Inc.

February 16, 2010

Note: All articles from medical journals and similar publications are reproduced with the required permissions and applicable royalties were paid. Special thanks are offered to the editors of *The Canadian Entomologist*, the *North American Bird Bander,* and the *Journal of the American Physicians and Surgeons* for waiving royalty fees. Thanks also to Dr. Dana Devine of the Canadian Blood Services for permission to reproduce her PowerPoint presentation of December 4, 2009, on blood safety measures.